Sleep Disorders: A Clinician's Guide

Sleep Disorders: A Clinician's Guide

Edited by Eric Stiles

hayle medical
New York

Hayle Medical,
750 Third Avenue, 9th Floor,
New York, NY 10017, USA

Visit us on the World Wide Web at:
www.haylemedical.com

ISBN: 978-1-63241-445-8

Printed in China.

Cataloging-in-Publication Data

Sleep disorders : a clinician's guide / edited by Eric Stiles.
p. cm.
Includes bibliographical references and index.
ISBN 978-1-63241-445-8
1. Sleep disorders. 2. Sleep disorders--Treatment. 3. Insomnia. 4. Clinical medicine. I. Stiles, Eric.

RC547 .S54 2017
616.849 8--dc23

Table of Contents

Preface

This book has been an outcome of determined endeavour from a group of educationists in the field. The primary objective was to involve a broad spectrum of professionals from diverse cultural background involved in the field for developing new researches. The book not only targets students but also scholars pursuing higher research for further enhancement of the theoretical and practical applications of the subject.

Sleep disorders are defined as the changes in sleeping patterns or habits that can negatively affect health. This book on sleep disorders aims to shed light on some of the unexplored aspects of this disorder and the recent researches in this field. It aims to provide its readers a wide spectrum of topics that are of utmost importance to sleep disorders. The causes of the disorder are elucidated so that the disorder could be understood in a better manner. This book also lays emphasis on the various techniques of treatment like different somatic treatment along with medicines. This book is an essential guide for both academicians, clinicians and those who wish to pursue this discipline further.

It was an honour to edit such a profound book and also a challenging task to compile and examine all the relevant data for accuracy and originality. I wish to acknowledge the efforts of the contributors for submitting such brilliant and diverse chapters in the field and for endlessly working for the completion of the book. Last, but not the least; I thank my family for being a constant source of support in all my research endeavours.

Editor

Violent Behaviour During Sleep

Scott G Williams[1,3]* and Christopher J Lettieri[2,3]

[1]Department of Medicine, Womack Army Medical Center, Fort Bragg, North Carolina, USA
[2]Pulmonary, Critical Care and Sleep Medicine, Walter Reed National Military Medical Center, Bethesda, Maryland, USA
[3]Department of Medicine, Uniformed Services University, Bethesda, Maryland, USA

Introduction

Sleep-related violence has been described as "aggressive behaviour arising out of disturbance or dysfunction during the sleep state that results in the physical harm of people or destruction of objects in the physical environment" [1]. A variety of medical, psychiatric and primary sleep disorders can manifest with potentially dangerous behaviour during the night. If not recognized and treated, serious harm or even death can result.

There are three main states of being: wake, Non-Rapid Eye Movement (NREM) sleep and Rapid Eye Movement (REM) sleep. Nocturnal violence can arise during any of these states. At times it can be difficult to determine whether an individual is awake and acting consciously, awake with some degree of cognitive impairment, or asleep with involuntary or unintended actions at the time of a violent act. Violence during sleep is, therefore, differentiated by the state of being during such actions and determined by whether the act was conscious or unconscious. Abnormal activities occurring during sleep, or parasomnias, are disruptive sleep disorders secondary to arousals or partial arousals from sleep or transitions among the different sleep stages. Sleep related violence is a unique, likely under-recognized parasomnia, which can manifest from aggressive gestures to significantly dangerous behaviours. The aim of this review is to provide an overview of violence during sleep and provide diagnostic and treatment strategies for these disorders.

Epidemiology

Although difficult to accurately assess due to under-reporting, violent acts are present in up to 3-5% of the general population. Of the epidemiologic studies that have assessed sleep-related violence, the one factor that seems to be consistent is that male gender is associated with an increased prevalence [2-4]. It is not well understood whether this is because sleep related violence truly occurs more often in men or if it is because men tend to experience more violent dreams and the resultant harm may be more significant. In the military population that we treat, sleep-related violence is almost exclusively a male phenomenon even though women are increasingly exposed to combat situations.

Ohayon et al. [5] conducted the two largest studies describing violence during sleep. In 1997, the authors reported that 2% of the 2078 men and 2894 women surveyed from a general population reported they had engaged in a violent act at least once when asleep [5]. Those who reported violent behaviours were also more likely to experience night terrors, daytime somnolence, somniloquy (sleep-talking), bruxism, hypnagogic hallucinations and hypnic jerks. Lifestyle factors associated with these events included an increased likelihood of smoking, caffeine use, and drinking alcohol close to bedtime. In 2010 the authors increased their sample size and conducted 19,961 telephone questionnaires in a general population. They discovered the reported prevalence of sleep related violence was 1.6%. Violent behaviours while asleep were more common in young adults less than 35 years of age. The majority (78.7%) of those with reported violent behaviours while asleep also reported vivid dream recall and 72.8% had other symptoms of parasomnias. Somnambulism (sleepwalking) and sleep terrors were commonly associated and had odds ratios of 2.0 and 4.2, respectively. Approximately 1/3 of those endorsing violent behaviours reported significant harm to themselves or others as a result of the act. A family history of violent behaviour during sleep was highly correlated with an odds ratio of 9.3 [6]. Only 12.3% consulted a physician for these behaviours.

NREM Disorders and Partial Arousals

NREM sleep is divided into stage 1 sleep (N1), stage 2 sleeps (N2), and slow wave sleep (SWS, N3). During stage 1 sleep, a patient can be easily awakened although they may seem confused or tired for a few seconds. Stage 2 sleep comprises a majority of the night and is associated with a higher arousal threshold than stage 1 sleep. Attempting to wake a patient from stage 2 sleep is more difficult and the post-arousal amnestic period is longer. SWS is a state of deep sleep and is the most difficult stage to arouse from. A partial awakening during SWS can results in a confusional arousal leading to unintentional or unconscious behaviour and activities, such as somniloqy (sleep talking), somnambulism (sleep talking), or night terrors.

Disorders of arousal have been described as an oscillation or dissociation between the wake and NREM state [7-9]. Other authors have used the terms "partial arousal" and "stuck between sleep and wakefulness". The American Academy of Sleep Medicine has defined these as "incomplete awakenings" from NREM sleep characterized by reduced vigilance, impaired cognition, retrograde amnesia for the event, and variable motor activity, ranging from repetitive and purposeless movements to more complex behaviours such as eating, drinking, driving, sexual intercourse and aggression [10]. They most commonly arise from SWS and, as such, typically occur during the first half of the night when the proportion of SWS is the highest. Confusional arousals are quite common in children, but may persist into adulthood. It is uncommon for SWS parasomnias to emerge during adulthood de novo, and precipitating factors, such as recreational drugs and alcohol, or alternative medical and psychiatric diagnoses should be considered in these cases [11,12]. Parasomnia events are often associated with predisposing and precipitating factors. Recent stress, sleep deprivation, alcohol use or erratic sleep-wake schedules may play a role in precipitating or exacerbating an event. Other sleep disorders that increase sleep fragmentation, such as Obstructive Sleep Apnea (OSA) or Restless Legs Syndrome (RLS) can also precipitate a confusional arousal.

***Corresponding author:** Scott G Williams, Department of Medicine, Womack Army Medical Center, Fayetteville, North Carolina, USA
E-mail: scott.g.williams@us.army.mil

NREM parasomnias with the potential for violence can be classified as either primary disorders of the sleep states or sleep state transitions, or secondary to pathologic conditions or external influences that emerge during sleep and/or disrupt normal sleep. Secondary parasomnias are typically a form of nocturnal frontal lobe epilepsy (NFLE) and are classified as "Parasomnias Due to Medical Condition" by the International Classification of Sleep Disorders [10]. Psychogenic dissociative states that occur during sleep may also result in parasomnia events [13].

For patients with a primary NREM parasomnia, violence tends to be uncommon unless the subject is provoked or suddenly awakened. A review of medical and legal case records from 1859 until 2007 concluded that reported violent behaviours were associated with provocations and/or close proximity in 100% of confusional arousal patients, 81% of sleep terror patients and 40-90% of sleepwalking patients [14].

In secondary NREM parasomnia events, violence may be an unintended consequence of the stereotyped behaviour common to NFLE or the result of activation of primitive defensive behaviours [15]. There are three subtypes of NFLE, nocturnal paroxysmal dystonia, paroxysmal arousals, and episodic nocturnal wanderings. Nocturnal paroxysmal dystonia can present with simple posturing but may also include more complex behaviours such as kicking or rhythmic core body motions. Paroxysmal arousals, on the other hand, tend to be less purposeful and can mimic night terrors. Episodic nocturnal wandering may include features of posturing, complex motor movement and can culminate with somnambulism [16]. NFLE is often successfully treated with anti-epileptic medication such as carbamazepine. However, despite adequate treatment up to 20 % of patients will have refractory seizures. Surgery may offer improved control of seizures in these individuals [17].

Given the potential complexity of the motor activity with some parasomnias events and the difficulty distinguishing these events from a wakeful state, disorders of arousal have been used as legal defense for violence occurring at night. During NREM sleep, there is a deactivation of the normal cortical regions responsible for monitoring and remembering behaviour despite preservation of motor activity. As stated, these patients lack the normal capacity to respond appropriately to the environment and their surroundings. This ability is the most useful means to differentiate parasomnias from a state of wakefulness [18]. Patients with NREM parasomnias may appear awake and can engage in complicated behaviours such as walking or even driving. However, they should not have appropriate interactions with their environment. Despite appearing awake, they are actually quite difficult to arouse and typically appear confused or even violent when awakened. They do not usually recall dreaming prior to their awakening.

Rapid Eye Movement Behaviour Disorder

Normal REM sleep produces skeletal muscle atonia. Rapid Eye Movement Behaviour Disorder (RBD) is a parasomnia characterized by the loss of normally occurring atonia during REM sleep accompanied by dream enacting behaviour [19]. The diagnosis of RBD requires both REM sleep without atonia (RSWA) during polysomnography as well as a clinical history consistent with dream enactment behaviour. Both criteria are required as RSWA in and of it may not produce complex behaviours, and dream enactment behaviour is present in a variety of disorders to include OSA, NREM parasomnias, Post-Traumatic Stress Disorder (PTSD) or as a consequence of alcohol use. Severe sleep deprivation may also precipitate dream enactment behaviour.

The lack of skeletal muscle atonia allows patients with RBD to act out their dreams without the normal inhibitory and defensive mechanisms present during the conscious state of wake. As such, both violent dreams, and those involving recreational activities and sports, can result in injury to self and others. The most common potentially lethal REM-related behavioural themes are choking or repeated striking of the bed partner. RBD may also co-exist with NREM parasomnias. This "overlap" syndrome can be complex and may result in severe injury [20]. RBD has been used successfully in numerous legal defenses and can be considered a "parasomnia with continuing danger" therefore classifying it a "non-insane automatism" [21].

Idiopathic RBD occurs in the absence of any identifiable underlying neurologic disease. Secondary, or symptomatic RBD results from, or occurs as part of an underlying neurodegenerative disorder. RBD can be precipitated by stroke and can be seen in narcolepsy patients. RBD is also reported as a side effect of SSRIs, mirtazapine, selegiline and cholinergic therapy in patients with pre-existing neurodegenerative conditions [4].

Among older adults, RBD has an estimated prevalence of 0.4-0.5%. However, the incidence is significantly greater in patients with neurodegenerative diseases such as Lewy body dementia, multiple system atrophy and Parkinson's disease [22]. Progressive supranuclear palsy has also been infrequently associated with REM behaviour disorder [23]. Multiple sclerosis is not commonly associated with RBD but can be seen when there are brainstem plaques. Over half of all RBD patients are eventually diagnosed with a neurological disease. A review of nearly 600 RBD cases since its formal classification in 1986 revealed a significant male predominance (80.8%) with a mean age of 65.6 years [4]. Other sources cite a slightly younger population (median onset 50-65 years) [24]. In comparison, NREM parasomnias are more common in younger men. The frequency of RBD episodes is highly variable, ranging from few lifetime occurrences to multiple events nearly every night [25].

In contrast to NREM parasomnias, RBD patients are usually easily awakened and can often recall dream content similar to the observed behaviour. Not all dreams occur during REM sleep, however. Dreaming can occur in all stages of sleep and dream enactment can be seen during somnambulism and sleep terrors. Oudiette et al. studied 43 patients with sleepwalking and observed that short, unpleasant dream-like mentations occurred in 71% of patients [11].

While not exclusive, the events typically occur in the latter part of the night when more REM sleep naturally predominates. Motor activity is usually less complex and shorter in duration than that seen with SWS parasomnias. Prolonged somnambulism is uncommon. RBD patients typically have their eyes closed during their episodes [26].

Post Traumatic Stress Disorder

Recurrent disturbing dreams are a common feature in PTSD. Sleep related violence is more common in patients with PTSD and its association is likely multifactorial. PTSD is associated with sleep fragmentation, and the psychoactive agents commonly used to treat PTSD cause disruption to normal sleep continuity and architecture. Some agents have, themselves, been shown to precipitate RBD events [4].

Violence during sleep often occurs following a particularly distressing dream or nightmare which can evoke a confusional arousal from NREM sleep or dream enacting behaviour during REM sleep. It is often difficult to determine if the physical behaviour manifests during sleep or if a patient wakes up and is confused by his/her surroundings, striking out at the nearest object. Given that a number of PTSD-related nightmares can arise from stage 2 NREM sleep [27,28] it may be more likely for disordered dreaming to result in a confusional arousal in this population. Confusional arousals, though typically seen during SWS, can also be seen during N2 sleep and may be present late into the sleep period [29]. Awakenings from N2 sleep are more abrupt than those occurring in SWS. And, unlike SWS which predominates in the early part of the night, N2 sleep occurs throughout the sleep period. As such, these events share many similar features with, and may be mistaken for RBD.

Common SWS parasomnias, such as somnambulism, may manifest differently in patients with PTSD. There is a paucity of data on the topic, but one study by Hartman et al. examined 22 patients with polysomnographically confirmed sleepwalking. Fourteen patients had no significant psychological trauma, while six had preceding traumatic events and symptoms consistent with PTSD. These patients differed from those without antecedent trauma in that they more commonly reported vivid, dreamlike mental content accompanying the parasomnia behaviour (83% vs. 25%). Those with a history of trauma also reported that the somnambulism was an attempt to flee from an attacker [30]. The inherently vulnerable state of sleep heightens primitive defensive mechanisms. It stands to reason, therefore, that the potential for violence is much greater if the patient feels as if he/she is being threated or has a pre-existing condition that makes them feel more vulnerable.

Other Causes of Sleep-Related Violence

Other conditions have the potential for sleep-related violence. Obstructive Sleep Apnea (OSA)-pseudo RBD is associated with violent dream enactment and may produce injury to the patient or bed partner. In a case report of OSA-pseudo RBD in which parasomnia behaviours manifested during abrupt respiratory-related arousals from REM and NREM sleep, CPAP was shown to significantly improve these symptoms[31]. Malingering, Munchausen Syndrome, and Munchausen Syndrome by proxy must also be considered in the differential diagnosis of violent sleep behaviours. Figure 1, reproduced from a recent review article by Siclari et al., lists the spectrum of medical and psychiatric disorders associated with sleep related violence [15]. If all other disease entities are ruled out, it is appropriate to consult with legal and forensic experts to determine the appropriate disposition [13].

Evaluation

The evaluation of nocturnal violence should begin with a thorough history. When evaluating patients with parasomnias, the first branch point is to distinguish NREM disorders from RBD. Table 1 summarizes the key clinical differences. Most parasomnias are non-violent, so if the only parasomnia behaviour reported is violent or the reason for the encounter is part of a forensic evaluation, the clinician should remain skeptical. Collateral information from the bed partner and other witnesses should always be obtained. Clinical tools such as the Nocturnal Frontal Lobe Epilepsy and Parasomnia Scale and the REM sleep behaviour disorder screening questionnaire can also be helpful [32,33]. Unexplained head trauma in an elderly individual should prompt questioning for RBD. Evaluation of underlying neurological conditions is also important. A detailed neurological exam with appropriate laboratory and radiographic studies may uncover subtle signs of a potentially treatable condition. Neuropsychological testing should be considered when any focal abnormality is discovered or if there are deficits on a mental status examination.

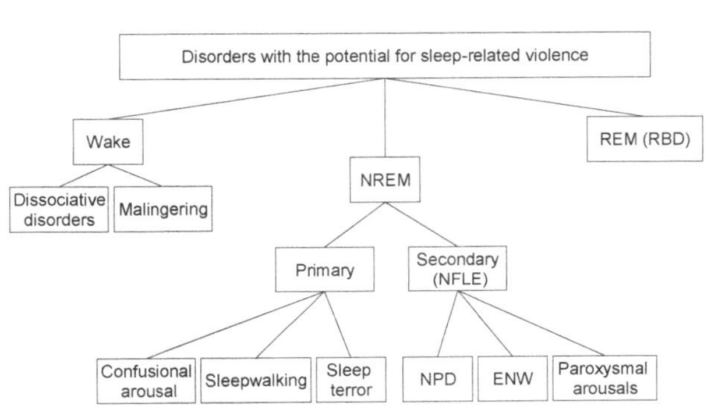

Figure 1: Disorders with the potential for sleep-related violence.

Polysomnography is an essential component in the evaluation of a patient with suspected violent behaviour during sleep. It can assess motor activity during different stages of sleep and help identify potential causes, such as OSA or nocturnal seizures. A polysomnographic evaluation must include multiple EEG channels to assess for seizure activity as well as video monitoring, and may be required over multiple nights. For RBD, RSWA should be a persistent abnormality. The sleep technologist should be instructed to take detailed notes regarding the patient's behaviour, especially if the patient moves out of the line of sight of the camera. As previously mentioned, laboratory staff should avoid touching the patient if possible since provocation may precipitate an attack. If the patient awakens, the technologist should ask the patient about any dreams that they can recall. This is helpful in correlating behaviour with dream-enactment. Though patients with NREM parasomnias have mostly normal sleep architecture, polysomnography (PSG) may also uncover a precipitating sleep disorder such as OSA. If there is a low concern for other sleep disorders, the PSG may be performed in the sleep-deprived state in order to uncover parasomnias [34]. If NFLE is suspected, additional daytime EEG may be considered after additional sleep deprivation. If in-lab PSG fails to capture any abnormal behaviour, a longer duration of nocturnal videography may be obtained using home videos [35].

Treatment

Non-pharmacologic therapies

Behavioural and environmental modifications are the mainstay of treatment for individuals with sleep-related violence. Due to the increased propensity for violent outbursts after sleep deprivation, it is essential to instruct patients on sleep hygiene and ensure that they adhere to a healthy sleep-wake routine. Avoidance of alcohol and other substances is also important in order to minimize violence while asleep. The bedroom should be made as a safe as possible. Particularly, for the NREM parasomnias, it may be necessary to put multiple locks on the bedroom and exterior doors of the house. Door alarms can be effective in alerting family members of a wandering individual. Potentially harmful objects or items that could be used as weapons should be removed. Padding the furniture, especially sharp corners, can also be helpful. Sleeping on the first floor may be required if there is the potential for defenestration. If a family member or caregiver encounters a wandering individual they should be cautious about approaching them due to the risk of a violent outburst upon awakening.

	NREM	RBD
Time	Early	Late
Memory of event	No	Yes
Arousability	Difficult	Easy
Post-event confusion	Yes	No
Age	Children/Young adults	Elderly
Genetic predisposition	Likely	Unlikely
Co-morbidities	Usually none	Neurodegenerative disorders
Treatment	BZD	BZD
Behaviours	More complicated, eyes open	Simple, eyes closed

Reproduced from: Lettieri CJ, **Williams SG** Sleep-related violence: what every clinician should know. MedScape Pulmonary Medicine, 2011

Table 1: Features of NREM vs. REM parasomnias.

Benzodiazepines

The most heavily prescribed medications for both NREM and REM parasomnias are benzodiazepines, particularly clonazepam. Although one recent retrospective chart review did showed a treatment response rate of 73.7%, [36] most of the data comes from clinical experience and there are few controlled trials to demonstrate the magnitude of the treatment effect.

N Serotonergic medications

It is postulated that serotonin is responsible for the increased muscle tone and inhibition of REM atonia due to actions at the pons or spinal cord. Serotonin reuptake inhibitors such as fluoxetine are associated with increased muscle tone during REM and theoretically may worsen RBD [37]. In contrast, sertraline and paroxetine have been effective treatments for disorders of arousal from NREM sleep [36,38].

Alpha-2-adrenoreceptor modulators

Alpha-2-adrenoreceptors are thought to mediate REM behaviour disorders. A case report by Onofrj et al. postulated that the alpha-2 antagonism of mirtazapine is implicated in REM behavioural disturbance [39]. Another group found that clonidine, an alpha-2 agonist, decreased the frequency of nocturnal outbursts in a case of treatment-refractory sleep-related violence [40].

High dose melatonin

Given that benzodiazepines can worsen sleep disorders such as OSA and can be dangerous in elderly patients at risk for falls, melatonin has been studied as an alternative and has been shown to be effective in retrospective studies [41-43] as well as in a small prospective cross-over study [44]. In many of these studies, doses from 3-12 mg per night were used. A recent survey compared the effectiveness of melatonin (mean dose 6mg per night) with clonazepam (mean dose 0.5 mg per night). Both medications were found to reduce injuries, with the melatonin group showing a more significant reduction. Melatonin also showed an improved safety profile compared with clonazepam. However, the majority of patients continued to have RBD symptoms and only 3 patients in each group reported complete resolution of nocturnal behaviours. (12% in the melatonin group vs. 16% in the clonazepam group). There were no differences in treatment retention, with 28% of melatonin patients and 22% of clonazepam patients discontinuing treatment [45].

Pramipexole

A few studies have shown that dopamine agonism may play a role in ameliorating RBD symptoms. Although the amount of RSWA did not change in these studies, patients did report symptomatic improvement [46,47]. In one study of 15 RBD patients, 80% reported improvement after 1 month of pramipexole therapy. Of the patients that reported improvement, most also reported a reduction or disappearance in nightmares. The authors hypothesized that reduction in REM density or alterations in dream content may have been partially responsible for the decrease in RBD severity [48]. Dopamine is highly linked to dreaming. High doses of dopaminergic drugs are known to induce vivid dreams or nightmares [49,50]. However, low doses of dopamine agonists such as pramipexole may actually reduce nightmares in patients with RBD. Clearly, more research is needed to identify optimal treatment strategies.

Conclusion

Violent behaviour resulting from primary sleep disorders is uncommon but potentially lethal. Recognizing the clinical differences between NREM parasomnias and RBD is important as it can impact both prognosis and treatment plans. Middle-aged or elderly patients with a suggestive history should have a comprehensive evaluation to include a neurologic exam and polysomnography to rule out RBD and potentially early signs of neurodegenerative disorders. Prompt identification of the etiology of the parasomnia, as well as initiation of safety precautions, can limit the morbidity associated with these disorders.

Evaluating patients for sleep related violence in response to criminal charges should not be immediately dismissed as an alibi. It is possible for the first reported event to result in significant injury or assault. However, these events are rarely isolated occurrences and the lack of a prior history of related events or identifiable precipitating factors should raise skepticism.

References

1. Leong G, Silva J (1999) Sleep-related violence. AAPL Newsl 24.
2. Moldofsky H, Gilbert R, Lue FA, MacLean AW (1995) Sleep-related violence. Sleep 18: 731-739.
3. Guilleminault C, Leger D, Philip P, Ohayon MM (1998) Nocturnal wandering and violence: review of a sleep clinic population. J Forensic Sci 43: 158-163.
4. Schenck CH, Lee SA, Bornemann MA, Mahowald MW (2009) Potentially lethal behaviors associated with rapid eye movement sleep behavior disorder: review of the literature and forensic implications. J Forensic Sci 54: 1475-1484.
5. Ohayon MM, Caulet M, Priest RG (1997) Violent behavior during sleep. J Clin Psychiatry 58: 369-376.
6. Ohayon MM, Schenck CH (2010) Violent behavior during sleep: prevalence, comorbidity and consequences. Sleep Med 11: 941-946.
7. Mahowald MW, Schenck CH (2004) Rem sleep without atonia--from cats to humans. Arch Ital Biol 142: 469-478.
8. Kotagal S (2009) Parasomnias in childhood. Sleep Med Rev 13: 157-168.
9. Fisher C, Kahn E, Edwards A, Davis DM (1973) A psychophysiological study of nightmares and night terrors. I. Physiological aspects of the stage 4 night terror. J Nerv Ment Dis 157: 75-98.
10. American Academy of Sleep Medicine. International classification of sleep disorders: diagnostic and coding manual, 2nd ed. Westchester, IL: American Academy of Sleep Medicine, 2005.
11. Oudiette D, Leu S, Pottier M, Buzare MA, Brion A, et al. (2009) Dreamlike mentations during sleepwalking and sleep terrors in adults. Sleep 32: 1621-1627.
12. Ohayon MM, Priest RG, Zulley J, Smirne S (2000) The place of confusional arousals in sleep and mental disorders: findings in a general population sample of 13,057 subjects. J Nerv Ment Dis 188: 340-348.

13. Mahowald MW, Bundlie SR, Hurwitz TD, Schenck CH (1990) Sleep violence--forensic science implications: polygraphic and video documentation. J Forensic Sci 35: 413-432.

14. Pressman MR (2007) Disorders of arousal from sleep and violent behavior: the role of physical contact and proximity. Sleep 30: 1039-1047.

15. Siclari F, Khatami R, Urbaniok F, Nobili L, Mahowald MW, et al. (2010) Violence in sleep. Brain 133: 3494-3509.

16. Provini F, Plazzi G, Tinuper P, Vandi S, Lugaresi E, et al. (1999) Nocturnal frontal lobe epilepsy. A clinical and polygraphic overview of 100 consecutive cases. Brain 122 : 1017-1031.

17. Nobili L, Francione S, Mai R, Cardinale F, Castana L, et al. (2007) Surgical treatment of drug-resistant nocturnal frontal lobe epilepsy. Brain 130: 561-573.

18. Bornemann MA, Mahowald MW, Schenck CH (2006) Parasomnias: clinical features and forensic implications. Chest 130: 605-610.

19. Boeve BF, Silber MH, Saper CB, Ferman TJ, Dickson DW, et al. (2007) Pathophysiology of REM sleep behaviour disorder and relevance to neurodegenerative disease. Brain 130: 2770-2788.

20. Schenck CH, Boyd JL, Mahowald MW (1997) A parasomnia overlap disorder involving sleepwalking, sleep terrors, and REM sleep behavior disorder in 33 polysomnographically confirmed cases. Sleep 20: 972-981.

21. Schenck CH, Mahowald MW (1995) A polysomnographically documented case of adult somnambulism with long-distance automobile driving and frequent nocturnal violence: parasomnia with continuing danger as a noninsane automatism? Sleep 18: 765-772.

22. Trotti LM (2010) REM sleep behaviour disorder in older individuals: epidemiology, pathophysiology and management. Drugs Aging 27: 457-470.

23. Compta Y, Martí MJ, Rey MJ, Ezquerra M (2009) Parkinsonism, dysautonomia, REM behaviour disorder and visual hallucinations mimicking synucleinopathy in a patient with progressive supranuclear palsy. J Neurol Neurosurg Psychiatry 80: 578-579.

24. Boeve B, Silber M, Ferman T (2003) REM sleep behavior disorder in Parkinson's disease, dementia with Lewy bodies, and multiple system atrophy. In: Bedard M, Agid Y, Chouinard S, Fahn S, Korczyn A, Lesperance P, editors Mental and behavioral dysfunction in movement disorders. Totowa: Humana Press, 383-397.

25. Olson EJ, Boeve BF, Silber MH (2000) Rapid eye movement sleep behaviour disorder: demographic, clinical and laboratory findings in 93 cases. Brain 123 : 331-339.

26. Schenck C. Paradox lost. Midnight in the battleground of sleep and dreams. Minneapolis, MN: Extreme-Nights, LLC, 2005.

27. van der Kolk B, Blitz R, Burr W, Sherry S, Hartmann E (1984) Nightmares and trauma: a comparison of nightmares after combat with lifelong nightmares in veterans. Am J Psychiatry 141: 187-190.

28. Kramer M, Kinney L (1988) Sleep patterns in trauma victims with disturbed dreaming. Psychiatr J Univ Ott 13: 12-16.

29. Naylor MW, Aldrich MS (1991) The distribution of confusional arousals across sleep stages and time of night in children and adolescents with sleep terrors. Sleep Res 20: 308.

30. Hartman D, Crisp AH, Sedgwick P, Borrow S (2001) Is there a dissociative process in sleepwalking and night terrors? Postgrad Med J 77: 244-249.

31. Iranzo A, Santamaría J (2005) Severe obstructive sleep apnea/hypopnea mimicking REM sleep behavior disorder. Sleep 28: 203-206.

32. Derry CP, Davey M, Johns M, Kron K, Glencross D, et al. (2006) Distinguishing sleep disorders from seizures: diagnosing bumps in the night. Arch Neurol 63: 705-709.

33. Stiasny-Kolster K, Mayer G, Schäfer S, Möller JC, Heinzel-Gutenbrunner M, et al. (2007) The REM sleep behavior disorder screening questionnaire--a new diagnostic instrument. Mov Disord 22: 2386-2393.

34. Joncas S, Zadra A, Paquet J, Montplaisir J (2002) The value of sleep deprivation as a diagnostic tool in adult sleepwalkers. Neurology 58: 936-940.

35. Nobili L (2009) Can homemade video recording become more than a screening tool? Sleep 32: 1544-1545.

36. Attarian H, Zhu L (2013) Treatment options for disorders of arousal: a case series. Int J Neurosci .

37. Winkelman JW, James L (2004) Serotonergic antidepressants are associated with REM sleep without atonia. Sleep 27: 317-321.

38. Lillywhite AR, Wilson SJ, Nutt DJ (1994) Successful treatment of night terrors and somnambulism with paroxetine. Br J Psychiatry 164: 551-554.

39. Onofrj M, Luciano AL, Thomas A, Iacono D, D'Andreamatteo G (2003) Mirtazapine induces REM sleep behavior disorder (RBD) in parkinsonism. Neurology 60: 113-115.

40. Nash JR, Wilson SJ, Potokar JP, Nutt DJ (2003) Mirtazapine induces REM sleep behavior disorder (RBD) in parkinsonism. Neurology 61: 1161.

41. Takeuchi N, Uchimura N, Hashizume Y, Mukai M, Etoh Y, et al. (2001) Melatonin therapy for REM sleep behavior disorder. Psychiatry Clin Neurosci 55: 267-269.

42. Boeve BF, Silber MH, Ferman TJ (2003) Melatonin for treatment of REM sleep behavior disorder in neurologic disorders: results in 14 patients. Sleep Med 4: 281-284.

43. Anderson KN, Shneerson JM (2009) Drug treatment of REM sleep behavior disorder: the use of drug therapies other than clonazepam. J Clin Sleep Med 5: 235-239.

44. Kunz D, Mahlberg R (2010) A two-part, double-blind, placebo-controlled trial of exogenous melatonin in REM sleep behaviour disorder. J Sleep Res 19: 591-596.

45. McCarter SJ, Boswell CL, St Louis EK, Dueffert LG, Slocumb N, et al. (2013) Treatment outcomes in REM sleep behavior disorder. Sleep Med 14: 237-242.

46. Fantini ML, Gagnon JF, Filipini D, Montplaisir J (2003) The effects of pramipexole in REM sleep behavior disorder. Neurology 61: 1418-1420.

47. Schmidt MH, Koshal VB, Schmidt HS (2006) Use of pramipexole in REM sleep behavior disorder: results from a case series. Sleep Med 7: 418-423.

48. Sasai T, Inoue Y, Matsuura M (2012) Effectiveness of pramipexole, a dopamine agonist, on rapid eye movement sleep behavior disorder. Tohoku J Exp Med 226: 177-181.

49. Kulisevsky J, Roldan E (2004) Hallucinations and sleep disturbances in Parkinson's disease. Neurology 63: S28-30.

50. Gjerstad MD, Boeve B, Wentzel-Larsen T, Aarsland D, Larsen JP (2008) Occurrence and clinical correlates of REM sleep behaviour disorder in patients with Parkinson's disease over time. J Neurol Neurosurg Psychiatry 79: 387-391.

2

Willis-Ekbomdisease (Restless Legs Syndrome) Pathophysiology: The Imbalance Between Dopamine and Thyroid Hormone Theory

José Carlos Pereira Jr[1]* and Marcia Pradella-Hallinan[2]

[1]*Departamento de Pediatria – Faculdade de Medicina de Jundiaí, Jundiaí, SP, Brazil*
[2]*Departamento de Psicobiologia - Universidade Federal de São Paulo, Brazil*

Abstract

Willis-Ekbom disease (WED), also known as restless legs syndrome, is generally accepted as a disease of unknown pathophysiology, though it is believed that dysfunctions in the dopaminergic system and iron metabolism may play a role. However, an increasing body of evidence points to the insufficient modulation of thyrotropin hormone by the neurohormone dopamine (DA) as the underlying mechanism of the disease pathology. Additionally, it has generally been accepted that the annoying symptoms of the disease are generated inside the Blood Brain Barrier (BBB). This assumption, which has little evidence supporting it, has been weakened by the recent observation that domperidone, a DA blocking agent that does not cross the BBB, worsens the severity of WED symptoms. In 1974, it was discovered that levodopa dramatically relieves WED symptoms, thus supporting the hypothesis that insufficient dopaminergic function contributes to WED pathogenesis. Earlier, in 1970, it was observed that venous infusion of DA diminishes thyrotropin levels, and from clinical studies, it is known that WED symptoms are worse in the evening and night, when thyrotropin activity increases. Furthermore, drugs that alleviate WED symptoms increase the DA activity or decrease the Thyroid Hormone (TH) activity, whereas drugs that worsen WED tend to have the opposite effects on DA and TH activity. In this article, we present robust evidence to support the hypothesis that WED is caused by an imbalance between DA and TH and that its symptoms are generated in the periphery of the somatosensory system. We theorize that WED should be considered a functional peripheral neuropathy.

Keywords: Willis-Ekbom disease; Restless legs syndrome; Restless legs syndrome pathophysiology; Dopamine; Thyroid hormone

Introduction

Willis-Ekbom disease (WED), also known as restless legs syndrome, is a common sensorimotor disorder characterized by a strong, nearly irresistible urge to move the legs when the patient is at rest [1]. The currently accepted definitions of adult RLS from the "International Restless Syndrome Study Group (IRLSSG)" and the "International Classification of Sleep Disorders, second edition (ICSD-2)", are described below (italic). All four features are necessary to make the diagnosis in adults and children [1,2].

1) An urge to move the legs is usually accompanied or caused by uncomfortable paresthesias and/or pain in the legs. When the paresthesias are not present, patients may only state that they are uncomfortable with inactivity, and as such, they have to move the legs. Many of these patients cannot precisely describe this inactivity or discomfort. Put simply, quietness drives the patient to move.

2) The urge to move or unpleasant sensations begin or worsen during periods of rest or inactivity, such as while lying or sitting. The urge to move may not be restricted to the legs but also extends to other parts of the body, mainly the arms.

3) The urge to move or unpleasant sensations are partially or totally relieved by movements such as walking or stretching, as long as the activity continues.

4) The urge to move or unpleasant sensations are worse in the evening or night than during the day or only occur during the evening or at night. This is considered the hard-rock criterion: if one subject has all of the first three criteria but not this fourth one, a WED diagnosis cannot be made, according to IRLSSG.

The main supportive clinical features of WED include a positive family history of WED, Periodic Limb Movements during Sleep (PLMS), and periodic limb movements during wakefulness (PLMW). An additional supportive clinical feature is the "improvement of RLS symptoms with dopamine (DA) therapy" [1-3].

As mentioned above, WED can be described as a sensorimotor disorder. As such, a better understanding of its pathogenesis may be obtained through separate analysis of its sensory and motor components. From clinical experience with WED, it is known that movements are caused by discomfort in the legs when the patient experiences a resting behavior. Movement tends to relieve the discomfort, thus suggesting that movement is a response to the discomfort. Although it is difficult for the patient to deliberately not move, he/she is able to remain still for a variable lapse of time, and additionally, the patient can stop moving when someone orders it. Likewise, the patient is able to move just one leg even when the desire is to move both. From these clinical observations, it is reasonable to suggest that the motor part of the disease most likely is not pathological by itself. Rather, the movements of a person during a typical WED symptom episode are entirely physiological, and they obey the normal mechanisms of movement physiology. Following this reasoning, the outstanding question is what causes the discomfort in WED patients.

Regarding the sensory part of WED clinical presentation, a question

***Corresponding author:** José Carlos Pereira Jr, Rua Isaí Leiner 54, Jundiaí - SP-13201 854, São Paulo, Brazil E-mail: joscarlospereirajr@gmail.com

must be addressed: Are WED symptoms generated in the periphery of the nervous system, or are they born centrally? [4]. Ekbom, who initiated studies on WED in 1945, was one of the first researchers to describe RLS in amputees (1961) [5,6]. In his paper [7], he hypothesized that the symptoms were generated in the periphery of the nervous system. There is currently no definitive proof of this hypothesis [8]; however, various clinical insights argue that WED symptoms are indeed generated in the periphery of the somatosensory system [9]. Recently, we hypothesized that stimuli of sensory receptors located deep inside the legs spread up to the somatosensory cortex and are felt as unpleasant WED symptoms when not appropriately modulated [9]. Frequently, applying massage or cold pads onto the legs or simply stretching them can relieve WED symptoms [8]. Commonsense reasoning indicates that these measures applied in the periphery would fail to relieve symptoms born centrally [4]. Furthermore, some patients who have had one leg amputated may have WED symptoms only in the missing limb (phantom WED) [7,10]. In addition, some patients who have undergone total knee arthroplasty surgery begin to experience WED symptoms only in the leg that underwent the operation [11]. Thus, many logical arguments suggest that the peripheral somatosensory system initiates WED symptoms. According to normal physiology, the peripheral somatosensory receptors deep inside the legs receive stimuli from the environment and send their signaling to the cortex. Regarding this function in WED sufferers, we have posited (2010) that WED symptoms may result when the threshold of sensory receptors is reduced and/or the strength of the neurotransmission is high enough to surpass the levels that can induce modulation by DA (and other modulation systems) [11,12]. If WED symptoms originated in the brain itself, then they would be hallucinations, which is an inappropriate hypothesis considering the clinical correlates of WED. Models of dopaminergic dysfunction in RLS focus on central dopaminergic neurons, meaning those inside the Blood Brain Barrier (BBB). However, recently it has been observed that domperidone, a peripheral dopamine blocker that cannot cross the BBB, dramatically worsens WED symptoms in Parkinson's disease patients [13]. This observation strongly challenges the hypothesis that WED symptoms are generated inside the brain. Of the four major neural DA systems, the only one where DA can be counteracted by domperidone is the tuberoinfundibular pathway. The hypothalamus releases DA as a neurohormone in the pituitary stalk, where it mainly functions as an inhibitor of thyrotropin and prolactin hormones.

Recently, we hypothesized that the neurohormone DA, released by the arcuate nucleus of the hypothalamus in the tuberoinfundibular pathway, is not sufficient to inhibit the release of thyrotropin by the thyrotrophs of the pituitary, causing WED symptoms to occur in some subjects. We refer to this as the imbalance between DA and thyroid hormones (TH) theory (IMBDA/TH) on WED pathophysiology [12]. Increased TH levels, secondary to an insufficient modulation of thyrotropin by DA, diminish the threshold for stimuli perception of somatosensory receptors located deep inside the leg and also increase the synaptic velocity of perceived stimuli on their way to the somatosensory cortex, where they are felt as unpleasant sensations [11].

In the 1970s, it was observed that the intravenous infusion of DA decreases thyrotropin levels [14]. DA does not cross the BBB, so its action on thyrotropin levels is exercised outside the BBB and likely in the DA tuberoinfundibular pathway, the most important site where thyrotropin is released. Additionally, it was observed that metoclopramide increases thyrotropin and TH levels [15,16], which is important because metoclopramide worsens the severity of WED symptoms [8]. Domperidone, which does not cross the BBB, acts as a DA blocker and equally worsens WED symptoms. These observations suggest that DA blocking agents worsen WED symptoms by acting in the tuberoinfundibular pathway, thus leading to impaired thyrotropin inhibition.

To summarize, DA diminishes thyrotropin levels (consequently, TH levels are also reduced) [14], and DA agonists mitigate WED symptoms [6]. DA blocking agents in the tuberoinfundibular pathway increase thyrotropin levels by impairing DA actions [14,15] and worsen the severity of WED [6]. Furthermore, elevated TH levels (e.g., Grave's disease) remarkably increase the incidence of WED symptoms [17,18]. Adding more plausibility to the IMBDA/TH, it is known that WED symptoms appear (or worsen) in the evening and night [6,8], a time when thyrotropin levels are increased compared to daytime levels [19]. Additionally, from clinical practice, it is known that many drugs that worsen WED symptoms increase TH activity by inhibiting the 3A4 isoform of cytochrome P450 where part of TH is degraded (e.g., calcium channel blockers; SSRIs) [8,12]; some drugs that relieve WED symptoms diminish TH activity by inducing the 3A4 isoform of cytochrome P450 (e.g., Saint John's Wort) [20]. Notably, it has been observed that the tuberoinfundibular and mesolimbic DA pathways in the brain regulate the expression of the cytochrome P450 system of enzymes in rats. Additionally, the DA agonist pramipexole decreases thyrotropin levels as a side effect after just a single oral administration [21-23].

Ultimately, it can be posited that WED is a very mild form of thyrotoxicosis with a circadian presentation, meaning that there is enhanced TH activity in the evening and night. Clinical observations demonstrate that patients in a thyrotoxicosis condition are characterized by nervousness and hyperkinesia. During a medical interview, these patients shift positions frequently and often without purpose. Fidgetiness is a hallmark characteristic of both WED and thyrotoxicosis patients [24] (Figure 1).

Thyroid Hormone Actions may Elicit WED Symptoms When Not Appropriately Modulated

TH affects virtually every organ system in the body, and it is crucial for the normal functioning of our sensory systems [25,26]. TH increases the basal metabolic rate, heat production, and oxygen consumption. It also alters cardiovascular and respiratory function to increase blood flow and oxygen delivery to the tissues. A vast array of proteins is synthesized under the direction of TH, including the NA+- K+ ATPase, the Ca^{2+} ATPase transport proteins, β-1-adrenergic receptors, lysosomal enzymes, and proteolytic enzymes [26]. Most TH actions are exercised by long-duration, slow-acting genomic effects [26]. Relative to the timescales of our circadian rhythms and to the fluctuation of symptoms of a typical WED patient over the course of a day, the genomic actions of TH are quite slow, which would suggest that these

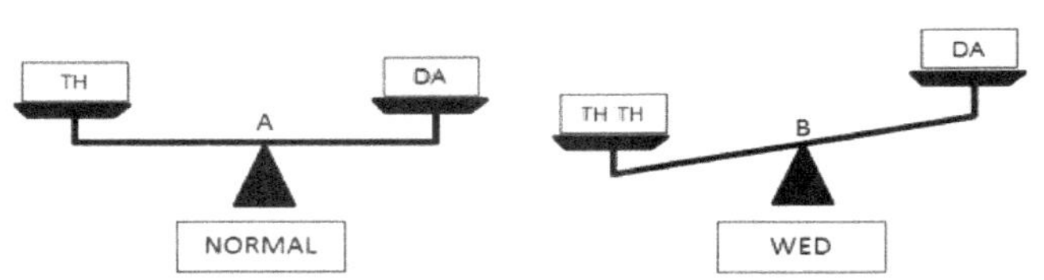

Figure 1: A representation of how Willis-Ekbom Syndrome (Restless legs syndrome) symptoms may occur when the "weight" of the TH axis is magnified compared to DA. A) The "weight" of DA is sufficient to counterbalance the excitatory effects of TH. B) WED may occur in prone subjects when the "weight" of the TH is magnified compared to DA. WED=Willis-Ekbom disease. TH=thyroid hormone. DA=dopamine.

mechanisms do not contribute to WED symptoms [27]. However, the actions of TH on mitochondria [26-29] may play an important role in the generation of WED symptoms and in their circadian aspects. Mitochondria are the organelles responsible for adenosine triphosphate (ATP) production, and TH increases their number and activity [26]. Throughout the nervous system, TH increases the strength and velocity of synaptic transmission [26]. In the CNS, an increase in TH levels enhances cognitive processes, and when levels of TH fall, these processes slow [26]. Burnstock et al. introduced the concept of purinergic neurotransmission, and it is now generally accepted that the multifunctional nucleoside ATP is also a neurotransmitter [30,31]. ATP acts mainly as an excitatory neurotransmitter [30,31] and may be the mechanism by which TH acts on alertness. It is common for WED patients to be in a state of hyper-arousal (increased level of alertness) [8]. We hypothesize that TH enhances synaptic transmission and, thus, causes increased vigilance and more WED symptoms in prone subjects.

Adenosine Triphosphate (ATP) acts as a fast excitatory transmitter in several regions of the Central Nervous System (CNS) [32]. In presynaptic terminals, ATP is accumulated and stored in the synaptic vesicles either alone or with other neurotransmitters (e.g., gamma-amino-butyric acid (GABA) or glutamate) [32]. Increasing evidence indicates a widespread role for glutamate as a fast-acting excitatory neurotransmitter at different levels in somatosensory pathways [33]. There is evidence that many different neuroactive substances are involved in the transmission and modulation of somesthetic information in the central nervous system, and additionally, there is evidence that glutamate, an excitatory neurotransmitter, has an important role in the ascending somatosensory pathways [33].

We hypothesize that TH acts on mitochondria to enhance ATP production, and then, ATP enhances transmission of the inputs that travel through the somatosensory pathways and glutamate neurotransmission. In this manner, stimuli received by the somatosensory receptors deep inside the leg are too strongly transmitted to the sensory cortex and are felt as unpleasant WED sensations. In this context, the diminished DA activity of the tuberoinfundibular pathway has a causative role in WED pathophysiology by not being able to sufficiently modulate TH actions on the mitochondria. Recently, it was observed that thalamic glutamate/glutamine activity is increased in WED patients, which increases arousal and shortens sleep [34]. This increased glutamate activity may be interpreted as a dense confluence of inputs that come from the peripheral somatosensory receptors, pass through the relay nuclei of the thalamus, and ultimately get to the somatosensory cortex. From the peripheral receptors, these sensory inputs travel in increased strength (secondary to increased TH activity), being facilitated mainly by glutamate and ATP. Together with paresthesias, pain is common in many WED patients [6]. Glutamate may be involved as a neurotransmitter, and most likely, the neuropeptide substance P plays a role [26].

The GABAergic system is the predominant inhibitory system in the CNS [26], and if a drug has the ability to enhance GABA signaling, it may alleviate WED symptoms. Drugs with this profile include the benzodiazepines, benzodiazepine-like drugs, and carbamazepine. Drugs that inhibit the excitability of the sensory neurons that convey messages to the cortex include many anticonvulsant drugs, such as gabapentin, an analog of GABA that is a highly efficient drug for ameliorating WED symptoms [35]. The pharmacological and therapeutic evidence highlight the importance of a strengthened neurotransmission of sensory inputs to the sensory cortex as the ultimate trigger of WED symptoms.

Iron Deficiency and Willis-Ekbom Disease

WED is more common or symptoms are more severe in iron deficient patients, and symptoms ameliorate when iron treatment is administered [6,8]. These facts imply that iron plays a central role in WED pathophysiology. These clinical and therapeutic observations may also be explained in terms of the IMBTH/DA as the main cause of WED [20].

Iron is a cofactor of many enzymatic systems [26], and it is reasonable to assume that when it is lacking in the enzymes of which it is part, these enzymes will experience a reduction in their activity, with the intensity correlating with the severity is the iron deficiency [20]. In the chain of reactions ending in the synthesis of DA, iron acts as a cofactor of the enzyme tyrosine hydroxylase (Thy) that catalyzes the conversion of tyrosine into L-DOPA. This step is the rate limiting stage in the synthesis of DA [36]; as such, we suggest that iron deficiency may result in less DA production. Additionally, iron is an integral part of all cytochromes [26], one of them being CYP450, which has a critical role in the degradation of TH (Figure 2).

As such, it is reasonable to assume that the lack of iron will impair the balance between TH and DA in two ways: (1) by decreasing DA synthesis and (2) by diminishing TH metabolism [20]. Many MRI and ultrasound observations have documented decreased brain iron in the substantia nigra [37]; however, it may be misleading to suggest that the DA dysfunction that causes WED exists in the dopaminergic system of the substantia nigra. It is reasonable to hypothesize that brain iron is scarce because some derangement impairs the brain's ability to acquire all of the iron it needs, but this is not clear evidence that deficient brain iron causes WED. If the overall levels of iron are deficient, then this deficiency will be observed ubiquitously throughout the brain. More importantly, the levels of ferritin (which is a measure of iron deposits) are low in some WED patients, and when these patients are treated with iron to increase their ferritin levels, they experience an improvement of their WED symptoms [6]. As it is improbable that the WED symptoms are generated inside the brain, it becomes unimportant to know if the brain iron is scarce or not. As iron is a cofactor for THy, iron scarcity may cause impaired synthesis of DA by low activity of the THy.

As dopaminergic agonists alleviate the symptoms of WED, it is

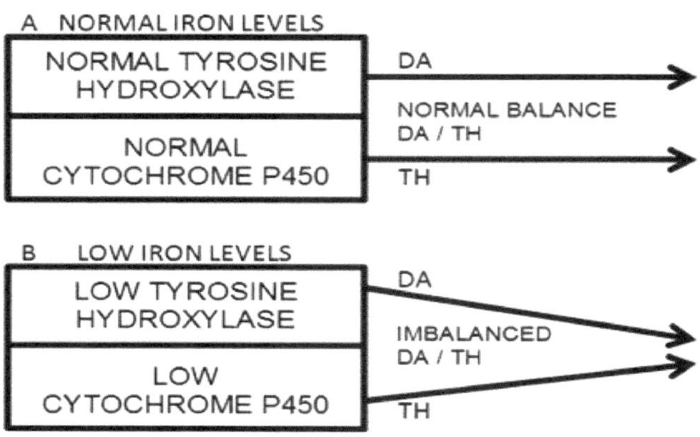

Figure 2: (A) Normal levels of iron correspond to normal expression of tyrosine hydroxylase and cytochrome P450, which results in normal DA synthesis and TH breakdown. (B) Low levels of iron correspond to the diminished expression of tyrosine hydroxylase and cytochrome P450, which leads to diminished DA synthesis and TH breakdown. This effect causes an imbalance in the interaction between TH and DA. DA=dopamine; TH=thyroid hormone. (With permission from Pereira et al. Clinics, 2010; 65(5): 547–54).

more likely that DA hypo function rather than DA dysfunction is the underlying cause of WED. A circadian insufficiency of DA is central to WED pathophysiology. The most significant DA system involved in WED pathophysiology is the tuberoinfundibular pathway, as mentioned above. Synthesized in the dopaminergic arcuate nucleus of the hypothalamus, DA reaches the pituitary portal blood supply. The half-life of DA is extremely short (2 minutes); thus, a dynamic iron supply is required for its synthesis so this trace element may quickly get connected to Thy and boost this enzyme that is so vital to DA production. The blood that bathes the arcuate nucleus is the more logical logistic mechanism to deliver iron for these DA neurons. If there is insufficient circulating iron to be delivered for the arcuate nucleus, the synthesis of DA may be delayed, and then, WED symptoms may ensue in prone subjects. From all this reasoning, it is possible to assert that the iron deficiency theory for WED pathophysiology is ultimately the DA hypo function theory. Recently, it was observed that there is increased THy activity in both WED autopsy and the rodent iron-deprivation model of WED, suggesting an increased DA synthesis in WED [38]. Our interpretation for this finding is that the increased presence of THy does not mean increased DA synthesis, as one cannot be certain that this is entirely functional. Iron is a cofactor for the THy protein, and thus if there is insufficient iron to be aggregated and to saturate the parent protein, then this enzyme will not be entirely functional. For DA metabolic production, this means that the enzyme is inappropriately produced and more parent enzymatic protein will be produced, although this excess of enzyme, lacking the cofactor iron, will not be entirely functional. For WED patients who do not have iron deficiency, the cause of the tuberoinfundibular DA hypo production is unknown. Primary WED is most frequently an inherited condition, and the inheritance of impaired enzymatic systems is a common cause of disease in humans, so it is reasonable to suggest that primary WED is a disease caused by some impairment in the enzymes involved in DA synthesis. Additionally, it is possible to speculate that primary WED patients are born with less DA neurons in the arcuate nucleus of the hypothalamus than normal individuals.

The Diencephalon-spinal Dopamine System

From the diencephalic dopamine A11 cell group, in the hypothalamus, dopaminergic neuron projections descend to the spinal cord and primarily reach the dorsal horns at all spinal levels and the associated parts of the intermediate and central gray matter [39]. There is evidence that favors the participation of the spinal dopaminergic system in pain modulation and autonomic and motor responses [40]. The dysfunction of spinal dopaminergic neurons could be involved in the pathophysiology of certain conditions, such as Parkinson's disease [40]. It appears possible that some beneficial effects of dopamine agonists in this condition as well as some of the side effects of neuroleptics are mediated through their actions on spinal dopaminergic mechanisms [40]. It has been hypothesized (2006) that the diminished activity of this dopaminergic tract is involved in WED pathophysiology [41]. This hypothesis seems well founded. From the somatosensory receptors in the legs, the inputs of unpleasant sensations reach the dorsal horn first and then ascend to the sensory cortex. Inhibitory systems in the dorsal horn modulate the excessive signaling of these sensory receptors to the cortex, which mainly include the GABA system and the mentioned DA system. Pain is common in WED patients, and as this diencephalon-spinal DA system is a pain modulator [40], it is likely that this system contributes to the pain and dysesthesia felt by WED sufferers when weakened [41]. In such a situation, dopaminergic modulation on the strong inputs from sensory receptors to the cortex would be diminished. As it is the DA neurotransmitter that plays a role in this mentioned tract, it is likely that DA hypo function underlies WED pathophysiology; DA, both as a neurohormone and neurotransmitter, acts on the hypothalamus to contribute to WED pathophysiology.

Drug-induced Willis-Ekbom Disease

Many drugs influence the severity of WED symptoms; some drugs alleviate, whereas others aggravate them. A study of pharmacological profiles suggests that drugs that alleviate WED tend to reduce TH activity, whereas drugs that aggravate WED tend to augment TH. One of these effects may actually be secondary to the diverse actions these drugs have on the Cytochrome P450 system (CYP450): the first induces the system (e.g., dopamine agonists), and the second inhibits it (e.g., SSRIs) [20].

Sequential deiodination degrades approximately 80% of the circulating pool of TH, and the remainder is mainly metabolized within the cytochrome P450 system, where TH is conjugated with glucuronides and sulfates. Glucuronides are then excreted into bile, where they participate as intermediates in the enterohepatic cycle and fecal excretion of TH [42]. Sulfation accelerates the deiodination of different iodothyronines by type I deiodinase and thus initiates the irreversible degradation of the hormone [20,42]. This second pathway is less prevalent and represents approximately 20% of the total TH metabolism [43]; however, for the pathophysiology of WED, it is of great significance. TH behaves similarly to a steroid hormone, and most steroid hormones are substrates for the CYP3A4 enzyme isoform [43]. There is strong evidence that when the CYP3A4 isoform is induced, TH glucuronidation and sulfation are also induced [20,43-45]. Notably, many drugs that relieve or worsen WED symptoms are inducers or inhibitors, respectively, of the CYP3A4 isoform (Table 1). Pramipexole is an effective treatment for WED that is a typical DA agonist with selective affinity for the D2 receptor subfamily [23,46]. Pramipexole also regulates the expression of many CYP450 enzymes through the tuberoinfundibular and mesolimbic dopaminergic pathways [22]. By inducing CYP4503A4 isoform, pramipexole increases TH metabolism. Furthermore, pramipexole administration decreases the release of TSH [47]. These two pharmacological actions of pramipexole may explain why it is effective as a WED treatment. Xenobiotic drugs may also aggravate WED symptoms through decreased dopaminergic signaling [8,20] (Table 1).

Regarding drugs that improve WED, there are four pharmacological targets for these drugs: 1) diminishing the TSH release (e.g., pramipexole); 2) enhancing theCYP3A expression (e.g., Saint John's wort); 3) modulating the WED sensation inputs on their pathway from the peripheral sensory receptors to the sensory cortex (e.g., gabapentin); and 4) diminishing the TH release from the thyroid gland by decreasing the SS activity (clonidine) [20]. The beneficial effects of clonidine on RLS symptoms highlight the importance of the connection between the Sympathetic System (SS) and the TH axis. Clonidine, which is an alpha-2 adrenergic receptor agonist, is a sympatholytic agent that relieves WED symptoms in many patients [35]. The SS has nerve projections to the thyroid gland and induces TH release [48] that, when excessive, may cause IMBTH/DA [20]. Clonidine targets the enhanced functioning of the SS, which makes it a useful drug for alleviating WED symptoms that are occasionally generated in response to an exacerbation of the SS tonus [20]. It is known that an enhanced tonus of the sympathetic nervous system impairs sleep [49]. As TH may inhibit sleep [27], we believe that one of the mechanisms by which an elevated sympathetic nervous tonus system hampers sleep is through releasing TH directly from the thyroid gland via its fibers directed to the gland.

Class of drugs	Examples	CYP3A4 substrates	CYP3A4 inhibitors	Effects on DA system
Calcium channel blockers	Verapamil Diltiazem	Yes +++ Yes +++	Yes ++ Yes ++	No
Selective serotonin reuptake inhibitors	Fluoxetine Paroxetine Sertraline Citalopram Escitalopram Fluvoxamine	Yes + No Yes + Yes +++ Yes +++ No	Yes + Yes + Yes ++ No No Yes +	No
Neuroleptics	Haloperidol Chlorpromazine Clozapine Pimozide Quetiapine	Yes +++ Yes + Yes + Yes +++ Yes +++	Yes ++ No Yes + Yes + No	Yes: block DA D2 receptors
Anti-nausea agents	Metoclopramide Domperidone	No Yes +	No	Yes: block DA D2 receptors
Lipid lowering agents	Atorvastatin Lovastatin Simvastatin	Yes +++ Yes +++ Yes +++	Yes + Yes + No	No
Non-steroidal anti-inflammatory drugs	Diclofenac	Yes +	Yes ++	No
Stimulants	Caffeine	Yes +	Yes ++	No

(+=mild, ++=moderate, and +++=strong), References: [20,44,45].

Table 1: Suggested mechanisms by which some drugs aggravate WED. The drugs listed in this table (substrates and/or inhibitors of CYP3A4) affect WED by inhibiting the CYP3A4 isoform, thereby decreasing TH metabolism. Some drugs are only substrates of the CYP3A4; nevertheless, they can diminish TH metabolism by competition with TH at sites of the enzyme. In addition, some drugs may cause a direct decline in dopaminergic signaling.

Periodic Limb Movements in Sleep

Periodic Limb Movements in Sleep (PLMS) consist of stereotypical, intermittent, and repetitive movements of the limbs that occur during sleep [49]. Up to 90% of the WED sufferers present PLMS [49], which is considered to be a supportive criterion for the diagnosis of WED. The concomitance between WED and PLMS is so great that it suggests a common causality between the two conditions, and our assumption is that both are engendered by the same mechanism: increased esthesia of the superficial and deep somatosensory receptors in the legs. The threshold for receiving stimuli from the environment by these receptors is reduced. Stimuli captured by these receptors are transduced and result in exaggerated action potentials and inputs, which strongly reach the spinal cord and then the somatosensory cortex. During wakefulness, these afferent signals prompt a response by the cortex to elicit conscious movements. Our assumption for this movement response is that activity incites a massage effect on the somatosensory receptors. During movement, leg muscles exert continuous and rhythmic pressure on the receptors so that they stop firing to the cortex, similar to what happens when massage is applied to the legs of a WED patient. The patient learns that movements relieve the ailment and movements thus become a conditioned reflex. During wakefulness, four neurons are responsible for the cortex to feel the WED sensation. During wakefulness, the cortex is activated by the reticular activating system, thus it is opened to stimuli that come from the periphery. The patient experiences the typical WED symptoms and consciously responds to them trying to obtain relief. During sleep, the cortex is relatively closed for stimuli that come from the periphery; the sensory cortex does not register WED symptoms. However, the spinal cord does register the inputs coming to it. These sensations are relayed by one of the two axon branches of the pseudo monosynaptic neuron that, located in the dorsal horn, is the neuron responsible by capturing stimuli from the periphery and transducing them into action potentials. As the patient is sleeping, the cortex is closed but the spinal cord is not, and a spinal reflex is triggered: the PLMS. PLMS usually involves the lower extremities, but arms can also be affected. The patient experiences partial flexion of the ankle, knee, and hip with extension of the big toe and fanning of the small toes [49]. PLMS resemble the pathologic slower spinal flexor nocifensive (protective) reflex, the triple flexion reflex. Dorsiflexion of the big toe and fanning of the other toes, found in PLMS, resembles the Babinski sign [50]. It is known that the Babinski sign can sometimes be elicited in normal subjects during sleep [50]. Regarding PLMS, our assumption is that the IMBDA/TH conditions enhance TH activity, which reduces the threshold for stimuli sensitivity of the nociceptors of the somatosensory system. Capturing nonspecific stimuli (allodynia), these receptors fire action potentials that trigger the PLMS, which resembles the triple flexion spinal reflex. Sensory receptors "adapt" to stimuli and for a variable lapse of time they silence, during which time the patient's limbs stay still. After this variable lapse of time, receptors recover their transduction capacity and fire action potentials again. As such, as their name implies, the PLMS are observed as periodic non-volitional movements. Periodic limb movements during wakefulness (PLMW), which some WED patients also present, most likely follow the same triggering mechanisms of PLMS. In our experience, PLMW are usually more prevalent in more severely affected WED patients; their IMBDA/TH most likely is more intense as the PLMW occur even though the wakefulness state is inhibiting spinal reflexes. Recently (2013), it was observed that RLS patients present a 3- to 4-fold increase in sensitivity to pinprick stimuli in both extremities, a sensory pathway involved in withdrawal reflexes [51]. This finding suggests that the somatosensory receptors of WED patients have a diminished threshold for nociceptive stimuli, when compared to normal subjects. This fact adds veracity to the "peripheral- engendered-symptoms" hypothesis, as well as the location where WED symptoms are generated, and also may explain why pain is common in WED patients.

Some Correlates of the Willis-Ekbom Disease

It is noteworthy that not only do many drugs worsen the severity of WED but also many clinical conditions increase the severity of existing WED, or even trigger a new WED episode. For the majority of the medical conditions in this category, there is a recognizable pathology that disrupts the fragile balance between DA and TH through impairing tuberoinfundibular DA release, or inducing an increase in TH levels that surpasses the counteracting capacity of DA in modulating TH actions.

WED during pregnancy is a straightforward example of impairment in DA release. Estradiol levels, mainly during the third trimester of pregnancy, increase considerably with the purpose of inhibiting the release of DA. DA inhibits prolactin, which must be counteracted once prolactin is needed to boost both enlargement of the mammary gland and milk production [9]. Estradiol accomplishes this function and thereby prepares the mother to breast feed the baby. If DA inhibition is too intense, the synthesis of thyrotropin by the pituitary increases too much, leading to WED symptoms [9].

The hyperthyroidism state of Grave's disease is an example of increased TH levels that surpass the counteracting capacity of DA in inhibiting TH actions, and thus cause WED. In Singapore, a cohort of Grave's disease patients presented with WED-like symptoms at a prevalence of 8,8% [18]. In Singapore, the prevalence of WED among the normal population is only of 0,9% [17,18]. These numbers support the notion that elevated TH levels can contribute to WED symptoms. However, the fourth diagnostic criterion (worsening of symptoms during evening and night) was not observed in those patients with WED- like symptoms, which precluded the authors from making a definitive WED diagnosis. However, it is known that the increased TH release in Grave's disease does not follow a circadian rhythm; TH release in Grave's patients is uniform along the day [52]. As the fourth WED diagnostic criterion is secondary to the circadian production of thyrotropin (increased at evening and night), it cannot be obtained in most Grave's disease patients with WED-like symptoms. However, in two Grave's disease patients in this study that previously presented with WED, the symptoms had previously been worse at night, before the onset of the hyperthyroidism. After the hyperthyroidism they started to have symptoms all day, but with worsening of the symptoms in the night.

Many neuropathies may present WED symptoms that fulfill all criteria to diagnosing a definite case, including diabetes neuropathy and some others [6,8]. In the affected patients, damage to their sensitive nervous fibers may expose the somatosensory receptors more overtly to the environment, and thus, stimuli are more intensely captured, transduced, and sent as inputs to the somatosensory cortex, where they will be felt as the annoying sensations of WED. Furthermore, when a denuded (due the neuropathy) nervous fiber is stimulated at any point of its path in the direction toward the cortex, an action potential may be triggered, which will be interpreted by the cortex as coming from the initial site of that fiber location, from the site nourished by that nervous fiber. This principle of labeled lines in the somatosensory system may explain phantom WED in amputees and in patients who have undergone total knee arthroplasty [11]. In this latter situation, the superficial fibular nerve is damaged at its path around the knee, a condition that may trigger action potentials at this site, which will be felt as paresthesias coming from the calf, a region nourished by the superficial fibular nerve. This principle may also explain the phantom limb pain phenomenon experienced by amputees [10,11]. Nerve fibers damaged by a neuropathy disease (not primary WED) may trigger inputs that will be turned into WED symptoms. These inputs follow the same basic transmission mechanisms that govern signals sent to the somatosensory cortex, whether they are conveyed from pathologically hyper sensitized somatosensory receptors or from demyelinated fibers that suffer damage (by the neuropathy) on their way to the cortex. WED symptoms are more common in diabetic patients than in normal subjects [8]. Most likely, neuropathy caused by the diabetic condition underpins the WED symptoms presented by these individuals.

In chronic renal failure, WED is more common than in normal subjects [53]. Most likely, this fact is conditioned by two relatively common complications of chronic kidney failure: 1) uremic neuropathy [54]; and 2) decreased activity of the cytochrome P450 superfamily of enzymes [55,56]. Both conditions are not as yet entirely understood. The first one may reduce the threshold for stimuli of the somatosensory receptors deep in the legs, what causes overwhelming signaling to the sensory cortex. The second may hamper the normal metabolism of TH, thus causing an imbalance between DA and TH.

Conclusion

A better understanding of the players involved in WED pathophysiology may contribute to a better treatment approach for this serious disturbance that affects so many people in the world and that causes much suffering.

The scientific community at large, including physicians of all specializations and health care providers, should be aware of the fragile equilibrium between DA and TH. Endocrinologists should not overlook the importance that DA has as a thyrotropin inhibitor. An appropriate balance between the DA of tuberoinfundibular pathway and the hypothalamus-pituitary-thyroid axis is essential for normal function of one of the most important aspects of our somatosensory system physiology: conveying refined messages from the periphery to the somatosensory cortex.

Primary WED, a sensorimotor disorder, may also be appropriately described as a functional peripheral neuropathy, or an endocrine disease. The first description because the symptoms of the disease are generated in the periphery of the somatosensory system and caused by a hypo function of the tuberoinfundibular dopaminergic system; the second, because the two most significant players in the disease are a classical hormone, and a neurohormone.

References

1. The International classification of sleep disorders, sec. edition. Diagnostic and coding manual. Wetchester, Illinois: American Academy of Sleep Medicine, 2005.
2. Allen RP, Picchietti D, Hening WA, Trenkwalder C, Walters AS, et al. (2003) Restless legs syndrome: diagnostic criteria, special considerations, and epidemiology. A report from the restless legs syndrome diagnosis and epidemiology workshop at the National Institutes of Health. Sleep Med 4: 101-119.
3. Walters AS (1995) Toward a better definition of the restless legs syndrome. The International Restless Legs Syndrome Study Group. Mov Disord 10: 634-642.
4. Pereira JC (2013) Are symptoms of restless legs syndrome generated in the periphery of the nervous system or are they born centrally? J Neurosci Rural Pract 4: 1-2.
5. Ekbom KA (1945) Restless legs: A clinical study. Acta Med Scand 158: 1-122.
6. Ekbom K, Ulfberg J (2009) Restless legs syndrome. J Intern Med 266: 419-431.
7. EKBOM KA (1961) Restless legs in amputees. Acta Med Scand 169: 419-421.
8. Hening WA, Allen RP, Walters AS, Chokroverty S (2009) Motor Functions and Dysfunctions of Sleep. In: Chokroverty S, editor. Sleep Disorders Medicine. Philadelphia: Saunders 397-435.
9. Pereira JC Jr, Rocha e Silva IR, Pradella-Hallinan M (2013) Transient Willis-Ekbom's disease (restless legs syndrome) during pregnancy may be caused by estradiol-mediated dopamine overmodulation. Mec Hypotheses 80: 205-208.
10. Pereira JC Jr, Alves RC (2011) The labelled-lines principle of the somatosensory physiology might explain the phantom limb phenomenon. Med Hypotheses 77: 853-856.
11. Pereira JC Jr, Silva Neto JL, Pradella-Hallinar M (2011) Restless legs syndrome in subjects with a knee prosthesis: evidence that symptoms are generated in the periphery. Clinics (Sao Paulo) 66: 1955-1959.

12. Pereira JC Jr, Pradella-Hallinan M, Lins Pessoa Hd (2010) Imbalance between thyroid hormones and the dopaminergic system might be central to the pathophysiology of restless legs syndrome: a hypothesis. Clinics (Sao Paulo) 65: 548-554.
13. Rios Romenets S, Dauvilliers Y, Cochen De Cock V, Carlander B, Bayard S, et al. (2013) Restless legs syndrome outside the blood-brain barrier--exacerbation by domperidone in Parkinson's disease. Parkinsonism Relat Disord 19: 92-94.
14. Delitala G (1977) Dopamine and TSH secretion in man. The Lancet 310: 760-761.
15. Feek CM, Sawers JS, Brown NS, Seth J, Irvine WJ, et al. (1980) Influence of thyroid status on dopaminergic inhibition of thyrotropin and prolactin secretion: evidence for an additional feedback mechanism in the control of thyroid hormone secretion. J Clin Endocrinol Metab 51: 585-589.
16. Scanlon MF, Weetman AP, Lewis M, Pourmand M, Rodriguez-Arnao MD, et al. (1980) Dopaminergic modulation of circadian thyrotropin rhythms and thyroid hormone levels in euthyroid subjects. J Clin Endocrinol Metab 51: 1251-1256.
17. Tan EK, Ho SC, Koh L, Pavanni R (2004) An urge to move with L-thyroxine: clinical, biochemical, and polysomnographic correlation. Mov Disord 19: 1365-1367.
18. Tan EK, Ho SC, Eng P, Loh LM, Koh L, et al. (2004) Restless legs symptoms in thyroid disorders. Parkinsonism Relat Disord 10: 149-151.
19. Pannain S, Van Cauter E (2007) Modulation of Endocrine Function by Sleep-Wake Homeostasis and Circadian Rhythmicity. Sleep Medicine Clinics 2: 147-59.
20. Pereira JC Jr, Pradella-Hallinan M, Alves RC (2013) Saint John's wort, an herbal inducer of the cytochrome P4503A4 isoform, may alleviate symptoms of Willis-Ekbom's disease. Clinics (Sao Paulo) 68: 469-474.
21. Wójcikowski J, Daniel WA (2009) The brain dopaminergic system as an important center regulating liver cytochrome P450 in the rat. Expert Opin Drug Metab Toxicol 5: 631-645.
22. WÃ³jcikowski J, GoÅ‚embiowska K, Daniel WA (2008) Regulation of liver cytochrome P450 by activation of brain dopaminergic system: physiological and pharmacological implications. Biochem Pharmacol 76: 258-267.
23. Schilling JC, Adamus WS, Palluk R (1992) Neuroendocrine and side effect profile of pramipexole, a new dopamine receptor agonist, in humans. Clin Pharmacol Ther 51: 541-548.
24. Davies T, Larsen PR (2008) Thyrotoxicosis. In Kronenberg HM, Melmed S, eds: Williams Textbook of Endocrinology, (11thedn), Saunders, Elsevier. Philadelphia, USA. 333-75.
25. Nunez J, Celi FS, Ng L, Forrest D (2008) Multigenic control of thyroid hormone functions in the nervous system. Mol Cell Endocrinol 287: 1-12.
26. Guyton AC, Hall JE (2006) Textbook of Medical Physiology, (11thedn). Elsevier Ltd, 2006.
27. Pereira Jr JC, Alves RC (2011) The "forbidden zone for sleep" might be caused by the evening thyrotropin surge and its biological purpose is to enhance survival: a hypothesis. Sleep Sci 4(2): 1-5.
28. Ly CV, Verstreken P (2006) Mitochondria at the synapse. Neuroscientist 12: 291-299.
29. Goglia F, Moreno M, Lanni A (1999) Action of thyroid hormones at the cellular level: the mitochondrial target. FEBS Lett 452: 115-120.
30. Burnstock G, Krügel U, Abbracchio MP, Illes P (2011) Purinergic signalling: from normal behaviour to pathological brain function. Prog Neurobiol 95: 229-274.
31. Purves D, Augustine GJ (2008) Neuroscience. (4thedn). Sunderland, MA, USA: Sinauer Associates Inc.
32. Pankratov Y, Lalo U, Verkhratsky A, North RA (2006) Vesicular release of ATP at central synapses. Pflugers Arch 452: 589-597.
33. Broman J (1994) Neurotransmitters in subcortical somatosensory pathways. Anat Embryol (Berl) 189: 181-214.
34. Allen RP, Barker PB, Horská A, Earley CJ (2013) Thalamic glutamate/glutamine in restless legs syndrome: increased and related to disturbed sleep. Neurology 80: 2028-2034.
35. Trenkwalder C, Hening WA, Montagna P, Oertel WH, Allen RP, et al. (2008) Treatment of restless legs syndrome: an evidence-based review and implications for clinical practice. Mov Disord 23: 2267-2302.
36. Rye DB, Freeman AAH (2008) Dopamine in behavioral state control, in Monti JM, Pandi-Perumal SR, and Sinton CM: Neurochemistry of Sleep and Wakefulness. Cambridge University press. Cambridge, 179-223.
37. Allen RP (2012) Restless legs syndrome (Willis-Ekbom disease) and periodic limb movements. In Morin CM, and Espie CA editors: The Oxford Handbook of Sleep and Sleep Disorders. Oxford University Press, Inc; New York, 707-725.
38. Allen RP, Connor JR (2009) Abnormally increased CSF 3-Ortho-methyldopa (3-OMD) in untreated restless legs syndrome (RLS) patients indicates more severe disease and possibly abnormally increased dopamine synthesis. Sleep Med 10(1): 123-128.
39. Skagerberg G, Björklund A, Lindvall O, Schmidt RH (1982) Origin and termination of the diencephalo-spinal dopamine system in the rat. Brain Res Bull 9: 237-244.
40. Lindvall O, Björklund A, Skagerberg G (1983) Dopamine-containing neurons in the spinal cord: anatomy and some functional aspects. Ann Neurol 14: 255-260.
41. Clemens S, Rye D, Hochman S (2006) Restless legs syndrome: revisiting the dopamine hypothesis from the spinal cord perspective. Neurology 67: 125-130.
42. Visser TJ (1996) Pathways of thyroid hormone metabolism. Acta Med Austriaca 23: 10-16.
43. Bruntom L, Parker K (2008) Goodman & Gilman's Manual of Pharmacology and Therapeutics. McGraw-Hill, New York.
44. Preissner S, Kroll K, Dunkel M, Senger C, Goldsobel G, et al. (2010) SuperCYP: a comprehensive database on Cytochrome P450 enzymes including a tool for analysis of CYP-drug interactions. Nucleic Acids Res 38: D237-243.
45. Thummel KE, Wilkinson GR (1998) In vitro and in vivo drug interactions involving human CYP3A. Annu Rev Pharmacol Toxicol 38: 389-430.
46. Antonini A, Calandrella D (2011) Pharmacokinetic evaluation of pramipexole. Expert Opin Drug Metab Toxicol 7: 1307-1314.
47. Shupnik MA, Greenspan SL, Ridgway EC (1986) Transcriptional regulation of thyrotropin subunit genes by thyrotropin-releasing hormone and dopamine in pituitary cell culture. J Biol Chem 261: 12675-12679.
48. Green ST (1987) Intrathyroidal autonomic nerves can directly influence hormone release from rat thyroid follicles: study in vitro employing electrical field stimulation and intracellular microelectrodes. Clin Sci 72(2): 233-238.
49. Lee-Chiong JRT (2008) Sleep Medicine Essentials and Review. Oxford University Press, Inc. New York.
50. Ropper AH, Samuels MA (2009) Adams' and Victor's Principles of Neurology, (9thedn). McGraw Hill.
51. Stiasny-Kolster K, Pfau DB (2013) Hyperalgesia and functional sensory loss in restless legs syndrome. Pain. 2013 May 10.
52. Schuppert F, Diegelmann B, Geest T, Wagner TO, von zur Mühlen A (1994) Loss of variability in Graves' disease: stimulatory TSH-receptor antibodies bind to the TSH-receptor in a continued, non-pulsatile and non-chaotic fashion. Chronobiologia 21: 21-32.
53. Araujo SM, de Bruin VM, Nepomuceno LA, Maximo ML, Daher Ede F, et al. (2010) Restless legs syndrome in end-stage renal disease: Clinical characteristics and associated comorbidities. Sleep Med 11: 785-790.
54. Ropper AH, Samuels MA (2009) Adams' and Victor's Principles of Neurology, (9thedn). McGraw Hill.
55. Dreisbach AW, Lertora JJ (2003) The effect of chronic renal failure on hepatic drug metabolism and drug disposition. Semin Dial 16: 45-50.
56. Dreisbach AW, Lertora JJ (2008) The effect of chronic renal failure on drug metabolism and transport. Expert Opin Drug Metab Toxicol 4: 1065-1074.

3

Changes of Procedural Memory in the Patients with Primary Insomnia

Yi-jun Ge[1], Lan Xia[2], Fang Wang[3] and Gui-hai Chen[1]*

[1]*Department of Neurology, the First People's Hospital of Chenzhou, China*
[2]*Department of Neurology, the Second Affiliated Hospital of Anhui Medical University, China*
[3]*Department of Neurology, the First Affiliated Hospital of Anhui Medical University, China*

Abstract

Objective: To explore changes of procedural memory in the patients with primary insomnia (PI) and its characteristics.

Methods: Thirty-six PI patients and 36 controls were enrolled. The procedural memory was respectively detected by category exemplar generation and motor sequence tasks respectively, and the declarative memory was assessed by free word task.

Results: Compared to the controls, the PI patients showed few correct numbers in the category exemplar generation (7.7 ± 2.1 vs. 9.9 ± 1.0, z = 5.247, P<0.001), motion sequence task (8.1 ± 3.3 vs 12.0 ± 3.0, z = 4.676, P<0.001) and the phases of immediate recall (3.3 ± 1.1 vs 6.0 ± 1.2, z=6.634, P<0.001), delayed recall (9.0 ± 2.2 vs. 11.2 ± 1.1, z=4.718, P<0.001) and delayed recognition (14.2 ± 1.0 vs. 15.0 ±0.0, z = 4.637, P<0.001) of the free word task. For the different subtypes of PI, the early morning awakening group had significantly worse performance in the motor sequence task compared to the difficulty initiating sleep (z=–2.768, P=0.006) and difficulty maintaining sleep (z=–2.502, P=0.012) groups, and less correct numbers of the word-delayed recognition compared to the difficulty maintaining sleep group too (z=–2.707, P=0.007).

Conclusion: The procedural and declarative memories are impaired in the PI patients, especially the early morning awakening insomniacs.

Keywords: Primary insomnia; Procedural memory; Declarative memory

Introduction

Insomnia refers to the difficulty in the sleep initiating maintaining of patients with adequate hours, good sleep environment and opportunities to sleep. As a result, the patients have a subjective experience of dissatisfied sleep time and/or quality, and daytime dysfunction, such as anxiety, depression, mental activity and cognitive (e.g. learning and memory) impairment in certain degree [1-4].

The imaging studies show that the insomnia patients had cerebral hypoper fusion of blood compared to the normal controls, and this change in the basal ganglia was more obvious than those in the frontal, occipital and parietal cortexes [5]. It is found by mean of magnetic resonance imaging that patients with insomnia had significantly reduced volume in the bilateral hippocampus [6]. In accordance with sleep deprivation experiments in animals, it is suggested that sleep deprivation leaded to decline of cognitive function in humans. Studies on memory with sleep deprivation model have shown that depriving different periods of sleep in the general population would make different impacts on learning and memory. For example, total sleep deprivation impairs semantic memory; slow wave sleep (SWS) deprivation without reducing total sleep time significantly affects declarative memory (DM) and coding related hippocampal activities; rapid eye movement sleep (REMS) deprivation influences the procedural memory (PM) rather than DM [7]. Polysomnography application has revealed some sleep characteristics of insomnia patients, such as the shortened total sleep time, extended sleep onset latency, decreased sleep efficiency, reductive SWS and incremental percentage of first-phase sleep [8]. The underlying mechanism of insomnia-related cognitive changes might be due to some kinds of sleep structure disorders or a specific SWS (0.5~2.0 Hz) defect, which is harmful to the brain protein synthesis, the establishment and consolidation of new synaptic connections and the recovery of synaptic homeostasis.

However, in the early stage of chronic insomnia patients, because of the mild condition, the body tends to have sufficient time to complete any compensation. So that, cognitive function changes between insomnia of the natural course and sleep deprivation are different. So far, memory impairment in patients with primary insomnia (PI) remains to be identified. A meta-analysis showed that patients with PI existed mild to moderate damage in working memory, episodic memory and certain aspects of attention, but there was no significant difference in perceptual processing, PM, speech and executive function [9,10]. PM impairment and its characteristics of patients with PI are inconclusive, which may be owing to different evaluation methods and sample sources. In the present, we observed the changes in PM and DM with three tasks (category exemplar generation, motor sequence tasks and free word task) in the patients whose symptoms met to the PI diagnostic criteria in the Diagnostic and Statistical Manual of Mental Disorders, Fourth Edition (DSM-IV) [11].

Materials and Methods

Study objects

PI group: Thirty-six patients were included, who went to the Sleep and Memory Disorders Clinic of the First Affiliated Hospital, Anhui

***Corresponding author:** Gui-hai Chen, Department of Neurology, the First People's Hospital of Chenzhou, Chenzhou, Hunan Province, PR 423000, China, E-mail: chenguihai1964@163.com

Medical University from September 2010 to May 2011 due to sleep difficulties. Their mean age was 37.0 ± 11.5 years, the illness duration ≥ 1 month and all of them met PI diagnostic criteria in the DSM-IV. All of them were right-handed, and were accepted high school education or above. Meanwhile, the Athens Insomnia Scale (AIS) [12] score was >6 and Montreal cognitive test scale (MoCA) [13] score was ≥ 26. Additionally, the following conditions were excluded: taking drugs (such as antidepressants, benzodiazepines, antiepileptics or other drugs/substances) possibly impacting on cognitive function past two weeks; suffering from other sleep disorders (such as sleep apnea syndrome, restless legs syndrome), medicine conditions (such as chronic obstructive pulmonary disease, chronic pain, or severe liver disease) and neuropsychiatric disorders (such as stroke, epilepsy, Parkinson's disease, dementia, depression and anxiety disorders, specifically, when 17-terms Hamilton Depression Rating Scale (HAMD-17) [14] score being ≥ 17); unable to complete the experiment; impaired visual acuity and audition. Furthermore, the patients were divided into several subgroups according to the type of insomnia: the difficultly initiating sleep group [7 males / 5 females; mean age 35.6 ± 13.2 years; education 12.5 ± 2.2 years], the early morning awakening group [6 males / 6 females; mean age 36.6 ± 10.2 years; education 12.7 ± 1.7 years] and the difficulty maintaining sleep group [5 males / 7 females; mean age 37.3 ± 11.0 years; education 13.2 ± 2.5 years]. There were no statistical differences among subgroups in gender, age and years of education (*Ps* > 0.05).

Healthy control group: A total of 30 cases consist of healthy adults who were subjected to health examination during the same period. The mean age was 37.3 ± 11.4 years. They were right-handed, and come from the comparable cities or countries with the similar habits, education, economics and other factors, in order to roughly match with the PI patients. Besides, they were required have no previous history of neuropsychiatric disorders and hypomnesis, and no obvious physical illness, with AIS score ≤ 4, MoCA score ≥ 26 and HAMD-17 score < 7.

This research was approved by the First Affiliated Hospital of Anhui Medical University Ethics Committee, and all participants signed informed consent.

Methods

Background information assessment: Background information, including AIS, Epworth Sleepiness Scale (ESS) [15], MoCA and HAMD-17, were completed by trained clinicians.

PM

Category exemplar generation task: Firstly, every subject was shown 10 randomized pictures of vegetables and household appliances, and then was required to name them. After 15 minutes, the subject was required to enumerate the name of vegetables and household appliances shown before as many as possible within 1 min successively, and the total correct numbers were recorded [16].

Motion sequence task: Subjects put their left fingers successively on the number keys of 1234 on the keyboard from little to index finger, and then entered a set of random sequences (such as 4-2-3-1-4) displayed on the computer screen as fast and accurate as possible within a certain period of time. After resting 24s, they would enter into the next round. They were required to complete 12 rounds in total consecutively. The average numbers of correct sequences in the last 3 rounds were counted [17].

DM

Words free recall task: Fifteen high-frequency Chinese notional words were selected in the test. Subjects were asked to read the words five times and recall them after reading immediately within 2 min. The correct number of first time recalling was defined as the immediate recall score. Then subjects recalled the free words after 15 min. The correct number of words was called the delayed recall score. After given another 15 new notional words, subjects were required to tell the word from old to new, the correct numbers of judgment of old words was called the delayed recognition score [18].

Statistical analysis

All statistical analyses were conducted by the SPSS 13.0. The data were expressed as mean ± standard deviation. The normal distribution data were analyzed by independent samples t test or ANOVA, and the non-normal distribution data were analyzed by Manne-Whitney U or Kruskal-Wallis H test.

Results

Background information

U or *t* test showed that there was no statistically difference in sex, age and years of education between the PI group and the control group (Table 1). There were no significantly difference in MoCA (z=1.781, P =0.075) and ESS (t=0.879, P=0.379) scores between the two groups, but the PI group had significantly higher scores of the AIS and HAMD-17 than the control group (z=7.345, P < 0.001; z=7.161, P < 0.001), indicating that the sample quality met requirement of the study (Table 1).

Memory testing

The U test showed that compared to the controls, the PI patients had worse performances in all measures of the immediate recall, delayed recall, delayed recognition, category generation and the motion sequence (z=6.634, 4.718, 4.637, 5.247 and 4.676, respectively, *Ps* <0.001) (Table 2).

Memories in the patients with different insomnia subtypes

The ANOVA or H test showed that there were significant or marginal differences among the three subgroups of difficultly initiating sleep, early morning awakening and difficultly maintaining sleep in the delay recall (F=3.264, P=0.051), delayed recognition (H=8.871, P=0.012) and exercise sequence (H=9.766, P=0.008) scores, but there were no significant differences in the immediate recall (H=0.840, P=0.657) and class generation (H=0.399, P=0.819) scores. Furthermore,

Groups	Gender (male/female)	Age (years)	Education Levels (years)	AIS	ESS	HAMD-17	MoCA
Insomnia	18/18	37.0 ± 11.5	13.0 ± 1.9	13.9 ± 3.1*	7.4 ± 3 .5	11.7 ± 3.9*	26.8 ± 1.2
Controls	14/16	37.3 ± 11.4	12.1 ± 2.7	2.5 ± 1.2	6.7 ± 2.1	2.6 ± 1.8	27.3 ± 1.5
Statistic	χ^2=0.073	t=0.378	z=1.262	z=7.345	z=0.879	z=7.161	z=1.781
P values	0.787	0.706	0.207	< 0.001	0.379	< 0.001	0.075

*Compare to the control group P<0.001

AIS: Athens Insomnia Scale; ESS: Epworth Sleepiness Scale; HAMD-17: 17-terms Hamilton Depression Rating Scale; MoCA: Montreal Cognitive Assessment

Table 1: Background information of the subjects (mean ± standard deviation).

Groups	Declarative memory			Procedural memory	
	Immediate recall	Delayed recall	Delayed recognition	Category generation	Motion sequence
Primary insomnia	3.3 ± 1.1*	9.0 ± 2.2*	14.2 ± 1.0*	7.7 ± 2.1*	8.1 ± 3.3*
Controls	6.0 ± 1.2	11.2 ± 1.1	15.0 ± 0.0	9.9 ± 1.0	12.0 ± 3.0
z	6.634	4.718	4.637	5.247	4.676
P values	<0.001	<0.001	<0.001	<0.001	<0.001

*Compare to the control group, $P<0.001$

Table 2: Memory test results of the subjects (the number of correct, mean ± standard deviation).

Groups	Declarative memory			Procedural memory	
	Immediate recall	Delayed recall	Delayed recognition	Category generation	Motion sequence
Difficultly initiating sleep	3.3 ± 1.1	9.3 ± 2.6	14.4 ± 0.8	7.9 ± 2.2	9.0 ± 2.7
Early morning awakening	3.2 ± 1.2	8.8 ± 2.0	13.4 ± 1.2#	7.2 ± 1.2	6.6 ± 2.6 *#
Difficultly maintaining sleep	3.4 ± 0.9	9.0 ± 2.2	14.7 ± 0.7	8.0 ± 2.7	8.6 ± 4.1
Statistic	*H* = 0.840	*F* = 0.101	*H* = 8.871	*H* = 0.399	*H* = 9.766
P values	0.657	0.904	0.012	0.819	0.008

*Compare to the difficultly initiating sleep group, $P<0.017$, # Compare to the difficulty maintaining sleep group, $P<0.017$

Table 3: Memory in the patients with different insomnia subtypes (correct number, mean ± standard deviation).

the U test for pair wise comparison (corrected size of the test: $\alpha=0.05 / 3=0.017$) showed the early morning awakening patients got worse scores in motion sequences and delay recall task than the difficulty maintaining sleep patients ($z=-2.502$, $P=0.012$ and $z=-2.707$, $P=0.007$, respectively, both P values < 0.017). However, when compared to the difficultly initiating sleep group, the worse performance in the early morning awakening group only occurred in the motion sequences task ($z=-2.768$, $P=0.006 < 0.017$), but not in delay recall task ($z = -2.157$, $P = 0.031 > 0.017$) (Table 3).

Discussion

One of the main functions of sleep is restoring brain synaptic plasticity and forming of new memories [19]. But previous studies have shown that patients with PI had generally no or slight damage in learning and memory [20], perhaps only in complex tasks memory [21]. An overview about the daytime function in PI patients has been exhibited i.e., no memory impairment was seen in simple tasks, such as audio verbal learning, Hopkins Verbal Learning, word matching, word recognition and visual recognition, however, the PI group had significantly worse performance than the control group in free word memory, the mirror image reading and phrase memory tasks [22]. Recent researches about mirror image reading (detecting PM) and visual verbal learning tasks (detecting DM) found that patients with PI showed decreased ability to complete these tasks [23]. In our study, the motion sequence and category generation tasks were respectively used to detect motor skill learning and priming effects on PM in the PI patients, while the free word recall task was used to detect DM. The results showed that compared to the control group, the motion sequence and category exemplar generation scores in the PI patients declined to certain degree, and three measures in the free word recall task were also damaged. Therefore, whether the PI patients have damaged PM or/and DM or not depended on a moderate difficulty of the tasks used.

Sleep plays an important role in the PM and DM, which is related to new memories and integration of existing knowledge [24]. Both REMS and SWS [25] would contribute to memory encoding, consolidation and neural plasticity. Studies on sleep deprivation have shown that the REMS deprivation only affected PM and SWS deprivation influenced DM [26]. However, the visual recognition task (a kind of DM) research found that the improved memory after sleep was only correlated to the amount of SWS in the first quarter of the night, but was also correlated to the amount of REMS in the last quarter. These results indicated that the consolidation of DM is connected with both SWS and REMS [27]. Actually, the data result from the PI patients indicated that PM also involved in the Stage 2 sleeps [28]. Relative to complex skills formation which relies more on REMS, the consolidation of existing skills and simple motor skills needs sleep spindles in Stage 2 [29]. Therefore, throughout the whole process of sleep, the memory consolidation of different types needs respectively unique pattern of sleep periods [28]. After comparison among diverse insomnia subtypes, the results showed that the early waking group had significantly impaired PM and DM when compared to the patients with difficultly maintenance sleep, and impaired PM when compared to ones with difficultly initiating sleep. We presumed that the reduction or changed percentage of REMS in early waking people may contribute to this result, because the patients with early waking mainly lose the sleep in the latter half of night, in which the REMS is predominant. Our results did not seem support the previous hypothesis that the SWS reduction in the difficultly initiating sleep patients should lead to DM damage. In fact, the difficultly initiating sleep patients often had earlier bedtime, but they don't always have reductive total sleep time or SWS. Furthermore, the changes of sleep architecture are not unitary in maintenance difficulties sleep patients, and some patients may be having a normal proportion of each phase. Without doubt, it is necessary to enlarge samples to certify our conclusion.

References

1. Schutte-Rodin S, Broch L, Buysse D, Dorsey C, Sateia M (2008) Clinical guideline for the evaluation and management of chronic insomnia in adults. J Clin Sleep Med 4: 487-504.
2. Pigeon WR (2010) Diagnosis, prevalence, pathways, consequences & treatment of insomnia. Indian J Med Res 131: 321-332.
3. Bastien CH (2011) Insomnia: Neurophysiological and neuropsychological approaches. Neuropsychol Rev 21: 22-40.
4. Varkevisser M, Kerkhof GA (2005) Chronic insomnia and performance in a 24-h constant routine study. J Sleep Res 14: 49-59.
5. Smith MT, Perlis ML, Chengazi VU, Pennington J, Soeffing J, et al. (2002) Neuroimaging of NREM sleep in primary insomnia: a Tc-99-HMPAO single photon emission computed tomography study. Sleep 25: 325-335.
6. Riemann D, Voderholzer U, Spiegelhalder K, Hornyak M, Buysse DJ, et al. (2007) Chronic insomnia and MRI-measured hippocampal volumes: a pilot study. Sleep 30: 955-958.
7. Roehrs T, Roth T (2000) Sleep-wake state and memory function. Sleep 23 Suppl 3: S64-68.

8. American Academy of Sleep Medicine (2005) The international classification of sleep disorders-Second edition (ICSD-2).
9. Li B (1999) The neural basis of learning and memory. World Sci Tech R & D 06: 47-50.
10. Fortier-Brochu E, Beaulieu-Bonneau S, Ivers H, Morin CM (2012) Insomnia and daytime cognitive performance: a meta-analysis. Sleep Med Rev 16: 83-94.
11. Ohayon MM, Reynolds CF 3rd (2009) Epidemiological and clinical relevance of insomnia diagnosis algorithms according to the DSM-IV and the International Classification of Sleep Disorders (ICSD). Sleep Med 10: 952-960.
12. Zhang ZJ (2005) Behavioral Medicine Scale Manual. Chinese Medical Multimedia Press.
13. Chen N, He L (2009) The research and application profiles of Montreal Cognitive Assessment. Chin J Nerv Ment Dis 35: 632-634.
14. Wang XD, Wang XL, Ma H (1990) Rating scales of mental health (Revised edition, in Chinese). Chin Ment Health J 13: 220-223.
15. Johns MW (1991) A new method for measuring daytime sleepiness: the Epworth sleepiness scale. Sleep 14: 540-545.
16. Fleischman DA, Wilson RS, Gabrieli JD, Schneider JA, Bienias JL, et al. (2005) Implicit memory and Alzheimer's disease neuropathology. Brain 128: 2006-2015.
17. Walker MP, Stickgold R, Alsop D, Gaab N, Schlaug G (2005) Sleep-dependent motor memory plasticity in the human brain. Neuroscience 133: 911-917.
18. Cheng HD, Wang K, Gong L, Yin CL, Meng Y (2010) The disorder of prospective memory in patients with amnesia mild cognitive impairment. Chin J Neurol 43: 174-177.
19. Walker MP, Stickgold R (2004) Sleep-dependent learning and memory consolidation. Neuron 44: 121-133.
20. Riedel BW, Lichstein KL (2000) Insomnia and daytime functioning. Sleep Med Rev 4: 277-298.
21. Altena E, Van Der Werf YD, Strijers RL, Van Someren EJ (2008) Sleep loss affects vigilance: effects of chronic insomnia and sleep therapy. J Sleep Res 17: 335-343.
22. Shekleton JA, Rogers NL, Rajaratnam SM (2010) Searching for the daytime impairments of primary insomnia. Sleep Med Rev 14: 47-60.
23. Nissen C, Kloepfer C, Feige B, Piosczyk H, Spiegelhalder K, et al. (2011) Sleep-related memory consolidation in primary insomnia. J Sleep Res 20: 129-136.
24. Tamminen J, Payne JD, Stickgold R, Wamsley EJ, Gaskell MG (2010) Sleep spindle activity is associated with the integration of new memories and existing knowledge. J Neurosci 30: 14356-14360.
25. Walker MP (2008) Sleep-dependent memory processing. Harv Rev Psychiatry 16: 287-298.
26. Roehrs T, Roth T (2000) Sleep-wake state and memory function. Sleep 23 Suppl 3: S64-68.
27. Stickgold R, Whidbee D, Schirmer B, Patel V, Hobson JA (2000) Visual discrimination task improvement: A multi-step process occurring during sleep. J Cogn Neurosci 12: 246-254.
28. Fogel SM, Smith CT, Cote KA (2007) Dissociable learning-dependent changes in REM and non-REM sleep in declarative and procedural memory systems. Behav Brain Res 180: 48-61.
29. Morin A, Doyon J, Dostie V, Barakat M, Hadj Tahar A, et al. (2008) Motor sequence learning increases sleep spindles and fast frequencies in post-training sleep. Sleep 31: 1149-1156.

Sleeping Pills and Quality of Wake Time: The Missing Link

Sohil A Khan[1,2,8]*, Treasure M McGuire[2-5] and Helen S Heussler[2,6,7]

[1]*School of Pharmacy, Griffith University, Gold Coast, Australia*
[2]*Mater Research Institute, Mater Health Services, South Brisbane, Australia*
[3]*Mater Pharmacy Services, Mater Health Services, South Brisbane, Australia*
[4]*Faculty of Health Sciences and Medicine, Bond University, Gold Coast, Australia*
[5]*School of Pharmacy, The University of Queensland, Woolloongabba, Australia*
[6]*Deparrment of Respiratory and Sleep Medicine, Mater Children's Hospital, Mater Health Services, South Brisbane, Australia*
[7]*School of Medicine, The University of Queensland, Herston, Australia*
[8]*Griffith Health Institute, Griffith University, Gold Coast, Australia*

Abstract

Background: The rising incidence of insomnia in a 24/7 global society quantifies the burden for the individual, in terms of reduced quality of life (QOL), and for society at large, in terms of work absenteeism, disability, and health care costs.

Aim: To evaluate research on hypnosedatives (benzodiazepines, non-benzodiazepines) and complementary medicines in paediatric insomnia where quality of wake time is one of the key efficacy outcomes.

Design and setting: Retrospective data analysis of clinical studies in paediatric insomnia

Methods: A systematic review of clinical studies of hypnosedatives and complementary medicines in paediatric insomnia was conducted. PubMed and Cochrane Central Register of Controlled Trials (January 2002- August 2013) were searched for studies in children aged 3 to18 years (male or female). Quality of wake time and/or health related QOL parameters were assessed as the outcomes.

Results: From 31 potentially relevant studies, only one, involving melatonin, met the inclusion criteria. One hundred and forty six children (aged 3 to15 years 8 months) diagnosed with insomnia were evaluated in a 12 week double masked randomised placebo controlled phase III multi-centre trial. Child behaviour and family functioning showed some improvement and favoured use of melatonin but was not statistically significant. There were no controlled clinical studies evaluating the impact of benzodiazepines and non-benzodiazepines hypnosedatives on quality of wake time in the management of paediatric insomnia.

Conclusion: Data on quality of wake time in children with insomnia are scarce. Research has focused on addressing the metrics of sleep, with quality of wake time notably ignored. QOL measurement provides valuable information about the psychological and social impact of treatment on children with insomnia. Complementary medicines such as melatonin appear to improve the quality of wake time in paediatric insomnia where there are co-morbid conditions; but further research is needed.

Keywords: Insomnia; Benzodiazepines; Non-benzodiazepines; Melatonin; Sleep; Children; Quality of life

Introduction

Human beings spend approximately one-third of their lifetime sleeping [1]. As one of the most fundamental processes of life, sleep has attracted a great deal of attention from ancient philosophers to present day biomedical researchers. The rising incidence of insomnia in a 24/7 global society continues to create increasing demands that pose significant challenges to sleep research and circadian physiology. A recently published epidemiological study [2] quantifies the burden of chronic insomnia for the individual, in terms of reduced Quality of Life (QOL), and for society at large, in terms of work absenteeism, disability and health care costs. The incidence is surprisingly high in the paediatric population, with a quarter of all children experiencing sleep problems. In children with visual impairment and neurodevelopmental disorders, the incidence is as high as 80% [3]. It is likely that this also has an impact on the carers of the affected child.

A sleep disorder exists when a lower quality of sleep results in impaired functioning or excessive sleepiness. For the past four decades, prescription hypnosedatives (benzodiazepine or non-benzodiazepine) have been widely used in the management of sleep disorders in adults and children. However, the risk associated with their chronic use (dependence, increased abuse potential, withdrawal symptoms) is alarming [4]. Recently, complementary medicines such as melatonin and valerian have gathered interest in sleep medicine. Prescriptions for sleep problems are common with melatonin, clonidine and antihistamines amongst the most frequent in paediatric practice [5]. There is significant variation in prescribing pharmacotherapeutic options in insomnia with lack of consensus based guidelines in diverse patient population. When novel hypnosedatives are developed, the focus tends to be on the statistically significant increase in total sleep time (marginal in minutes) during the night instead of the effects on the quality of wakefulness [1]. Pharmaceutical companies are focussed heavily on the metrics of sleep; and have neglected quality of wake time as a key measure of hypnosedatives efficacy, yet quality of wake

***Corresponding author:** Sohil A Khan, School of Pharmacy, Griffith University, Gold Coast, Australia E-mail: s.khan@griffith.edu.au

time is an integral domain in the definition of insomnia disorders in the Diagnostic and Statistical Manual of Mental Disorders, 5th edition, described as "... causing clinically significant distress or impairment in social, occupational or other important areas of functioning" [6].

Poor sleep can exacerbate medical, psychiatric or developmental conditions; and insomnia has been a contributing factor in traffic and work-related accidents [2]. High risk patients, with underlying co-morbidities such as anxiety, depression and chronic pain, are more prone to impaired daytime function. However, there are few studies involving currently marketed hypnosedatives that evaluate the extent of improvement (if any) in daytime functioning or the consequences of disrupted sleep. This is not surprising, as the cohort of primary insomniacs selected for clinical trials tend to be without co-morbid conditions. This differs significantly from the 'real world' scenario where people with multiple co-morbidities are more likely to suffer from, and be adversely affected by insomnia. This review aims to evaluate research on hypnosedatives (benzodiazepines, non-benzodiazepines) and complementary medicines (e.g. melatonin) in paediatric insomnia where quality of wake time is one of the key efficacy outcomes.

Method

This systematic literature review included clinical trials that evaluated quality of wake time in paediatric insomnia. Participants included were children aged 3 to 18 years (male or female) on hypnosedatives [benzodiazepines or non-benzodiazepines (zolpidem, zaliplon, zopiclone, eszopiclone)] or complementary medicine for the management of insomnia. Both typically developing children with no co-morbidities and those with existing co-morbidities were included. PubMed and the Cochrane Central Register of Controlled Trials (January 2002 to August 2013) were searched using the following Medical Subject Heading [MeSH] terms: 'quality of life' AND [exp] 'child' AND 'sleep initiation and maintenance disorders'. Studies were then filtered to retrieve any involving a pharmacotherapeutic intervention - benzodiazepine, non-benzodiazepine or complementary hypnosedatives. The following string of terms was used: 'hypnotics and sedatives' OR [exp] 'plants' OR 'homeopathy' OR 'naturopathy' OR [exp] 'phytotherapy' OR [exp] 'medicine, traditional' OR 'horticultural therapy' OR 'melatonin' OR 'drugs chinese herbal OR 'plant extracts' OR 'complementary' (mp) OR 'herb' (mp). Only studies published in English language were included. An extended search (hand search) technique was applied to retrieve any relevant cross-references (Table 1).

Results

Of 31 potentially relevant studies retrieved, 26 were excluded as cohorts included adults or insomnia was not the primary diagnosis. The remaining five were selected for detailed evaluation. Four studies were excluded as they lacked a pharmacotherapeutic intervention, leaving one study for inclusion in this systematic review (Figure 1).

A recently published, randomised controlled trial [11] of the complementary medicine – melatonin was included for evaluation in the systematic review. This trial assessed the effectiveness and safety of melatonin in treating severe sleep problems in children with neurodevelopmental disorders. One hundred and forty-six children (aged 3 to 15 years and 8 months) were studied in a double masked randomised placebo controlled phase III multi-centre trial in 19 hospitals across England and Wales. Immediate release melatonin or matching placebo capsules were administered 45 minutes before the child's bedtime for a 12 week period. All children started with a 0.5 mg capsule in a dose escalation design to 2 mg, 6 mg, and 12 mg depending on their response to treatment. Total sleep time comprised the primary outcome. Secondary outcomes included sleep onset latency, assessments of child behaviour, family functioning, and adverse events. Sleep was measured with diaries and actigraphy. Melatonin increased total sleep time by 22.4 minutes (95% confidence interval 0.5 to 44.3 minutes) measured by sleep diaries (n=110) and 13.3 (−15.5 to 42.2) measured by actigraphy (n=59).

Quality of wake time was evaluated as a secondary outcome. Child behaviour and family functioning showed some improvement and favoured use of melatonin. Four questionnaires were administered: the Composite Sleep Disturbance Index (CSDI), Aberrant Behaviour Checklist (ABC) to assess behavioural problems, the family impact module of the Paediatric Quality of Life inventory (PedsQL) to assess the quality of life of the care giver; and the Epworth Sleepiness Scale (ESS) to assess the daytime sleepiness of the care giver. The ESS scale showed a clinically small but statistically significant improvement of 1.6 points on the 24 point scale for melatonin compared with placebo. The results of the PedsQL and ABC tended to favour melatonin but were not statistically significant.

A summary of the commonly used tools to evaluate QOL in

Study	N	Age (yrs) Mean	Objective	Study design	Medical co-morbidity	Type of sleep disorder	HRQOL tool	Study outcome
de Serres et al. (2002) [7]	101	6.2	Impact of adenotonsillectomy on HRQOL in children with OSDs	Prospective observational study	OSD	OSD with restless sleep	Obstructive Sleep Disorders-6 survey (OSD-6)	Sleep disorder – an important domain that directly affects QOL
Rosen et al. (2002) [8]	298	11.1	Extent of SDB with impairment of HRQOL	Longitudinal genetic-epidemiologic cohort study	Obesity, Asthma	SDB	Child Health Questionnaire (CHQ-PF50)	Decrements in HRQOL were measurable even with mild SDB; Increasing effects with more severe SDB
Hart et al. (2005) [9]	80	11.2	Assess relationship between sleep disturbance and HRQOL	Retrospective review of a clinical database	Obesity, pulmonary and neurologic disorders	Behaviour and biological origin	Child Health Questionnaire (CHQ-PF50)	Variety of HRQOL decrements experienced that may benefit from intervention
Díez-Montiel et al. (2006) [10]	101	4.1	Long term impact of tonsillectomy/ adenoidectomy in children with OSA	Prospective controlled study	SDB, OSA	SDB, OSA	OSDs-6 survey	Long term improvement in HRQOL after surgery in children with OSA

Key: OSD: Obstructive Sleep Disorders, SDB: Sleep disordered breathing ; OSA: Obstructive sleep apnoea

Table 1: Characteristics of excluded studies (after detailed evaluation).

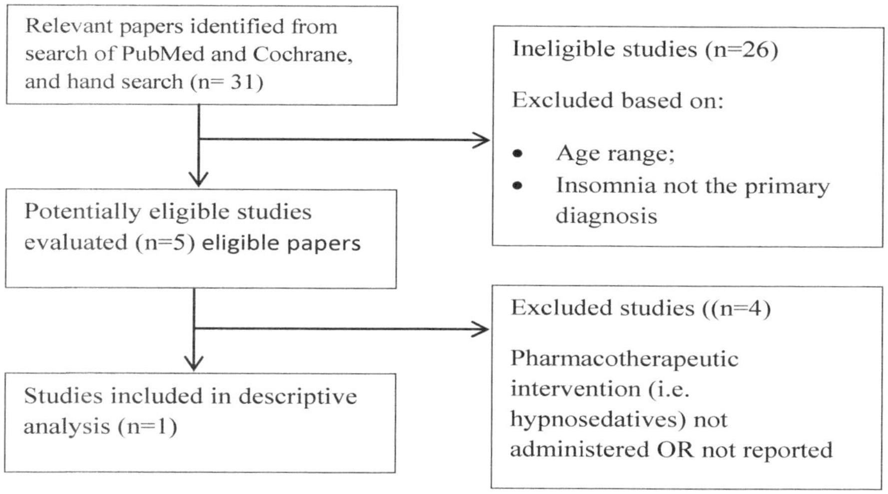

Figure 1: Flow chart of study selection process. The characteristics of the excluded studies (after detailed evaluation) are provided in Table 1. The participants' mean age was 8 years. These studies highlighted the impact of sleep problems on health related QOL (HRQOL) in children with various co-morbid conditions (not primary insomniacs).

insomnia and other sleep problems in children are presented in Table 2. It should be noted that administration of such tools in children less than 5 years needed to be completed by their parents/care givers.

Discussion

In recent times, measurement of QOL has added a new dimension to clinical trials and the drug development process. Results of epidemiological studies have demonstrated the increasing burden of chronic disease and its social impact, based on disability and not mortality. QOL measurement provides valuable information about the psychological and social impact of treatment on children, especially where differences in survival rates are anticipated. Despite the lack of a pharmacotherapeutic intervention in the four studies excluded from this systematic review, they serve to highlight the adverse impact of paediatric sleep disorders on HRQOL.

To the best of our knowledge, there is only one controlled trial that has evaluated the impact of a pharmacotherapeutic intervention on quality of wake time in paediatric insomnia. This study assessed the impact of melatonin on QOL and daytime functioning in children with neurodevelopmental disorders suffering from severe sleep problems [11]. Findings from measures of child behaviour and family QOL tended to favour melatonin but were not statistically significant. The authors justify this as the outcome measures were not sensitive enough over the study time period (12 weeks). The lack of studies addressing this issue with benzodiazepine or non-benzodiazepine hypnosedatives is surprising, considering their extensive use. Nonetheless, the melatonin study provides a baseline for future trials to focus on this neglected but an important parameter in sleep medicine – the quality of wake time.

A similar search in adult insomniacs with co-morbid conditions also retrieved only one placebo-controlled trial [18]. Claimed to be the first of its kind, the study demonstrated that long-term nightly treatment of primary insomnia with eszopiclone was able to enhance QOL, reduce work limitations, and reduce global insomnia severity, in addition to improving patient-reported sleep variables. Patient-reported sleep and daytime function were improved more with the hypnosedative than with placebo at months 1-6 (duration: 6 months) ($P<0.001$). Furthermore, statistically significant improvements were observed with eszopiclone compared with placebo for the SF-36 domains of Physical Functioning, Vitality, and Social Functioning ($P<0.05$), and all domains of the work limitations questionnaire ($P<0.05$). As this trial was conducted in primary insomniacs, impact of quality of wake time from the findings may not be extrapolated to patients with co-morbid conditions.

The use of medication to manage insomnia often follows a 'one-size-fits-all' approach. Yet the nature of the sleep problem experienced by those with insomnia varies. At present, daytime performance is considered as an absence of impairment — improvement of function with benzodiazepines or benzodiazepine receptor agonists has never been demonstrated. There are a number of barriers in evaluating quality of wake time. One is the lack of subjective and objective parameters to evaluate the clinical effect. Validated tools designed to assess HRQOL (Table 2) would be suitable for evaluating daytime performance and QOL in paediatric sleep pharmacotherapy.

Insomniacs with co-morbid conditions (e.g. neurodevelopmental disorders or circadian rhythm sleep disorders) are presented with challenging therapeutic decisions. A recently published therapeutic guideline [19] highlighted the need for studies to identify how to optimally manage insomnia in patients with co-morbid conditions. Newer strategies such as chronobiotic therapies are under trial. Melatonin seems one of the promising options to address this unexplored yet an important clinical domain of sleep medicine.

Implications for practice and research

- Despite their long history in the management of sleep disorders, there are no controlled clinical studies evaluating the impact of benzodiazepines and non-benzodiazepines hypnosedatives on quality of wake time in the management of paediatric insomnia.
- Complementary medicines such as melatonin appear to improve the quality of wake time in paediatric insomnia where there are co-morbid conditions (e.g. neurodevelopmental disorders, visual impairment and circadian rhythm sleep disorders). Further long term studies (more than 6 months) are needed.

Measure	Age range (years)	Concept	Child (self) Report	Parent (proxy) Report	Domain	Time to complete (min)	Reliability data	Validity data
Child Health and Illness Profile [12]	6-11 and 12-17	Measure based on a broad concept that includes evaluation of perception of well being and illness, participation in developmentally appropriate tasks, and activities or behaviours that promote or threaten health	X		6 domain; Child edition (6-11 years); Adolescent edition (12-17 years)	30	X	X
Child Health Questionnaire [13]	5-18	Measures health with regard to physical, psychological and social domains	X	X	11 domains; Self and Parent version	20	X	X
Dartmouth Coop Functional Health Assessment Charts [14]	15 (median)	Measures exclusive dimensions of health and social problems through picture/word charts	X		6 charts (pictures and words)	15-20	X	
KINDL [15]	4-16	Describes physical, psychological, social, and functional aspects of well-being and functioning from patient's perspective	X	X	6 domains	10	X	X
Pediatric Quality of Life Questionnaire [16]	2-18	Evaluates physical, mental and social health of children and adolescents	X	X	4 domain, 23 items	5-10	X	X
Quality of Life Profile – Adolescent Version [16]	14-20	Evaluates physical, psychological and spiritual parameters through being, belonging and becoming options	X		3 domains, 54 items	40	X	
Warwick Child Health and Morbidity Profile [17]	0-5	Evaluates general, acute, chronic and functional health status and QOL	X	X	10 domains	10	X	

Table 2: Summary of generic measures of health-related QOL used in paediatric sleep disorders.

- Inclusion of quality of wake time as a secondary outcome in pharmacotherapeutic studies will be a key step in addressing this neglected but significant aspect of sleep medicine.

There are number of good quality validated tools (outcome measures) to study the quality of wake time for therapeutic trials in insomnia although some of these may not be suitable where children are affected by disability.

References

1. Wafford KA, Ebert B (2008) Emerging anti-insomnia drugs: tackling sleeplessness and the quality of wake time. Nat Rev Drug Discov 7: 530-540.
2. Morin C, Jarrin DC (2013) Epidemiology of insomnia: prevalence, course, risk factors, and public health burden. Sleep Medicine Clinics.
3. Khan S, Heussler H, McGuire T, Dakin C, Pache D, et al. (2011) Melatonin for non-respiratory sleep disorders in visually impaired children. Cochrane Database Syst Rev: CD008473.
4. Glass J, Lanctôt KL, Herrmann N, Sproule BA, Busto UE (2005) Sedative hypnotics in older people with insomnia: meta-analysis of risks and benefits. BMJ 331: 1169.
5. Heussler H, Chan P, Price AM, Waters K, Davey MJ, et al. (2013) Pharmacological and non-pharmacological management of sleep disturbance in children: an Australian Paediatric Research Network survey. Sleep Med 14: 189-194.
6. American Psychiatric Association (2013) Diagnostic and Statistical Manual of Mental Disorders (5thedn.). Arlington, VA: American Psychiatric Publishing: 5–25.
7. De Serres LM, Derkay C, Sie K, Biavati M, Jones J, et al. (2002) Impact of adenotonsillectomy on quality of life in children with obstructive sleep disorders. Arch Otolaryngol Head Neck Surg 128: 489-496.
8. Rosen CL, Palermo TM, Larkin EK, Redline S (2002) Health-related quality of life and sleep-disordered breathing in children. Sleep 25: 657-666.
9. Hart CN, Palermo TM, Rosen CL (2005) Health-related quality of life among children presenting to a pediatric sleep disorders clinic. Behav Sleep Med 3: 4-17.
10. Díez-Montiel A, de Diego JI, Prim MP, Martín-Martínez MA, Pérez-Fernández E, et al. (2006) Quality of life after surgical treatment of children with obstructive sleep apnea: long-term results. International Journal of Pediatric Otorhinolaryngology 70: 1575-1579.
11. Gringras P, Gamble C, Jones AP, Wiggs L, Williamson PR, et al. (2012) Melatonin for sleep problems in children with neurodevelopmental disorders: randomised double masked placebo controlled trial. BMJ 345: e6664.
12. Child health and illness profile – a comprehensive assessment of health and functioning for children and adolescents.
13. Waters E, Salmon L, Wake M, Hesketh K, Wright M (2000) The Child Health Questionnaire in Australia: reliability, validity and population means. Aust N Z J Public Health 24: 207-210.
14. Dartmouth COOP functional health assessment charts: brief measures for clinical practice (1995) Quality of life and pharmacoeconomics. In: Spilker B, editor Clinical Trials 2nd edition Philadelphia, PA: Lippincott-Raven Publishers, 161-168.
15. KINDL: Information. Available from http://kindl.org/english/information/.
16. The PedsQL: Measurement model for pediatric quality of life inventory.
17. Spencer NJ, Coe C (2000) Validation of the Warwick Child Health and Morbidity profile in routine child health surveillance. Child Care Health Dev 26: 323-336.
18. Walsh JK, Krystal AD, Amato DA, Rubens R, Caron J, et al. (2007) Nightly treatment of primary insomnia with eszopiclone for six months: effect on sleep, quality of life, and work limitations. Sleep 30: 959-968.
19. Minkel J, Krystal AD (2013) Optimizing the Pharmacologic Treatment of Insomnia: Current Status and Future Horizons. Sleep Med Clin 8: 333-350.

5

Sleep Disordered Breathing after Stroke: Clinical Profile of Patients with Obstructive- as Opposed to Central-Sleep Apnea

Maria Luisa Sacchetti[1]*, Maria Teresa Di Mascio[1], Giacomo Della Marca[2], Antonio Minni[3], Silvia Ottaviani[1], Danilo Toni[1] and Marco Fiorelli[1]

[1]Department of Neurology and Psychiatry, Sapienza University, Rome, Italy
[2]Sleep Unit, Institute of Neurology, Catholic University, A. Gemelli, Rome, Italy
[3]Department of Sensory Organs, Sapienza University of Rome, Rome, Italy

Abstract

Aim: In order to define the clinical and instrumental profile of patients with Obstructive Sleep Apnea/Hypopnea (OSAH) and to compare them with that of cases with Central Sleep Apnea/Hypopnea (CSAH), a series of stable strokes were studied.

Methods: Thirty four patients were submitted to both clinical and polisomnographyc study (PSG) after 4 months of stroke. A Sleep Disordered Breathing (SDB) was diagnosed in all cases with an AHI>5. Patients were classified as affected by predominantly OSAH (*p*OSAH*)*, predominantly CSAH (*p*CSAH*)*, or normal patients. Comparisons were made among the groups and correlation analyses were done in each group. Significance was set at p<0.005.

Results: Thirty-four ischemic strokes were enrolled (55% embolic, 6% large artery, 32% lacunar, 9% with undetermined cause). The 76% of them had a SDB (pOSAH=61%; pCSAH=39%). Nearly the 47% of cases had an obstruction of the upper airways alone or combined with an increase in pharyngeal tissue. No significant differences were found between *p*OSAH and *p*CSAH. In *p*OSAH cases, 8 cases (50%) had an obstruction of the upper airways; in 4 of them it was combined with an increase in pharyngeal tissue; the time interval from stroke to PSG (Δ t), was inversely related to both TST (p 0.017) and TSP (p 0.039); the NIH-SS at entry was directly related to the number of arousals /h of sleep (p 0.044); the more severe AHI the higher is ODI (p 0.000). In the pCSAH group, 4 cases (40%) had an obstruction of the upper airways combined with an increase in pharyngeal tissue; two of these 4 cases had also a BMI>30. In CSAH, Δt was inversely related to SE Index (p 0.021), and directly related to both the number of arrhythmias/h sleep (p 0.016) and ODI (p 0.033). No correlations were found between the number of arrhythmias/h sleep and causes of stroke both in *p*OSAH and in *p*CSAH groups.

Conclusions: Our data suggest a direct effect of stroke on the peripheral breathing system with subsequent alteration of loop gain and CSAH phenotype, at least in a subgroup of cases. To confirm this hypothesis multicenter clinical sleep studied are needed.

Keywords: Sleep apnea; Stroke; Loop gain; Cycling alternating patterns

Introduction

Prevalence of Sleep-Disordered Breathing (SDB) in patients with first-ever stroke or TIA is higher than in normal populations [1]. The disturb more frequently recognized in these cases is a 'mixed' rather than purely obstructive or central disorder [1,2]. In some cases, what starts as clearly obstructive disease, evolves into predominantly central by the end of the recording [3,4]. This phenomenon has been reported to frequently occur in patients affected by Congestive Heart Failure (CHF) [4,5]; more often it is precipitated by the Continuous Positive Airway Pressure (CPAP) treatment of an obstructive sleep apnea/hypopnea (OSAH) [6-8]. Characteristics of SDB in patients with stable stroke have not been studied jet.

In order to define the clinical and instrumental profile of patients affected by OSAH and to compare them with the profile of cases affected by a Central Sleep Apnea/Hypopnea (CSAH), we report here data on a series of 34 cases with stable stroke, studied at Sapienza, University of Rome.

Methods

Patients

A consecutive series of patients with acute stroke, admitted to the Stroke Unit of Policlinico Umberto I University Hospital, were screened. After the exclusion of patients who did not consent to enter the study, elected cases were submitted to both clinical and instrumental diagnostic tests at 4 months of stroke onset. Stroke risk profile was assessed, and then classified, according to the Italian SPREAD guidelines [9]. Participants were visited firstly at stroke onset and at discharge from the Stroke Unit, and then on the day of the polisomnographic Study (PSG). The severity of neurological deficit was assessed by means of NIH-SS [10,11]. Causes of stroke were classified as to TOAST criteria [12]. Daytime sleepiness was estimated with the Epworth Sleepiness Scale questionnaire (ESS) [13]. The presences of symptoms other than daytime sleepiness have also been investigated, and classified so as: choking, gasping, fragmented sleep, unrefreshing sleeps, reported daytime sleepiness, inattention, accordingly with guidelines [13,14]. In order to identify conditions predisposing to OSAHS, an otorhinolaryngology's (ORL) evaluation was performed.

***Corresponding author:** Maria Luisa Sacchetti, Department of Neurology and Psychiatry, Sapienza University, Rome, Italy
E-mail: marialuisa.sacchetti@uniroma1.it

Sleep studies and polysomography

The ambulatory PSG study was performed by the hand-held 34 channel Morpheus Ambulatory recorder by Micromed® S.r.l. Ambulatory 34 Channels PSG was preferred to standard laboratory recording in order to allow the patients to sleep in their home setting, without needs of adaptation. The following parameters were recorded: 1) body position; 2) rib-gage and abdominal respiratory efforts (Dual thoracoabdominal RIP -respiratory inductance Plethysmography-belts by Micromed® S.r.l. Accessories EPM 915x A); oro-nasal airflow (thermistor transducer by Micromed® S.r.l. Accessories EPMs 1450-S); 4) haemoglobin saturation (finger pulse oximeter sensor); 5) 8 EEG channels (2 frontal, 2 central, 2 temporal, 2 occipital); 6) right and left electrooculography, and 7) sub mental electromyography from surface electrodes; 8) Electrocardiogram (EKG). Morpheus was retrieved the following morning the sensors were attached; data were downloaded to the SystemPlus Evolution software, and subsequently analyzed with dedicated software Rembrandt Sleep View, by a sleep expert. Were considered adequate only PSGs with a total recording time >4 hours and a Total Sleep Time (TST) >2 hours, with presence of both NREM and REM sleep episodes. Sleep-stage scoring was done visually according to standard criteria [15].

Definitions

Apnea was defined as the cessation of airflow for at least 10 seconds. Hypopnea was defined a reduction less than a 50% from baseline of a valid measure of breathing during sleep, associated with an arousal or with an oxygen desaturation of >3%. Apnoea-Hypopnoea Index (AHI) was the sum of all apneas and hypopneas occurring per hour of sleep. Sleep Disordered Breathing (SDB), either central or obstructive, was diagnosed in presence of an Apnea/Hypopnea Index (AHI) value>5 [13]. Three different degrees of severity were outlined: Mild SDB: AHI value > 5 ≤ 15; Moderate SDB: AHI value >15 ≤ 30; Severe SB: AHI value >30 [16]. Each event without associated chest wall movement was considered as central in origin (CSAH). A diagnosis of OSAHS was set in cases in whom at least 50% of the total respiratory events showed a clear dissociation between preserved chest wall movement and airflow pattern with a decrease in the amplitude >50% from baseline, and lasting at least 10 seconds (*p*OSAH). A CSAHS was instead diagnosed when at least 50% of the total respiratory events were central in origin (*p*CSAH). Central Periodic Breathing (CPB) was defined so as recommended [17]. Arousals were defined as "an abrupt change from a "deeper" stage of non-REM (NREM) sleep to a "lighter" stage, or from REM sleep toward wakefulness, with the possibility of awakening as the final outcome" [18]. Arrhythmias were defined as any disturbances of the normal rhythmic beating of the heart.

Statistical analysis

On the bases of PSG study, 3 groups were identified: patients with normal sleep study, cases with predominantly OSAHS (*p*OSAH), and cases with predominantly CSAHS (*p*CSAH). Groups were compared in terms of: age, sex, time from stroke to PSG evaluation (days); NIH-SS at entry and at discharge from Stroke Unit; Body Mass Index (BMI), ESS, TST; Total Sleep Period (TSP); Sleep Efficiency Index; arousal /h sleep; sleep phases; number and type of apneas and hypopneas; arrhythmias of sleep; total number of central apneas-hypopneas per hour of sleep; total number of obstructive apneas-hypopneas per hour of sleep; and Oxygen Desaturation Index (ODI). Patient's demographic data, risk factors for stroke, and sleep study data are expressed as mean and SD or percentages. Statistical comparisons between groups were made using ANOVA, χ^2 or Fisher exact test, depending on which was more appropriate. Correlation analyses were done with non-parametric tests (Spearman's rho). Statistical significance was set at $p<0.05$. Statistical analysis was performed with Statistical Package of Social Sciences (SPSS) version 18.0 for Windows.

Results

After the exclusion of patients who did not consent, 34 cases entered the study. All had an ischemic stroke. The 55% (n=18) were embolic in nature, the 32% (n=11) were lacunar, in the 9 % (n=3) of cases the cause of stroke was undetermined, and in 6% (n=2) a large artery cause was revealed. Patients' mean age was 62.4 ± 14.6. Sixteen cases had a mild (AHI value>5 ≤ 15), 8 had a moderate (AHI value>15 ≤ 30) and 2 cases a severe SDB (AHI value > 30). Sixteen out of the 26 cases with an AHI ≥ 5 (61.5%) had a predominantly OSAH (*p*OSAH), and 10 cases (38.5%) had a predominantly CSAH (*p*CSAH). None of the patients affected by *p*CSAH presented central periodic breathings during sleep (CPBS). The BMI was 28 ± 6 kg/m^2 (range 21 to 47; median 26.5). The mean AHI was 12 ± 9 (range 1 to 35; median 10.5). The PSG study was performed 126.4 ± 49 days after stroke onset (range: 66-282; median 113,5 days). The ORL evaluation was performed in 32 cases and was abnormal in 15 of them. Fourteen cases had an obstruction of the upper airways and in 8 of them the obstruction was combined with an increase in pharyngeal tissue. Eight patients with positive ORL evaluation had a *p*OSAH at the PSG and 4 were affected by *p*CSAHS. All these 4 cases who presented at PSG a *p*CSAH had an obstruction of the upper airways combined with an increase in pharyngeal tissue; two of them had a BMI>30.

The profile of cases respectively affected by *p*OSAH and *p*CSAH are reported in table 1.

No significant difference was found between *p*OSAH and *p*CSAH cases (Table 1). In the group of cases with *p*OSAH the PSG study was performed 147.1 ± 63,2 days after stroke onset (range: 92-282; median 124,5 days). Correlation analysis highlighted that the time interval from stroke to PSG (Δ t) was inversely correlated with both TST (p=0.017) and TSP (p 0.039); the NIH-SS score at entry significantly correlated to the number of arousals /h of sleep (p=0.044); finally, the more severe AHI the higher is ODI (p=0.000). In the group of cases with *p*CSAH the PSG study was performed 113.5 ± 18,5 days after stroke onset (range: 87-140; median 110,5 days). In this group the only significant correlations found were between Δ t and SE Index (inverse correlation; p 0.021) and between Δ t and both arrhythmias/h sleep (p=0.016) and ODI (direct correlation; p=0.033). No significant correlation was found between the number of arrhythmias/h sleep and causes of stroke as to the TOAST criteria (p=0.164) either in the group of cases with *p*OSAH and *p*CSAH.

Discussion

In our series of cases, nearly the 76% of patients had an abnormal breathing during sleep; the 61% of them were predominantly obstructive, and the 39% were predominantly central events.

Patients with predominantly CSAH did not differ significantly to OSAH in demographic characteristics, stroke risk profile, and sleep study parameters. Paradoxically, some of cases with predominantly CSAH are affected also by conditions that would better explain a severe OSAH. In fact, 4 out of 10 cases with *p*CSAH had an obstruction of the upper airways combined with an increase in pharyngeal tissue; in two of them also a BMI higher than 30 was documented. This result may indicate that the predominance of CSAH over OSAH is just phenotypical and that in certain cases, stroke itself is responsible

		Controls	pOSAH	pCSAH	p values
		n=8	n=16	n= 10	
Demographics	Age mean ± SD	55.1 ± 19	60.2 ± 12.4	72 ± 11*	0.032
	Males n (%)	6 (75)	8 (50)	8 (80)	0.233
Clinical	NIH-SS at entry mean ± SD	3 ± 3	5.1 ± 3.6	3.6 ± 2.5	0.780
characteristics	NIH-SS at discharge mean ± SD	1.5 ± 1.4	2.2 ± 1.9	1.3 ± 1.8	0.740
	BMI mean ± SD	28.5 ± 7.8	27.41 ± 5.3	28.4 ± 4	0.976
	AHI mean ± SD	2.3 ± 0.9	15.3 ± 8.7*	15.3 ± 8.2*	0.001
	BMI ≥ 30 n (%)	2 (5.9)	3 (8.8)	4 (11.8)	0.480
	ESS mean ± SD	1.9 ± 2.5	7.7 ± 4.6*	6.8 ± 4.9	0.013
	Obstruction of the upper airways n (%)	2 (6.7)	8 (26.7)	4 (13.3)	0.050
	Increase in pharyngeal tissue n (%)	0 (0)	4 (11.8)	4 (11.8)	0.333
Risk factors	Hypertension n (%)	5 (62.5)	11 (68.8)	8 (80.0)	0.703
for stroke	Smoke n (%)	4 (50.0)	5 (31.1)	5 (50)	0.540
	Atrial fibrillation n (%)	1 (12.5)	5 (31.3)	5 (50)	0.237
	ICA stenosis n (%)	2 (25.0)	7 (43.8)	2 (20)	0.397
	Diabetes n (%)	0 (0)	5 (31.3)	2 (20)	0.203
	Previous TIA n (%)	0 (0)	3 (18.8)	2 (20)	0.404
	Ischemic heart disease n (%)	0 (0)	5 (31.3)	3 (30)	0.199
	Patent foramen ovale n (%)	3 (37.5)	4 ((25)	1 (10)	0.385
	Hyperomocisteinemia n (%)	0 (0)	2 (12.5)	1(10)	0.558
	Hypercholesterolemia n (%)	6 (75)	12 (75)	6 (60)	0.682
	Congestive heart failure n (%)	0 (0)	2 (12.5)	0 (0)	0.302
PSG data	Days between stroke and PSG (Δ t) mean ± SD	100.9 ± 18.7	147.1 ± 63.2	113.5 ± 18.5	0.701
	Total Sleep Time (in minutes) mean ± SD	414.4 ± 85.9	344.4 ± 134.3	333 ± 122	0.182
	Total Sleep Period (in minutes) mean ± SD	488 ± 87.9	427.7 ± 137.1	496.5 ± 96.4	0.783
	Sleep Efficiency Index mean ± SD	81.3 ± 13	74.3 ± 19	63.6 ± 26.5	0.073
	Arousals/h sleep (in thousands) mean ± SD	32 ± 16	39 ± 18	42.5 ± 14.8	0.205
	Arrhythmias /h sleep mean ± SD	15.3 ± 37	73.8 ± 167.8	238 ± 272.9*	0.020
	ODI mean ± SD	7.4 ± 14	15.6 ± 11	13.9 ± 6.5	0.240
	Symptoms other than Daily Sleepiness n (%)	1 (12.5)	10 (62.5)	7 (70)*	0.030
	OSAHS before stroke n (%)	0 (0)	1 (6.3)	1 (10)	0.666

Fisher exact Test, or Anova as appropriate. Significance is set at 0.05
*=significant difference with controls

Table 1: Patients demographic data, clinical characteristics, risk factors for stroke, PSG data, and comparisons respectively between OSAHs, CSAHs, and controls.

for the new onset of an OSAH (or of the worsening of a pre-existing one); in a group of those cases, cause of complex, and only partially understood pathophysiological mechanism (loop gain >1, altered chemo sensitivity), the central drive to breathe may be altered so as to result in the absence of efforts to breath, i.e. central sleep apnea [19,20]. In *p*OSAH cases, the NIH-SS score at entry significantly correlated to the number of arousals of sleep. Given that one of the most significant indicators of sleep efficiency is the number of arousals per hour of sleep, it seems as if the more severe the neurological deficit at the onset of stroke, the less efficient the breathing at the long term. One possible explanation of this phenomenon is that stroke affects airways anatomy or function proportionally to the severity of neurological deficit. The tendency toward a significant correlation between stroke severity at entry and the total number of OSAH events (p 0.080), allows not deny this hypothesis. In the group of cases with *p*OSAH, the more severe AHI the higher is ODI; not the same in *p*CSAH. Actually cases affected by central apnea are able to maintain the O2 saturation within normal values more easily than *p*OSAHs. Nonetheless, this datum conflicts with interpreting *p*CSAHs as more severe *p*OSAHs with altered loop gain, and goes instead in the direction of a role of stroke on patients' CAP (Cycling Alternating Patterns). In this case, the lack of differences between *p*OSAH and *p*CSAH events may consist in the fact that stroke causes the fragmentation of sleep and of altered CAP; in order to elucidate differences in *p*OSAH and *p*CSAH CAP's, more insights into the relationship between the microstructure of sleep and the sleep disordered breathing after stroke are required [21].

Correlation analysis highlighted that the longer the time interval from stroke to PSG the higher AHI and ODI, the shorter both the TST and TSP, the lower the Sleep Efficiency index, as if time has a negative influence both on the quality of sleep and on its duration. Also this result goes in the direction of SDB as a consequence of stroke on the microstructure of sleep [22]. Given the influence of depression on CAP, of great interest would be to elucidate its role on stroke patients' CAP, either affected by *p*OSAH or *p*CSAH.

Sleep studies on stroke populations demonstrate they are affected by some mix of OSAH and CSAH, as if these disturbances are the result of an interaction between the patients' primary breathing condition and some of the long term consequences of stroke on the breathing system (altered loop gain), or on the microstructure of sleep (i.e. CAP system) [1,2,23-25].

The presence of patients affected by obstruction of the upper airways combined with an increase in pharyngeal tissue and a higher than 30 BMI, among cases with predominantly central sleep apnea, goes in the direction of an altered loop gain, probably in cases with severe OSA. This might explain the higher rates of predominantly central sleep apnoea-hypopneas of our series.

Many questions about the SDB profile after stroke are unanswered. Multicenter clinical sleep studied, properly designed to answer these questions are needed.

Acknowledgement

Funded by Sapienza, University of Rome on year 2010. Grant n. C26A10E3ST.

References

1. Johnson KG, Johnson DC (2010) Frequency of sleep apnea in stroke and TIA patients: a meta-analysis. J Clin Sleep Med 6: 131-137.
2. Bassetti C, Aldrich MS (1999) Sleep apnea in acute cerebrovascular diseases: final report on 128 patients. Sleep 22: 217-223.
3. De Paolis F, Colizzi E, Milioli G, Grassi A, Riccardi S, et al. (2013) Complex sleep apnea syndrome in stroke patients. Sleep Med 14: 224.
4. Tkacova R, Niroumand M, Lorenzi-Filho G, Bradley TD (2001) Overnight shift from obstructive to central apneas in patients with heart failure: role of PCO2 and circulatory delay. Circulation 103: 238-243.
5. Ryan CM, Bradley TD (2005) Periodicity of obstructive sleep apnea in patients with and without heart failure. Chest 127: 536-542.
6. Morgenthaler TI, Kagramanov V, Hanak V, Decker PA (2006) Complex sleep apnea syndrome: is it a unique clinical syndrome? Sleep 29: 1203-1209.
7. Gilmartin GS, Daly RW, Thomas RJ (2005) Recognition and management of complex sleep-disordered breathing. Curr Opin Pulm Med 11: 485-493.
8. KuÅºniar TJ, KovaÄ eviÄ‡-RistanoviÄ‡ R, Freedom T (2011) Complex sleep apnea unmasked by the use of a mandibular advancement device. Sleep Breath 15: 249-252.
9. Gensini GF, Dilaghi B, Zaninelli A (2006) Italian SPREAD Guidelines: from past to future. Neurol Sci 27 Suppl 3: S254-257.
10. Pezzella FR, Picconi O, De Luca A, Lyden PD, Fiorelli M (2009) Development of the Italian version of the National Institutes of Health Stroke Scale: It-NIHSS. Stroke 40: 2557-2559.
11. Muir KW, Weir CJ, Murray GD, Povey C, Lees KR (1996) Comparison of neurological scales and scoring systems for acute stroke prognosis. Stroke 27: 1817-1820.
12. Madden KP, Karanjia PN, Adams HP Jr, Clarke WR (1995) Accuracy of initial stroke subtype diagnosis in the TOAST study. Trial of ORG 10172 in Acute Stroke Treatment. Neurology 45: 1975-1979.
13. Johns MW (1991) A new method for measuring daytime sleepiness: the Epworth sleepiness scale. Sleep 14:540-545.
14. Thorpy MJ. American Academy of Sleep Medicine.ICSD-2(2005)-International Classification of Sleep Disorders, 2nd edition:Diagnostic and coding Manual American Academy of Sleep Medicine. 2005.
15. Kushida CA, Littner MR, Morgenthaler T, Alessi CA, Bailey D, et al. (2005) Practice parameters for the indications for polysomnography and related procedures: an update for 2005. Sleep 28: 499-521.
16. Epstein LJ, Kristo D, Strollo PJ Jr, Friedman N, Malhotra A, et al. (2009) Clinical guideline for the evaluation, management and long-term care of obstructive sleep apnea in adults. J Clin Sleep Med 5: 263-276.
17. Berry RB, Budhiraja R, Gottlieb DJ, Gozal D, Iber C, et al. (2012) Rules for scoring respiratory events in sleep: update of the 2007 AASM Manual for the Scoring of Sleep and Associated Events. Deliberations of the Sleep Apnea Definitions Task Force of the American Academy of Sleep Medicine. J Clin Sleep Med 8: 597-619.
18. (1992) EEG arousals: scoring rules and examples: a preliminary report from the Sleep Disorders Atlas Task Force of the American Sleep Disorders Association. Sleep 15: 173-184.
19. Younes M, Ostrowski M, Thompson W, Leslie C, Shewchuk W (2001) Chemical control stability in patients with obstructive sleep apnea. Am J Respir Crit Care Med 163: 1181-1190.
20. Younes M (2008) Role of respiratory control mechanisms in the pathogenesis of obstructive sleep disorders. J Appl Physiol 105: 1389-1405.
21. Thomas RJ, Terzano MG, Parrino L, Weiss JW (2004) Obstructive sleep-disordered breathing with a dominant cyclic alternating pattern-a recognizable polysomnographic variant with practical clinical implications. Sleep 27: 229-234.
22. Parrino L, Ferri R, Bruni O, Terzano MG (2012) Cyclic alternating pattern (CAP): the marker of sleep instability. Sleep Med Rev 16: 27-45.
23. Parra O, Arboix A, Bechich S, García-Eroles L, Montserrat JM, et al. (2000) Time course of sleep-related breathing disorders in first-ever stroke or transient ischemic attack. Am J Respir Crit Care Med 161: 375-380.
24. Dziewas R, Humpert M, Hopmann B, Kloska SP, Lüdemann P, et al. (2005) Increased prevalence of sleep apnea in patients with recurring ischemic stroke compared with first stroke victims. J Neurol 252: 1394-1398.
25. Bassetti CL (2005) Sleep and stroke. Semin Neurol 25: 19-32.

6

Nurse Practitioners (NPs) as Cognitive Behavioral Treatment for Insomnia (CBT-I) Providers: An Underutilized Resource

Barry G Fields[1], Sharon Schutte-Rodin[1*], Megin Myers[1] and Michael L. Perlis[1,2]

[1]*Center for Sleep and Circadian Neurobiology, Division of Sleep Medicine, University of Pennsylvania, USA*
[2]*Department of Psychiatry, University of Pennsylvania Medical Center, Philadelphia, Pennsylvania, USA*

Abstract

Cognitive Behavioral Therapy for Insomnia (CBT-I) is an effective treatment for chronic insomnia, but it remains underutilized. Lack of appropriately-trained CBT-I providers is a major reason. Nurse Practitioners (NPs) may, in addition to psychologists, be uniquely positioned to fill this role, based not only on their professional training but also given a handful of studies showing these individuals' care outcomes meet or exceed standard outcomes. Questions as to how to attract NPs to the field, credential them, and incorporate them into established practices remain unanswered.

The Scope of the Problem

If safe, effective, non-medication based therapy existed for any chronic disorder affecting up to 1/3 of the population, widespread implementation would be expected. If that disorder resulted in more than $100 billion in direct and indirect costs [1], foregoing such therapy would seem ill-advised. Yet, such is the case for cognitive behavioral therapy for insomnia (CBT-I). More than three decades of research support its utility in treating chronic insomnia, with several meta-analyses showing both short-term and long-term efficacy [2-5]. One comparative meta-analysis showed that CBT-I is as at least as efficacious as treatment with benzodiazepine receptor agonists [6]. In the 2005 NIH Consensus and State-of the Science Statement, the NIH panel recognized CBT-I as a first-line therapy for insomnia [7]. In 2008, the Chronic Insomnia Task Force of the American Academy of Sleep Medicine published practice guidelines for the treatment of chronic insomnia that confirmed CBT-I and behavioral therapies as first line therapy for primary and comorbid insomnias [8]. Nevertheless, CBT-I is generally underutilized.

There are many possible reasons as to why CBT-I is not prescribed more frequently. They include both patient-centered and systems-based barriers to CBT-I delivery. Some patient-centered issues include: patients' inability to make time for 4-8 sessions lasting 30–60 minutes each, visit costs or insurance co-pays, difficulties maintaining the strict wake/sleep regimen prescribed, the stigma of psychotherapy, and patient desires for a simple pill to "cure" insomnia without behavioral changes. Some systems-based issues include: providers' lack of awareness regarding CBT-I's effectiveness, limitations on physician time and patient visit length typically needed to deliver behavioral therapies, limited availability of CBT-I trained specialists to perform the therapy, and CBT-I insurance coverage difficulties.

How Should CBT-I be Provided?

Despite enormous growth in sleep medicine practices, the substantial increase in the number of Behavioral Sleep Medicine (BSM) training programs, and the establishment of a BSM credentialing process via the American Board of Sleep Medicine (ABSM), the number of certified BSM (CBSM) specialists and/or CBT-I providers remains insufficient. In 2007, less than one hundred PhDs, PsyDs, nurses, and physicians were BSM certified [9]. While these numbers have increased to over 200 [10], the number and access to the certified specialists remains notably inadequate for millions of chronic insomnia patients [11].

How can this supply-and-demand gap be narrowed? There is essentially 3 approaches:

1) Minimize or eliminate the need for therapists by encouraging the use of self help approaches including patient manuals and/or web based CBT-I.

2) Enable the available clinicians to treat more patients. This could be accomplished by providing CBT-I in group format, by utilizing an abbreviated form of CBT-I (i.e., "BBT-I), and/or by extending the reach of individual clinicians via telemedicine (site to site) or Skype type technology (one to one).

3) Broaden the provider base so that clinicians other than Clinical Psychologists provide CBT-I.

Each of these approaches represent possible pathways towards universal coverage (provision of CBT-I) and may, in the end, all be deployed within a stepped care model. For the purposes of the present analysis, we will focus on how to expand the provider base.

Who Should Provide CBT-I?

Identifying potential clinicians who can provide CBT-I, when indicated, is essential. Critical to their effectiveness is recognizing when and when not to proceed with therapy, a key component of BSM education and training. Providers must have reasonable familiarity with sleep medicine differential diagnoses (such as sleep apnea, restless legs syndrome, and other sleep disorders) as well as other comorbid psychological and medical disorders that frequently accompany insomnia. Patients with chronic insomnia often have related but

***Corresponding author:** Sharon Schutte-Rodin, Center for Sleep and Circadian Neurobiology, Division of Sleep Medicine, University of Pennsylvania, USA, E-mail: Sharon.Schutte-Rodin@uphs.upenn.edu

separate comorbid sleep, psychiatric, substance, and/or medical disorders which also require identification and treatment.

Some have argued that the contingent of doctoral-level clinicians should be expanded and that this could and should be accomplished by increasing the availability of graduate and post graduate educational offerings. Others have argued that "opening the pipe" in such a manner will not produce the number of clinicians needed in the short or long term, and that the clinician base needs to be expanded to include clinical psychologists currently in practice in other specialty areas and/or master's level healthcare workers with mental health skills, specific training in CBT-I, and the proviso that care be provided with supervision. With respect to the last consideration, some view supervision as an on-going component of practice (akin to nurse-physician practice agreements) while others view supervision as a training component that is time limited.

Some sleep clinicians propose that CBT-I can be provided successfully by clinicians who are not BSM certified, or that a doctoral level background is not necessary for BSM eligibility or CBT-I delivery. These clinicians believe that those with master's level background can be equally trained in BSM, particularly in the very specific skill set of CBT-I delivery. The ideal master's level healthcare workers to fill the gap are nurse practitioners (NPs) [9]. NPs appear strategically positioned for this role for several reasons including their ability to: 1) conduct medical assessments, develop differential diagnoses, and evaluate response to initial treatment; 2) provide care for both general medicine and specialty disorders; 3) conceptualize their assessment and treatment using a biopsychosocial approach which is essential in insomnia evaluation and treatment; and 4) be easily integrated into sleep centers because of their primary care skills and because their care is covered under a medical rather than mental health coverage umbrella.

The sleep community, however, has divided opinions as to whether NPs and other non-doctorate clinicians should be trained or certified to provide CBT-I. Advocates argue that a distinct CBT-I skill set could be delivered without complete BSM training, as long as proper BSM evaluation has been done prior to ordering CBT-I therapy and that supervision by a CBSM is provided on an on-going basis (for either a prescribed training period or for on-going practice). Opponents express concern that appropriate BSM evaluation (before CBT-I) cannot be ensured and that continuing education training is not sufficient to allow for the management of the complex cases that typically present with chronic insomnia. The traditional response to this point of view is that a "stepped care" approach be utilized whereby the NP triages the most complex cases (cases that also present with other medical and/or psychiatric and/or sleep disorders) to doctoral-level credentialed specialists [12].

Beyond the arguments "for and against" NPs having a role in CBT-I delivery is a small evidence base including at least three studies that speak to the potential for NPs to conduct CBT-I. In 2007, Espie et al. showed initial and sustained (6 month) improvements in objective and subjective sleep quality indicators after a course of CBT-I therapy [13]. Providers were primary care NPs who received specialized CBT-I training and ongoing supervision. Jungquist et al. found significant improvements in sleep and chronic pain using Masters-level CBT-I practitioners who received similar training and ongoing supervision [14]. Buysse et al. recently published promising findings in a geriatric population, where a short version of CBT-I (brief behavioral treatment for insomnia; BBTI) provided by NPs produced significant remission in insomnia symptoms up to 6 months after treatment [15]. The studies referenced above not only demonstrate that NPs can deliver effective CBT-I, but also that general medicine providers (vs. Psychiatric NPs) can do so successfully when provided adequate training and supervision.. Of note, there are no direct studies assessing NP or master's level versus doctoral-level provider care (MD, PhD, PsyD) in terms of treatment outcomes, patient adherence and retention, and the occurrence of adverse events. Such studies are needed before a decision can be reached regarding unsupervised practice.

How do We Train CBT-I providers?

Although there are similarities between CBT and CBT-I training and practice, CBT-I training and certification is distinct from CBT. General CBT training and certification are traditionally obtained through two pathways: Psychologists through the American Psychological Association credentialed programs (e.g., PhD in Clinical Psychology) and Psychiatrists through the American Psychiatric Association credentialed programs (Psychiatry Residency). Distinct from these CBT training pathways, formal CBT-I training is obtainable within a select few Psychology Internships, Psychiatric Residencies Nursing, and/or Sleep Medicine Fellowship programs. More recently, training is available through SBSM accredited fellowship and mini-fellowship programs, through the Veterans Administration CBT-I dissemination and implementation program (for VA employees only), and through a variety of continuing education (CE)/continuing medical education (CME) offerings through the American Academy of Sleep Medicine, The Society of Behavioral Sleep Medicine, through University-based programs, and finally through private educational offerings (e.g., Sleep Medicine Schools; see Box 1). Burden, in terms of both time and cost, varies greatly among options. Some online courses offer maximum scheduling flexibility (University of Massachusetts), while live CBT-I seminars offer more intensive 2-3 day experiences in various cities (University of Pennsylvania). Training costs vary from free (e.g., within the VA system), to $200-$700 for multi-day trainings, to $1000-$5000 for mini-fellowships, certificate and diploma programs (See, Box 1).

Eventually, such educational opportunities may not only provide NPs the requisite education to provide CBT-I but also establish eligibility for a BSM credentialing exam offered by the American Board of Sleep Medicine. Potential credentialing pathways could be based on those currently in place for doctoral-level clinicians. NPs would obtain eligibility for the exam through either (1) completion of a BSM-accredited training program ('standard track') or (2) demonstration

Overview

SBSM accredited Programs: www.behavioralsleep.org/FellowshipPrograms.aspx

The American Board of Sleep Medicine: www.absm.org/bsmcertification.aspx

Clinician Training

University of Massachusetts: www.umassonline.net/degrees/Online-Graduate-Certificate-Sleep-Disorders-Health-Disease.cfm

University of Pennsylvania: www.med.upenn.edu/cbti/index.html

University of Glasgow: http://www.gla.ac.uk/media/media_145680_en.pdf
The Atlanta School of Sleep Medicine & Technology: www.sleepschool.com

The School of Sleep Medicine: www.sleepedu.net

Sleep School: www.freesleepschool.com
Center for Sleep Counseling Studies: http://sleepcounseling.org/training-certification-program/overview

Box 1: Educational and Credentialing Resources.

of significant clinical experience ('alternative track'). Upon providing appropriate documentation of these prerequisites, they could then sit for a standardized BSM licensing examination. This formalized credentialing model could help ensure uniform competence among NP CBT-I providers.

In addition to training established NPs, other approaches are still needed. Nursing programs can help address the shortage of CBT-I providers by increasing access to training. Historically, nursing schools have failed to offer CBT-I training as one of their educational offerings. Development of improved nursing education curricula to address these potential shortcomings began in 2000 and culminated in 2004, with an Association of Professional Sleep Societies Nursing Task Force publishing their "Recommendations for Nursing Education." [16] Undergraduate sleep education and specific sleep training for NP's were encouraged, but CBT-I was not highlighted as an integral part of the training. Including CBT-I training as a regular offering in nursing curricula will allow greater numbers of providers to be trained while improving visibility and awareness of this treatment.

How Should CBT-I Services be Reimbursed?

One final obstacle to increasing the number of CBT-I clinicians is appropriate reimbursement. Despite insurers' recognizing insomnia as a (sleep) medical disorder, they may carve out coverage for CBT-I as a mental health service, leaving the patient in a self-pay situation. When coverage is provided, it is often covered as either a medical or a mental health benefit. In the case of the former, millions of insomnia patients without anxiety, depression, or other psychiatric disorders may be required to see a medical provider who cannot offer CBT-I. In the case of the latter, the patient may be referred to a mental health provider who is trained in CBT but not BSM or CBT-I. Compounding the problem, many sleep centers do not offer CBT-I, partly because they are often credentialed as medical practices without mental health services. As such, these sleep centers are unable to bill insurance companies that follow older coding of insomnia treatment(s) as exclusively mental health disorders. While these reimbursement considerations are daunting, here again, the provision of CBT-I by NPs may represent a solution. Since NPs may have within their scope of practice the provision of both medical and psychiatric services, this could allow CBT-I to be reimbursable when delivered as part of their sleep disorders practice. The NPs' unique position to practice CBT-I, which incorporates both medical and mental health services, may motivate them to seek this additional CBT-I training. Further, sleep and general practices may encourage NPs to pursue this additional training in order to improve patient care and to expand billable services.

Moving Forward

We need multiple pathways for CBT-I training, including expanded offerings within existing nursing, graduate and medical programs, additional post graduate offerings with a special emphasis on both residency and fellowship training, and CE/CME educational offerings. Finally, the success of the Veterans Administration (VA) CBT-I training program has much to teach us. The question moving forward is how to export this level of dissemination from a self contained system like the VA to the open access Health care system that exists throughout the U.S [17].

In sum, our challenge is to increase CBT-I treatment accessibility while maintaining standardization of training and quality in delivery. The major approach to date has been to expand the availability of training opportunities, and to do so across the educational spectrum. The next step is likely to be a vigorous discussion/evaluation about who can and should provide CBT-I, and under what conditions. The position propounded here is that NPs represent an underutilized resource and should be considered the next professional group to target for the provision of CBT-I. This position is founded not only on "goodness of professional fit" and practical and logistical considerations, but on good preliminary evidence that quality of these individuals' care meets or exceeds standard outcomes [13,15]. What remains for the development of an NP model for CBT-I delivery is: 1) what practice approach to adopt (such as supervised practice vs. independent practice); 2) how to attract NPs to seek out training; and ultimately 3) how to credential these clinicians.

References

1. Matteson-Rusby SE, Pigeon WR, Gehrman P, Perlis ML (2012) Why treat insomnia? Prim Car Companion J Clin Psychiatry 12: e1-e9.
2. Okajima I, Komada Y, Inoue Y (2011) A meta-analysis on the treatment effectiveness of cognitive behavioral therapy for primary insomnia. Sleep Biol Rhythms 9: 24-34.
3. Morin CM, Culbert JP, Schwartz SM (1994) Nonpharmacological interventions for insomnia: a meta-analysis of treatment efficacy. Am J Psychiatry 151: 1172-1180.
4. Murtagh DR, Greenwood KM (1995) Identifying effective psychological treatments for insomnia: a meta-analysis. J Consult Clin Psychol 63: 79-89.
5. Irwin MR, Cole JC, Nicassio PM (2006) Comparative meta-analysis of behavioral interventions for insomnia and their efficacy in middle-aged adults and in older adults 55+ years of age. Health Psychol 25: 3-14.
6. Smith MT, Perlis ML, Park A, Smith MS, Pennington J, et al. (2002) Comparative meta-analysis of pharmacotherapy and behavior therapy for persistent insomnia. Am J Psychiatry 159: 5-11.
7. National Institutes of Health (2005) National Institutes of Health State of the Science Conference statement on Manifestations and Management of Chronic Insomnia in Adults, June 13-15, 2005. Sleep 28: 1049-1057.
8. Schutte-Rodin S, Broch L, Buysse D, Dorsey C, Sateia M (2008) Clinical guideline for the evaluation and management of chronic insomnia in adults. J Clin Sleep Med 4: 487-504.
9. Perils ML, Smith MT (2008) How can we make CBT-I and other BSM services widely available? J Clin Sleep Med 4: 11-13.
10. American Board of Sleep Medicine.
11. McKay GD, Grandner MA, Gehrman P, Brember EM, Perlis ML. Where are the CBSMs and where are they needed? [Abstract]. Sleep 2012; 35: A446.
12. Neylan TC (2011) Time to disseminate cognitive behavioral treatment of insomnia: comment on "Efficacy of brief behavioral treatment for chronic insomnia in older adults". Arch Intern Med 171: 895-896.
13. Espie CA, MacMahon KM, Kelly HL, Broomfield NM, Douglas NJ, et al. (2007) Randomized clinical effectiveness trial of nurse-administered small-group cognitive behavior therapy for persistent insomnia in general practice. Sleep 30: 574-584.
14. Jungquist CR, O'Brien C, Matteson-Rusby S, Smith MT, Pigeon WR, et al. (2010) The efficacy of cognitive-behavioral therapy for insomnia in patients with chronic pain. Sleep Med 11: 302-309.
15. Buysse DJ, Germain A, Moul DE, Franzen PL, Brar LK, et al. (2011) Efficacy of brief behavioral treatment for chronic insomnia in older adults. Arch Intern Med 171: 887-895.
16. Lee KA, Landis C, Chasens ER, Dowling G, Merritt S, et al. (2004) Sleep and chronobiology: recommendations for nursing education. Nurs Outlook 52: 126-133.
17. Manber R, Carney C, Edinger J, Epstein D, Friedman L, et al. (2012) Dissemination of CBTI to the non-sleep specialist: protocol development and training issues. J Clin Sleep Med 8: 209-218.

Association between Subjective Sleep Quality, Hypertension, Depression and Body Mass Index in a Nigerian Family Practice Setting

Shittu RO[1]*, Issa BA[2], Olanrewaju GT[2], Odeigah LO[3], Sule AG[4], Sanni MA[5], Aderibigbe SA[6], Uthman MB[6] and Nyamngee AA[7]

[1]Department of Family Medicine, Kwara State Specialist Hospital, Nigeria
[2]Department of Behavioral Sciences, University of Ilorin Teaching Hospital, Nigeria
[3]Department of Family Medicine, University of Ilorin Teaching Hospital, Nigeria
[4]Department of Family Medicine, Ahmadubello University, Teaching Hospital, Nigeria
[5]Department of Hematology, Kwara State Specialist Hospital, Nigeria
[6]Department of Epidemiology and Community Health, University of Ilorin Teaching Hospital, Nigeria
[7]Department of Medical microbiology and parasitology, College of Health, Sciences, University of Ilorin, Nigeria

Abstract

Objectives: Poor subjective sleep quality in primary care has not been widely studied in Nigeria; hence this study was aimed to evaluate the subjective sleep quality and to find the association with blood pressure, depression and body mass index.

Methodology: Pittsburg Sleep Quality Index (PSQI) questionnaire was administered. Good sleep quality was defined as PSQI less than 5. The level of depression was assessed using the Patient Health Questionnaires (PHQ–9).

Results: The sample consisted of 400 subjects in the age group 18-70years. The overall mean age did 48.0 + 13.2 years, with the age group 41-50years constitute 29.5% of the studied subjects. Whilst 240 (60%) had normal blood pressure, 29(7.5%) had stage 1 and 43 (10.8%) had stage 2 hypertension. One hundred and thirty eight (34.5%) had normal weight, while 108 (27.0%) were obese. Overall sleep quality was very good, fairly good, fairly bad, and very bad in, 30.8%, 33.2%, 19.5%, and 16.5% of the respondents respectively. The prevalence of poor sleep quality was 44.0%. There was strong statistical association between poor sleep quality, blood pressure (p-value 0.002), depression (p-value 0.000) and body mass index (p-value 0.05).

Conclusion: A substantial proportion of the subjects had poor sleep quality associated with high blood pressure, increased body mass index and depression.

Keywords: Sleep quality; Hypertension; Depression; Body mass index

Introduction

Sleep is a vital reparative, restorative and physiological phenomenon, and impaired sleep has significant negative impact on health [1]. The quality of sleep is a measure of both the quantitative and qualitative component of sleep. The quantitative component involves the duration of sleep whereas the qualitative components is a subjective measure of the depth and feeling of restfulness upon awakening [2]. Sleep quality is an important clinical entity for two major reasons. In the first instance, complaints about sleep quality are common; epidemiological surveys indicate that 15-35% of the adult population complain of frequent sleep quality disturbance, such as difficulty falling asleep or difficulty maintaining sleep [3]. In addition, poor sleep quality can be an important symptom of many sleep and medical disorders. One frequently measured component of sleep quality, sleep duration, may even have a direct association with mortality [4]. According to the National Sleep Foundation adults should get between 7 and 9 hours of sleep each night [5].

Sleep quality complaints are particularly relevant to physicians. Factors relating to anxiety and stress are one of the most important concomitants of sleep complaints in the general population [6]. Sleep quality represents a complex phenomenon that is difficult to define and measure objectively. It varies with sex and age. Females have higher risk of poor sleep quality [7]. Increased age is also associated with indices of poor sleep quality [8]. Bansil et al. reported that combinations of sleep disorders short sleep duration and quality of sleep were associated with increased risk in the prevalence of hypertension [9]. In another study, subjective sleep duration was negative related to depressive state [10].

The largest and longest study on adult sleep habits and weight was the Nurses' Health Study, which followed 68,000 middle-age American women for 16 years [11]. Compared to women who slept seven hours a night, women who slept five hours or less were 15 percent more likely to become obese over the course of the study. Abdulsalam et al. [12] found no significant correlation between age, weight, height, BMI and sex of students.

Subjective Sleep quality had been associated with hypertension, depressive symptoms and higher body mass index (BMI) with paucity of data in Nigeria, hence the need for this study.

Methodology

This study was conducted at the General Outpatients Clinic

***Corresponding author:** Shittu RO, Department of Family Medicine, Kwara State Specialist Hospital, Nigeria E-mail: oorelopehospital@gmail.com

(GOPD) of Kwara State Specialist Hospital, Ilorin, and north Central Nigeria. The target populations were the newly registered patients attending the clinic.

The sample size was estimated using the Fisher's Formula [13], $n = \frac{Z^2p(1-p)}{e^2} = \frac{(1.96)^2 0.325(1-0.325)}{(0.05)^2} = 337.1$ using 32.5% from a previous study [14], as the best estimate of poor sleep quality among medical students at a Nigerian University, a minimum sample size of 337.1 was calculated, but 400 was used to increase the reliability of the study.

A systematic random sampling method was used in recruiting respondents for this study, from the period of study from October 30 to November 30, 2013. Already identified depressed subjects who were on treatment and those who refused to give consent were excluded from the study. Pretesting was carried out at the Kwara State Civil Service Hospital, using 40 respondents (10% of the sample size). Ethical approval was obtained from the Ethical Review Committee of the Kwara State Ministry of Health before the commencement of the study.

The Pittsburgh Sleep Quality Index (PSQI) was used for the subjective assessment of sleep quality [2]. The PSQI is a questionnaire consisting of 19 items which are coded on a 4-point scale (0-3) to obtain seven sub-categories, including sleep duration, sleep efficiency, sleep satisfaction, and medication use. The sum of all sub scores represents the total sleep quality score, ranging between 0-21, with higher scores representing lower sleep quality. The individuals were categorized as follows: good sleep quality (less than 5) and poor sleep quality (greater than or equal to 5). Psychometric properties have demonstrated good reliability internal consistency 0.89; test retest reliability 0.85) and good construct validity for the English language version [15].

The Patients Health Questionnaire (PHQ-9) [16] is a brief, 9 - item, patients self-report depression assessment tool that was derived from the interview-based PRIME-MD [17]. It was specifically developed for use, in primary care. It is the only tool that was specifically developed for use as a patient self-administered depression diagnostic tool, rather than as a severity or screening tool. It is the only short self-report tool that can reasonably be used both for diagnosis of DSM-4 major depression as well as for tracking of severity of major depression over time [18]. Psychometric evaluation of the PHQ-9 revealed a sensitivity ranging from 62%-92% and a specificity between 74%-88% [16-18]. All subjects screened positively for depression using Patients Health Questionnaire - 2 (PHQ-2), which was the first two questions of PHQ-9, triggered full diagnostic interviews by the behavioral scientists. Respondents who scored one and more were assessed clinically for depression. Scoring and level of depression was assessed viz: (1-4) minimal depression, (5-9) mild depression, (10-14) moderate depression, (15-19) moderately severe depression, and (20-27) severe depression. Some direct depression care, such as care support, coordination, case management, and treatment was embarked on.

Height and weight were measured according to standardized procedures. Body Mass Index (BMI) was calculated as weight in Kg divided by height in m^2 (kg/m^2). The international classification of BMI was used. The principal cut-off points were as follows: moderate thinness (16.00-16.99), mild thinness (17.00-18.49), normal (18.50-24.99), pre-obese (25.00-29.99), obese class I (30.00-34.99), obese class II (35.00-39.99), obese class III (>40.00).

An Accosson Mercury sphygmomanometer was used to measure the resting blood pressure of the subjects in a sitting position. Classification of hypertension was made according to the seventh report of the Joint National Committee on Prevention, Detection, Evaluation and Treatment of high blood pressure (JNC 7) [19] recommends the following classification of blood pressure for adults aged ≥ 18 years

Normal: Systolic: <120 mm Hg Diastolic: <80 mm Hg

Pre-hypertension: Systolic: <120-139 mm Hg Diastolic: <80-89 mm Hg

Stage 1 hypertension: Systolic: <140-159 mm Hg Diastolic: <90-99 mm Hg

Stage 2 hypertension: Systolic: ≥ 160 Hg Diastolic: ≥ 100 mm Hg

Completed questionnaire and measurements were entered into a computer data base. The data were analyzed using the epidemiological information (Epi-info) 2005 software package of Center for Disease Control and Prevention (CDC).Stepwise multiple regression analysis was conducted and poor sleep quality was significantly correlated with hypertension, depression and body mass index, the level of significance and values less than 0.05 were regarded as statistically significant.

Results

Table 1 displays the socio-demographic characteristics of the respondents. 400 newly registered patients were recruited. Subject with the age group 41-50 constituted 29.5% of the respondents with an overall mean age of 48.0 + 13.2. Female outnumbered males. The respondents were predominantly Yoruba, 384 (96.0%) and Muslims, 354 (88.5%). Majority, 238 (59.5%) had no formal education; they were mostly traders, 156 (39.0%). Thirty (7.5%) agreed to alcohol intake. Thirty six (9.0%) formerly engaged in smoking, while 8 (2.0%) were currently smoking Table 2 shows the association between socio-demographic factors and PSQ 1 scores. Marital status (p-value .020) and ethnicity (p-value .053) were significant.

Table 3 shows that the overall sleep quality was very good, fairly good, fairly bad, and very bad in 30.8%, 33.2%, 19.5%, and 16.5% of the subjects respectively.

Table 4 shows the association between blood pressure, depression, body mass index and psqi among the subjects, at the family practice clinic.

Figure 1 evaluates the Pittsburgh Sleep Quality Index Score. Two hundred and twenty four (56%) scored ≤ 5 indicating good sleepers, while 176 (44.0%) scored >5 indicated poor sleepers.

Discussion

The prevalence of poor sleep quality among the subjects was 44%. This was consistence with Suen and co-workers [20], in the US, who reported 42% and also similar to the findings of Krishna and colleagues with the prevalence of 42% [21], but higher than the CDC surveillance report of 35.3% [22] and the findings of Bawo and co-workers, at a Nigerian University with 32.5% [14], On the other hand, the result was lower than Seblewngel and colleagues [23], who found that the prevalence of poor sleep quality was 55.8%, Cheng et al. [24], who reported 54.7% and Adewole et al. while studying sleep disorders and sleep quality among adult's patients presenting at the General Outpatients Department in ObafemiAwolowo University Teaching Hospital Complex (OAUTHC) in Nigeria, who reported prevalence of 50% [25].

The apparently high prevalence in this study may be attributed to lower health-related quality of life, low socio-economic status

Variable	Frequency	(%)	Mean	Std. Deviation
Age				
≤ 20	4	1.0		
21-30	58	14.5		
31-40	64	16.0	48.0	13.16
41-50	118	29.5		
51-60	100	25.0		
≥ 61	59	14.0		
Gender				
Male	96	24		
Female	304	76		
Ethnicity				
Hausa	8	2.0		
Yoruba	384	96.0		
Igbo	6	1.5		
Others	2	0.5		
Religion				
Christianity	46	11.5		
Islam	354	88.5		
Marital Status				
Married	250	62.5		
Single	24	6.0		
Divorced	14	3.5		
Separated	26	6.5		
Widow	82	20.5		
Widower	4	1.0		
Educational Level				
Non-formal	238	59.5		
Primary	48	12.0		
Secondary	62	15.5		
Tertiary	52	13.0		
Occupation				
Trader	156	39.0		
Civil Servant	56	14.0		
Self Employed	126	31.0		
Unemployed	50	24.0		
Student	12	76.0		
Alcohol Intake				
Yes	30	7.5		
No	370	92.5		
Smoking Status				
Never	356	89.0		
Former	36	9.0		
Current	8	2.0		

Table 1: Socio-Demographic Characteristics of The Respondents.

and concomitant poor medical conditions, and to snoring which is common among hypertensive subjects in South Western Nigeria [26]. In addition, it could also results from Obstructive sleep apnea (OSA) was high in Nigeria [27]. In this study, the overall sleep quality was very good, fairly good, fairly bad, very bad in 30.8%, 33.2%, 19.5%, and 16.5% of the subjects respectively. This result was higher than that of Vivek et al. [28], in Banasthali University Rajasthan, India, where distribution of sleep quality were excellent 20.4%, good 38.5%, satisfactory 35.8%, poor 4%, very poor, 1.3%.

Seblewengel et al. found out that approximately 25% had very good and 60% fairly good overall sleep quality [23].

Consistent with previous studies [29,30], poor sleep quality was associated with depression [31,32]. Depression was significantly associated with sleep complaints; a finding that was consistent with previous reports [33]. The relationship between depression and sleep disturbances was so strong that it was one of the diagnostic criteria of major depression [34]. High degree of depression and anxiety were found to be the influencing factors of poor sleep among Chinese adolescents [35].

There was a strong statistical association between body mass index and PSQI Score. Obese class 3 was poor sleepers. This was similar to the finding of Pearson et al. [36] who found that obese patient had difficulty with sleep. This result was consistence to the findings of Anne et al. [37]. However Abdul Salam et al. [12] found no significant correlation between age, weight, height and BMI.

Several studies had indicated that insufficient sleep, less than five or six hours were associated with weight gain [38]. The result of this study contrasted with Watson et al. [38] who found no relationship between subjective sleep quality and BMI and to Aylin et al. [30] who found no significant relationship between body measurement and PSQI scores

Variables	PSQI SCORES		Total	p-value
	<=5	>5		
Age Groups				
<=20	3	1	4	.775
21-30	35	23	58	
31-40	33	31	64	
41-50	62	56	118	
51-60	59	41	100	
>=61	32	24	56	
Total	224	176	400	
Sex				
Male	48	48	96	.174
Female	176	128	304	
Total	224	176	400	
Ethnicity				
Hausa	3	5	8	.053
Yoruba	220	164	384	
Igbo	1	5	6	
Others	0	2	2	
Total	224	176	400	
Religion				
Christianity	22	24	46	.235
Islam	202	152	354	
Total	224	176	400	
Marital Status				
Married	149	101	250	.020
Single	7	17	24	
Divorced	11	3	14	
Separated	11	15	26	
Widow	44	38	82	
Widower	2	2	4	
Total	224	176	400	
Level of Education				
Non-formal	135	103	238	.547
Primary	23	25	48	
Secondary	38	24	62	
Tertiary	28	24	52	
Total	224	176	400	
Occupation				
Trader	94	62	156	.398
Civil Servant	27	29	56	
Self Employed	68	58	126	
Unemployed	30	20	50	
Student	5	7	12	
Total	224	176	400	

Table 2: Association between Socio Demographic Factors and Psqi Scores at the Family Practice Clinic.

Sleep Quality	Frequency	(%)
Very good	123	30.8
Fairly good	133	33.2
Fairly bad	78	19.5
Very bad	66	16.5
Total	400	100

Table 3: Subjective Sleep Quality.

Variables	PSQI SCORES		Total	p-value
	<=5	>5		
Blood Pressure				
Normal	150	90	240	.002
Pre-HTN	46	42	88	
Stage 1	9	20	29	
Stage 2	19	24	43	
Total	224	176	400	
Depression				
Minimal Depression	212	129	341	.000
Mild Depression	12	42	54	
Moderate Depression	0	2	2	
Severe Depression	0	3	3	
Total	224	176	400	
Body Mass Index				
Moderate thinness	0	4	4	.045
Mild thinness	9	11	20	
Normal	84	54	138	
Pre-obese	72	58	130	
Obese class 1	38	34	72	
Obese class 2	15	5	20	
Obese class 3	6	10	16	
Total	224	176	400	

Table 4: Association between Blood Pressure, Depression, Body Mass Index and Psqi among the Subjects, At the Family Practice Clinic.

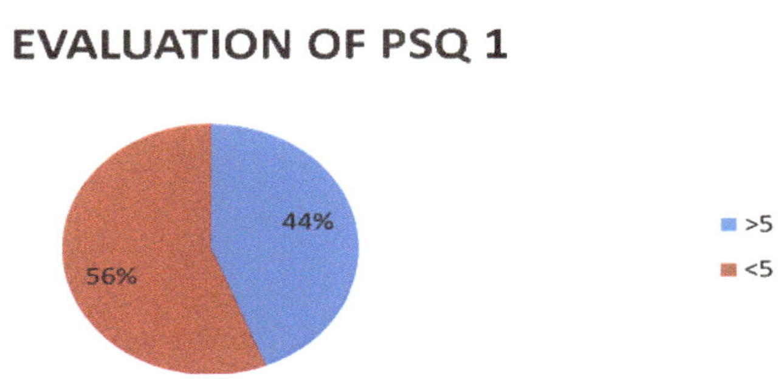

Figure 1: Evaluation of Psq 1.

[39]. Also, Van and Knutson [40] found no association between sleep quality and BMI.

In this study, there was statistical association between high blood pressure and PSQI (p-value = .002). Pooja et al. [9] found out that among people with both sleep disorder and short sleep, the likelihood of hypertension was slightly more than twice that for people with no sleep problems. This relationship may, in part, be the result of biologic mechanisms, suggesting that sleep deprivation may alter cortisol stress hormones and the sympathetic nervous system, resulting in elevated BP. In the sleep Heart Health Study, subjects sleeping ≤5 h/night had a higher frequency of prevalent hypertension [41] The Whitehall II [42] study also found that, women sleeping ≤ 5h/night had a higher risk of hypertension compared with those sleeping 7 h/night.

Conclusion

A large proportion of adults, attending the Kwara State Specialist Hospital, Ilorin Nigeria are poor sleepers with associated hypertension, depression and increased body mass index. Taking into account that poor sleep quality has major negative long term impact on health, prevention programs should be put in place.

References

1. Guilleminault C, Brooks SN (2001) Excessive daytime sleepiness: a challenge for the practicing neurologist. Brain 124: 1482-1491.
2. Buysse DJ, Reynolds CF 3rd, Monk TH, Berman SR, Kupfer DJ (1989) The Pittsburgh Sleep Quality Index: a new instrument for psychiatric practice and research. Psychiatry Res 28: 193-213.
3. Mellinger GD, Balter MB, Uhlenhuth EH (1985) Insomnia and its treatment. Prevalence and correlates. Arch Gen Psychiatry 42: 225-232.
4. Kripke DF, Simons RN, Garfinkel L, Hammond EC (1979) Short and long sleep and sleeping pills. Is increased mortality associated? Arch Gen Psychiatry 36: 103-116.
5. National sleep foundation (2012) How much sleep do we need? And how much sleep are we getting?
6. Karacan I, Thornby JI, Williams RL (1983) Sleep/Wake Disorders: natural History, Epidemiology, and Long-Term Evolution. New York: Raven Press, 37-60.
7. Oluwole OS (2010) Sleep habits in Nigerian undergraduates. Acta Neurol Scand 121: 1-6.
8. Dregan A, Armstrong D (2010) Adolescence sleep disturbances as predictors of adulthood sleep disturbances--a cohort study. J Adolesc Health 46: 482-487.
9. Bansil P, Kuklina EV, Merritt RK, Yoon PW (2011) Association between sleep disorders, sleep duration, quality of sleep and hypertension: results from the National Health and Nutrition Examination Survey, 2005 to 2008. J Chin Hypertens (Greenwich) 13:739-743.
10. Kawada T (2012) Quality of sleep, Sleep duration and depressive state. The Journal of Clinical Hypertension14: 479-82.
11. Patel SR, Malhotra A, White DP, Gottlieb DJ, Hu FB (2006) Association between reduced sleep and weight gain in women. Am J Epidemiol 164: 947-954.
12. Abdulsalam, Salman MT, Gupta S, Trivedi M, Farooqi M (2013) Poor quality of sleep and its relationship with depression in first year medical students. Advances in life science and technology 12: 17-21.
13. Araoye MO (2003) Data Collection in: Research methodology with statistics for health and social sciences. Nathadex Publishers130-159.
14. James BO, Omoaregba JO, Igberase OO (2011) Prevalence and correlates of poor sleep quality among medical students at a Nigerian university. Annals of Nigerian Medicine 5:1-4.
15. Shochat T, Tzischinsky O, Oksenberg A, Peled R (2007) Validation of the Pittsburgh Sleep Quality Index Hebrew translation (PSQI-H) in a sleep clinic sample. Isr Med Assoc J 9: 853-856.
16. Kroenke K, Spitzer RL, Williams JB (2003) The Patient Health Questionnaire-2: validity of a two-item depression screener. Med Care 41: 1284-1292.
17. Spitzer RL, Williams JB, Kroenke K, Linzer M, deGruy FV 3rd, et al. (1994) Utility of a new procedure for diagnosing mental disorders in primary care. The PRIME-MD 1000 study. JAMA272: 1749-1756.
18. Kroenke K, Spitzer RL, Williams JB (2001) The PHQ-9: validity of a brief depression severity measure. J Gen Intern Med 16: 606-613.
19. Chobanian AV, Bakris, GL, Black HR, Cushman WC, Green LA, et al. (2003) The Seventh Report of the Joint National Committee on Prevention, Detection, Evaluation and Treatment of High Blood Pressure: the JNC 7 report. JAMA 289: 2560-2572.
20. Suen LK, Hon KL, Tam WW (2008) Association between sleep behavior and sleep-related factors among university students in Hong Kong. ChronobiolInt 25:760-775.

21. Pushpa K, Shwetha S (2008) Sleep quality and correlates of sleep among medical students. The Indian Journal of Sleep Medicine. 3: 58-61.

22. CDC (2014) Youth Risk Behaviour Surveillance (YRBSS).

23. Lemma S, Gelaye B, Berhane Y, Worku A, Williams MA (2012) Sleep quality and its psychological correlates among university students in Ethiopia: a cross-sectional study.BMC Psychiatry 12: 237.

24. Cheng SH, Shih CC, Lee IH, Hou YW, Chen KC, et al. (2012) A study on the sleep quality of incoming university students. Psychiatry Res 197: 270-274.

25. Adewole TO, KuteyiBA,Ezeoma I, Bello I (2013) Sleep disorders and sleep quality among adults patients presenting at a General Outpatient Department in Ile Ife, Nigeria- A preliminary report. European Respiratory Society. 12: 50-54.

26. Alebiosu OC, Ogunsemi OO, Familoni OB, Adebayo PB, Ayodele OE (2009) Quality of sleep among hypertensive patients in a semi-urban Nigerian community: a prospective study. Postgrad Med 121: 166-172.

27. Akintunde AA, Okunola OO, Oluyombo R, Oladosu YO, Opadijo OG (2012) Snoring and obstructive sleep apnoea syndrome among hypertensive Nigerians: prevalence and clinical correlates. Pan Afr Med J 11: 75.

28. Jain V, Tomar R, Jha J, Pareek A, Ratan Y, et al. (2013) Sleep quality and sleep associated problems in female pharmacy students. Chronicles of young scientists 4: 138-143.

29. Moo-Estrella J, Pérez-Benítez H, Solís-Rodríguez F, Arankowsky-Sandoval G (2005) Evaluation of depressive symptoms and sleep alterations in college students. Arch Med Res 36: 393-398.

30. Eller T, Aluoja A, Vasar V, Veldi M (2006) Symptoms of anxiety and depression in Estonian medical students with sleep problems. Depress Anxiety 23: 250-256.

31. Breslau N, Roth T, Rosenthal L, Andreski P (1996) Sleep disturbance and psychiatric disorders: a longitudinal epidemiological study of young adults. Biol Psychiatry 39: 411-418.

32. Sahraian A, Javadopur A (2010) Sleep disruption and its correlation to psychological distress among medical students. Med J 11: 12-17.

33. Ford DE, Kamerow DB (1989) Epidemiologic study of sleep disturbances and psychiatric disorders. An opportunity for prevention? JAMA 262: 1479-1484.

34. American Psychiatric Association (1994) Diagnostic and statistical manual of mental disorders, (4thedn), Text Revision (DSM-IV-TR).

35. Xu Z, Su H, Zou Y, Chen J, Wu J, et al. (2012) Sleep quality of Chinese adolescents: distribution and its associated factors. J Paediatr Child Health 48: 138-145.

36. Pearson NJ, Johnson LL, Nahin RL (2006) Insomnia, trouble sleeping, and complementary and alternative medicine: Analysis of the 2002 national health interview survey data. Arch Intern Med 166: 1775-1782.

37. Hayley AC, Williams LJ, Berk M, Kennedy GA, Jacka FN, et al. (2013) The relationship between excessive daytime sleepiness and depression and anxiety disorders in women. Aust NZ J Psychiatry 47: 772-778.

38. Watson NF, Harden P, Buchwald D, Schur E, Goldberg J (2011) Sleep duration modifies the heritability of body mass index. Poster presented at the Annual Meeting of the association Professional Sleep Societies.

39. Aylin A, Esra AK, Duygu O (2012) Pittsburgh sleep quality index score and its relationship between body measurements in late menopause patients.

40. Van Cauter E, Knutson KL (2008) Sleep and the epidemic of obesity in children and adults. Eur J Endocrinol 159 Suppl 1: S59-66.

41. Gottlieb DJ, Redline S, Nieto FJ, Baldwin CM, Newman AB, et al. (2006) Association of usual sleep duration with hypertension: the Sleep Heart Health Study. Sleep 29: 1009-1014.

42. Cappuccio FP, Stranges S, Kandala NB, Miller MA, Taggart FM, et al. (2007) Gender-specific associations of short sleep duration with prevalent and incident hypertension: the Whitehall II Study. Hypertension 50: 693-700.

Revision of Estimation Method for an Established Morphometric Model for Prediction of Obstructive Sleep Apnea

Oommen Nainan[1]*, Jayan B[2], Chopra SS[3] and Mukherjee M[4]

[1]*Graded Specialist-Orthodontics & Dentofacial Orthopedics, Naval Institute of Dental Sciences, India*
[2]*Department of Dental Surgery, Armed Forces Medical College, India*
[3]*Classified Specialist-Orthodontics & Dentofacial Orthopedics, Corps Dental Unit, India*
[4]*Classified Specialist-Periodontology, Military Dental centre, India*

Abstract

Background: The morphometric model (MM) provides a rapid, accurate and reproducible method for predicting whether patients in an ambulatory setting are at risk for obstructive sleep apnea (OSA).

Introduction: The aim of this study was to estimate mean MM scores in a mixed Indian population and to test a revision of the method for making intraoral measurements.

Methods: A total of 60 subjects were included in the study and were divided into two groups of 30 subjects each; Group 1: Patient group; Group 2: Control group. A comparative cross-sectional study design was employed and MM value as suggested by Kushida was estimated by applying their clinical rule. The measurements in our study were made on study models to ensure precise and accurate measurement of these anatomic distances, thus ensuring a greater accuracy for the morphometric model.

Results: The comparison of morphometric model values between OSA and non OSA groups showed an extremely statistically significant difference. The average predictive morphometric model value for OSA in this sample of Indian patients is only slightly lesser than that observed by Kushida

Conclusions: The results of this study could facilitate the early recognition of OSA and support the available diagnostic setup. This revised methodology may be used to widen the reach of the morphometric model from the sleep physician's clinic to the Dental operatory.

Keywords: Obstructive sleep apnea; Morphometric model; Polysomnography; Predictors; Clinical rule

Introduction

Obstructive sleep apnea (OSA) is characterized by repetitive obstruction of the upper airway during sleep, resulting in oxygen desaturation and sleep fragmentation. Even though OSA is fairly common, it often remains undiagnosed in primary care practice. While overnight polysomnography (PSG) is considered the 'gold standard' for the diagnosis of OSA, the need for accurate, quantitative diagnostic criteria is further compounded by the significant cost incurred with routine PSG. However, the lack of a simple, non-invasive, repeatable method has been an obstacle for the early recognition of OSA patients. The limited number of sleep laboratories available restricts the proper identification of OSA and may lead to underestimation of the magnitude of the problem and under-treatment, with undesirable public and personal health consequences.

Common symptoms of the condition have limited predictive value in identifying patients with OSA [1]. The morphometric model is a useful screening test to investigate the possibility of OSA in patients during initial office visits. The most commonly used predictive model is the morphometric model given of the Stanford Sleep Disorders Clinic and Research Centre, California (hereafter referred to as the Stanford Morphometric Model-SMM), which provides a rapid, accurate and reproducible method for predicting whether patients in an ambulatory setting are at risk for OSA [2]. This clinical morphometric model combines measurements of the oral cavity with body mass index and neck circumference and was tested on Caucasian patients, where it was found that patients with values equal to or more than 70, typically had OSA. There is no data available on the applicability of the predictive model to Indian subjects.

The key step in the management of OSA is to firmly establish the diagnosis. The Dental Practitioner in general and the Orthodontist in particular, now has an ever increasing role in the recognition of a patient who may be at risk for a sleep disorder. We carried out a pilot study with the aim of estimating mean SMM scores in a mixed Indian population. The method used in the original study by Kushida for intra-oral measurements, was found to be subjective and difficult to standardize for a group. A revision of the method for making intraoral measurements was also tested with an objective to provide increased usefulness to clinicians tackling this significant disorder, in many countries. The results of this study could facilitate the early recognition of OSA and support the available diagnostic setup. Based on the intra oral findings, orthodontists may request a polysomnographic evaluation when OSA is suspected and the final diagnosis of sleep disorder, its severity and the evaluation of comorbidities are made by a physician according to polysomnographic findings.

***Corresponding author:** Oommen Nainan, Graded Specialist-Orthodontics & Dentofacial Orthopedics, Naval Institute Of Dental Sciences, INHS Asvini Campus, Colaba, Mumbai 400005, Maharashtra, India
E-mail: droommennainan@yahoo.in

Material and Methods

This multi-disciplinary study was undertaken at the Division of Orthodontics and Dentofacial Orthopedics, Armed Forces Medical College, Pune, India. The research protocols were reviewed and approved by the Institutional Ethical Committee of the hospital. Informed consent under witness was obtained from each participant at enrollment after each subject was explained the nature and purpose of the study. To detect a clinically significant difference with 80% power, α=0.05 and a ratio between two groups of 1:1, 60 adult Indians aged 18 years and above were recruited for this study [3]. A comparative cross-sectional study design was employed. The total of 60 subjects included in the study was divided into two groups of 30 subjects each; Group 1: Patient (test) group; Group 2: Control group.

The patient sample (test group) consisted of 30 randomly selected PSG diagnosed OSA patients referred by the Department of Respiratory Medicine, Military Hospital, Cardio-Thoracic Centre, Pune, India, for the analysis of craniofacial morphology. PSG performed was level I, using a 16-channel polygraph (Sleep Scan Analysis VISION, Bio-logic Systems Corp, USA). For the purpose of this study, only one variable-the number of apneas and hypopneas was utilized. There was no prior knowledge of the patient to be seen and there was no regular pattern of days to examine the patients. For the test group, the patients who satisfied the following criterion were included in the study: age - 18 years and above; polysomnographic evidence of OSA (defined as an apnea/hypopnea index (AHI) of $\geq$ 5/hour of sleep) and the presence of at least ten teeth in each arch. AHIs were calculated using using the "recommended" (AHI_{Rec}) AASM hypopnea scoring criteria. Apnoea was defined as cessation of airflow for atleast 10 seconds with oxygen desaturation of more than 3%. Hypopnoea was defined as a reduction of 30% or greater in airflow from baseline for more than 10 seconds with associated drop in oxygen saturation of 4% or more and arousal as per the recommendations of American Academy of Sleep Medicine Task Force, 2001.

The control group consisted of 30 randomly selected adults attending the dental outpatient department, with an Angle's Class I molar relation and no history of sleep obstructed breathing. The control group was matched with the patient sample to the best extent possible for age, gender, height and weight. For the control group, the subjects who satisfied the following criterion were included in the study: age - 18 years and above; subjects with Angle's Class I occlusion, Epworth Sleepiness Scale (ESS) score <9 (to exclude daytime sleepiness); no reported snoring by family members and the presence of at least ten teeth in each arch. Snoring frequency, snoring intensity and ESS was used as a questionnaire for selection of subjects in the control group.

The exclusion criteria for both groups were: edentulous subjects; subjects with hypothyroidism; subjects with history of orthodontic treatment; subjects with history of reconstructive/orthognathic surgery; subjects with craniofacial deformity, such as cleft lip and/or palate; subjects with history of pharyngeal surgery and subjects with patient-specific disorders (such as neuromuscular disorders).

Each of the groups consisted of 19 men and 11 women. Data collection was divided into three sections as follows:

a. Medical and sleep history including an ESS.

b. Clinical examination with anthropomorphic recordings of the subject's height, weight and neck circumference. Neck circumference (NC) in centimetres, was measured with a tape measure, at the level of the cricothyroid cartilage in upright awake subjects. For each subject, obesity was expressed as body mass index (BMI) [4].

c. Study model analysis: Measurements were taken from the maxillary and mandibular study models using a pair of digital callipers (Workzone, Global tronics GmbH & Co, Germany), with a resolution of 0.01 mm.

Upper and lower dental arch study models were obtained with alginate dental impression material and dental stone. The following measurements were recorded on the study models [2,5]. All the measurements were carried out by the principal investigator.

1. Maxillary intermolar width [Mx]: Distance between the mesiobuccal cusp tips of the crowns of the maxillary right and left permanent first molars (Figure 1).
2. Mandibular intermolar width I [Mn]: Distance between the mesiobuccal cusp tips of the crowns of the mandibular right and left permanent first molars (Figure 2).
3. Overjet [OJ]: Horizontal overlap of the crowns of the maxillary and mandibular central incisors, in millimetres.
4. Palatal height [P]: To standardize measurement of palatal depth/height, models were trimmed until the distal contact point of the upper first molars showed up on the edge. Distance from the mid-deepest part of the palate to the line connecting the left and right distolingual cusp tips of the upper first molars was taken as palatal depth (Figure 3).

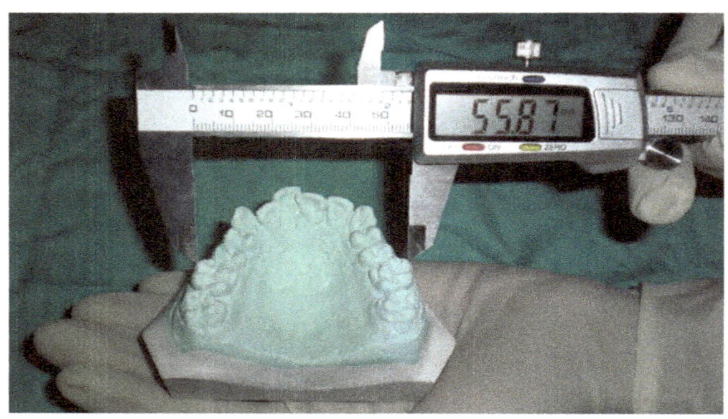

Figure 1: Measurement of maxillary intermolar width on study model.

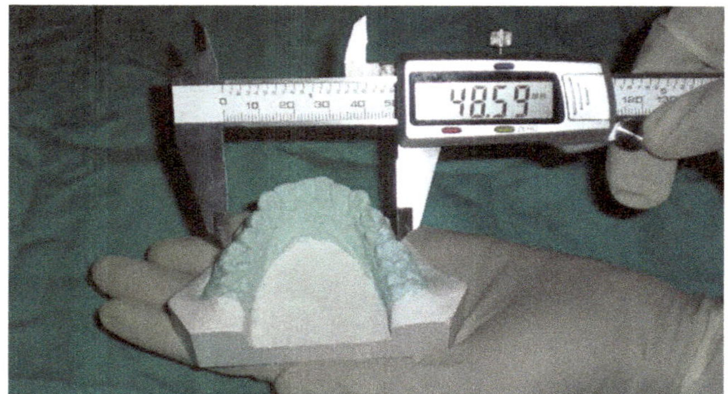

Figure 2: Measurement on mandibular intermolar width on study model.

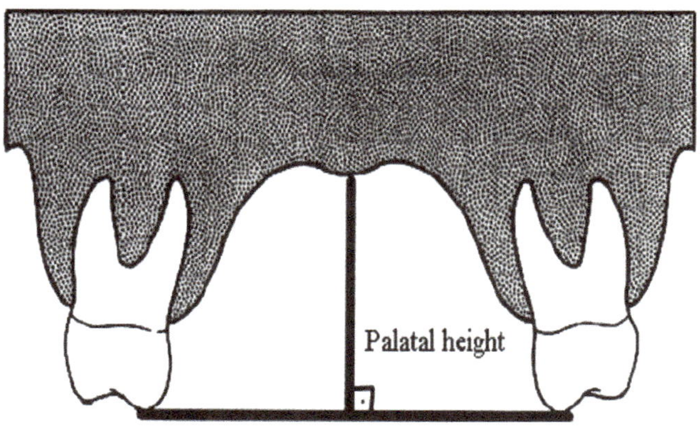

Figure 3: Measurement of palatal height/depth.

SMM score was calculated by applying the clinical rule as follows:

P+ (Mx-Mn) + 3 x OJ + 3 x (BMI – 25,0) x (NC / BMI)

where P=palatal height in millimeters, NC=neck circumference in centimetres, measured at the level of cricothyroid membrane, Mx=distance between the mesial surfaces of the crowns of the maxillary molars in millimetres, MN=distance between the mesial surfaces of the crowns of the mandibular molars in millimeters, OJ=overjet, horizontal overlap of the crowns of the maxillary and mandibular central incisors in millimeters, BMI=body mass index (kg/m^2).

Data compilation and statistical analysis

The readings were tabulated separately for the OSA (test) group and control group. The measurement of 20 randomly selected casts was repeated on separate occasions with a 2-week interval, for evaluation of intra-operator error. The difference between the first and second measurements was not significant. All measurements obtained in the study were expressed as mean ± standard deviation (SD). The data was analysed using MATLAB version 1.0 and Excel 2007. To determine the correlation between OSA severity as indicated by apnea/hypopnea index [AHI] and Stanford morphometric model, linear and multiple regression models were applied.

Results

Stanford morphometric model values were calculated for all the subjects. The comparison of morphometric model values between OSA and non OSA groups showed an extremely statistically significant difference (P<0.0001) with the OSA group having an average morphometric model value of 67.30 ± 11.95 while in the control group, it was 55.43 ± 7.80, as shown in Table 1. The results of the regression analysis showed that there was no significant correlation between the severity of OSA as indicated by AHI and Stanford morphometric model value in this sample of Indian OSA patients (Table 1). The results of the regression analysis indicate that there is no significant correlation between AHI and Stanford morphometric model in this sample of Indian OSA patients. The line diagram for the distribution of patient's AHI versus the calculated Stanford morphometric model value is depicted graphically in Chart 1.

The average age was 53.6 ± 9.42 years. While the two groups had no significant difference in terms of height, the OSA patients were found to be significantly heavier than control subjects with a resulting statistically significant increase in BMI (P<0.05), as shown in Table 2. The patients in the test group also had a statistically significant increase in neck circumference (P<0.05), when compared to the controls. The neck circumference in the test group ranged from 34 to 45 cms with an average of 41.11 ± 2.05 cms for men and 37.55 ± 3.53 cms for women. Table 2 presents the mean of general physical examination measurements of the two groups. All patients in the test group had varying degree of OSA, as confirmed by overnight polysomnography and symptoms of snoring and excessive daytime sleepiness. OSA severity was defined by the AHI. The AHI ranged from 5.6 per hour to 86.4 per hour with an average of 42.04 ± 26.14 events per hour. In the test group, the ESS recorded a statistically significant increase (P<0.05) and ranged from 9 to 20 with an average of 13 ± 2.85 events per hour.

The comparison of mean intraoral values between OSA and controls is summarised in Table 3. Overjet was found to be larger in the controls when compared with the OSA sample, but analyses failed to detect

S No	Parameter	Patients with OSA (Test Group) (n=30)	Patients without OSA (Control Group) (n=30)	P value (<0.05)
1	Age,yrs	53.6 ± 9.42	53.6 ± 9.422	—
2	ESS score	13 (± 2.85)	3.26 (± 0.94)	<0.0001*
3	Weight,kg	80.10 (± 12.5)	67.13 (± 6.78)	<0.0001*
4	Height,mtrs	1.64 (± 0.01)	1.64 (± 0.09)	1
5	Body Mass Index, kg/m2	29.47 (± 4.57)	24.84 (± 1.87)	<0.0001*
6	Neck Circumference, cm	39.80 (± 3.16)	36.10 (± 2.59)	<0.0001*
7	Maxillary intermolar distance, mm	53.05 (± 3.57)	51.58 (± 3.26)	<0.01*
8	Mandibular intermolar distance, mm	46.51 (± 3.93)	44.48 (± 2.87)	0.208
9	Palatal Height, mm	24.1 (± 1.74)	20 75 (± 2.01)	<0.05*
10	Overjet,mm	1.97 (± 1.92)	2.30 (± 1.76)	0.086
11	AHI, events/hr	42.04 (± 26.14)		
12	Morphometric Model Value	67.30 (± 11.95)	55.43 (± 7.80)	<0.0001*
13	Corelation between AHI & SMM			0.209

Table 1: Comparison of Study Group Characteristics & Correlation Between Smm Values & Ahi.

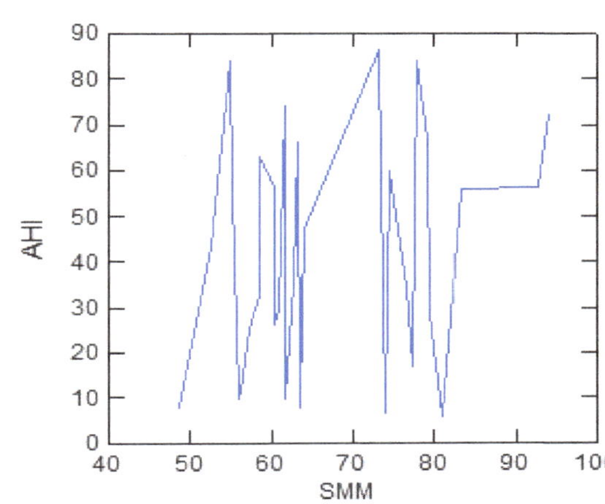

Chart 1: Line Diagram For The Distribution of Patient's Ahi Versus Calculated Stanford Morphometric Model Values.

S no	Parameter	Test Group (n=30)		Control Group (n=30)		df (n-1)	P value (<0.05)
		Mean	SD	Mean	SD		
1	Ht in mtrs	1.64	0.01	1.642	0.09	29	1
2	Wt in kgs	80.1	12.5	67.13	6.78	29	<0.0001*
3	BMI(kg/m^2)	29.47	4.57	24.84	1.87	29	<0.0001*
4	NC in cms	39.8	3.16	36.1	2.59	29	<0.0001*
5	ESS	13	2.85	3.26	0.94	29	<0.0001*
6	AHI	42.04	26.14			29	

Ht - height; Wt - weight; BMI - body mass index; NC - neck circumference; ESS - Epworth sleepiness scale; AHI - apnoea hypopnoea index.
*P ≤ 0.05 = statistically significant.

Table 2: Comparison of Mean of General Physical Characteristics between Test and Control Groups.

S no	Parameter	Test Group (n=30)		Control Group (n=30)		df (n-1)	Regression coefficient	P value (<0.05)	R value (<0.01)
		MEAN	SD	MEAN	SD				
	Column 1	Column 2	Column 3	Column 4	Column 5	Column 6	Column 7	Column 8	Column 9
1	Mx	53.05	3.57	51.58	3.26	29	0.061	<0.05*	<0.01**
2	Mn	46.51	3.93	44.48	2.87	29	-1.875	0.208	≥ 0.01
3	OJ	1.97	1.92	2.8	1.76	29	0.06	0.086	≥ 0.01
4	P	24.1	1.74	20.75	2.01	29	0.043	<0.05*	<0.01**

Mx - maxillary intermolar width; Mn - mandibular intermolar width; OJ - overjet;
P - depth of palate;
*P ≤ 0.05 = statistically significant.
**R < 0.01 = statistically significant.

Table 3: Comparison of Mean of Intraoral Measurements between Test and Control Groups.

statistically significant differences (P>0.05). Statistically significant differences were found between the groups for the measurements of palatal height/ depth (P<0.05).

Discussion

Different clinical prediction rules have been described in the literature. Scientists have used various factors to predict a person's risk of having OSA, based on their demographics, symptoms and body-mass index. Using these factors, scientists have been able to correctly identify 76% to 96% of patients who have OSA and 13% to 54% of patients who do not have OSA [6]. A comprehensive comparative effectiveness review carried out by the U.S. Department of Health and Human Services has concluded that of the available models, the morphometric model by Kushida gave near perfect discrimination between OSA and non-OSA subjects [7].

Sleep problems are common among primary care patients. A study conducted in an Indian population estimated the prevalence of sleep-disordered breathing (SDB) among middle-aged urban Indian men to be at 19.5% and that of obstructive sleep apnea-hypopnea syndrome (SDB with excessive daytime sleepiness), to be 7.5% [8]. Many studies have been done assessing craniofacial characteristics in OSA patients using cephalometrics, computed tomography, magnetic resonance imaging and acoustic reflection. Although there is controversy in the results, craniofacial alterations most closely related to the occurrence and severity of OSA are: retroposition of the maxilla, shortening of the mandibular body, inferiorly displaced hyoid bone, retrognatism, dental occlusion class II and narrow, arched hard palate [9,10].

No data are available on the applicability of the predictive SMM in patients with OSA from the Indian subcontinent and a Medline search confirms that this is the first study evaluating the correlation between SMM values and the severity of OSA, from this country. There has been only one previous Indian study in which a diagnostic model was derived and validated for the prediction of OSA in subjects presenting with non-sleep-related complaints [11]. The results of our study indicate that the relatively easier morphometric measurements afforded by the SMM enable faster screening for OSA in a primary health care setting. Other studies worldwide have also validated the applicability of SMM in identifying OSA in clinical practice, with the separation value between subjects with or without OSA being 70 [12,13].

An important aspect in medical research is to understand and improve existing measurement frameworks and methodology. In the original study, measurements were made in the mouth. The measurements in our study were made on study models to ensure precise and accurate measurement of these anatomic distances, thus ensuring a greater accuracy for the morphometric model. Plaster study models were used for the intraoral measurements in this study, since they are a standard component of orthodontic records and they are fundamental to diagnosis and treatment planning, case presentations, evaluation of treatment progress and results, besides record keeping [14]. The dental arch dimensions were measured on study models made of dental stone, by means of digital vernier callipers. Compared to dividers, studies have shown that by using sliding manual/digital vernier callipers, accurate measurements could be made from the study models in all three dimensions [15]. Although some new methods like geometric morphometrics provide excellent possibilities for morphological analysis, distance measurements on dental casts were calculated because most dental practitioners are familiar with the method used in this study.

On comparing the SMM values in this pilot study, we have been able to demonstrate statistically significant differences between the two groups. The comparison of morphometric model values between OSA and non-OSA groups showed a highly statistically significant difference, with the OSA group having an average SMM value of 67.30 while in the control group, it was 55.43. The average morphometric model value in this sample of Indian OSA patients is only slightly lesser than that observed by Kushida who found that patients with values equal to or more than 70, typically had OSA [2]. The fact that the populations under study in our group and in the study by Kushida, belong to different origins (Indian and North-Americans) and that there was no standardization to account for ethnicity may explain the differences between both studies.

The method used by Kushida and in subsequent studies for measurement of palatal depth was found to be subjective and difficult to standardize for a large group. The palatal height as suggested in the study by Kushida was measured with the tongue in a relaxed position and the maxillary and mandibular incisor tips subtending an angle of 20 degrees from the mandibular condyle. A new method for measurement of palatal depth was resorted to, because it is difficult to measure palatal depth with 20 degrees mouth opening and from the dome of the tongue in all cases. In order to standardize the measurement of palatal depth in this study, the study models were trimmed until the distal contact point of the upper first molars showed up on the edge. Distance from the mid-deepest part of the palate to the line connecting the left and right distolingual cusp tips of the upper first molars was taken as palatal depth. In the present study, statistically significant differences were found between the two groups for the measurements of palatal height/ depth ($P<0.05$) with the mean palatal depth in patients being greater than the mean palatal depth of the controls.

The minimum age of the subjects in this study was chosen on the basis of previous studies which have reported that molar and canine arch widths do not change after 13 years of age in females and 16 years of age in males [16]. Therefore, it was assumed that the arch widths of the subjects studied were fully developed. The strength of the present study is the inclusion of a relatively large group of Indian patients with OSA, who underwent a limited hospital-based sleep study, matched with control subjects for age and gender. This study highlights the importance of matching subjects for age to prevent any age-related morphological changes from confounding the results.

Study Limitations

This is a cross-sectional study based on enrolment of patients attending one hospital clinic. As expected, the patients in this study only represent at best the patients attending this clinic. Further research is necessary to generalise the results to the general population and other ethnicities. Another limitation of this study was that PSG was not carried out for the controls, due to ethical considerations and the prohibitive expense of the procedure. This is usually the case with studies incorporating normal controls who do not exhibit any symptoms of OSA.

Conclusion

1. The SMM proposed by Kushida is applicable to this selected sample in clinical practice.
2. The average predictive morphometric model value for OSA in this sample of Indian patients is slightly lesser than that observed by Kushida.
3. The revised approach for making intraoral measurements was tested and validated in this case study, performed in a real and mature measurement framework.

Our immediate objectives were to better formalize the use of the morphometric model by restructuring existing measurement frameworks and to augment the existing approach. This revised methodology may be used to widen the reach of the morphometric model from the sleep physician's clinic to the dental operatory.

References

1. Hoffstein V, Szalai JP (1993) Predictive value of clinical features in diagnosing obstructive sleep apnoea. Sleep 16: 118-122.
2. Kushida CA, Efron B, Guilleminault C (1997) A predictive morphometric model for the obstructive sleep apnoea syndrome. Ann Intern Med 127: 581-587.
3. Dupont WD, Plummer WD (1997) PS power and sample size program available for free on the internet. Controlled Clin Trials 18: 274
4. Revicki DA, Israel RG (1986) Relationship between body mass indices and measures of body adiposity. Am J Public Health 176: 992-994.
5. Sayin MO, Turkkahraman H (2004) Comparison of dental arch and alveolar widths of patients with Class II division 1 malocclusion and subjects with Class I ideal occlusion. Angle Orthod 74: 356-360.
6. Lee RW, Chan AS, Grunstein RR, Cistulli PA (2009) Craniofacial phenotyping in obstructive sleep apne--a novel quantitative photographic approach. Sleep 32: 37-45.
7. Ethan M Balk, Denish Moorthy, Ndidiamaka Obadan (2011) Diagnosis and treatment of obstructive sleep apnea in adults. Agency for Healthcare Research and Quality.
8. Udwadia ZF, Doshi AV, Lonkar SG, Singh CI (2004) Prevalence of sleep-disordered breathing and sleep apnea in middle-aged urban Indian men. Am J Respir Crit Care Med 169: 168-173.
9. Lowe AA, Santamaria JD, Fleetham JA, Price C (1986) Facial morphology and obstructive sleep apnea. Am J Orthod Dentofac Orthop 90: 484-491.
10. Jayan B, Prasad BNBM, Kotwal A, Kharbanda OP, Chowdhury SKR, et al. (2007) The role of cephalometric analysis in obese and non obese urban Indian adults with obstructive sleep apnea syndrome: A Pilot Study. Indian J Sleep Med 2: 59-63.
11. Sharma SK, Malik V, Vasudev C, Banga A, Mohan A, et al. (2006) Prediction of obstructive sleep apnea in patients presenting to a tertiary care center. Sleep Breath 10: 147-154.
12. Soares MC, de Azeredo Bittencourt LR, Zonato AL, Gregorio LC (2006) Application of the Kushida morphometric model in patients with sleep-disordered breathing. Bras J Otorrinolaringol 72: 541-548.
13. Jung DG, Cho HY, Grunstein RR, Yee B (2004) Predictive value of Kushida Index and acoustic pharyngometry for the evaluation of upper airway in subjects with or without obstructive sleep apnea. J Korean Med Sci 19: 662-667.
14. Santoro M, Galkin S, Teredesai M, Nicolay OF, Cangialosi TJ (2003) Comparison of measurements made on digital and plaster models. Am J Orthod Dento facial Orthop 124: 101-115.
15. Singh SP, Goyal A (2006) Mesiodistal crown dimensions of the permanent dentition in North Indian children. J Indian Soc Pedod Prev Dent 24: 192-196.
16. Knott VB (1972) Longitudinal study of dental arch widths at four stages of dentition. Angle Orthod 42: 387-394.

Quality of Life and Public Health Issues in Patients Suffering from Obstructive Sleep Apnea Syndrome

Athanasia Pataka*

Department of Respiratory Medicine, Respiratory Failure Unit, G. Papanikolaou Hospital, University of Thessaloniki, Thessaloniki, Greece

Abstract

Quality of Life (QoL) in patients with Obstructive Sleep Apnea Syndrome (OSAHS) is substantially reduced. OSAHS is as an important cause of morbidity and mortality as it is associated with a wide range of medical consequences (hypertension, cardiovascular diseases, psychological effects) and also accidents. Sleepiness, depression, fatigue and obesity have an important impact on QoL. Patients report problems in their social, professional and sexual relationships. Effective treatment of sleep apnea can improve the QoL of the patients and their families. As we live in an era of economic crisis cost effectiveness is crucial and in OSAHS the application of treatment with Continuous Positive Airway Pressure (CPAP) results in a significant reduction in healthcare costs, accidents and in an improvement of QoL of individuals and of society. This review focuses on the impact of OSAHS on quality of life and public health issues and the effectiveness of OSAHS treatment in these aspects.

Keywords: QoL; Public health issues; OSAHS

Introduction

Obstructive Sleep Apnoea/Hypopnoea Syndrome (OSAHS) is characterised by repetitive episodes of complete or partial airway obstruction leading to nocturnal sleep fragmentation and daytime symptoms (sleepiness). The prevalence of OSAHS in the middle-aged population ranges from 1-4% depending on research methods, equipment and study location. As obesity is increasing worldwide, the prevalence of OSAHS will probably also increase [1].

OSAHS has been recognized as an important cause of morbidity and mortality as it is associated with a wide range of medical consequences (hypertension, cardiovascular diseases, psychological effects) and accidents [2,3]. Sleepiness, depression, fatigue and obesity have an important impact on the person's quality of life. Patients report problems in their social, professional and sexual relationships, as well as concerns about poor memory and a fear of dying [4]. One of the most important complications of OSAHS which has the greatest impact from the public health perspective is driving accidents. Additionally OSAHS patients have an increased risk of work place accidents [5,6]. In this review we will focus on the impact of OSAHS on quality of life and public health issues.

Quality of Life and OSAHS

The term quality of life (QoL) refers to the general well-being of individuals and societies. Health-related QoL usually refers to the patients' perception of performance in somatic sensation, physical function, emotional state and social interaction.

Sleepiness, cognitive performance, and quality of life are interrelated aspects of daytime function for patients with OSAHS. Sleep apnea is the most common cause of excessive daytime sleepiness leading to significant impairments in QoL, cognitive performance and social functioning. The daytime consequences of OSAHS are usually more important to the patient than the nocturnal events on which clinicians tend to focus on [7]. Patients may be unaware of their nocturnal symptoms as snoring and breathing pauses, but they are aware of OSAHS consequences when awake as daytime sleepiness, decreased concentration, memory loss, impaired work performance, irritability, moodiness, depression, decreased libido and impotence, marital disharmony, reduced participation and enjoyment of everyday activities [8]. Over 2/3 of patients with severe OSAHS have problems in their social and interpersonal function, especially in the areas of work performance, marital and family relationships [9].

OSAHS has independently been related to lower general health status before and after adjustment for age, sex, BMI, smoking status, alcohol usage and cardiovascular disease [10]. Many different instruments have been used to assess QoL of OSAHS patients [11]. Instruments have included the Nottingham Health Profile (NHP) [12], the medical outcomes study short form-36 questionnaire (SF-36), illness-specific scales as the Calgary sleep apnoea quality of life index (SAQLI) [13] and the functional outcomes of sleepiness questionnaire (FOSQ).

The American Academy of Sleep Medicine has recommended the Medical Outcomes Study Short-Form-36 (SF-36) as the most widely used instrument [14]. Even mild OSAHS was associated with decrements in SF-36 comparable to the magnitude of decrements linked to other chronic conditions such as arthritis, diabetes, and back problems [10]. QoL in OSAHS is substantially reduced, with limitations occurring both in mental and physical function. OSAHS patients have significant impairments in every domain of health-related QoL, with the most consistent impairments in the domains of sleep and vitality/energy. Sleep fragmentation may have an important role in the impaired aspects of QoL. Fatigue and excessive daytime sleepiness (EDS) may be partially associated with diminished QoL [15].

One of the chief consequences of impaired QoL may be minor psychiatric illness such as anxiety and depressive disorders. Depression is commonly reported in OSAHS and is a major component of

***Corresponding author:** Athanasia Pataka, Lecturer of Respiratory Medicine, Medical School, Aristotle University of Thessaloniki, Respiratory Failure Unit, G. Papanikolaou Hospital, 57010 Exohi, Thessaloniki, Greece
E-mail: patakath@yahoo.gr

impaired QoL. Patients with OSAHS who have depressive symptoms have particularly impaired emotional QoL scores and clinical interventions for mood symptoms may be warranted to improve their emotional QoL [16,17]. Patients with worse cognitive performance are more vulnerable to impairments in the physical domain of QoL as well and impairments in sustained attention and vigilance may be particularly determinative of impairments in the physical domain of QoL [18]. Inflammation in OSAHS patients may be an important factor to cognitive functioning and markers of chronic inflammation have been associated with diminished neuropsychological functioning in patients with OSAHS [19].

Patients with OSAHS (but also snorers) have more daytime sleepiness at work and worse performance in questionnaires concerning learning new tasks, concentration and performing monotonous tasks than subjects without OSAHS or snoring [20]. Work limitations were more present in the more sleepy patients compared to the less sleepy. This was independent from the severity of OSAHS but depended solely on the daytime sleepiness [21]. Sleepiness and hypoxaemia contribute to cognitive deficit. Patients with OSAHS and hypoxaemia had impaired mean performance scores on measures of attention, concentration, complex problem-solving and short-term recall of verbal and spatial information whereas patients who had OSAHS without hypoxaemia had no impaired scores. CPAP treatment may improve cognitive performance [22].

Studies have not consistently demonstrated a linear relationship between physiologic measures of OSAHS severity (i.e., apnea hypopnea index [AHI] or degree of nocturnal oxygen desaturation [ODI]) and the degree of impairment in health-related QoL. The limited correlation between the impairment of QoL and the severity of OSAHS reinforces the need for direct measurement of health status in OSAHS [16,23-25].

Bed partners of individuals with OSAHS also have impaired QoL due to sleep disruption from the patient's snoring, gasping, or choking respirations, or because of the bed partner's own concern about the patient's abnormal breathing [26,27]. The changes in patients' mood or character and decreased libido may also cause problems in relationships.

Treatment of OSAHS

Continuous Positive Airway Pressure (CPAP) has been the first-line treatment for OSAHS. Several studies have shown that CPAP decreases EDS, while improving neuropsychological function and QoL [28]. CPAP has beneficial effects on excessive daytime sleepiness and on self-reported functioning and well-being, affecting QoL. The low scores of SF-36 especially in the vitality/energy, role-emotional, mental health, and social functioning domains, improved after continuous positive airway pressure (CPAP) treatment. The use of CPAP in elderly patients reduced oxidative stress and improved their quality of life [29]. CPAP reduces subjective sleepiness and improves QoL of both patients and bed partners [24,30-35].

Other treatment options as the systematic use of mandibular repositioners improved the global quality of life (Calgary SAQLI) of patients with mild to moderate OSAHS [36]. Regular physical activity may help in the improvement of QoL as it has been found that OSAHS patients who performed regular physical activity for at least 2 h/week or more scored higher on all eight QoL domains of SF-36 than patients that were non-physically active [25].

Social Aspects of OSAHS

OSAHS represents not only a medical but also a social problem. OSAHS is characterised by some degree of daytime sleepiness and this affects tasks requiring sustained attention, such as driving. Patients with OSAHS have more motor vehicle accidents than drivers in the general population. Motor vehicle crashes correlate with the degree of sleepiness and not the AHI. OSAHS represents a risk factor for road accidents which is estimated to be three to seven-fold of that of the general population. Almost 35.4% of male and 14.7% of female frequent drivers was found to have severe OSAHS [37]. This excess is negated when patients start and remain on treatment with CPAP [38-44].

A unified European Directive seems desirable as within the European Union there is still a lack of uniformity concerning driving license regulations. Despite the available scientific evidence, most countries in Europe do not include OSAHS or excessive daytime sleepiness among the specific medical conditions to be considered when judging whether or not a person is fit to drive. Drivers with undiagnosed OSAHS may freely drive within Europe. The basic legislation on driving and health was documented in Annex III of Directive 91/439/CEE which included a list of diseases that should be taken into account when someone was administering for a driving license. Annex III did not include OSAHS and the next amendment of the Directive (possibly nto effect in 2013), remains silent about OSAHS. Rare conditions (e.g., narcolepsy) were considered a driving safety risk more frequently than OSAHS [44]. Non-governmental consensus conference had made recommendations for sleep apnea and commercial motor vehicle operators and when to allow drivers under evaluation to return to work [45]. These recommendations have high positive predictive value but have not been adopted by federal regulators and thus do not have the weight of law. Drivers with positive screening for OSAHS often fail to proceed for additional testing in the absence of legal requirements for follow-up and treatment [46].

Monitoring for patients with known OSAHS is controversial. Obtaining an EEG assessment for "microsleeps" during testing on a driving simulator has been suggested but is expensive and time consuming. Patients with OSAHS might use in-vehicle detection and alerting systems to help prevent crashes due to waning driver attention and alertness.

OSAHS also represents a causal factor for occupational and domestic accidents that decreased after CPAP use [47].

Public Health Issues

Patients with OSAHS have increased utilization of health resources with higher healthcare costs. Costs increase over time until diagnosis, decrease after the administration of an effective treatment and are related to the severity of the disease. Sleep apnea not only increases the actual number of road traffic accidents but also has an impact in with a wide range of medical consequences (hypertension, cardiovascular diseases, diabetes, metabolic syndrome, depression). Patients with more severe OSAHS spend more than less affected patients [48,49]. These increased costs may be attributable to cardiovascular, metabolic diseases and accidents [50].

OSAHS increases health costs when not been diagnosed but the cost-effectiveness improves after CPAP treatment as the cost remains stable but the benefits increase year after year. CPAP was found to be more effective than no treatment and proved to be a cost-effective strategy after a minimum of 2 years of treatment [51]. The cost of road accidents is an indirect health cost of OSAHS and their rate has been reduced with treatment, resulting in a further reduction of the indirect economic costs due to the disease [52].

Conclusion

OSAHS affects the QoL of patients, their families and the society and represents a major public health problem. Current available resources allow only a minority of affected patients to be assessed and treated. The application of treatment results in a significant reduction in healthcare costs, accidents and in an improvement of QoL of individuals and of society.

References

1. Young T, Palta M, Dempsey J, Skatrud J, Weber S, et al. (1993) The occurrence of sleep-disordered breathing among middle-aged adults. N Engl J Med 328: 1230-1235.
2. Marshall NS, Wong KK, Liu PY, Cullen SR, Knuiman MW, et al. (2008) Sleep apnea as an independent risk factor for all-cause mortality: the Busselton Health Study. Sleep 31: 1079-1085.
3. Young T, Finn L, Peppard PE, Szklo-Coxe M, Austin D, et al. (2008) Sleep disordered breathing and mortality: eighteen-year follow-up of the Wisconsin sleep cohort. Sleep 31: 1071-1078.
4. Veale D, Poussin G, Benes F, Pepin JL, Levy P (2002) Identification of quality of life concerns of patients with obstructive sleep apnoea at the time of initiation of continuous positive airway pressure: a discourse analysis. Qual Life Res 11: 389-399.
5. George CF (2007) Sleep apnea, alertness, and motor vehicle crashes. Am J Respir Crit Care Med 176: 954-956.
6. Accattoli MP, Muzi G, dell'Omo M, Mazzoli M, Genovese V, et al. (2008) Occupational accidents, work performance and obstructive sleep apnea syndrome (OSAS). G Ital Med Lav Ergon 30: 297-303.
7. Engleman HM, Douglas NJ (2004) Sleep. 4: Sleepiness, cognitive function, and quality of life in obstructive sleep apnoea/hypopnoea syndrome. Thorax 59: 618-622.
8. Jean-Louis G, Kripke DF, Ancoli-Israel S (2000) Sleep and quality of well-being. Sleep 23: 1115-1121.
9. Grunstein RR, Stenlöf K, Hedner JA, Sjöström L (1995) Impact of self-reported sleep-breathing disturbances on psychosocial performance in the Swedish Obese Subjects (SOS) Study. Sleep 18: 635-643.
10. Finn L, Young T, Palta M, Fryback DG (1998) Sleep-disordered breathing and self-reported general health status in the Wisconsin Sleep Cohort Study. Sleep 21: 701-706.
11. Jenkinson C, Stradling J, Petersen S (1997) Comparison of three measures of quality of life outcome in the evaluation of continuous positive airways pressure therapy for sleep apnoea. J Sleep Res 6: 199-204.
12. Fornas C, Ballester E, Arteta E, Ricou C, Diaz A, et al. (1995) Measurement of general health status in obstructive sleep apnea hypopnea patients. Sleep 18: 876-879.
13. Flemons WW, Reimer MA (1998) Development of a disease-specific health-related quality of life questionnaire for sleep apnea. Am J Respir Crit Care Med 158: 494-503.
14. (1999) Sleep-related breathing disorders in adults: recommendations for syndrome definition and measurement techniques in clinical research. The Report of an American Academy of Sleep Medicine Task Force. Sleep 22: 667-689.
15. Moore P, Bardwell WA, Ancoli-Israel S, Dimsdale JE (2001) Association between polysomnographic sleep measures and health-related quality of life in obstructive sleep apnea. J Sleep Res 10: 303-308.
16. Baldwin CM, Griffith KA, Nieto FJ, O'Connor GT, Walsleben JA, et al. (2001) The association of sleep-disordered breathing and sleep symptoms with quality of life in the Sleep Heart Health Study. Sleep 24: 96-105.
17. Fornas C, Ballester E, Arteta E, Ricou C, Diaz A, et al. (1995) Measurement of general health status in obstructive sleep apnea hypopnea patients. Sleep 18: 876-879.
18. Lee IS, Bardwell W, Ancoli-Israel S, Natarajan L, Loredo JS, et al. (2011) The Relationship between psychomotor vigilance performance and quality of life in obstructive sleep apnea. J Clin Sleep Med 7: 254-260.
19. Haensel A, Bardwell WA, Mills PJ, Loredo JS, Ancoli-Israel S, et al. (2009) Relationship between inflammation and cognitive function in obstructive sleep apnea. Sleep Breath 13: 35-41.
20. Ulfberg J, Carter N, Edling C (2000) Sleep-disordered breathing and occupational accidents. Scand J Work Environ Health 26: 237-242.
21. Mulgrew AT, Ryan CF, Fleetham JA, Cheema R, Fox N, et al. (2007) The impact of obstructive sleep apnea and daytime sleepiness on work limitation. Sleep Med 9: 42-53.
22. Findley LJ, Barth JT, Powers DC, Wilhoit SC, Boyd DG, et al. (1986) Cognitive impairment in patients with obstructive sleep apnea and associated hypoxemia. Chest 90: 686-690.
23. Fornas C, Ballester E, Arteta E, Ricou C, Diaz A, et al. (1995) Measurement of general health status in obstructive sleep apnea hypopnea patients. Sleep 18: 876-879.
24. D'Ambrosio C, Bowman T, Mohsenin V (1999) Quality of life in patients with obstructive sleep apnea: effect of nasal continuous positive airway pressure--a prospective study. Chest 115: 123-129.
25. Lopes C, Esteves AM, Bittencourt LR, Tufik S, Mello MT (2008) Relationship between the quality of life and the severity of obstructive sleep apnea syndrome. Braz J Med Biol Res 41: 908-913.
26. McArdle N, Kingshott R, Engleman HM, Mackay TW, Douglas NJ (2001) Partners of patients with sleep apnoea/hypopnoea syndrome: effect of CPAP treatment on sleep quality and quality of life. Thorax 56: 513-518.
27. Parish JM, Lyng PJ (2003) Quality of life in bed partners of patients with obstructive sleep apnea or hypopnea after treatment with continuous positive airway pressure. Chest 124: 942-947.
28. Jenkinson C, Davies RJ, Mullins R, Stradling JR (1999) Comparison of therapeutic and subtherapeutic nasal continuous positive airway pressure for obstructive sleep apnoea: a randomised prospective parallel trial. Lancet 353: 2100-2105.
29. Yagihara F, Lucchesi LM, D'Almeida V, Mello MT, Tufik S, et al. (2012) Oxidative stress and quality of life in elderly patients with obstructive sleep apnea syndrome: are there differences after six months of Continuous Positive Airway Pressure treatment? Clinics (Sao Paulo) 67: 565-572.
30. Derderian SS, Bridenbaugh RH, Rajagopal KR (1988) Neuropsychologic symptoms in obstructive sleep apnea improve after treatment with nasal continuous positive airway pressure. Chest 94: 1023-1027.
31. Sánchez AI, Buela-Casal G, Bermúdez MP, Casas-Maldonado F (2001) The effects of continuous positive air pressure treatment on anxiety and depression levels in apnea patients. Psychiatry Clin Neurosci 55: 641-646.
32. Millman RP, Fogel BS, McNamara ME, Carlisle CC (1989) Depression as a manifestation of obstructive sleep apnea: reversal with nasal continuous positive airway pressure. J Clin Psychiatry 50: 348-351.
33. Montserrat JM, Ferrer M, Hernandez L, Farré R, Vilagut G, et al. (2001) Effectiveness of CPAP treatment in daytime function in sleep apnea syndrome: a randomized controlled study with an optimized placebo. Am J Respir Crit Care Med 164: 608-613.
34. Barnes M, McEvoy RD, Banks S, Tarquinio N, Murray CG, et al. (2004) Efficacy of positive airway pressure and oral appliance in mild to moderate obstructive sleep apnea. Am J Respir Crit Care Med 170: 656-664.
35. Siccoli MM, Pepperell JC, Kohler M, Craig SE, Davies RJ, et al. (2008) Effects of continuous positive airway pressure on quality of life in patients with moderate to severe obstructive sleep apnea: data from a randomized controlled trial. Sleep 31: 1551-1558.
36. Machado MA, Prado LB, Carvalho LB, Francisco S, Silva AB, et al. (2004) Quality of life of patients with obstructive sleep apnea syndrome treated with an intraoral mandibular repositioner. Arq Neuropsiquiatr 62: 222-225.
37. P3851 ERS 2012 Vienna Professional and frequent driving habits detected in the ESADA – Call for a safety alert
38. George CF (2007) Sleep apnea, alertness, and motor vehicle crashes. Am J Respir Crit Care Med 176: 954-956.
39. Engleman HM, Asgari-Jirhandeh N, McLeod AL, Ramsay CF, Deary IJ, et al. (1996) Self-reported use of CPAP and benefits of CPAP therapy: a patient survey. Chest 109: 1470-1476.

40. Cassel W, Ploch T, Becker C, Dugnus D, Peter JH, et al. (1996) Risk of traffic accidents in patients with sleep-disordered breathing: reduction with nasal CPAP. Eur Respir J 9: 2606-2611.

41. Krieger J, Meslier N, Lebrun T, Levy P, Phillip-Joet F, et al. (1997) Accidents in obstructive sleep apnea patients treated with nasal continuous positive airway pressure: a prospective study. The Working Group ANTADIR, Paris and CRESGE, Lille, France. Association Nationale de Traitement à Domicile des Insuffisants Respiratoires. Chest 112: 1561-1566.

42. George CF (2001) Reduction in motor vehicle collisions following treatment of sleep apnoea with nasal CPAP. Thorax 56: 508-512.

43. Strohl KP, Bonnie RJ, Findley L (1994). Sleep apnea, sleepiness and driving risk. Am J Respir Crit Care Med 1994; 150: 1463–1473.

44. Alonderis A, Barbé F, Bonsignore M, Calverley P, De Backer W, et al. (2008) Medico-legal implications of sleep apnoea syndrome: driving license regulations in Europe. Sleep Med 9: 362-375.

45. Hartenbaum N, Collop N, Rosen IM, Phillips B, George CF et al.(2006) Sleep apnea and commercial motor vehicle operators: statement from the joint Task Force of the American College of Chest Physicians, American College of Occupational and Environmental Medicine, and the National Sleep Foundation. J Occup Environ Med 48:S4

46. Parks P, Durand G, Tsismenakis AJ, Vela-Bueno A, Kales S (2009) Screening for obstructive sleep apnea during commercial driver medical examinations. J Occup Environ Med 51: 275-282.

47. Krieger J, Meslier N, Lebrun T, Levy P, Phillip-Joet F, et al. (1997) Source Working Group ANTADIR, Paris, France Accidents in obstructive sleep apnea patients treated with nasal continuous positive airway pressure: a prospective study. The Working Group ANTADIR, Paris and CRESGE, Lille, France. Association Nationale de Traitement à Domicile des Insuffisants Respiratoires. Chest 112:1561-1566.

48. Kapur VK, Alfonso-Cristancho R (2009) Just a good deal or truly a steal? Medical cost savings and the impact on the cost-effectiveness of treating sleep apnea. Sleep 32: 135-136.

49. Wittmann V, Rodenstein DO (2004) Health care costs and the sleep apnea syndrome. Sleep Med Rev 8: 269-279.

50. Tarasiuk A, Greenberg-Dotan S, Brin YS, Simon T, Tal A, et al. (2005) Determinants affecting health-care utilization in obstructive sleep apnea syndrome patients. Chest 128: 1310-1314.

51. Guest JF, Helter MT, Morga A, Stradling JR (2008) Cost-effectiveness of using continuous positive airway pressure in the treatment of severe obstructive sleep apnoea/hypopnoea syndrome in the UK. Thorax 63: 860-865.

52. Sassani A, Findley LJ, Kryger M, Goldlust E, George C, et al. (2004) Reducing motor-vehicle collisions, costs, and fatalities by treating obstructive sleep apnea syndrome. Sleep 27: 453-458.

10

Emerging Adult Sleep Quality: Health and Academic Performance Factors of Assessment

Kathy Sexton Radek[1]* and Julie Kaprelian[2]

[1] *Suburban Pulmonary and Sleep Associates, 700 E Ogden Avenue, Suite 201, Westmont, IL 60559 Elmhurst College, USA*
[2] *The Chicago School of Professional Psychology, Merchandise Mart, 13th Floor, Chicago, IL, USA*

Abstract

It is estimated that approximately 10% of "emerging" adults (18-25 years) report significant sleep disturbance. Academic stress and social schedule demands characteristic of this population contribute to compromised sleep. Further, cognitive functions such as attention and concentration are negatively influenced by compromised sleep. The need to address compromised sleep schedules in emerging adults as they are significantly impacted by social schedules. Sleep disturbances/disorders such as insomnia and delayed sleep phase onset are represented.

Emerging Adult sleep was measured in this intense assessment study of sleep, health, and academic performance. Consistent with previous research, we found that poor sleep contributes to poor health and academic performance. This indicates a need for further research that identifies what education and services emerging adults will benefit from in order to implement healthier sleep practices that will positively impact on health and academic performance.

Keywords: Sleep quality; Young adult sleep; Sleep disorders; Adolescent sleep; Academic performance; Health

Introduction

The National Sleep Foundation acts as clearing house of general and empirically based information about sleep. Their annual "Sleep in America" poll indicted a serious sleep deprivation problem in our country [1]. A closer inspection of their data reveals particular cohorts of the elderly and adolescent/emerging adults as most sleep deprived. Adolescent sleep has received considerable focus from the scientific community [2] as well as the elderly [3]. Sleep disturbances in both populations are prevalent. Young adults have typically served as a control group in many sleep studies; however few studies have descriptively examined young adult sleep. It is the case that sleep disturbances are prevalent in young adults primarily shortened sleep periods, increased traffic accidents secondary to sleep deprivation, and undiagnosed sleep disorders [4].

The emerging adult sleep population is defined as those between the ages of 18 and 25 years. Over 50% are enrolled at least part time in college level education [4]. This developmental period is further described as a period of transition to adulthood responsibilities with mounting social pressures and expectations such as advanced education and professional training, establishment of an independent self, and the setup of social support systems with the newly established autonomy. With these changes, emerging adults have to determine their knowledge, skills and abilities within their identity context as well as their social self to the world around them. College students underestimate their need for sleep; with the stresses related to classes, jobs and the independence of living away from home, coupled with an active social life, many fall into the pattern of poor sleeping habits. In addition, emerging adults are determining their health habits within their independent lifestyle which are essential to cognitive, emotional, and social performance.

Female emerging adults report more daytime sleepiness [5,6] These general findings about college student sleep quality have generated additional research to evaluate specific sleep quality factors in young adults [7]. For example, positive health behaviours of exercise and food choices have not often been assessed in sleep studies despite their relation to good sleep quality.

Research has indicated that emerging college students are at risk for engaging in unhealthy sleep practices. Insufficient sleep and daytime sleepiness have been found to be the highest ranking sleep problem within this population [6]. This is a concern for today's emerging adults, as sleep deprivation and poor sleep quality have been found to be associated with lowered cognitive performance and decreased physical and psychological well-being.

Emerging Adult College Student Sleep Studies

A median of 6 hours and 39 minutes of sleep from a student young adult population [8]. The student population, as a group, reported increased dissatisfaction with their sleep. The increased social, academic and occupational demands may lead to the variable sleep pattern choice of emerging adults [4,9]. Adolescents require approximately 8.5 hours of sleep although less than 20% accomplish this [1]. Emerging adults require 7.5 to 8 hours and less than 20% accomplish this [4]. This sleep problem of loss is escalated by changing sleep patterns typical of the poor sleepers [4]. That is, sleeping later on the weekends and daytime napping, both of which substantially disturb sleep determinants, are used frequently as compensation for poor sleep during the week and late weekend nights. While a causal relationship has not been found, an association between poor sleep, low grades and poor school performance, in adolescents, has been identified [2,4].

***Corresponding author:** Kathy Sexton Radek, Suburban Pulmonary and Sleep Associates, 700 E Ogden Avenue, Suite 201, Westmont, IL 60559, Elmhurst College, 190 Prospect Avenue, Elmhurst, IL 60126, USA
E-mail: ksrsleep@aol.com

Emerging adults' sleep patterns per survey reports sometimes reached criteria for delayed sleep phase [4]. Situational factors that initially start this condition may serve to sustain the pattern. For many emerging adults, strategies to alleviate their poor sleep quality often worsen the problem. Investigations in this area have examined emerging adults' sleep time (i.e., bedtime, wake time, during weekdays and weekend days) [4].

In college students, the behavioral deficits are evident but the acknowledgement of their significance by students seems to be lacking [4]. Some research has indicated that a period of 20 hours of sleep deprivation (i.e., an all-nighter) may be equal to a blood alcohol level of 0.08 [1]. College students have a large work load and nearly 50% are also employed at least part time - which is often masked by excessive activity and social/personal scheduling of events. Excessive worry about relationships was highly reported on surveys [10-12]. A seminal study in this area that collected performance data of college students on exams given on a daily basis for a six week period, across a 12 hour day revealed mental efficiency, as measured by performance scores, was best at mid-week (Wednesdays) with a steady decline each day from 8 am until the period of 4 to 5 pm [13]. In this study of 112 college student, there was a rise from 8 pm until 10 pm that did not, however, exceed the average for the day. It was also reported that a decrease from 10 to 11 pm occurred on a daily basis. Hourly measures over a six week period on tasks similar to academic work were not compromised; these data highlight the natural tendencies of mental deficiency that is assumed to be modified by sleep loss.

Cognitive and Academic Performance

College students are also at risk for poor sleeping behaviors due to their academic load [14] Students who carried a full course load and reported poor sleep quality performed less well within academic majors when compared to those students who reported better sleep quality [15].

Measurements of student performance on cognitive tasks declined with increasing sleep deprivation. As compared to non-sleep deprived students, the sleep deprived students were more willing to give up on difficult tasks, or express unrelated thoughts such as "I wonder what I should have for lunch today".

Oversleeping is found to be significantly correlated with the lowered grade point average [16]. It has been found that students with a grade point average below 2.0 reported more unhealthy sleep behaviors that put them at risk for a sleep disorder [16]. College students often believe that they will be able to catch up on sleep that they missed during the week on weekends, but this has not been shown to be the case. Research has shown that differences between weekend and weekday sleep duration and bedtimes lead to sleep wake problems [17].

In one study it was reported findings about sleep quality with sleep logs, journals of emotional memory measures administered in the morning and evening. Participants with good sleep quality reported 58% recollections of judgments made on the morning task after sleep. They concluded that sleep facilitates the consolidation of emotional declarative memory.

Health, Sleep Quality and Academic Performance

Reporting's from stable subjective measurements of sleep, health and well-being over a three month period in young adult college students indicated that with decreased sleep quality, participants also reported psychological and physical health complaints, feelings of tension, decreased positive affect and life satisfaction over the semester-long measurement [18]. Poor sleep quality has also been associated with decreased fitness levels in female college students as measured by lower levels of muscular endurance, flexibility, and cardiovascular fitness [19]. Regardless of the extent or type of sleep disturbance, a clear association consistently appears in the co-descriptions of findings in the literature—health and academic performance vary as a function of sleep quality. Trockel et al. [16] report negative effects of sleep deprivation on college students' cognitive performance. Further, the weekend sleeping intervals were reported to be significantly delayed compared to weeknight sleeping times [4,17]. The irregular sleep patterns, impaired driver safety (dozing while driving), poor time management and not eating breakfast or taking vitamins were other health related factors associated with poor sleep. Greater variability in rise time, consuming a morning beverage, and later bedtimes were found in those participants with more disturbed sleep. When academic examination stress in emerging adults was measured with randomized conditions of exam-stress and stress-free intervals, significant increases in perceived stress and emotional distress; increase in smoking and caffeine consumption; decrease in healthy eating, emotional control, frequency and duration of physical activity; and deterioration in sleep patterns and study habits were found in controlled conditions [20].

In an odds ratio analysis, sleep was reported as higher in those that participated in regular vigorous/moderate physical activity, were not employed and who had not experienced anxiety. Emerging adults in the A and B grade range were more likely to report good sleep [21]. Interestingly, the strongest predictor of grade point average reported in the study was Body Mass Index (BMI) [21]. Those classified with a normal BMI were more likely to earn a grade of A or B according to the results [21]. Thus, sleep quality is associated with grade point average, a primary measure of academic productivity among college students [21].

The current study was designed to re examine the issues related to academic performance and sleep quality in a contemporary sample of emerging adult college students. It was hypothesized that a significant positive correlation would be found between the variables measuring sleep quality, academic performance, and health.

Method

Participants

College students enrolled in psychology undergraduate courses at a Mid western liberal arts college were invited to participate in an assessment study that entailed 2 weeks of sleep logging and the completion of several self-report measures about the quality of their sleep and wake experiences. The information specifically indicated that changing one's sleep or a diagnosis of sleep disturbance/disorder was not the focus of the study.

Nineteen subjects signed up for the study and 16 participants completed the study. The attrition of 3 was related to the students conveying disinterest in spending time logging sleep for the full 2 weeks and preferred to be a part of a study that was a one time only survey. 16 participants were within the ages of 18 to 23 years. Males (N=4, mean age=19) reported on average completing 11 hours of employment per week. Females (n=12, mean age=20) reported a mean of 17 hours of work per week. All participants were Caucasian

Measures

A standard structured sleep interview (Pittsburgh Sleep Quality

Index) was used along with several measures rating sleep quality, health, study habits, and mood. A standard sleep log form was used by each participant for six days following the assessment period. A questionnaire composed of general health questions germane to the emerging adult population was constructed. Each question was coded as a separate variable.

Procedure

Students that signed up for the study were provided with full information about the specific extent of the study and reasons for the importance of logging their sleep. They were provided with full information about each measure with the exception of the research hypothesis. Every subject signed an informed consent form and agreed to be a participant in the study in exchange for extra credit or psychology laboratory coursework credit.

A time period that fell two weeks before the midterm exams was chosen as the schedule was deemed to be the most balanced with academic assignment deadlines and exams than other periods during the term. Thus, students were required to participate in the study only during that specified 2 weeks. All participants were free of sleep disorders and in good academic standing per interview findings by the first author. The proposal for this study had received approval from the Internal Review Board of the College.

All participants were requested to come at the same appointment time where a general overview of the investigator's research program and the intent of the study were presented. Following this, a full explanation of sleep measures and the log was given. All questions were answered. Participants were then asked to complete the materials with the investigator and trained assistants available to manage any questions or need for further information. Following this, all participants handed in their materials and were given an additional, brief explanation of the sleep log and the importance of tracking their sleep. The first author met with each participant individually and went over the rationale and procedure for completing the sleep log and self-assessment measures. Participants were telephoned by the first author every other day to see if they had any questions and to provide any further information about the measurements they were doing. Semester grade point averages were obtained from the registrar for all participants.

Results

All data responses from the sleep logs and surveys were treated as separate variables and descriptive statistical analyses using SPSS PC was conducted. The grades recorded in each students class at the time of the sleep study and that were summated into an overall grade point average by the college registrar were correlated with the sleep log and health survey responses.

Tables 2 and 3 illustrate median values of the sleep variables during the weekdays and weekends, and daily ratings, on average, for the group, of the sleep variables. There were a moderate number of endorsed health factors. Table 3 summarizes the average daily rating of the sample on health factors.

The participants' ratings emotions experienced each day were also recorded. The averaged values by emotion rating appear in table 4. Of note, the participants' highest ratings were for "irritable", "poor concentration" and "tired". Cross tabulation analyses of the emotion ratings, sleep efficiency and grade point average were non-significant.

Correlational analyses of the health variables and grade point average resulted in a statistically significant relationship between "dozing off during an activity" and lowered grade point average. These findings are illustrated in table 5.

Discussion

The findings are consistent with the literature in indicating a relationship between poor health, low grades and poor sleep quality. The disturbance in each category appears to be sufficient to impact the other area yet the interrelationship is unknown. We have an ongoing investigation at present to examine wake day activity levels, health and sleep quality in the college student that addresses the interrelationship question we identified [4,21].

The irregularity of sleep for weekdays and compared to weekends has been noted in the sleep literature. Variable sleep patterns sustain poor sleep quality with sleep deprivation accumulated during the week that is met by extended sleep intervals and napping on weekends [4]. We think our findings on this aspect points to the need for quality psychosocial intervention delivered in effective small group workshop fashion. The patterned behavior can be restructured efficiently, we think, with a small scale workshop approach combined with online resources for this population. It is clear that emerging adults need

Median	**Weekday Sleep**	**Weekend**
Total Sleep Time (TST)	5 h 46 m	7 h 8 m
Total Time in Bed (TiB)	7 h 33 m	8 h 27 m
Sleep Efficiency (TST/TiB)	76.37%	84.42%
Number Awakenings	1.0	1.0
Sleep Quality*	2.71	2.50
Time Until Sleep (minutes)	15	10
Nap		
Wakeup Prompts Needed	$\bar{x}$ = 2	1.98

*= 1-5 scale where 1=poor, 5=excellent.

Table 1: Sleep variables.

	$\bar{x}$	
Number of activities dozed off in today	1.13	(1.36)
Number of hours dozing off during the day	1.31	(2.44)
Number of planned naps* today	.31	(.479)
Amount of time spent in daylight	15 minutes	(39.94 minutes)
Difficulty waking up (1=easy, 5= hard)	3	(1.81)
Use of sleep aid	1.94	(.250)

Note: Nap time reported as 2 p.m., for thirty minutes.

Table 2: Sleep experience.

	$\bar{x}$	SD
Headache	1.75	.447
G/I Upset	1.94	.250
Cold/Allergy Symptoms	1.75	.447
# Caffeine Use	.56	.73
Muscle/Joint Pain	1.75	.447
Exercise	1.75	1.44
Light Exposure*	15 minutes (0-45 min range)	—
Medication Use	0	—
Stomach Ache	0	—
Tobacco Use	2	.32

Note: The mean and standard deviation summarize the frequency endorsement of these behaviors by the participants in one week's time.

Table 3: Health disturbing behaviors report by young adults.

Emotions	$\bar{x}$	SD
Happy – Sad	2.44	1.09
Tense – Relaxed	2.81	0.834
Sleepy – Alert	2.81	1.424
Even tempered – Mood swings	2.25	0.931
Irritable – Easy going	3.75	1.065
Poor conc. – Good conc.	3.00	1.033
Tired – Energetic	2.75	1.00
Worried – Carefree	2.69	1.014
Calm – Jittery	2.56	0.964

Note = Ratings were 1=none to 5=very much so. Higher scores are indicative of the first term in the description.

Table 4: Emotions ratings.

Grade Point Average	
Typical week	ns
Headache	ns
Gastrointestinal symptoms	ns
Cold/Allergy Symptoms	ns
Planned naps	ns
Number of activities dozed off in	6.38*
Use of tobacco	ns

Table 5: Correlational analysis of academic performance, health and sleep factors.

more education and information on the importance of sleep and ways to increase their sleep quality and efficiency.

Furthermore, the findings of inadequate sleep efficiencies (Table 1, weekday sleep efficiency = 76.37%; weekend sleep efficiency = 84.42%) denote poor sleep in a context of high sleep need. The prolonged times in bed despite not sleeping reflect, we believe, sleep deprivation/disturbance. Investigations and subsequent psychosocial interventions in this area are needed to examine sleep perception, pre-sleep behaviors, and wake day behaviors of health and academic activity that influence sleep in the college student. The need for intervention is blatant. Our findings reflected in Table 3 present varied behaviors such as dozing off in activities during the day, napping and use of sleep aids that can be addressed. Controlled treatment interventions to measure behaviors before and after a psychosocial intervention are paramount to addressing this need. The number of times during the week that participants endorsed a health disturbing behavior is of clinical note as there are comparable weekly tabulation data sets. Current sleep courses need to continue to be refined in order to create long-lasting change in sleep patterns of emerging adults. The effect of a "sleep management" course on sleep patterns over 18 weeks found that the students' sleep quality increased throughout the semester when compared to controls, these were mild and limited findings [18]. Intervention programs need to be further developed and implemented into colleges because poor quality sleepers report more than decreased academic functioning; they also report significantly more problems with physical and psychological health [21]. The sleep factors and moderate number of endorsed health factors by our sample indicate, collectively, life adjustment issues co-occur with sleep disturbances. These findings are parallel to nationwide studies of sleep in emerging adults. A summarization of the data from the National College Health Assessment that was based on students' responses from 78 United States institutions (N=56,637) indicated that more students reported having poor sleep (affirmative response to "haven't gotten enough sleep over the last 7 days to feel rested") than good sleep [21].

This study also highlights that an emerging adult's health and emotional state impacts sleep. Poor sleep was found to be related to wake-day emotional changes. It is likely that an individual experiencing negative emotions has additional difficulty with completing and attending to academic work, as well as difficulties with obtaining quality sleep. Our findings of endorsements of "irritableness", require, we feel, intervention with education about getting good quality sleep.

In future research, it will be important to consider wake-day activities with wake-day emotions. This will lead to a broadened understanding of how an individual's 24-hour complete day impacts sleep quality. Additionally, further research should be done with within subjects groups and longitudinal designs in order to reveal emerging adult sleep patterns more fully. This will allow for a better understanding of what information and education these emerging adults need in order to implement healthier sleep practices that subsequently affect overall health and academic progress.

In conclusion, we feel we have measured support for the relationship between poor sleep quality, health disturbing behaviors and poor academics. The specific measurements of sleep and health provide evidence for mismanagement of these behaviors. A short-term psycho educational intervention with online resources for the college student about sleep and health would be of potential benefit and would likely contribute to better academic outcomes.

References

1. Sleep in America Poll 2013. National Sleep Foundation.
2. Carskadon MA (1999) When world collide: Adolescent need for sleep versus societal demands. Phi Delta Kappan 80: 348-349.
3. Morin CM (1993) Insomnia: Psychological Assessment and Management. The Guilford Press, New York.
4. Sexton-Radek K (2004) Sleep Quality in Young Adults. Mellon Press, New York.
5. Wolfson AR (2010) Adolescents and emerging adults' sleep patterns: New developments. J Adolesc Health 26: 97-99.
6. Lin HH, Tsai PS, Fang SC, Liu JF (2011) Effect of kiwi fruit consumption on sleep quality in adults with sleep problems. Asia Pac J Clin Nutr 20: 169-174.
7. Brooks PR, Girgenti AA, Mills MJ (2009) Sleep patterns and symptoms of depression in college students. Coll Stud J 43: 464.
8. Hicks RA, Fernandez C, Pelligrini RJ (2001) The changing sleep habits of university students: An update. Percept Mot Skills 93: 648.
9. Pichler JJ, Ginter DR, Sadowsky B (1997) Sleep quality versus sleep quantity: Relationship between sleep and measures of health, well-being and sleepiness in college students. J Psychosom Res 42: 583-596.
10. Kelly WE (2003) Worry content associated with decreased sleep length among college students -sleep deprivation leads to increased worry. J Genetic Psychol (in press).
11. Kelly WE, Kelly KE, Clanton RC (2001) The relationship between sleep length and grade-point average among college students. Coll Stud J 35: 84.
12. Kelly WE (2004) Sleep length and life satisfaction in a college student sample. Coll Stud J 38: 428-430.
13. Laird DA (1906) Relative Performance of College Students as Conditioned by Time of Day and Day of Week. J Exp Psychol 8: 50-63.
14. Machado ERS, Varella BRV, Andrade MM (1998) The influence of study schedules and work on The sleep –wake cycle of college students. Biological Rhythms Research 29: 578-584.
15. Meilman PW, Manley C, Gaylor MS, Turco JH (1992) Medical withdrawals from college for mental health reasons and their relation to academic performance. J Am Coll Health 40: 217-223.
16. Trockel MT, Barnes MD, Egget DL (2000) Health-related variables and academic performance among first-year college students: Implications for sleep and other behaviors. J Am Coll Health 49: 125-131.

17. Sexton-Radek K, Graci G (2008) Combating your sleep problems. New York: Prager Press.

18. Lee AJ, Lin WH (2007) Association between sleep quality and physical fitness in female young adults. J Sports Med Phy Fitness 47: 462-467.

19. Oaten M, Cheng K (2005) Academic examination stress impairs self-control. J Soc Clin Psychol 24: 254-279.

20. Becker CM, Adams T, Orr C, Quilter L (2008) Correlates of quality sleep and academic performance. The Health Educator 40: 82-89.

21. Val-Smith K, Felts MW, Becker C (2009) Relationship between sleep quality and health risk behaviors in undergraduate college students. Coll Stud J 43: 924-930.

Hypothesizing that Putative Dopaminergic, Melatonin, Benzodiazepine Reward Circuitry Receptor(s) Activator Provides Sleep Induction Benefits

Kenneth Blum[1,3]*, Marlene-Oscar-Berman[2], William Downs B[3], Eric R Braverman[1,4], Florian Kreuk[4], Kristina Dushaj[4], Courtney Truesdell[4], Mona Li[4], John Giordano[5], Joan Borsten[6], Thomas Simpatico[7], Debmayla Barh[8], Margaret A Madigan[3,4,9], Scott Jones[5] and Stephen Schoenthaler[5,10]

[1]Department of Psychiatry, University of Florida, McKnight Brain Institute, USA

[2]Departments of Psychiatry and Anatomy & Neurobiology, Boston University School of Medicine, and Boston VA Healthcare System, Boston, USA

[3]Impact genomics, Inc., Lederoch, Pennsylvania, USA

[4]Department of Clinical Neurology, Path Research Foundation, USA

[5]Department of Holistic Medicine, National Institute for Holistic Addiction Studies, USA

[6]Department of Addiction Research & Therapy, Malibu Beach Recovery Center, USA

[7]Human Integrated Services Unit University of Vermont Center for Clinical & Translational Science, College of Medicine, USA

[8]Institute of Integrative Omics & Applied Biotechnology, India

[9]Department of Personalized Genomics, IGENE LLC., USA

[10]Department of Sociology, California State University, USA

Abstract

The issue of insomnia is a global phenomenon which requires additional in-depth research. Insomnia especially in alcohol-dependent patients, for example, may lead to suicide. It is noteworthy that childhood sleep problems predict the onset of drinking in boys. We now know that while there are multi-faceted reasons for sleep problems and disturbances (e.g. sleep drive homeostasis, circadian rhythm physiology, and genetic influences), the scientific community has not been able to deliver an appropriate solution. Some benefit has been noted with cognitive behavioral therapy, but it has minimal effects in patients relapsing from drugs especially alcohol, cocaine and opiates. While there are a number of pharmaceutical drugs developed to treat insomnia, most have associated side effects and even addiction liability. We do know that benzodiazepines hijack the midbrain dopamine system leading to addiction. Finally, it has been proposed that dopamine D2 receptors are involved in rapid eye movement sleep, suggesting as proposed herein that dopaminergic activation is a worthwhile mechanism to explore in the future. The concepts presented herein on potential nutrigenomic therapy warrants further in-depth analysis. In this regard we hypothesize based on both literature review and empirical data that a putative dopaminergic, melatonin, benzodiazepine reward circuitry receptor(s) activator provides sleep induction benefits.

Keywords: Insomnia; Reward circuitry; Reward Deficiency Syndrome (RDS); Melatonin; Benzodiazepines, Nutrigenomics; Rapid-eye movement; Sleep

Introduction

Considering the benefits provided by typical hypnotic and non-hypnotic medication for the treatment of chronic insomnia such as barbiturates, benzodiazepines, as well as Zolpidem, versus the risk of both abuse liability and toxicity is a challenging calculation. The calculation is confounded by the paucity of evidence-based data on the hypnotic efficacy of sleep inducing pharmacological and non pharmacological treatments for chronic insomnia. While inducing sleep, many hypnotic-type medications may also induce potential abuse liability for the patient and other side effects. For example, benzodiazepines, prescription drugs remedying anxiety and insomnia, are recreationally abused; the number of individuals abusing the benzodiazepines is on the rise [1]. Importantly, the mechanism of benzodiazepine activation of midbrain dopamine neurons is well-known, with the mesocorticolimbic reward system affected by benzodiazepine [1].

Others have suggested that non-pharmacological approaches can facilitate sleep and reduce sleep disruption without the specter of side effects and may be a satisfactory regimen in the potential of regaining restorative sleep patterns. In this hypothesis paper, we attempt to show certain neurological mechanisms involved in normal sleep patterns may provide a blueprint to the development of a non-pharmacological treatment for chronic insomnia.

Insomnia Definition and Prevalence

Sleep disorders affect one fifth of Americans [2] and manifest in impaired function or excessive sleepiness due to reduced sleep quality [3]. For persons with sleep disorders, quality of life is greatly affected, for example, attention is reduced, concentration limited, memory negatively affected, reasoning and problem solving skills decreased, and reaction time to emotional and physical pain worsened in persons with insomnia compared to matched controls [4]. Classified by the International Classification of Sleep Disorders (ICSD) as a dyssomnia [5], insomnia is the chief sleep disorder [6].

A condition which negatively affects the ability of an individual to fall asleep or maintain desirable sleep duration or quality, insomnia has

***Corresponding author:** Kenneth Blum, Department of Psychiatry, University of Florida, McKnight Brain Institute, Gainesville, Florida, USA
E-mail: drd2gene@gmail.com

several risk factors. Age and gender have been implicated as risk factors for insomnia, with the elderly more likely to experience insomnia and women more likely to experience difficulties sleeping than men [7]. Older individuals have trouble maintaining sleep, while falling asleep is the primary sleep issue in younger individuals [8]. 95% of adults had experienced insomnia in 1979, according to a Gallup poll survey, indicating that most people are vulnerable to some instances of sleep disorder [8].

The range of adults with chronic insomnia, ~10% to 15%, and the range of adults with transient insomnia, 25% to 35%, can be explained by the variable diagnostic measures and differing definitions in the study of sleep disorders [7]. Recent changes in the definitions of insomnia now reflect perceptions of sleep problems in patients and include the effect poor quality sleep has on daily function [8]. The constantly evolving definitions in the study of sleep disorders limit the potential for determining the scope of the problem. However, comprehensive surveys in large cohorts provide opportunities to measure this scope-one third of all people experiencing sleep issues annually, half of which seek medical advice for the issue, with only 15% of people actually reported as having sleep disorders [8]. To effectively treat a sleep disorder, the differences between sleep disorders must be understood fully and undoubtedly, such that diagnosis is accurate and treatment is pointed and geared specifically to each respective condition.

According to a 1995 report from the National Sleep Foundation, in a primary care population study, only 6% of insomniacs had gone to their physician specifically for this complaint. Additionally, insomnia in psychiatric patients is under-recognized [9]. While insomnia has been investigated in depth, insomnia is still not completely understood, the study hindered by inconsistent diagnostic criteria and variable definitions.

Insomnia and Sleep Disorder Comorbidities

Primary sleep disorders, not accompanied by other conditions, occur in some cases; however, many sleep disorders occur concomitantly with other medical and/or psychiatric conditions [10]. Latest sleep surveys indicate that of the general adult population, insomnia affects 10% to 17%, and increased rates of insomnia occur in patients with psychiatric conditions [11]. In example, Okuji et al. [11] determined that 69% of patients with mood disorder spectrum, 63% of patients with anxiety disorder, and 50% of patients with an ICD-10 schizophrenia spectrum complained of insomnia.

It is well known that insomnia commonly occurs concomitantly with depression, and it is generally thought of as a symptom in mood disorder [12]. Some studies, however, have claimed that depression and insomnia are disorders distinct in etiology and of genetic influences [13]. Utilizing a 15,000 subject European cohort and longitudinal study, in 40% of cases insomnia occurred before depression and in 56% of cases insomnia occurred before recurrent depression [13]. Insomnia has been implicated as a risk factor for depression. Individuals with a history of insomnia have four times the risk for depression as those that do not [14]. Moreover, the Breslau et al. [14] study also found that prior insomnia history significantly correlated with substance use disorder (S.U.D.), smoking, and risk for anxiety. Finally, following successful treatment for depressive symptoms, as measured with the Hamilton Rating Scale for Depression (HAM-D) scores, patients still reported sleeping difficulties [14].

Many of the symptoms that occur in insomniacs also occur in other sleep disorders; furthermore, sleep disorders, in general, are associated with a myriad of additional co morbidities. For example, the relationship of sleep and suicide has been investigated. A 1997 study conducted by Ağargün determined that persons with the worst quality of sleep, as measured through the Pittsburgh Sleep Quality Index (PSQI), consequently scored the highest suicide subscale scores, indicating an inverse relationship between suicide and sleep quality [15].

In regards to stress, numerous anxiety disorder patients report problems falling and staying asleep; in support, polysomnographic tests of panic disorder patients indicate a reduced efficiency in sleep patterns when compared to normal controls-with increased time awake and increased time before falling asleep [16]. Interestingly, REM sleep measures do not differ significantly nor does sleep architecture for panic disorder patients and normal subjects [16]. For patients with generalized anxiety disorder, 60% to 70% complain that they have issues sleeping; polysomnographs of these patients showed an increase in the time it took to fall asleep as well as a reduction in ability to maintain sleep [16]. Similarly, the REM sleep measures and sleep architecture were not significantly different from controls. Obsessive-compulsive disorder (OCD) patients, though reporting poor sleep, did not show significant difference from controls; patients with social phobias have not been shown to differ in sleep parameters from controls [16].

More recently, utilizing a cohort of 375,653 US adults ($\geq$ 18 years of age) in a 2013 study, Liu et al. [17] investigated the relationship between chronic disease and insufficient sleep. Controlling for various demographics and adjusting for covariates, a significant positive relationship ($p<0.0001$) was observed between six chronic diseases and insufficient sleep [17]. These relationships were modestly explained by frequent mental distress; the relationships between both high blood pressure and diabetes and insufficient sleep were modestly explained by obesity [17]. While the relationship between insufficient sleep and chronic diseases has been investigated, the comprehensive cause-and-effect relationship is impossible to infer from such studies; thus, relationships between these conditions remains unclear [7].

Post-traumatic Stress disorder (PTSD) has also been associated with degradation in sleep quality, 70% to 91% of patients with PTSD have reported issues falling to and maintaining sleep, and 19% to 71% of patients report nightmares, dependent on PTSD severity and physical aggression exposure [18]. The studies relating sleep patterns of PTSD patients and controls are presently inconclusive; however, for PTSD patients the system of REM sleep control seems to be dysregulated [18]. Interestingly, PTSD patients are more predisposed to sleep disordered breathing (SDB) and disorders involving movement during sleep; these comorbidities have been implicated as playing roles in the sleep deficiencies of PTSD patients [18].

Other conditions associated with insomnia are Chronic Obstructive Pulmonary Diseases, Obstructive Sleep Apnea, and Restless Leg Syndrome (RLS).

Insomnia and Sleep Disorder Management

Sleep disorders are presently managed with pointed and treat-to-target techniques depending on condition, with the type and etiology of the condition influencing ideal management [19]. The initial treatment regimen for sleep disorders involves improving sleep hygiene; this is completed by utilizing routine strategies to promote a healthy and silent sleep situation, reducing caffeine or alcohol consumption prior to bed, adhering to a non-disruptive exercise schedule, limiting exposure to stimulates, and employing wind-down sessions prior to sleep [20].

Determined through a comprehensive 59 trial meta-analysis, sleep induction and sleep maintenance have both been improved by non-pharmacological treatments for insomnia [21]. In these studies, sleep restriction therapy and stimulus control therapy were associated with the strongest evidence [21]. Moreover it was found that an average of 5 hours of intervention was shown to reduce time of onset latency and time awake after sleep onset [21].

Furthermore, cognitive behavioral therapy is utilized to treat insomnia and nightmares in PTSD patients by utilizing specialized strategies such as the imagery rehearsal therapy (IRT), a technique in which alternate positive endings are imagined and discussed for nightmares of the patient between a therapist and the patient [18]. While there have been only a few studies on the matter, significant reductions in insomnia and nightmares have been demonstrated through IRT therapy in PTSD patients [18]. Some uncontrolled experiments implicate continuous positive airway pressure as also improving sleep quality, with reduction in nightmare incidence, insomnia and other PTSD symptoms [18]. Continued research is necessary to determine the value of behavioral therapies for sleep disorders.

Additional sleep disorder treatment techniques include behavioral therapy such as biofeedback, as well as light therapy, chronotherapy, and pharmacotherapy, using sedatives and/or hypnotics [19,22-24]. Relaxation therapy, stimulus control therapy [25], sleep restriction therapy [26], and cognitive behavioral therapy (CBT) [27] are other interesting non-pharmacological techniques utilized to treat sleep disorders.

Pharmacotherapeutic Intervention

In the search for a drug which induces sleep without the usual hypnotic–abuse liability and toxicity has been a real challenge for the pharmaceutical industry. Griffiths et al. [28] evaluated 19 hypnotic drugs for both abuse liability and toxicity and found that Phenobarbital has the highest abuse liability and toxicity and Trazodone (a non-approved anti-insomniac drug) while having no abuse liability potential does have significant toxicity [28]. However, one drug, ramelteon, was found not to have any abuse liability or toxicity. This is quite interesting considering that this substance does not bind to the typical GABA receptor. Unlike all other hypnotic drugs used to treat insomnia, ramelteon is amelatonin receptor agonist acting at MT1 MT2 receptors located at/in the superachiasmatic nucleus, which affects the circadian sleep-wake cycle. The MT1 receptor seems to be associated with direct promotion of sleep. This receptor is believed to play a role in helping to quiet down arousal and allow sleepiness to take over. The MT2 receptor seems to be acting primarily with respect to the reinforcement of the whole 24-hour cycle. Ramelteon has negligible affinity for the MT3 receptors, which are widely distributed throughout the body, or for other major neurotransmitter receptors such as GABA, histamine, opioid, dopamine, or acetylcholine. A recent PubMed search revealed a total of 1,138 papers regarding pharmacological and non-pharmacological treatment of chronic insomnia of which 755 were pharmacological.

Hypothesis

It is hypothesized that measurement of various genetic mutations through gene expression, single nucleotide polymorphisms, as well as additional phenotypic and genetic diagnostics, with the interest of changing the makeup and creation of nutritional supplements, will shift the diagnostic, stratification, prognostic, and treatment paradigm for sleep in humans. Furthermore, mesolimbic neurochemical reward circuitry manipulation inducing dopamine release at the Nucleus accumbens will offer benefits in stress and pain relief, both major factors in sleep processes [29]. Specifically, the present theoretical notion includes proprietary algorithms that combine genetic mutations into index values, referred to as Genoscores, to represent specific pre-defined formulations. We hereby propose that a number of experiments be performed to further our scientific credibility. The experiments will include both genetic and non-genetic subjects and the formulations will include both "one-size-fits all" as well as DNA-based customized formulations to induce sleep. The trials will also include comparisons with known FDA approved sleep medications. The protocol will consist of a double-blind randomized placebo-controlled cross-over study. The measurement scales will include one of the following instruments: Fatigue Severity Scale (FSS); Stanford Sleepiness Scale (SSS); Epworth Sleepiness Scale (ESS) and/or Chalder Fatigue Scale (CFS) or Empirical Sleepiness & Fatigue Scales developed by Bailes and associates.

EZ-Sleep™

EZ-sleep™ is a unique formula and method to safely and naturally induce effective sleep. This novel technology contrasts with existing tactics to manipulate three important pathways in sleep induction. Moreover we are hypothesizing that EZ-Sleep™, a putative dopaminergic, melatonin, benzodiazepine reward circuitry receptor(s) activator, may become an important front-line non-pharmacological treatment for chronic insomnia. We further hypothesize that utilization of this nutraceutical may result in significant reduction of hypnotic medication abuse and toxicity liability thereby increasing benefit over risk.

Rationale

This novel approach utilizes synergistic nutraceutical components to exploit symbiotic mechanisms stimulating metabolism and healthy sleep through:

1. Pleasure mechanisms that effect stress

2. The metabolic and immunological mechanisms that effect sleep induction.

3. The neuroendocrine system that affects circadian rhythm

Importantly, these three systems are homeostatic and compensatory, intimately interactive and interdependent in ensuring optimal sleep and metabolic function. This novel nutraceutical technology optimizes sleep mechanisms especially those tied to stress. Table 1 lists the ingredients in EZ-Sleep™. A careful review of the existing literature reveals that the ingredients in EZ-Sleep™ should lead to enhance sleep function. In the arsenal of nutrients, EZ-Sleep™ primarily contains sleep inducing ingredients.

Ingredients & Scientific Explanation

EZ-Sleep™ complex: stress reduction components

Manipulation of pleasure mechanisms that effect stress is exploited by some of the ingredients of EZ-Sleep™, especially through promotion of dopamine release at the Nucleus accumbens, stimulating stress reduction and pain reduction.

In humans, an imaging study by Hilker and associates (2006) found that marked striatal dopamine depletion was demonstrated in patients with REM sleep behavior disorder utilizing functional MRI [30]. Dopamine is also involved in other sleep disorders including Restless Leg syndrome (RLS). A neurological disorder affecting 1-10% of the population, RLS induces urges to move ones extremities in an effort to address paraesthetic sensations [31]. RLS symptoms are heightened when going to sleep in the evening and interrupt/delay desired sleeping

Supplement Facts
Serving Size: 1 Tablet, 45 minutes before bedtime without food
Serving per container: 60
Amount per Serving
Vitamin B6 (as Pyridoxine HCL, Pyridoxal-5-Phosphate)
Calcium (as hydroxycitrate)
Magnesium (as magnesium citrate and oxide) (aspartate is better!)
Manganese (ascorbate)
Potassium (as hydroxycitrate)
Synaptamine Proprietary Complex
Chromium picolinate
DL-phenylalanine (D-PhenEze™)
L-Glutamine
Rhodiola rosea Extract (3%)‡ (RhodiGen™
Grifonia simplicifolia Extract (5-HTP)
**EZ Sleep™ Proprietary Calming blend
Passiflora incarnata L. Extract Δ (EM103 Passiflora incarnata)
Protykin (50% trans-resveratrol)
Melatonin
* Daily Value not established.
**Chamomile, Valerian, and Hops Flower (33 mg each)
TOTAL MGs

Table 1: Ingredients of EZ-Sleep™: the putative dopaminergic, melatonin, benzodiazepine reward circuitry receptor(s) activators that enable sleep induction benefits.

and waking times. While the etiopathogenesis of RLS remains unknown, a dopaminergic system is hypothesized to play an important role in RLS manifestation-the use of dopamine agonists in treatment, such as 2005 FDA approved ropinirole, offer valuable therapeutic solutions to RLS [31].

Dopaminergic involvement of sleep and wakefulness is very complex, and exact mechanisms are still unclear. The various receptors of dopamine (D1-D5) all have very distinct properties and may interact at different sleep processes. While dopamine agonists seem to induce sleep interaction of dopamine at various dopamine receptor sites, there may be differential sleep induction and wakefulness depending on the dopamine receptor targeted. For example, recent hypotheses implicate D3 receptor involvement in pramipexole stimulated sleep increase and locomotor activity reduction [32]. Furthermore, high dose pramipexole stimulated postsynaptic D2 receptor activation has been hypothesized to increase motor behavior and wakefulness [32]. REM latency has been increased in rats that were administered a dopamine D4 receptor antagonist (L-741,741), and these results suggest a role for D4 receptors in the regulation of wake and sleep [33].

Lima et al. [34] following animal experimentation, proposed that blockage of dopaminergic D2 receptors produce a decrease of REM but not of slow wave sleep in rodents after REM sleep deprivation [34]. This work suggests that in regards to sleep and wake state maintenance and regulation, dopamine acts as a key substance [34].

While there is sufficient evidence for serotonergic involvement in stress induced insomnia and SSRI's may work in certain instances, long term treatment of insomnia with these agents have been somewhat disappointing, in spite of significant animal work suggestive of serotonin involvement in sleep disorders.

The serotonergic synthesis inhibitor para-chlorophenylalanine, p-CPA, pretreatment has been studied in a murine model, utilizing young male Charles Foster rats subjected to acute immobilization stress, to investigate their resultant sleep-wake patterns [35]. Three groups of rats, subjected to (i) acute immobilization stress, (ii) p-CPA pretreatment and acute immobilization stress, and (iii) neither p-CPA pretreatment nor acute immobilization stress, were monitored in their sleep quality and resultant wakefulness [35]. As a result, p-CPA pretreatment successfully reversed the detrimental effects following acute immobilization stress, including changes in total sleep time and total time of REM sleep [35]. Other work from the laboratory of Geller and Blum initially showed that p-CPA caused an enhancement of stress related conflict in rats [36].

The following ingredients promote stress manipulation through synergistic and symbiotic mechanisms.

Passiflora incarnate: Passionflower is the name of several plants stemming from the Passiflora genus [37]. The origin of Passiflora is in the tropical and subtropical regions of the western hemisphere, and there are over 40 different species in the genus. First transported by Spanish conquerors from Mexico to Europe in the sixteenth century, Passionflower has been utilized as a calming tea remedying menstrual pain, conjunctivitis, hemorrhoids, diarrhea, colic, dysentery, skin eruptions, and muscle spasms and is now a worldwide medical herb. The inclusion of Passionflower in sleep inducing formulas exploits its effect on the central nervous system (CNS) and its stress reduction effects [38]. When in a comfortable sleep environment a reduction in stress should be associated with sleepiness.

A problem with Passionflower is its identity since a number of alkaloids have been sold under its name; however, *Passiflora incarnate* (P. incarnata) stands out as the most important, being the most consistently effective. The total alkaloid content of P. incarnate, as listed on the U.S. Agricultural Research Service's ethno botanical database, is 100 to 900 ppm, and it has a 1.2% to 3.9% total flavonoid content. In P. incarnata, there are twenty flavonoids, amongst them gynocardine and cyanogenic glycoside, as well as six alkaloids, and some researchers have attributed the sedative effects from *P. incarnatato* the alkaloids: Harmane and relatives, harmol and harmaline. In contrast, other researchers have attributed CNS bioactivity to flavonoids such as luteolin, apigenin, or their glycosides, stating that the alkaloid content of P. incarnatais not high enough to cause CNS effects.

Most recently, a highly anxiolytic, tri substituted benzoflavone moiety has been isolated from a P. incarnata extract. P. incarnata extract has effectively restored the libido of older male rats [39]; restored fertility and libido previously compromised by tetra hydro cannabinol, nicotine and alcohol addiction [40]; and compared to oxazepam, double-blind randomized studies have indicated that Passiflora extract has been proven to be a fairly effective means for managing generalized anxiety [39]. Interestingly, other double-blind randomized controlled trials have suggested the potential for Passiflora extract as a valuable adjuvant for managing opiate withdrawal [41]. In a mice model, Passiflora has been shown to decrease benzodiazepine dependence. Moreover, the sedative effects of P. incarnata have been verified in numerous pharmacological investigations. EZ-Sleep™ was formulated with information from Euro med (source of dried aerial EM103 P. incarnata parts, cut or fragmented). Separated leaves have been demonstrated as affording the highest possible CNS results, and excluding the flowers, the usage of all aerial parts may prove to be the best method for maximizing bioactive EM103 P. incarnata plant parts. Passiflora preparation standardization has been studied actively, in special regard to its relation on anxiolytic activity.

It was suggested in the early 1970's, by one of us (KB), that serotonin was a biological substrate of stress. Through injections of p-CPA, a serotonin chemical synthesis depletor in rodents, the initiation of stress in rodents was attenuated. Other researchers have also recognized and shown serotonin and dopamine involvement in the production of stress in humans and other animals. By comparing skin conductance levels in a double-blind randomized controlled human trial, stress levels have been shown to be reduced by amino acid and enkephalinase inhibition therapy. These results support Passiflora extract use for anxiety disorder treatments, especially for serotonin mediated disorders. Interestingly, this is homologous to a Passiflora extract phyto constituentindole.

The genus Passiflora comprises about 500 species [37]. The substance Passiflora incarnata and its benzoflavone isolate binds to the benzodiazepine receptor [42]. As such, it has many biological effects including promotion of sleep, anxiolytic activity [43], anti-alcohol and opiate craving activity [40], promotion of sexual appetite [39], and hypnotic activity [44].

11.1.2 DL-Phenylalanine (validated via FTIR verified reference standard D-PhenEze™): DL-phenylaline (DLPA) inhibits the breakdown of the opioid peptides and has been shown to reduce stress in a double blind placebo controlled study. DLPA has been found to reduce stress by anti-craving reward mechanism.

D-phenylalanine inhibits the enzyme enkephalinase, which metabo¬lizes or breaks down enkephalins, thereby increasing enkephalins availability and, most likely, increasing dopamine availability at reward sites (under stressful conditions especially) [45-47].

Furthermore, L-phenylalanine is utilized to stimulate dopamine production and/or increase brain reward neither area nor epinephrine levels. A significant problem with L-phenylalanine is potential competition with other amino-acids, i.e. blood born L-tyrosine and L-tryptophan at the large neutral amino–acid brain carrier system. However, for the first time, other data has demonstrated synthesis and release responses to several dopaminergic agents may be stemming from synaptosomal dopamine, a product of the hydroxylation of phenylalanine. Dopamine created from 14C-phenylalanine in the Caudate nucleus of a rat through synaptosomal preparation was increased and concomitantly stimulated by Cogentin and Amphetamine. A net increase in dopamine also occurs due to amfoelic acid. In this regard, synaptosomal particles are potential components that can synthesize dopamine from L-phenylalanine; synthesis from L-phenylalanine potentially under regulatory control by synaptosomal particles.

L-Tyrosine: L-tyrosine is utilized to increase dopamine levels in the brain as an amino-acid synthesis promoter, direct precursor. L-tyrosine is used for repletion of metabolized neurotransmitters (i.e. dopamine).

EZ Sleep™ Proprietary Calming Blend: The following ingredients constitute the calming blend to promote sleep: Chamomilia flower, hops flower, valerian root extract, Jamaican dogwood extract, valanic acid, and kava kava. Chamomile extract leads to a significant decrease in sleep latency in rats [48]. Kava Kava reduced generalized anxiety disorder in humans [49,50]. A combination of Valerian–Hops is used as a sleep aid [51]. Binding affinities were observed for this combination of serotonin receptor subtypes including 5-HT7 that promotes sleep. Valerian and valanic acid are partial agonists of the 5-HT5A receptor, a substrate involved in insomnia. Valanic acid enhances the sedative effects of Valarian. Trends toward increase in slow-wave sleep and lack of effect on REM sleep were observed in 1994. There have been studies on Hops that show a sedative effect [52].

Pyridoxal-5-phosphate: Pyridoxal-5-phosphate is the active ingredient of vitamin B_6, important as a co-factor in neurotransmitter production and gastrointestinal amino acid absorption improvement.

Calcium: Calcium promotes release of neurotransmitters. Many metabolic events require calcium, and calcium nutrient inclusion is therefore proposed by the authors to promote sleep. Calcium in a number of species induces a sleep-like state [53,54].

EZ-Sleep™ complex: sleep induction enhancement components

While stress-reduction plays an important role in enabling sleep induction, other components of EZ-Sleep™ directly promote sleep induction through various other mechanisms. Most of the hypnotic drugs on the market are central nervous depressants acting at the gamma- aminobutyric acid $(GABA)_A$ receptor. In this regard, wisdom dictates that only a few hypnotic–like drugs have been approved to treat insomnia, but not beyond short term therapy because of the abuse liability. The benzodiazepine hypnotics are only approved for short term use, as are zolpidem immediate-release (Ambien) and zaleplon (Sonata) the non-benzodiazepine agents that act at the same benzodiazepine-activated $GABA_A$ receptor complex. The following ingredients make use of the GABA complex and serotonergic mechanisms to aid sleep induction.

L-Glutamine: L-glutamine, a precursor amino-acid for GABA, is utilized to increase GABA levels in the brain at anxiety associated receptors. L-glutamine maintains balance in case of D-phenylalanine over-inhibition. The inhibitory action of GABA on brain function is tied to integrated sleep processes [55]. GABA shuts off the neurotransmitters that induce wakefulness. Chronic excess of GABA in the brain induces increased slow–wave sleep [56]. Studies have shown that Adenosine A2A receptor agonist induced sleep by inhibiting the histaminergic system through increasing GABA release in the tuberomammillary nucleus [57]. GABA is linked to the benzodiazepine receptor. The sedative hypnotic benzodiazepine–GABA receptor agonist (BzRas) Zaleplon induces a long-term anti-insomnia effect in older patients [58]. The $GABA_A$ receptor is the target for most widely prescribed sleep medications [59]. The stimulation of the benzodiazepin–GABA site induces sedation, hypnosis, and anxiolytic activity.

Grifoniasimplicifolia Extract, 5-HTP (optional): 5-HTP is an amino acid precursor to brain serotonin. Serotonin levels rise during sleep stages. Sleep is a problem with age and many old people complain about insomnia. It is known that age induces a decrease in serotonergic receptors. The serotonin precursor 5-HTP causes a reversal of insomnia by para-chlorophenylalanine induced serotonin brain depletion [60]. While Serotonin-2A and 2C receptor gene polymorphisms may associate with sleep problems in Japanese patients, these polymorphisms did not associate with apnea [61]. However, both age and BMI did associate. Sleep apnea syndrome is associated with serotonin transporter gene polymorphism [62]. While the 5-HT2A receptor may be involved in insomnia (whereby antagonists may be helpful), 5-HT7 promotes REM sleep [63,64]. Injection of a 5-HT1A –receptor agonist directly into the dorsal midbrain promotes sleep.

Utilizing brain micro dialysis, lateral hypothalamus serotonin release was examined following systemic administration of 5-hydroxy-1-tryptophan in an in vivo rat model [65]. A long lasting, dose-dependent and immediate increase in dialysates 5-HT is observed with the administration of 5-HTP. The 5-HTP- induced response of 5-HT was significantly attenuated and levels of basal 5-HT decreased significantly, when calcium was not included in the perfusion medium, thereby limiting exocytosis.

Chromium Salts (Nicotinate and Picolinate): Chromium is a tryptophan enhancing substance, which increases the brain content of serotonin. Serotonin is involved in the natural sleep process [66]. Brain serotonin production has been shown to be promoted by an oxygen-coordinated chromium nicotinate. Picolinate, another chromium salt, effects the production of serotonin. Since brain serotonin is important as a sleep neurotransmitter, the EZ–sleep™ formula will contain this salt [67].

Rhodiola rosea Extract (3%) (validated via FTIR verified reference standard RhodiGen™): As demonstrated in several clinical trials with double–blind placebo controls, Rhodiola rosea (R. rosea) positively enhances mood, reduces stress and has no detectable toxicity levels. R. rosea extract positively influences the higher nervous system, improving memory and attention span. Where lower dopamine and serotonin brain levels are observed, it is hypothesized that R. rosea can potentially act as a COMT inhibitor. COMT activity has been decreased by 60% and neurotransmitter levels by 30% by R. rosea. This phenomenon will assist in sleep induction. Moreover, the plant adaptogen R. rosea promotes positive effects on sleep [68]. R. rosea has a positive effect on paradoxical sleep deprivation [69]. R. rosea improves endurance exercise in healthy young adults [70]. R. rosea reduces stress and improves sleep [71]. R. rosea improves mental capacity in a double–blind study [72]. R. rosea was effective in improving sleep quality in young men living in high altitudes [73].

Manganese (ascorbate) (ManganEze™): Manganese is found in a large variety of minerals, sea and fresh water, marine and land plants, and animals [74]. Manganese is an essential trace element, human requirements being estimated at between 3 and 9 mg per day. 15 studies have described the adverse mood effects of Manganese (Mn) overexposure, specifically in six dimensions of mood: (i) irritability, nervousness and anxiety; (ii) emotional disturbance; (iii) psychotic experiences; (iv) sleep disturbance, lack of vigor and fatigue; (v) aggression hostility; (vi) compulsive and/or impulsive behavior [75]. 1:15 studies utilized standardized measures of mood. When the Brief Symptom Inventory (BSI) and Profile of Moods State (POMS) standardized mood scales were used to evaluate low Mn levels of exposure and its consequence on mood, results indicated that older men with higher Mn levels showed significant disturbances on four of the six mood dimensions relative to men with lower MN levels, including irritability, nervousness and anxiety; aggression hostility; and emotional disturbance [75]. The POMS and BSI are useful standardized mood scales for the assessment of Mn/mood effects [75]. However, optimal doses produce health benefits. Mn has hypnotic-like effects and as such, enhances alcohol-induced sleeping time in mice. There are no human studies directly involving the effects of Mn on sleep performance, but it has been considered as a sedative inducing nutrient for years.

EZ-Sleep™complex: neuroendocrine circadian rhythm manipulation components

Circadian rhythm, created by molecular mechanisms, is considered a biological property universal to the majority of living things on earth; in which, the regulation of clock genes through a transcription feedback loop is vital to all studied species [76]. The clock genes observed in insects and mammals have been remarkably alike, indicating genetic level, evolutionary circadian rhythm conservation [76]. Homeostasis and circadian rhythms work concomitantly to regulate arousal and sleep in mammals; however, the underlying genetic pathway through which sleep is regulated is not readily understood. Similarities in the molecular arousal regulation pathways between insects and mammals have been discovered; in example, dopamine has been implicated as a key player in the regulation of arousal and sleep-like behavior in ants [76].

Interestingly there is strong evidence for the interaction of melatonin and dopamine D2 receptor. Both the melatonin and dopaminergic systems regulate the light/dark cycles in the animal as well as in the human [77].

Acknowledged to play a role in numerous mammalian brain regions such as the retina, hypothalamus, and nigrostriatal system, the presence of a dopamine-melatonin association is of particular interest. For example, in C57BL/6 mice nigrostriatal damage is caused by the effect of melatonin on 1 methyl-4-phenyl-1, 2, 3, 6-tetrahydropyridine [78]. In C57BL/6 mice, however, the interaction between striatal dopamine and melatonin rhythmic production is not readily understood [77].

Work utilizing the C57BL/6 mice model has investigated circadian rhythm variations in striatal dopamine levels and pineal production of melatonin [78]. This work has indicated the possibility for a series of significant dopamine and melatonin interactions. In mice controls, melatonin has a narrow circadian rhythm peak at midnight, striatal dopamine reaches a low-point at midnight, and 3,4-dihydroxyphenylacetic acid (DOPAC) levels, a primary dopamine metabolite, increase shortly after a decrease in striatal dopamine levels [78]. Following pineal gland removal, the cyclic changes in dopamine and DOPAC levels were less pronounced; however, administration of melatonin over a 6 day period to pinealectomized mice dose-dependently repaired this rhythm [78]. This suggests a potential murine linkage between pineal melatonin secretion and dopamine circadian rhythm [78].

Ramelteon, approved by the Food and Drug Administration (FDA) in 2005, is presently the only medication utilized for long-term insomnia treatment and works by exploiting the soporific property of melatonin; it works as a melatonin receptor agonist [79]. The efficacy of ramelteon is not presently known, although findings have been promising; the efficacy will rely on the results of additional placebo-controlled trials [79]. The effectiveness of melatonin and ramelteon in treating insomnia requires further attention, as present data on the topic is based on studies with several limitations, and there have been only three control trials for ramelteon [79]. It is important to note that sleep maintenance has not been shown to improve with zolipidem controlled–release or eszopiciline, a GABAA agonist. In fact, according to Johnson and Griffiths (2005) subjective comparisons have characterized the hypnotic effect of ramelteon relative to the benzodiazepine and non-benzodiazepine $GABA_A$ active agents as "more subtle" and "less prominent" [28]. Furthermore, post –sleep questionnaires have indicated that ramelteon's hypnotic effect may be experienced as less robust than could be expected from polysomnography data [80].

The following EZ-Sleep™ ingredients affect circadian rhythms, promoting improved sleep quality and improved duration.

Melatonin: Existing as a hormone, endogenous melatonin is secreted by the pineal gland and linked to circadian rhythm [81]. A study of melatonin in the 1970's and 1980's revealed sedative/hypnotic effects of this compound [82,83]. In a recent meta–analysis of 16 studies by Buscemi et al. [84]. It has been concluded that while melatonin may not be effective in primary sleep disorder treatment, it is potentially useful in short term DSPS treatment [84]. The use of melatonin for a short period, 3 months or less, has been implicated as safe.

The pineal gland hormone melatonin improves sleep quality [85]. A recent meta–analysis reveals melatonin treatment significantly reduced sleep onset latency and increased total sleep duration [86]. Melatonin secretion helps regulate sleep and circadian rhythms [87]. Beta-Methyl-6 chloromelatonin significantly decreases sleep latency in insomnia

[88]. Melatonin improves sleep behavior in children with epilepsy [89]. While one study was negative with respect to the effectiveness in melatonin versus placebo with regard to sleep deprivation of winter depression, other studies are positive in terms hypnotic actions [90]. It seems that the effects of melatonin on sleep works best in patients that have abnormal sleep patterns compared to health individuals [91, 92].

Magnesium (ligand? aspartate?) (MagNezyum™?): Chronic stress reduces intracellular magnesium [93]. Aging effects sleep and magnesium reverses these age-related effects and promotes sleep [94]. EEG blood magnesium levels are under strong genetic control, whereas brain magnesium levels are not [95]. Optimal levels of magnesium are required for normal sleep regulation [96].

INGREDIENT	DOSE	FINDING
Pyridoxine HCL Pyridoxal 5-Phosphate	20 mg (20% PHCL; 80% P-5-P	Catalyst for synthesis of neurotransmitters
Chromium[a,b]	400 mcg	Chromium is a tryptophan enhancing substance, which increases the brain content of serotonin. Serotonin is involved in the natural sleep process [66].
DL-phenylalanine[c,d,e,f]	2000 mg	DLPA inhibits the breakdown of the opioid peptides and has been shown to reduce stress in a double blind placebo controlled study. DLPA has been found to reduce stress by anti-craving reward mechanism.
L-Glutamine[g,h,i,j,k]	150 mg	L-Glutamine is the precursor amino-acid for GABA. The inhibitory action of GABA on brain function is tied to integrated sleep processes [55]. GABA shuts off the neurotransmitters that induce wakefulness. Chronic excess of GABA in the brain induces increased slow–wave sleep [56]. Studies have shown that Adenosine A2A receptor agonist induced sleep by inhibiting the histaminergic system through increasing GABA release in the tuberomammillary nucleus [57]. GABA is linked to the benzodiazepine receptor. The sedative hypnotic benzodiazepine–GABA receptor agonist (BzRas) Zaleplon induces a long-term anti-insomnia effect in older patients [58]. The GABAA receptor is the target for most widely prescribed sleep medications [59]. The stimulation of the benzodiazepin –GABA site induces sedation, hypnosis, and anxiolytic activity.
Grifoniasimplicifolia Extract (5-HTP)[l,m,n,o,p,q,r,s,t,u]	100 mg	5-HTP is an amino acid precursor to brain serotonin. Serotonin levels rise during sleep stages. Sleep is a problem with age and many old people complain about insomnia. It is known that age induces a decrease in serotonergic receptors. The serotonin precursor 5-HTP causes a reversal of insomnia by para-chlorophenylalanine induced serotonin brain depletion [60]. While Serotonin-2A and 2C receptor gene polymorphisms may associate with sleep problems in Japanese patients, these polymorphisms did not associate with apnea [61]. However, both age and BMI did associate. Sleep apnea syndrome is associated with serotonin transporter gene polymorphism [62]. While the 5-HT2A receptor may be involved in insomnia (whereby antagonists may be helpful), 5-HT7 promotes REM sleep [63,64]. Injection of a 5-HT1A –receptor agonist directlyinto the dorsal midbrain promotes sleep.
Melatonin	10 mg	The pineal gland hormone melatonin improves sleep quality [85]. A recent meta-analysis reveals melatonin treatment significantly reduced sleep onset latency and increased total sleep duration [86]. Melatonin secretion helps regulate sleep and circadian rhythms [87]. Beta-Methyl-6 chloromelatonin significantly decreases sleep latency in insomnia [88]. Melatonin improves sleep behavior in children with epilepsy [89]. While one study was negative with respect to the effectiveness in melatonin versus placebo with regard to sleep deprivation of winter depression, other studies are positive in terms hypnotic actions [90]. It seems that the effects of melatonin on sleep works best in patients that have abnormal sleep patterns compared to health individuals [91,92].
Rhodiola rosea	100 mg	The plant adaptogen rhodiola rosea promotes positive effects on sleep [68]. Rhodiola rosea has a positive effect on paradoxical sleep deprivation [69]. Rhodiola rosea improves endurance exercise in healthy young adults [70]. Rhodiola rosea reduces stress and improves sleep [71]. Rhodiola rosea improves mental capacity in a double-blind study [72]. Rhodiola was effective in improving sleep quality in young men living in high altitudes [73].
Passion Flower	300 mg	The genus Passiflora comprises about 500 species [37]. The substance Passifloraincarnita and its benzoflavobe isolate binds to the benzodiazepine receptor [42]. As such, it has many biological effects including promotion of sleep, anxiolytic activity [43], anti-alcohol and opiate craving activity [40], promotion of sexual appetite [39], and hypnotic activity [44].
Calming Blend		
(The following ingredients constitute the calming blend to promote sleep: Chamomilia flower, hops flower, valerian root extract, Jamaican dogwood extract, valanic acid, and kava kava)	200 mg	Chamomiles extract lead to a significant decrease in sleep latency in rats [48]. Kava Kava reduced generalized anxiety disorder in humans [49,50]. A combination of Valarian–Hops is used as a sleep aid [51]. Binding affinities were observed for this combination of serotonin receptor subtypes including 5-HT7 that promotes sleep. Valarian and Valanic acid are partial agonists of the 5-HT5A receptor a substrate involved in insomnia. Valanic acid enhances the sedative effects of Valarian. Trends toward increase in slow-wave sleep and lack of effect on rapis eye movement (REM) sleep were observed in 1994. There have been studies on Hops that show a sedative effect [52].
Magnesium	270 mg	Chronic stress reduces intracellular magnesium [93]. Aging effects sleep and magnesium reverses these age-related effects and promotes sleep [94]. EEG blood magnesium levels are under strong genetic control, whereas brain magnesium levels are not [95]. Optimal levels of magnesium are required for normal sleep regulation [96].
Calcium	555 mg	Calcium in a number of species induces a sleep-like state [53, 54].
Manganese ascorbate	13.25 mg	Manganese is found in a large variety of minerals, sea and fresh water, marine and land plants, and animals [74]. Manganese is an essential trace element, human requirements being estimated at between 3 and 9 mg per day. 15 studies have described the adverse mood effects of Manganese (Mn) overexposure, specifically in six dimensions of mood: (i) irritability, nervousness and anxiety; (ii) emotional disturbance; (iii) psychotic experiences; (iv) sleep disturbance, lack of vigor and fatigue; (v) aggression hostility; (vi) compulsive and/or impulsive behavior [75]. 1:15 studies utilized standardized measures of mood. When the Brief Symptom Inventory (BSI) and Profile of Moods State (POMS) standardized mood scales were used to evaluate low Mn levels of exposure and its consequence on mood, results indicated that older men with higher Mn levels showed significant disturbances on four of the six mood dimensions relative to men with lower MN levels, including irritability, nervousness and anxiety; aggression hostility; and emotional disturbance [75]. The POMS and BSI are useful standardized mood scales for the assessment of Mn/mood effects [75]. However, optimal doses produce health benefits. Mn has hypnotic-like effects and as such, enhances alcohol sleeping time in mice. There are no human studies directly involving the effects of Mn on sleep performance, but it has been considered as a sedative inducing nutrient for years.

Table 2: Clinical support for ingredients of EZ-Sleep™: the relative dosage and scientific findings in clinical support of various ingredients to be utilized in the EZ-Sleep™ formula.

EZ-Sleep™ complex: additional components

The final components of EZ-Sleep™ are supplements and proprietary complexes involved in antioxidant support and sleep mechanism facilitation.

Protykin (50%): Protykin is an extract of Polygonumcuspidatum which supplies antioxidant and hormone support.

Potassium

Synaptamine Proprietary Complex: Table 2 lists the relative dosages and summarizes the clinical support for the ingredients of EZ-Sleep™.

Conclusion

The issue of insomnia is a global phenomenon which requires additional in-depth research. Insomnia especially in alcohol-dependent patients, for example, may lead to suicide. It is noteworthy that childhood sleep problems predict the onset of drinking in boys [97]. We now know that while there are multifaceted reasons for sleep problems and disturbances (e.g. sleep drive homeostasis, circadian rhythm physiology and genetic influences), the scientific community has not been able to deliver and appropriate solution. Some benefit has been noted with cognitive behavioral therapy, but it has minimal effects in patients relapsing from drugs especially alcohol, cocaine and opiates. While there are a number of pharmaceutical drugs developed to treat insomnia, most have associated side effects and even addiction liability. We do know that benzodiazepines hijack the midbrain dopamine system leading to addiction. Finally, Lima et al. [34] proposed that dopamine D2 receptors are involved rapid eye movement sleep, suggesting as we have proposed herein that dopaminergic activation is one mechanism worthwhile exploring in the future [34]. The concepts presented herein on potential nutrigenomics therapy warrants further in-depth analysis [98-105].

Acknowledgement

The writing of this paper was supported in part by funds from the National Institutes of Health, NIAAA (RO1-AA07112 and K05-AA00219) and the Medical Research Service of the US Department of Veterans Affairs (MOB). TS is partially support by SAHMSA grants as well. The writing of this paper was funded in-part by a grant awarded to Kenneth Blum and Eric R. Braverman from Life Extension Foundation, Ft. Lauderdale, Florida to PATH Foundation NY.

Conflicts of Interest

Kenneth Blum, PhD, holds US and foreign patents on nutraceutical complex. Kenneth Blum, Bernard W. Downs, Margaret Madigan are owners and employees of IGENE and Impact Genomics. There are no other conflicts.

References

1. Lalive AL, Rudolph U, Lüscher C, Tan KR (2011) Is there a way to curb benzodiazepine addiction? Swiss Med Wkly 141: w13277.
2. National Institute of Health (2003) National Sleep Disorders Research Plan.
3. Roller L (2002) Treating sleep disorders. Australian Journal of Pharmacy 83: 443-447.
4. Zammit GK, Weiner J, Damato N, Sillup GP, McMillan CA (1999) Quality of life in people with insomnia. Sleep 22 Suppl 2: S379-385.
5. Cartwright R (2000) Sleep-related violence: does the polysomnogram help establish the diagnosis? Sleep Med 1: 331-335.
6. Grunstein R (2002) Insomnia. Diagnosis and management. Aust Fam Physician 31: 995-1000.
7. Doghramji K (2006) The epidemiology and diagnosis of insomnia. Am J Manag Care 12: S214-220.
8. Rosekind MR (1992) The epidemiology and occurrence of insomnia. J Clin Psychiatry 53 Suppl: 4-6.
9. Berlin RM, Litovitz GL, Diaz MA, Ahmed SW (1984) Sleep disorders on a psychiatric consultation service. Am J Psychiatry 141: 582-584.
10. American Psychiatric Association (1994) American Psychiatric Task Force on DSM-IV Diagnostic and Statistical Manual of Mental Disorders: DSM IV (4thedn), American Psychiatric Association, Washington, DC.
11. Okuji Y, Matsuura M, Kawasaki N, Kometani S, Shimoyama T, et al. (2002) Prevalence of insomnia in various psychiatric diagnostic categories. Psychiatry Clin Neurosci 56: 239-240.
12. Jindal RD, Thase ME (2004) Treatment of insomnia associated with clinical depression. Sleep Med Rev 8: 19-30.
13. Ohayon MM, Roth T (2003) Place of chronic insomnia in the course of depressive and anxiety disorders. J Psychiatr Res 37: 9-15.
14. Breslau N, Roth T, Rosenthal L, Andreski P (1996) Sleep disturbance and psychiatric disorders: a longitudinal epidemiological study of young adults. Biol Psychiatry 39: 411-418.
15. AÄŸargÃ¼n MY, Kara H, Solmaz M (1997) Subjective sleep quality and suicidality in patients with major depression. J Psychiatr Res 31: 377-381.
16. Papadimitriou GN, Linkowski P (2005) Sleep disturbance in anxiety disorders. Int Rev Psychiatry 17: 229-236.
17. Liu Y, Croft JB, Wheaton AG, Perry GS, Chapman DP, et al. (2013) Association between perceived insufficient sleep, frequent mental distress, obesity and chronic diseases among US adults, 2009 behavioral risk factor surveillance system. BMC Public Health 13: 84.
18. Maher MJ, Rego SA, Asnis GM (2006) Sleep disturbances in patients with post-traumatic stress disorder: epidemiology, impact and approaches to management. CNS Drugs 20: 567-590.
19. Reite M, Ruddy J, Nagel K (2002) Evaluation and Management of Sleep Disorders (3rdedn), American Psychiatric Publishing Inc., Washington, DC.
20. Neubauer DN (2003) Pharmacologic approaches for the treatment of chronic insomnia. Clin Cornerstone 5: 16-27.
21. Morin CM, Culbert JP, Schwartz SM (1994) Nonpharmacological interventions for insomnia: a meta-analysis of treatment efficacy. Am J Psychiatry 151: 1172-1180.
22. Wagner DR (1999) Circadian Rhythm Sleep Disorders. Curr Treat Options Neurol 1: 299-308.
23. Czeisler CA, Kronauer RE, Allan JS, Duffy JF, Jewett ME, et al. (1989) Bright light induction of strong (type 0) resetting of the human circadian pacemaker. Science 244: 1328-1333.
24. Reiter RJ (2003) Melatonin: clinical relevance. Best Pract Res Clin Endocrinol Metab 17: 273-285.
25. Bootzin RR, Perlis ML (1992) Nonpharmacologic treatments of insomnia. J Clin Psychiatry 53: 37-41.
26. Spielman AJ, Saskin P, Thorpy MJ (1987) Treatment of chronic insomnia by restriction of time in bed. Sleep 10: 45-56.
27. Smith MT, Neubauer DN (2003) Cognitive behavior therapy for chronic insomnia. Clin Cornerstone 5: 28-40.
28. Griffiths RR, Johnson MW (2005) Relative abuse liability of hypnotic drugs: a conceptual framework and algorithm for differentiating among compounds. J Clin Psychiatry 66 Suppl 9: 31-41.
29. Brown RJ, Blum K, Trachtenberg MC (1990) Neurodynamics of relapse prevention: a neuronutrient approach to outpatient DUI offenders. J Psychoactive Drugs 22: 173-187.
30. Hilker R, Burghaus L, Razai N, Jacobs AH, Szelies B, et al. (2006) Functional brain imaging in combined motor and sleep disorders. J Neurol Sci 248: 223-226.
31. Fulda S, Wetter TC (2005) Dopamine agonists for the treatment of restless legs syndrome. Expert Opin Pharmacother 6: 2655-2666.
32. Lagos P, Scorza C, Monti JM, Jantos H, Reyes-Parada M, et al. (1998) Effects of the D3 preferring dopamine agonist pramipexole on sleep and waking, locomotor activity and striatal dopamine release in rats. Eur Neuropsychopharmacol 8: 113-120.
33. Canvas M, Navarro JF (2006) Effects of selective dopamine D4 receptor antagonists, L-741,741, on sleep and wakefulness in rats. Prog Neuropsychopharmacol Biol Psychiatry 30: 668-678.

34. Lima MM, Andersen ML, Reksidler AB, Silva A, Zager A, et al. (2008) Blockage of dopaminergic D(2) receptors produces decrease of REM but not of slow wave sleep in rats after REM sleep deprivation. Behav Brain Res 188: 406-411.

35. Sinha RK (2006) P-CPA pretreatment reverses the changes in sleep and behavior following acute immobilization stress rats. J Physiol Sci 56: 123-129.

36. Geller I, Blum K (1970) The effects of 5-HTP on para-Chlorophenylalanine (p-CPA) attenuation of "conflict" behavior. Eur J Pharmacol 9: 319-324.

37. Dhawan K, Dhawan S, Sharma A (2004) Passiflora: a review update. J Ethnopharmacol 94: 1-23.

38. Dhawan K, Kumar S, Sharma A (2001) Anti-anxiety studies on extracts of Passiflora incarnata Linneaus. J Ethnopharmacol 78: 165-170.

39. Dhawan K, Sharma A (2003) Restoration of chronic-Delta 9-THC-induced decline in sexuality in male rats by a novel benzoflavone moiety from Passiflora incarnata Linn. Br J Pharmacol 138: 117-120.

40. Dhawan K, Kumar S, Sharma A (2002) Suppression of alcohol-cessation-oriented hype-anxiety by the benzoflavone moiety Passiflora incarnate Linneaus in mice. J Etnopharmacology 81: 239-244.

41. Akhondzadeh S, Kashani L, Mobaseri M, Hosseini SH, Nikzad S, et al. (2001) Passionflower in the treatment of opiates withdrawal: a double-blind randomized controlled trial. J Clin Pharm Ther 26: 369-373.

42. Dhawan K, Dhawan S, Chhabra S (2003) Attenuation of benzodiazepine dependence in mice by a tri substituted benzoflavone moiety of Passiflora incarnate Linneasus: a non-habit forming anxiolytic. J Pharm Pharm Sci 6: 215-222.

43. Dhawan K, Kumar S, Sharma A (2001) Anxiolytic activity of aerial and underground parts of Passiflora incarnata. Fitoterapia 72: 922-926.

44. Krenn L (2002) [Passion Flower (Passiflora incarnata L.)--a reliable herbal sedative]. Wien Med Wochenschr 152: 404-406.

45. Blum K, Briggs AH, Trachtenberg MC, Delallo L, Wallace JE (1987) Enkephalinase inhibition: regulation of ethanol intake in genetically predisposed mice. Alcohol 4: 449-456.

46. Blum K, Trachtenberg MC, Ramsay JC (1988) Improvement of inpatient treatment of the alcoholic as a function of neurotransmitter restoration: a pilot study. Int J Addict 23: 991-998.

47. Blum K, Trachtenberg MC, Elliot CE, Dingler ML, Sexton RL, et al. (1988) Enkephalinase inhibition and precursor amino acid loading improves inpatient treatment of alcohol and polydrug abusers: Double-blind placebo-controlled study of the nutritional adjunct SAAVE. Alcohol 5: 481-493.

48. Shinomiya K, Inoue T, Utsu Y, Tokunaga S, Masuoka T, et al. (2005) Hypnotic activities of chamomile and passiflora extracts in sleep-disturbed rats. Biol Pharm Bull 28: 808-810.

49. Cauffield JS, Forbes HJ (1999) Dietary supplements used in the treatment of depression, anxiety, and sleep disorders. Lippincotts Prim Care Pract 3: 290-304.

50. Boerner RJ, Sommer H, Berger W, Kuhn U, Schmidt U, et al. (2003) Kava-Kava extract LI 150 is as effective as Opipramol and Buspirone in Generalized anxiety Disorder--an 8 week randomized, double –blind multicentre clinical trial in 129 out patients. Phytomedicine 4: 38-49.

51. Fernández S, Wasowski C, Paladini AC, Marder M (2004) Sedative and sleep-enhancing properties of linarin, a flavonoid-isolated from Valeriana officinalis. Pharmacol Biochem Behav 77: 399-404.

52. Abourashed EA, Koetter U, Brattström A (2004) In vitro binding experiments with a Valerian, hops and their fixed combination extract (Ze91019) to selected central nervous system receptors. Phytomedicine 11: 633-638.

53. Veale WL, Myers RD (1971) Emotional behavior, arousal and sleep produced by sodium and calcium ions perfused within the hypothalamus of the cat. Physiol Behav 7: 601-607.

54. Erickson CK, Tyler TD, Beck LK, Duensing KL (1980) Calcium enhancement of alcohol and drug-induced sleeping time in mice and rats. Pharmacol Biochem Behav 12: 651-656.

55. Gottesmann C (2004) Brain inhibitory mechanisms involved in basic and higher integrated sleep processes. Brain Res Brain Res Rev 45: 230-249.

56. Arnulf I, Konofal E, Gibson KM, Rabier D, Beauvais P, et al. (2005) Effect of genetically caused excess of brain gamma-hydroxybutyric acid and GABA on sleep. Sleep 28: 418-424.

57. Hong ZY, Huang ZL, Qu WM, Eguchi N, Urade Y, et al. (2005) An adenosine A receptor agonist induces sleep by increasing GABA release in the tuberomammillary nucleus to inhibit histaminergic systems in rats. J Neurochem 92: 1542-1549.

58. Ancoli-Israel S, Richardson GS, Mangano RM, Jenkins L, Hall P, et al. (2005) Long-term use of sedative hypnotics in older patients with insomnia. Sleep Med 6: 107-113.

59. Bateson AN (2004) The benzodiazepine site of the GABAA receptor: an old target with new potential? Sleep Med 5 Suppl 1: S9-15.

60. Petitjean F, Buda C, Janin M, Sallanon M, Jouvet M (1985) [Insomnia caused by administration of para-chlorophenylalanine: reversibility by peripheral or central injection of 5-hydroxytryptophan and serotonin]. Sleep 8: 56-67.

61. Sakai K, Takada T, Nakayama H, Kubota Y, Nakamata M, et al. (2005) Serotonin-2A and 2C receptor gene polymorphisms in Japanese patients with obstructive sleep apnea. Intern Med 44: 928-933.

62. Ylmaz M, Bayazit YA, Ciftci TU, Erdal ME, Urhan M, et al. (2005) Association of serotonin transporter gene polymorphism with obstructive sleep apnea syndrome. Laryngoscope 115: 832-836.

63. Fish LR, Gilligan MT, Humphries AC, Ivarsson M, Ladduwahetty T, et al. (2005) 4-Fluorosulfonylpiperidines: selective 5-HT2A ligands for the treatment of insomnia. Bioorg Med Chem Lett 15: 3665-3669.

64. Hedlund PB, Sutcliffe JG (2004) Functional, molecular and pharmacological advances in 5-HT7 receptor research. Trends Pharmacol Sci 25: 481-486.

65. Levkovitz Y, Richter-Levin G, Segal M (1994) Effect of 5-hydroxytryptophane on behavior and hippocampal physiology in young and old rats. Neurobiol Aging 15: 635-641.

66. Evans GW (1993) Chromium picolinate is an efficacious and safe supplement. Int J Sport Nutr 3: 117-122.

67. Jha SK, Ross RJ, Morrison AR (2005) Sleep-related neurons in the central nucleus of the amygdala of rats and their modulation by the dorsal raphe nucleus. Physiol Behav 86: 415-426.

68. Panossian A, Wagner H (2005) Stimulating effect of adaptogens: an overview with particular reference to their efficacy following single dose administration. Phytother Res 19: 819-838.

69. Provalova NV, Skurikhin EG, Pershina OV, Suslov NI, Minakova MY, et al. (2002) Mechanisms underling the effects of adaptogens on erythropoiesis during paradoxical sleep deprivation. Bull Exp Biol Med 133: 428-432.

70. De Bock K, Eijnde BO, Ramaekers M, Hespel P (2004) Acute Rhodiola rosea intake can improve endurance exercise performance. Int J Sport Nutr Exerc Metab 14: 298-307.

71. Earnest CP, Morss GM, Wyatt F, Jordan AN, Colson S, et al. (2004) Effects of a commercial herbal-based formula on exercise performance in cyclists. Med Sci Sports Exerc 36: 504-509.

72. Shevtsov VA, Zholus BI, Shervarly VI, Vol'skij VB, Korovin YP, et al. (2003) A randomized trial of two different doses of a SHR-5 Rhodiola rosea extract versus placebo and control of capacity for mental work. Phytomedicine 10: 95-105.

73. Ha Z, Zhu Y, Zhang X, Cui J, Zhang S, et al. (2002) [The effect of rhodiola and acetazolamide on the sleep architecture and blood oxygen saturation in men living at high altitude]. Zhonghua Jie He He Hu Xi Za Zhi 25: 527-530.

74. Hine CH, Pasi A (1975) Manganese intoxication. West J Med 123: 101-107.

75. Bowler RM, Mergler D, Sassine MP, Larribe F, Hudnell K (1999) Neuropsychiatric effects of manganese on mood. Neurotoxicology 20: 367-378.

76. Kume K (2006) [Molecular biology of biological clock--genetic regulation of circadian rhythm and sleep]. No To Hattatsu 38: 247-252.

77. Sumaya IC, Byers DM, Irwin LN, Del Val S, Moss DE (2004) Circadian-dependent effect of melatonin on dopaminergic D2 antagonist-induced hypokinesia and agonist-induced stereotypies in rats. Pharmacol Biochem Behav 78: 727-733.

78. Khaldy H, León J, Escames G, Bikjdaouene L, García JJ, et al. (2002) Circadian rhythms of dopamine and dihydroxyphenyl acetic acid in the mouse striatum: effects of pinealectomy and of melatonin treatment. Neuroendocrinology 75: 201-208.

79. Bellon A (2006) Searching for new options for treating insomnia: are melatonin and ramelteon beneficial? J Psychiatr Pract 12: 229-243.

80. Roth T, Stubbs C, Walsh JK (2005) Ramelteon (TAK-375), a selective MT1/MT2-receptor agonist, reduces latency to persistent sleep in a model of transient insomnia related to a novel sleep environment. Sleep 28: 303-307.

81. Reiter RJ (2003) Melatonin: clinical relevance. Best Pract Res Clin Endocrinol Metab 17: 273-285.

82. Cramer H, Rudolph J, Consbruch U, Kendel K (1974) On the effects of melatonin on sleep and behavior in man. Adv Biochem Psychopharmacol 11: 187-191.

83. Arendt J, Borbely AA, Franey C, Wright J (1984) The effects of chronic, small doses of melatonin given in the late afternoon on fatigue in man: a preliminary study. Neurosci Lett 45: 317-321.

84. Buscemi N, Vandermeer B, Hooton N, Pandya R, Tjosvold L, et al. (2005) The efficacy and safety of exogenous melatonin for primary sleep disorders. A meta-analysis. J Gen Intern Med 20: 1151-1158.

85. España RA, Scammell TE (2004) Sleep neurobiology for the clinician. Sleep 27: 811-820.

86. Brzezinski A, Vangel MG, Wurtman RJ, Norrie G, Zhdanova I, et al. (2005) Effects of exogenous melatonin on sleep: a meta-analysis. Sleep Med Rev 9: 41-50.

87. Burch JB, Yost MG, Johnson W, Allen E (2005) Melatonin, sleep, and shift work adaptation. J Occup Environ Med 47: 893-901.

88. Zemlan FP, Muchahey JJ, Scharf MB, Mayleben DW, Rosenberg R, et al. (2005) The efficiency and safety of the melatonin against beta-methyl-6 chloromelatonin in primary insomnia: a randomized, placebo-controlled, crossover clinical trial. J Clin Psychiatry 66: 384-90.

89. Gupta M, Aneja S, Kohli K (2005) Add-on melatonin improves sleep behavior in children with epilepsy: randomized, double-blind, placebo-controlled trial. J Child Neurol 20: 112-115.

90. Danilenko KV, Putilov AA (2005) Melatonin treatment of winter depression following total sleep deprivation: waking EEG and mood correlates. Neuropsychopharmacology 30: 1345-1352.

91. Zhdanova I (2005) Reply to the comment on Melatonin as a hypnotic: Pro. J smrv 9: 69-70.

92. Dolberg OT, Hirschmann S, Grunhaus L (1998) Melatonin for the treatment of sleep disturbances in major depressive disorder. Am J Psychiatry 155: 1119-1121.

93. Tanabe K, Osada N, Suzuki N, Nakayama M, Yokoyama Y, et al. (1997) Erythrocyte magnesium and prostaglandin dynamics in chronic sleep deprivation. Clin Cardiol 20: 265-268.

94. Chollet D, Franken P, Raffin Y, Henrotte JG, Widmer J, et al. (2001) Magnesium involvement in sleep: genetic and nutritional models. Behav Genet 31: 413-425.

95. Held K, Antonijevic IA, Künzel H, Uhr M, Wetter TC, et al. (2002) Oral Mg(2+) supplementation reverses age-related neuroendocrine and sleep EEG changes in humans. Pharmacopsychiatry 35: 135-143.

96. Takase B, Akima T, Uehata A, Ohsuzu F, Kurita A (2004) Effect of chronic stress and sleep deprivation on both flow-mediated dilation in the brachial artery and the intracellular magnesium level in humans. Clin Cardiol 27: 223-227.

97. Brower KJ (2013) Treating Insomnia in alcohol-dependent patients. Presented at Omics 2nd International Conference on addiction research & Therapy, July 22-24, Las Vegas, NV, USA

98. Wyatt JK (2004) Delayed sleep phase syndrome: pathophysiology and treatment options. Sleep 27: 1195-1203.

99. Dulcis D, Jamshidi P, Leutgeb S, Spitzer NC (2013) Neurotransmitter switching in the adult brain regulates behavior. Science 340: 449-453.

100. Comings DE, Muhleman D, Gysin R (1996) Dopamine D2 receptor (DRD2) gene and susceptibility to posttraumatic stress disorder: a study and replication. Biol Psychiatry 40: 368-372.

101. Anderson RA (1998) Recent advances in the clinical and biochemical manifestation of chromium deficiency in human and animal nutrition. Journal of Trace Elements in Experimental Medicine 11: 2-3.

102. Petijean F, Buda C, Janin M, Touret M, Salvert D, et al.(1978) Sleep and monoamines: differential radioautography of central neurons after systematic injection of tritiated 5-hydroxytryptophane (5 hTP 3H) or of dihydroxyphenylalanine (DOPA 3H). C R Acad Sci Hebd Seances Acad Sci D 287: 1135-1139.

103. Capasso A, Sorrentino L (2005) Pharmacological studies on the sedative and hypnotic effect of Kava kava and Passiflora extracts combination. Phytomedicine 12: 39-45.

104. Akhondzadeh S, Naghavi HR, Vazirian M, Shayeganpour A, Rashidi H, et al. (2001) Passionflower in the treatment of generalized anxiety: a pilot double-blind randomized controlled trial with oxazepam. J Clin Pharm Ther 26: 363-367.

105. Lechin F, Pardey-Maldonado B, van der Dijs B, Benaim M, Baez S, et al. (2004) Circulating neurotransmitters during the different wake-sleep stages in normal subjects. Psychoneuroendocrinology 29: 669-685.

12

Treatment for Insomnia in Depressed Adolescents

Deirdre A. Conroy* and Edward D. Huntley

University of Michigan, Department of Psychiatry, 4250 Plymouth Road, Ann Arbor, MI 48109, USA

Abstract

Objective: Sleep undergoes dramatic changes during the adolescent years due to biological, circadian, and psychosocial influences. It is now known that sleep loss, both acute and chronic, can affect emotion regulation and can increase the likelihood of developing depression and risky behaviors.

Method: The authors carried out a systematic review utilizing the PubMed database by using the search terms including: "adolescence, depression, sleep, and insomnia." The present review covers manuscripts accepted up to the year 2013. The following review discusses findings on the bidirectional relationship between insomnia and depression and will cover current evaluation and treatment options.

Results: Depression can be present in up to 20 percent of adolescents and most of these children will have some form of sleep disturbance. The etiology of sleep disturbances may reflect insomnia, circadian rhythm sleep disorder, sleep apnea, or other factors. Pharmacological and cognitive behavioral therapy approaches are common, but may result in limited gains due to persistent insomnia. Antidepressant medications may be lessened and relapse may be higher in those with insomnia. Treatment monitoring may be helped by motivational interviewing techniques and examining the teen's self-report over parental sleep reports.

Conclusion: Sleep disturbances that are identified, addressed, and appropriately monitored may result in improved sleep and mood. Active involvement of the teen in the therapy process may improve outcomes. Further research is needed to develop non-pharmacological strategies that are acceptable and sustainable for adolescents.

Keywords: Adolescents; Sleep and mood; Antidepressant medications; Circadian rhythm; Insomnia

Introduction

Sleep undergoes dramatic changes during the adolescent years due to biological, circadian, and psychosocial influences[1]. While there is a wide range of individual variability, there is a consistent trend in a decrease of total sleep time in healthy children between the ages of 11 and 15 [2]. In addition to a reduction in the number of hours teens sleep, there are also age-related changes in the quality and timing of sleep. For example, deep slow wave sleep duration, (a proxy for sleep quality and restorative sleep) which makes up nearly half of the sleep period in childhood, declines by 27% from early adolescence to late adolescence [3]. While it is not yet clear whether these declines are associated with functional outcomes during adolescence, it is a critical time for emerging psychiatric disorders.

Additionally, the body's internal clock—which regulates sleep (also called circadian rhythm)—shifts to a later clock time. This delay in the timing of the sleep/wake cycle during adolescence is across-cultural phenomenon [4] and is theorized to potentially be caused by a change in the circadian timekeeping mechanism due to pubertal hormones [5].

Regulation of the circadian rhythm is highly dependent upon exposure to bright light. Depending on the timing and the level of light, this exposure can reset the timing of sleep. For example, light exposure at night can cause the synthesis of the "night hormone" melatonin to be suppressed and shift the circadian rhythm to a later time [6].

As the circadian rhythm drifts to a later time, teens may prefer to interact socially (either in person or online) at night and delay the start of sleep. In fact, weekend bedtimes have been found to be delayed by approximately three hours between the ages of 11 to 18 [4].

Essentially, the circadian timing and quality of sleep in healthy teens undergo changes during adolescence, which may increase vulnerability to depression or chronic sleep disturbances like insomnia. Depression is diagnosed in up to 20 percent of adolescents, [7] and up to 90 percent of those adolescents also have sleep complaints. Adolescents with depression may experience exacerbation of sleep problems as well as the consequences of poor sleep. Insomnia can be a symptom of depression and can also be a distinct co-occurring illness with a chronic course in depressed youth. This becomes important as depression is a predictor of depression relapse. According to a meta-analysis of 21 longitudinal epidemiological studies investigating sleep complaints and depression, even healthy individuals with insomnia were found to be twice as likely(confidence interval [CI]: 1.98-3.42) to become depressed compared to people without sleep complaints [8]. This review will focus on understanding the complexity of sleep complaints in the context of depression during the teen years, along with diagnostic assessments, clinical decision making, and treatment interventions for insomnia in depressed adolescents.

Methods

The authors carried out a systematic review utilizing the PubMed database by using the search terms including: "adolescence, depression, sleep, and insomnia." The present review covers manuscripts accepted up to the year 2013. The following review discusses findings on the bidirectional relationship between insomnia and depression and will cover current evaluation and treatment options.

***Corresponding author:** Deirdre A. Conroy, Ph.D. University of Michigan, Department of Psychiatry, 4250 Plymouth Road, Ann Arbor, MI 48109, USA
E-mail: daconroy@umich.edu

Results

The bidirectional relationship between depression and insomnia during adolescence

The directionality of the relationship between depression and insomnia across the lifespan is complicated; it is a topic that is under investigation by a number of research groups.

It is now known that sleep loss, both acutely and chronic, can affect emotion regulation and can increase the likelihood of developing depression [9] and risky behaviors [10,11]. Depression and risky behaviors, such as substance use may also lead to insomnia. The relationship between sleep hours and risky behaviors was examined in a 2007 survey entitled the "National Youth Risk Behavior Survey." This population survey analyzed reports of the sleep and behaviors of approximately 12,000 US high school students. The study revealed that teenagers who obtained insufficient sleep ("insufficient sleep" defined as less than 8 hours a night; 69% of the sample) were almost twice as likely to drink alcohol(AOR, 1.64; 95% CI, 1.46-1.84);, use marijuana(AOR, 1.52; 95% CI, 1.31-1.76),, be sexually active(AOR, 1.41; 95% CI, 1.25-1.59);, to seriously consider attempting suicide(AOR, 1.86; 95% CI, 1.60-2.16),as well as feel sad or hopeless(AOR, 1.62; 95% CI, 1.43-1.84) [12].

Another large scale study utilizing data from 700 teenage participants examined both cross-sectional and longitudinal components contributing to the bidirectional nature of sleep and substance use. The study adjusted for the presence of depression, socio demographic characteristics, pubertal status, and body mass index. In adolescents between 11 and 18 years of age, shorter sleep periods during the school week were related to greater likelihood of alcohol use. Longitudinal follow up after two years revealed that achieving more sleep during the week predicted lower cigarette and marijuana use [13].

Insomnia symptoms may begin early in life and may increase risk for depression. Two studies have highlighted this issue. In an epidemiological study, lifetime questionnaire data about insomnia was collected in approximately 1,000 adolescents between 13 and 16 years of age. Results showed that the median age of insomnia onset was during the 11th year of life. In girls, onset of menses was associated with an onset of insomnia; yet, in boys, maturational development was not a factor. Over half of the adolescents with insomnia in that sample also had a comorbid psychiatric disorder [14].

In a prospective study depression and insomnia scores were examined in approximately 3,000 youths between ages of 11 through 17. Researchers found that baseline insomnia (either with or without daytime impairment) increased risk for major depression 2- to 3-fold. Given that the presence of daytime impairment caused by insomnia is a diagnostic necessity, this suggests that even those without insomnia diagnosis, but with sleep symptoms only may still be at risk for depression. The reverse was also true;i.e., major depression increased the risk for symptoms of insomnia, with and without impairment [15].

Studies comparing the sleep of depressed children and adolescents to healthy control children and adolescence suggest that there are differences in sleep that can be measured objectively. These objective differences may influence clinical outcome. In one study, researchers investigated the relationship between sleep polysomnography (PSG) in depressed children and adolescents and the clinical course of the disorder. Depressed adolescents with decreased sleep efficiency (defined as a measure of total sleep time divided by time in bed) and a "delayed" sleep onset (defined as >10 minutes) had a probability of recurrence of depression at 12 months of 0.39 compared to 0.15 in subjects with non-delayed sleep onset (p=0.005) [16]. More sophisticated analyses of the sleep electroencephalogram—such as temporal coherence (the degree of synchrony between all night EEG rhythms) was significantly lower in adolescents with MDD, compared to healthy controls [17]. These studies raise the question of whether temporal coherence is a state or trait feature of depression and the clinical correlates of low coherence [18]. Lastly, a study using actigraphy to measure sleep patterns in depressed adolescents showed that there were differences in the rest/activity cycles. For example, lower activity levels, lower light exposure, and less time spent in bright light (>1000 lux) were found in depressed adolescents compared to healthy controls. Depressed girls, in particular, were prone to having a dampened circadian amplitude, thought to reflect weak entrainment to a 24-hour day [19].

The natural preference to initiate sleep at a later time may provide more time for teens to socialize or use electronics. This may unintentionally precipitate/contribute to and perpetuate symptoms of depression. For example, frequent use of social media at night may contribute to increased anxiety or cognitive rumination. A recent study found an association between social networking and higher depression scores [20]. Unresolved anxiety and guilt about the day's events may also interfere with sleep onset. Catastrophic worry has been found to partially mediate the relationship between adolescent sleep disturbances and depressive symptoms [21]. In high school students with early school start times the next day, this may limit the opportunity to meet ones physiological sleep need [22]. While this is highly individual and difficult to determine [23], this can result in chronic sleep deprivation during a time when sufficient sleep is essential for physician and emotional maturation. Clinical interventions, such as establishing a "worry time" has been shown to be effective in decreasing pre-sleep cognitive arousal in a college student population [24].

In summary, to date, research suggests an association between sleep disturbances and depression. Short sleep time, subjective sleep complaints, and/or objective signs (PSG) of sleep disturbance may lead to increased risk of the onset or recurrence of depression. On the other hand, insomnia is common in depression. The cognitive, behavioral, and biological rhythm changes associated with depression may exacerbate the sleep disturbance.

The Consequences of sleep disturbance during adolescence

According to the National Sleep Foundation, 61%of teenagers are chronically sleep deprived [25]. Sleep deprivation at any age can impair one's ability to regulate emotions and can also impair judgment. As a result, chronic sleep deprivation in healthy teens has been associated with unintentional injuries, poor school performance [26], substance use [27], obesity [28], and the risk for suicide [29-31]. Adolescents with a preexisting history of major depressive disorder may be at even greater risk for these outcomes.

In 1998, researchers found that high school students who were struggling academically reported that they slept 25 minutes less and went to bed 40 minutes later than those getting As and Bs [32]. Approximately fifteen years later, adolescents are likely either sleeping the same or fewer minutes [2]. This negative trajectory may be associated with other academic, emotional and physical changes in adolescent health [33].

In addition to poor school performance, sleep deprivation in teens has been shown to be associated with depression in cross-sectional studies [34]; further, in a longitudinal study, it has been found to exacerbate depression symptoms in middle school students [35]. In addition to short total sleep time, "chronotype" (which refers to the time at which a person prefers to be awake and asleep according to their body's internal clock) may be playing an interactive role. Teens who categorize themselves as having an evening preference have more daytime complaints (such as attention problems, poor school achievement, and becoming emotionally upset) than other non-evening types [34]. Self-described "morning -type" adolescents have shown fewer waking problems and female morning types appear to show less externalizing and internalizing problems [36]. Furthermore, when examining the role of both sleep deprivation and chronotype on emotions (e.g. positive affect vs. negative affect), all participants reported lower positive affect when sleep deprived, but evening types reported less positive affect regardless of being sleep deprived or rested. The authors suggest that evening chronotype be a marker of emotional vulnerability [37].

Studies have now found that sleep disturbance (e.g. typically defined generally as "trouble sleeping" by a parent) plays a significant role in suicidal ideation, self-harm, and completed suicide. In 2010, researchers examined the subjective sleep reports from approximately 16,000 adolescents who participated in the National Longitudinal Study of Adolescent Health. The sample included teens in grades 7 through 12 in the United States between 1994 and 1996. The researchers found that adolescents with later bedtimes had greater likelihood of suicidal ideation and the perception that they were not getting enough sleep [38]. Two studies by Wong and Brower [39,40] examined whether sleep problems were prospectively associated with reports of suicidal ideation and self-harm. The investigators controlled for depression at baseline. Those who had trouble sleeping between ages 12-14 were four-times more likely to deliberately harm themselves or attempt suicide by 15-17 years of age (OR=10.4, 95% CI=3.9 to 27.8, $p<.01$) [40]. A third study examined retrospective reports found that adolescents who completed suicide were ten-times (OR = 10.4, 95% CI = 3.9 to 27.8, $p< .01$) more likely to have been experiencing sleep problems prior to suicide compared to controls [41,42].

Diagnostic Assessment

Depression

In the diagnostic assessment of depression in an adolescent, the clinician will typically use a combination of a semi-structured clinical interview **(Children's Depression Rating Scale, Revised (CDRS-R),** self-report symptom inventories (e.g. CDI, Reynolds Adolescent Depression Scale, BDI, Center for Epidemiological Studies-Depression Scale for Children) and rating scales completed either by the patient or by an observer, such as a parent or teacher. See Table 1. The diagnosis of depression is made based on a set of symptoms outlined in the Diagnostic and Statistical Manual of Mental Disorders (DSM).It is worthy of note that in the latest version of DSM, DSM –V, differs from DSM-IV as anxiety symptoms such as irrational worry or preoccupation with unpleasant worries may also indicate depression. In addition, new disorders have been included such as disruptive mood dysregulation disorder and premenstrual dysphoric disorder. Dysthymia in DSM-IV now falls under the category of persistent depressive disorder, which includes both chronic major depressive disorder and the previous dysthymic disorder [43].

While the criteria for the diagnosis of major depression in adolescents do not differ from the criteria used in adults, certain symptoms of depression may be more prominent at certain young ages (e.g. irritability in children or adolescents) [44]. The adolescent must meet at least five of nine symptoms of depression to meet diagnosis. These symptoms must represent a change from prior functioning, be present for two weeks or longer, and be present for most of the time almost every day. See Table 2.

Insomnia

According to the diagnostic criteria outlined in the International Classification of Sleep Disorders, Second Edition, [45] insomnia is defined by difficulty falling asleep, staying asleep, waking too early, and having non-restorative sleep. This difficulty must be present despite adequate opportunity to sleep and must be associated with next-day impairment. The fact that the sleep difficulty must occur despite adequate opportunity to sleep distinguishes insomnia from behaviorally-induced insufficient sleep syndrome. Both disorders, however, can result in short sleep periods and an accumulation of sleep debt.

Assessment for insomnia begins with a full clinical evaluation. The clinician takes a thorough history of the insomnia from the patient, which may include information about the primary symptoms, frequency, and duration of the insomnia, as well as triggers or precipitants of the sleep disturbance. Information about the individual's sleep prior to the onset of the insomnia helps to provide baseline sleep information. Obtaining a medication list, their doses, and their previous effectiveness is helpful. For example, stimulants and steroids can contribute to insomnia symptoms.

It can be difficult to ascertain whether the insomnia is associated only with the underlying depression (as insomnia is one of the symptoms of depression), or whether it reflects an independent sleep disorder. An understanding of the relationship between the insomnia and depression over time is warranted. For example, did the insomnia begin coincidently with the onset of depression? What has been the course of the two disorders? Does the insomnia wax and wane in unison with the depression over time? Use of a timeline may be helpful but may still be difficult to discern from the patient. Therefore, use of collateral information from parent/caregiver would be helpful.

The next step of the assessment includes the patient's description of their current sleep pattern. This may include obtaining information such as typical bedtime, how long it takes to fall asleep, how many awakenings occur, how long the individual spends awake during the night, and wake time. A distinction between the time the individual awakens in the morning and what time they physically get out of bed (also called "rise time") provides information about early morning awakenings. Typically this information is collected each day in a sleep diary [46] and patients meet either weekly or biweekly with their therapist. Sleep diaries in addition to actigraphy, a watch-like device to monitor daily activity patterns, can provide valuable information.

Measure Children and Adolescents	Age appropriateness (approximate years)
Beck Depression Inventory (BDI)[92]	14 and older
Children's Depression Inventory (CDI)[93]	7 to 17
Center for Epidemiological Studies-Depression Scale for Children (CES-DC) [94]	12 to 18
Center for Epidemiological Studies-Depression Scale (CES-D)[95]	14 and older
Reynolds Adolescent Depression Scale[96]	13 to 18

Table 1: Scales for Measuring Mood in Children and Adolescents.

1.	Depressed mood [b]
2.	Significant reduction in the level of interest or pleasure in most or all activities[b]
3.	Loss or gain of weight, characterized by a change of more than 5 percent of body weight in a month or failure to make expected weight gains
4.	Insomnia or hypersomnia is present nearly every day
5.	Behavior may be agitated or slowed down
6.	Adolescents may report diminished energy or fatigue
7.	Thoughts of worthlessness or guilt
8.	Reduced ability to think, concentrate, or make decisions
9.	Frequent thoughts of death or suicide, or a suicide attempt

[a]These symptoms cannot be attributed to another cause such as drugs or another medical condition . [b]Required for diagnosis

Table 2: Depressive symptomatology a depression in adolescents[a]

Understanding the impact of the sleep problem on next-day functioning is important. Examples of common daytime disturbances may include impaired concentration or memory, fatigue, daytime sleepiness, or excessive sleep concerns.Ohayon et al. (2102) found that global sleep dissatisfaction is the symptom most helpful in identifying daytime consequences [47].

Concerns about sleep are common;they characterize a specific type of insomnia known as psychophysiological insomnia. Adolescents with depression may present with features of this type of insomnia [21]. In adult patients with psychophysiological insomnia, there is "hyperarousal" about sleep—that is, they have excessive focus and heightened anxiety about sleep. Often, they will report mind racing in bed or an inability to relax their body in bed. Sleeping better away from home can sometimes be present, suggesting that the patient's bed or bedroom have become a source of anxiety.

Clinical Decision Making: Differential Diagnoses

Behaviorally induced insufficient sleep syndrome (BIISS)

BIISS is a common phenomenon for adolescents. Insufficient sleep can result when one does not allow adequate opportunity for sleep. It is typically characterized by excessive daytime sleepiness, short habitual sleep time, and sleeping longer than usual during weekends or vacations. In a large study of approximately 1200 Norwegian adolescents, BIISS was associated with poor grades, alcohol use, and symptoms of depression and anxiety [48].

Delayed Sleep Phase Syndrome

During adolescence, there is a natural tendency for the underlying biological rhythm to drift to a later clock time. This developmental shift in circadian rhythm phase can cause sleep difficulty and impair daytime functioning. Delayed sleep phase syndrome is a mismatch between the internal biological rhythm and preferred schedule. The complaints typically include difficulty falling asleep when attempting to go to sleep at an earlier clock time than usual. Once sleep is initiated, however, the amount and quality of sleep is normal for the individual's age.Difficulty waking at planned rise time is also not unusual and can result in high conflict with caregiver.

When these complaints begin to interfere with daily functioning, this may be diagnosed as a sleep disorder called delayed sleep phase syndrome (DSPS).Rates of this disorder range between 0.2 percent and 10 percent [49,50] of the population butis more common in adolescents [14]. Delayed circadian sleep phase may increase the risk of developing depression [51] and people who prefer to be awake at night (or "night owls") have greater incidence of depression [52].

Differentiating whether an adolescent has sleep onset insomnia versus a delayed circadian sleep phase can be tricky. It is also possible that there are components of both disorders at play. The use of a questionnaire, such as the Horne-ÖstbergMorningness-Eveningness Questionnaire (MEQ), [53] may be of benefit because it may highlight a mismatch between internal clock and preferred schedule.

Sleep Apnea

The complaint of insomnia may reflect an underlying primary sleep disorder. In the process of taking a thorough clinical history, clinicians should inquire about symptoms of sleep-disordered breathing and sleep apnea. These symptoms may include loud snoring, pauses in breathing while sleeping, gasping or choking in sleep. A dry mouth and a headache may be present upon morning awakening.

There is a line of research suggesting that Sleep-Related Breathing Disorders (SRBD) play a key role in the development of depression. Children with SRBD have shown higher scores on depression scales [54,55].

A correlation was also found in this population between severity of the apnea-hypopnea index, oxygen desaturation values, and depression scores [56]. Treatments for sleep-disordered breathing may be of benefit. Treatments can include nasal Positive Airway Pressure (PAP) therapy, an oral appliance, or upper airway surgeries.

In a case report, an 18 year old with treatment-resistant depression who underwent a procedure to widen the upper airway (a procedure called rapid palatal expansion) to treat his upper airway resistance syndrome resulted in marked improvement in mood and sleep. Two years after his last ECT treatment, the patient was in remission and maintained improvement off all psychotropic medications [57]. A questionnaires—such as the "STOP [58] questionnaire" (which is a four item scale that asks about snoring, daytime tiredness, stopping breathing during sleep, and high blood pressure)—may be of benefit.

Other Considerations

There are a number of other sleep and psychiatric disorders that may be considered. Here, some additional differential diagnoses are discussed. When insomnia is temporally associated with use or abuse of the substance or its withdrawal, insomnia due to a drug or substance may be considered [45]. Information regarding the use of substances—such as alcohol, recreation drugs, or prescription drug abuse (for example, taking medications in a way that was not prescribed or taking medications that were not prescribed to that individual) or other risky behaviors[59]—will help guide the clinical interview.

When substances such as alcohol, nicotine, or caffeine are used just before bedtime, the patient may have inadequate sleep hygiene. Inadequate sleep hygiene can accompany a diagnosis of insomnia and typically includes practices such as a variable sleep schedule, spending excessive amount of time in bed, use of mentally stimulating activities (such as video games or social media) close to bedtime, or failure to maintain a comfortable sleeping environment [45].

Other primary sleep disorders might also be considered in the context of insomnia complaints in an adolescent. If they are available to the clinician, it is helpful to review any previous sleep studies that the patient might have undergone. The sleep study will provide information about sleep continuity (for example, latency to sleep and wakefulness during the night) and will describe any sleep pathology (for example, sleep apnea or periodic limb movements in sleep).

If the patient has not undergone a sleep study and suspicion of other occult sleep pathology is present (such as snoring or choking in sleep), a referral for a diagnostic polysomnogram (PSG) at an accredited sleep disorders center is warranted.

If the adolescent reports restlessness at night, further inquiry about symptoms of restless legs syndrome (RLS) or periodic limb movement disorder may be warranted.Obtaining a thorough family history of sleep disorders may help provide additional information as RLS may have a genetic component. RLS might also be associated with diet, so asking teens about diet (e.g. green leafy vegetables) is important.

Finally, if the teen reports significant daytime sleepiness for at least three months with or without episodes of cataplexy, one may consider referring for an evaluation for narcolepsy In this case, however, the excessive daytime sleepiness must not be due to a medical, psychiatric, medication, or substance-use problem. If suspicion is high for any primary sleep disorder, a referral for a diagnostic PSG is recommended. If there is suspicion of narcolepsy, a PSG followed by a next-day Multiple Sleep Latency Test (MSLT) may is indicated.

Administering Treatment Interventions

If, after the clinical interview, the insomnia appears to be associated in time with the depression, a referral to initiate psychological intervention or to continue psychological follow up may be indicated. If the underlying mood disorder improves with psychological or psychopharmacological treatment, the insomnia may improve as well. Cognitive Behavioral Therapy (CBT) for depression and antidepressant therapy are common treatments.

While these treatments independently or in combination may be helpful for some teens, data from a large study on this topic suggests that CBT plus a selective Serotonin Reuptake Inhibitor (SSRI) was only minimally effective in helping teens fully remit from depression (a 37 percent remission rate) after three months [60]. This may be due, in part, to sleep disturbance, as insomnia is one of the most common residual symptoms in teens with low response rates [60,61] to CBT and SSRI therapy for depression. For this reason, addressing the sleep disturbance directly may be beneficial. Pharmacological and nonpharmacological options are available. A referral to a board certified behavioral sleep medicine specialist for nonpharmacological treatment delivery is best if there is a clinician with this distinction the area.

A Nonpharmacological Option

Cognitive Behavioral Therapy for Insomnia (CBT-I) is the current recommended approach for nonpharmacological treatment of chronic insomnia [62]. This multicomponent therapy, which includes behavioral and cognitive strategies to improve sleep quality and daytime functioning, benefits 70 to 80 percent of insomnia patients and has more sustained benefits than medications in adults [63-66].

Components of CBT-I include a combination of behavioral techniques (including stimulus control, sleep restriction, and relaxation) combined with sleep hygiene education and cognitive therapy.

There are four main components of CBT-I:

1. Stimulus control: The primary goals of stimulus control therapy for insomnia are to help the insomnia patient establish a consistent sleep/wake rhythm, reestablish the bed and bedroom as cues for sleep and sleepiness, and reduce the bedroom's association with sleep-incompatible activities.
2. Sleep restriction: Sleep restriction therapy is based on the clinical observation that insomnia patients spend excessive amounts of time in bed to compensate for sleep loss. The therapy is designed to have patients limit the amount of time they spend in bed to approximate the amount that they are actually sleeping, as ascertained by baseline sleep logs. The major goal of this strategy is to build the "drive for sleep" by restricting sleep to shorter periods of time spent in bed and by prohibiting sleep at times outside of this restricted sleep schedule.
3. Sleep hygiene education: Sleep hygiene education is a set of guidelines about health practices and environmental considerations that can either aid or disturb the quality and quantity of sleep. Sleep hygiene is recommended as part of a comprehensive treatment approach. It is considered a second-line intervention because there are insufficient data supporting its use as a stand-alone treatment for insomnia.
4. Cognitive therapy: Cognitive therapy for insomnia alters the dysfunctional beliefs about sleep which perpetuate insomnia; further, it helps patients develop realistic expectations about their sleep. The best candidates are those patients who worry about how much sleep they need (such as a patient saying "I need eight hours of sleep"), the consequences of their insomnia (as with a patient saying "Without adequate sleep, I can barely function the next day"), the predictability of their sleep ("I'm losing control of my sleep"), or strategies used to promote sleep ("I should stay in bed and try harder to fall asleep").

Other adjunctive therapies may include relaxation therapy for patients who "cannot relax" or who report feeling too "keyed up." There are several types of relaxation, including progressive muscle relaxation, diaphragmatic breathing, autogenic training, guided imagery, and biofeedback.

Adding CBT-Ito depression therapy

In adults, adding an insomnia treatment component to antidepressant therapy can improve both depression and insomnia outcomes. For example, in a 2008 study, depressed participants with insomnia were randomly assigned either to take escitalopramplus a CBT-I or to anescitalopram plus a control condition. Rates of remission for both depression and insomnia weremarkedly higher for those treated with the escitalopramplus CBTI compared to those treated with escitalopram and the control condition [67].

Another group compared antidepressant therapy plus placebo to antidepressant therapy plus the hypnotic medicationeszopiclone. They found that the treatment with the added hypnotic improved depression response and remission [68].

Unfortunately, few randomized, controlled studies of nonpharmacological treatment options for depressed adolescents with sleep disturbances have been conducted. One study utilized cognitive behavioral therapy for insomnia in adolescents in substance abuse treatment and foundimproved sleep [69]. Other adjunctive treatment options are described below.

Behavioral activation

Behavioural Activation (BA) can be a powerful compliment to sleep restriction and stimulus control. This brief psychotherapeutic approach aims to increase engagement in adaptive activities, decrease engagement in activities that maintain depression or increase risk for depression, as well as solve problems that limit access to reward. [70] Including behavioral activation and exercise into one's therapy approaches can be powerful adjuncts [71,72].

Bright light therapy

Light therapy can be used to treat both mood and sleep disorders at any age. Seasonal Affective Disorder (SAD) occurs in approximately 2% of adolescents and is higher in adolescent females [73]. Commons symptoms of season affective disorder may include fatigue, irritability, and school problems that are confined to the winter months. Light therapy for SAD has been successfully utilized as a therapeutic approach in adults [74], but few studies have been conducted utilizing bright light therapy in SAD in adolescents. Additional randomized controlled trails on morning light therapy for depression in a teenage population are underway [75]. In one of the first randomized controlled trials of light therapy in children (ages 7-17) with SAD, participants who received 1 hour of bright-light therapy plus 2 hours of dawn simulation had significant improvements in their Hamilton Depression Rating Scale, Seasonal Affective Disorders version (SIGH-SAD) compared to those in a placebo condition [76]. Similar findings were revealed in a 14-17 year old sample who underwent light therapy in a randomized cross-over trial. Beck's depression inventory scores improved significantly [77].

Circadian rhythm sleep disorders, e.g. delayed sleep phase syndrome (DSPS) also reponds well to bright light therapy. Delayed circadian sleep phase occurs in 7-16% of adolescents and young adults [78]. If it is suspected that the patient has a circadian rhythm sleep disorder, they may benefit from sleep scheduling combined with bright light therapy. The time of day that the light is delivered and the light level is important to consider in the treatment of circadian rhythm disorder.

In adolescents with DSPS, teens can begin the light therapy after their normal wake-up time and then shift it about 15 to 30 minutes earlier every day or every few days. The light shifts the internal clock to an earlier time and helps the teen initiate sleep at an earlier bedtime.

Bright light plus a CBT-Icondition has been shown to be effective. When in 23 healthy adolescents with delayed sleep phase received bright light and CBT-I (the CBT-I consisted of six sessions and included education, sleep hygiene, and plans for morning bright light)results showed that compared to waitlist control groups, teens in the treatment condition showed improvements in sleep and an earlier sleep onset time [79]. Adherence over time to this treatment can be challenging in teenagers.

Pharmacological Options

Residual symptoms are common in adolescents who respond to antidepressant treatment interventions. Research findings from the Treatment for Adolescents with Depression Study reveal that residual sleep disturbances, mood problems, and fatigue are some of the most common residual symptoms [60]. These symptoms can increase the likelihood of a relapse to depression.

To determine the influence of insomnia on acute treatment intervention for depression, a large study was conducted on 309 depressed children and adolescents between 7 to 18 years of age with insomnia. Children were defined as 11 years of age and younger; adolescents as 12 years of age and older. Insomnia was defined as a score of greater than four on the sleep item on the Children's Depression Rating Scale. One hundred fifty-seven participants were randomized to receive fluoxetine and one hundred fifty two participants were randomized to placebo for 8-9 weeks.

Adolescents with insomnia were less likely to respond to fluoxetine (39.2%; 20/51) than those without (65.9%; 27/41; p=0.013), whereas children on fluoxetine with insomnia were more likely to respond (69.4%; 25/36) than those without insomnia (41.4%; 12/29; p=0.027). [80] This study suggests that insomnia may interfere with the response to antidepressant medications and highlights the need for targeted insomnia treatment in adolescent depression.

To obtain a better understanding of the prescribing practices in child psychiatry, in 2010, a large survey was sent out to approximately 6,000 members of the American Academy of Child and Adolescent Psychiatry. Child psychiatrists said that they were more likely to use sleep medications in children with mood and anxiety disorders, particularly for the more severe disorders (such as bipolar disorder and PTSD). Clinicians typically prescribed pharmacological therapies to improve daytime functioning—but also added that they were concerned about side effects and lack of empirical support regarding efficacy.

Non-Benzodiazepine Receptor Agonists

The commonly-used hypnotics in adults—such as benzodiazepine receptor agonists like zolpidem, eszopiclone, and zaleplon have limited research studies on their use in teenagers. In adolescents who had attention-deficit hyperactivity disorder-associated insomnia, a double-blind, placebo-controlled, parallel-group study was conducted. Zolpidem (at a maximum of 10 mg) failed to reduce the latency to persistent sleep on polysomnographic recordings after 4 weeks of treatment in children and adolescents 6 through 17 years of age [81].

Some clinicians may be reticent about prescribing these medications in this population amid concerns of illicit use or misuse. The 2009 National Survey on Drug Use and Health, which included a sample of more than 17,000 adolescents (ages 12 to 17), had a 1.4 percent lifetime prevalence of misusing zolpidem. Older and white adolescents were at an increased risk for zolpidem misuse. Those who reported a major depressive episode (OR=4.16) had four-times the risk of misusing zolpidem [82].

Melatonin

Melatonin is a hormone naturally produced by the pineal gland in the brain. It plays an important role in the regulation of sleep through a feedback system controlled by the suprachiasmatic nuclei—also known as the body's master clock.

In the American Academy of Child and Adolescent Psychiatry Survey, approximately one-third of respondents said they recommended melatonin to adolescents with sleep problems. However, there is concern about the use of melatonin in children and adolescents because of the role it plays in the reproductive systems in animals [83].

For other clinicians, melatonin is considered to be a safe treatment with the appropriate dosage and timing of administration. A recent study on prepubertal children (ages 6 through 12) who had been taking melatonin for difficulty initiating sleep at an average dose of 2.69 mg for 3.1 years did not find any changes in pubertal development or mental health changes [84].

In most European countries, melatonin is a prescription-only medication. Among hypnotic prescriptions written for children in Norway (ages 0 to 17), melatonin was dispensed in the highest annual amount of all hypnotic drugs. Between 2004 and 2011, melatonin use increased steadily from 6 to 12 years of age, and this was most pronounced in males [85].

While more than one-third of clinicians recommend melatonin for insomnia in pediatric populations, the research regarding melatonin in pediatric sleep disorders is somewhat limited [86]. Melatonin does have empirical supports for its use as a "chrono-biotic;"i.e., as an agent that helps shift one's internal circadian clock. However, it is important to note that in the US, melatonin is a hormone that is not a Food and Drug Administration- approved medication.

In one study, researchers administered melatonin 1 mg in the evening to adolescents 14 to 19 years old with sleep onset insomnia. In this placebo-controlled crossover study, teenagers received the melatonin in the evening for five weeks between 4:30 pm and 6:00 pm. Results showed that after five weeks, teens reported earlier sleep-onset times and sleep length was longer compared with the baseline week [87].

Trazodone

Trazodone is a commonly-prescribed medication for the treatment of insomnia in both the adult and pediatric populations. According to a survey of the American Academy of Child and Adolescent Psychiatry members, trazodone was the most commonly-prescribed insomnia medication for children with mood disorders (78%) and anxiety disorders (72%) [88].

In 2008, a large, randomized, controlled trial called the Treatment of Resistant Depression in Adolescents (TORDIA) study was conducted by Brent and colleagues. Approximately 300 adolescents who did not respond to SSRI therapy were studied. Patients were randomized to one of four categories: (1) they were switched to another SSRI;(2) they were prescribed venlafaxine XR; (3) they were prescribed another SSRI plus CBT; or (4) they were prescribed venlafaxine plus CBT.

After 3 months, 55 percent of the adolescents in the CBT plus medication responded—compared to only 40 percent of those who received medication alone. Patients who had also been prescribed a medication for insomnia at the treating clinician's discretion, had even lower response rates to treatment [89].

A separate study reporting a more detailed analysis of the Brent 2008 study revealed that adolescents who were prescribed trazodone were six-times less likely to respond to treatment (adjusted odds ratio [OR]=0.16, 95% confidence interval [CI]: 0.05-0.50, p=0.001) than those with no sleep medication. In addition, they were three-times more likely to engage in self-harming behaviors(OR=3.0, 95% CI: 1.1-7.9, p=0.03).Adolescents treated with other sleep medications (such as antihistamines and non-benzodiazepines) did not fare much better and still had greater likelihood of self-harming behavior [90].

In summary, prescribing practices for adolescents may differ by clinician preference. To date, few studies have explored the use of non-benzodiazepine receptor agonists (e.g. zolpidem, escopiclone) in adolescents. Recommendations to use melatonin are common, however data is lacking to support its use as a hypnotic in teens; there is some evidence to support its use as a chronobiotic. Trazodone is a commonly prescribed medication for insomnia in teens with mood disorders, but has been shown to be associated with decrease response rate to depression treatment and an increased likelihood of self-harming behaviors.

Treatment Monitoring

Treatment monitoring for sleep disorders typically includes completing a daily sleep diary. Actigraphy may also be used to collect information about sleep/wake patterns, although the use of actigraphy is more often utilized in research studies. In this analysis, the patient wears a wrist watch-like device on their nondominant hand called an actigraph—a device that is placed generally where a wristwatch is worn to collect daily patterns of motor activity. Actigraphy is most informative when used in conjunction with the sleep diary.

There are some barriers that may arise with treatment monitoring with adolescents with depression and sleep disturbance. First, motivational issues may limit the patient's ability to engage in and benefit from therapy. Even when an adolescent has achieved therapeutic gains during the therapy process (such as sleeping better), the maintenance of those treatment gains may drop once the adolescent has left therapy [91-95].

Treatments may be improved with motivational interviewing or motivational enhancement techniques. Another barrier may arise if the clinician chooses to obtain a parental report of the adolescent's sleep pattern instead of or in addition to direct reporting from the adolescent. Parents may either provide socially-desirable reports or report on the time the adolescent goes into their room intending to sleep, but might not actually be sleeping.

To explore this phenomenon, researchers obtained parental reports of adolescent sleep patterns and compared them to the adolescent's personal reports of sleep habits and to actigraphy [91]. The study revealed that parents estimated that their adolescent went to bed significantly earlier and woke up significantly later in the morning than was captured by actigraphy and by adolescent self-report.This was true on both school nights and weekends. This study suggests that more a more accurate picture of the adolescent's sleep patterns may be obtained from the adolescent themselves as opposed to parental report.

In conclusion, depression can be present in up to 20 percent of adolescents and most of these children will have some form of sleep disturbance. The etiology of the sleep disturbances can be multifactorial, including (but not limited to) insomnia, circadian rhythm sleep disorder, sleep apnea, or other factors. These sleep disturbances can play either a precipitating or perpetuating role in depression during these years. Pharmacological and cognitive behavioral therapy approaches are common but may result in limited gains. The limitation in gains may be associated, at least in part, to the presence of insomnia. If insomnia is present, the effectiveness of the antidepressant medications may be lessened and relapse may be higher. Unfortunately, few nonpharmacological treatment studies for insomnia have been conducted in depressed teens. Treatment monitoring may be helped by motivational interviewing techniques and examining the teen's self-report over parental sleep reports.

Sleep disturbances that are identified, addressed, and appropriately monitored may result in improved sleep and mood. Active involvement of the teen in the therapy process may improve outcomes. Further research is needed to develop non-pharmacological strategies that are acceptable and sustainable for adolescents.

Conclusion

Depression is common during the adolescent years, occurring in up to 20% of adolescents. Mostof these children have some form of sleep disturbance. Research studies have revealed that insomnia in teens may precipitate or perpetuate depression. Untreated sleep disturbances in adolescents may to lead to negative consequences, such as academic problems, substance abuse, and risk for suicide. The etiology of sleep disturbances may reflect insomnia, circadian rhythm sleep disorder, sleep apnea, or other factors. Treatment interventions may include pharmacological or non-pharmacological options (e.g. cognitive behavioral therapy, bright light therapy, behavioral activation). Pharmacological approaches have been found to be helpful in some studies, but other studies suggest that they may result in limited gains if insomnia persists. Treatment monitoring may be helped by motivational interviewing techniques and examining the teen's self-report over parental sleep reports.

In summary, sleep disturbances that are identified, addressed, and appropriately monitored may result in improved sleep and mood. Active involvement of the teen in the therapy process may improve outcomes. Further research is needed to develop non-pharmacological strategies that are acceptable and sustainable for adolescents.

References

1. Carskadon MA (2011) Sleep in adolescents: the perfect storm. Pediatr Clin North Am 58: 637-647.
2. Leger D, Beck F, Richard JB, Godeau E (2012) Total sleep time severely drops during adolescence. PLoS One 7: e45204.
3. Tarokh L, Van Reen E, LeBourgeois M, Seifer R, Carskadon MA (2011) Sleep EEG provides evidence that cortical changes persist into late adolescence. Sleep 34: 1385-1393.
4. Gradisar M, Gardner G, Dohnt H (2011) Recent worldwide sleep patterns and problems during adolescence: a review and meta-analysis of age, region, and sleep. Sleep Med 12: 110-118.
5. Carskadon MA, Vieira C, Acebo C (1993) Association between puberty and delayed phase preference. Sleep 16: 258-262.
6. Czeisler CA, Gooley JJ (2007) Sleep and circadian rhythms in humans. Cold Spring Harb Symp Quant Biol 72: 579-597.
7. Lewinsohn PM, Hops H, Roberts RE, Seeley JR, Andrews JA (1993) Adolescent psychopathology: I. Prevalence and incidence of depression and other DSM-III-R disorders in high school students. J Abnorm Psychol 102: 133-144.
8. Baglioni C, Battagliese G, Feige B, Spiegelhalder K, Nissen C, et al. (2011) Insomnia as a predictor of depression: a meta-analytic evaluation of longitudinal epidemiological studies. J Affect Disord 135: 10-19.
9. Johnson E: Epidemiology of Insomnia: from Adolescence to Old Age. In Sleep Medicine Clinics. Volume 1. Edited by Roth T. Philadelphia: Elsevier Saunders; 2006:305-317.
10. O'Brien EM, Mindell JA (2005) Sleep and risk-taking behavior in adolescents. Behav Sleep Med 3: 113-133.
11. Pasch KE, Laska MN, Lytle LA, Moe SG (2010) Adolescent sleep, risk behaviors, and depressive symptoms: are they linked? Am J Health Behav 34: 237-248.
12. McKnight-Eily LR, Eaton DK, Lowry R, Croft JB, Presley-Cantrell L, et al. (2011) Relationships between hours of sleep and health-risk behaviors in US adolescent students. Prev Med 53: 271-273.
13. Pasch KE, Latimer LA, Cance JD, Moe SG, Lytle LA (2012) Longitudinal bi-directional relationships between sleep and youth substance use. J Youth Adolesc 41: 1184-1196.
14. Johnson EO, Roth T, Schultz L, Breslau N (2006) Epidemiology of DSM-IV insomnia in adolescence: lifetime prevalence, chronicity, and an emergent gender difference. Pediatrics 117: e247-256.
15. Roberts RE, Duong HT (2013) Depression and insomnia among adolescents: a prospective perspective. J Affect Disord 148: 66-71.
16. Emslie GJ, Armitage R, Weinberg WA, Rush AJ, Mayes TL, et al. (2001) Sleep polysomnography as a predictor of recurrence in children and adolescents with major depressive disorder. Int J Neuropsychopharmacol 4: 159-168.
17. Armitage R, Hoffmann R, Emslie G, Rintelmann J, Robert J (2006) Sleep microarchitecture in childhood and adolescent depression: temporal coherence. Clin EEG Neurosci 37: 1-9.
18. Armitage R, Hoffmann RF, Rush AJ (1999) Biological rhythm disturbance in depression: temporal coherence of ultradian sleep EEG rhythms. Psychol Med 29: 1435-1448.
19. Armitage R, Hoffmann R, Emslie G, Rintelman J, Moore J, et al. (2004) Rest-activity cycles in childhood and adolescent depression. J Am Acad Child Adolesc Psychiatry 43: 761-769.
20. Pantic I, Damjanovic A, Todorovic J, Topalovic D, Bojovic-Jovic D, et al. (2012) Association between online social networking and depression in high school students: behavioral physiology viewpoint. Psychiatr Danub 24: 90-93.
21. Danielsson NS, Harvey AG, Macdonald S, Jansson-Fröjmark M, Linton SJ (2013) Sleep disturbance and depressive symptoms in adolescence: the role of catastrophic worry. J Youth Adolesc 42: 1223-1233.
22. Iglowstein I, Jenni OG, Molinari L, Largo RH (2003) Sleep duration from infancy to adolescence: reference values and generational trends. Pediatrics 111: 302-307.
23. Jenni OG (2013) How much sleep is "normal" in children and adolescents? JAMA Pediatr 167: 91-92.
24. Carney CE, Waters WF (2006) Effects of a structured problem-solving procedure on pre-sleep cognitive arousal in college students with insomnia. Behav Sleep Med 4: 13-28.
25. Sleep in America Poll. Washington, DC: National Sleep Foundation; 2006.
26. Adolescent Sleep Needs and Patterns: Research Report and Resource Guide. Washinton DC: National Sleep Foundation Sleep and Teens Task Force; 2000.
27. Wong MM, Brower KJ, Zucker RA (2009) Childhood sleep problems, early onset of substance use and behavioral problems in adolescence. Sleep Med 10: 787-796.
28. Kong AP, Wing YK, Choi KC, Li AM, Ko GT, et al. (2011) Associations of sleep duration with obesity and serum lipid profile in children and adolescents. Sleep Med 12: 659-665.
29. Weissman MM, Bland RC, Canino GJ, Greenwald S, Hwu HG, et al. (1999) Prevalence of suicide ideation and suicide attempts in nine countries. Psychol Med 29: 9-17.
30. Li S, Lam S, Yu M, Zhang J, Wing Y: Nocturnal sleep disturbances as a predictor of suicide attempts among psychiatric outpatients: a clinical, epidemiologic, prospective study.J Clin Psychiatry 2010 71(11):1440-1446.
31. Lee YJ, Cho SJ, Cho IH, Kim SJ (2012) Insufficient sleep and suicidality in adolescents. Sleep 35: 455-460.
32. Wolfson AR, Carskadon MA (1998) Sleep schedules and daytime functioning in adolescents. Child Dev 69: 875-887.
33. George NM, Davis JE (2013) Assessing sleep in adolescents through a better understanding of sleep physiology. Am J Nurs 113: 26-31.
34. Giannotti F, Cortesi F, Sebastiani T, Ottaviano S (2002) Circadian preference, sleep and daytime behaviour in adolescence. J Sleep Res 11: 191-199.
35. Fredriksen K, Rhodes J, Reddy R, Way N (2004) Sleepless in Chicago: tracking the effects of adolescent sleep loss during the middle school years. Child Dev 75: 84-95.
36. Gelbmann G, Kuhn-Natriashvili S, Pazhedath TJ, Ardeljan M, Wöber C, et al. (2012) Morningness: protective factor for sleep-related and emotional problems in childhood and adolescence? Chronobiol Int 29: 898-910.
37. Dagys N, McGlinchey EL, Talbot LS, Kaplan KA, Dahl RE, et al. (2012) Double trouble? The effects of sleep deprivation and chronotype on adolescent affect. J Child Psychol Psychiatry 53: 660-667.
38. Gangwisch JE, Babiss LA, Malaspina D, Turner JB, Zammit GK, et al. (2010) Earlier parental set bedtimes as a protective factor against depression and suicidal ideation. Sleep 33: 97-106.
39. Wong MM, Brower KJ (2012) The prospective relationship between sleep problems and suicidal behavior in the National Longitudinal Study of Adolescent Health. J Psychiatr Res 46: 953-959.
40. Wong MM, Brower KJ, Zucker RA (2011) Sleep problems, suicidal ideation, and self-harm behaviors in adolescence. J Psychiatr Res 45: 505-511.

41. Bailly D, Bailly-Lambin I, Querleu D, Beuscart R, Collinet C (2004) [Sleep in adolescents and its disorders. A survey in schools]. Encephale 30: 352-359.

42. Goldstein TR, Bridge JA, Brent DA (2008) Sleep disturbance preceding completed suicide in adolescents. J Consult Clin Psychol 76: 84-91.

43. Highlights of changes from DSM-IV-TR to DSM-5

44. Carlson G: The challenge of diagnosing depression in childhood and adolescence. Journal of Affective Disorders 2000, 61:S1-S8.

45. Scharf SM, Tubman A, Smale P (2005) Prevalence of concomitant sleep disorders in patients with obstructive sleep apnea. Sleep Breath 9: 50-56.

46. Carney C, Ancoli-Israel S, Buysse D, Edinger J, Krystal A, Lichstein K, Morin C: An update from the Sleep Log Standardization Workgroup. In Associated Professional Sleep Societies Annual Meeting: 2008; Baltimore, MD; 2008.

47. Ohayon MM, Riemann D, Morin C, Reynolds CF 3rd (2012) Hierarchy of insomnia criteria based on daytime consequences. Sleep Med 13: 52-57.

48. Pallesen S, Saxvig I, Molde H, Sørensen E, Wilhelmsen-Langeland A, et al. (2011) Brief report: behaviorally induced insufficient sleep syndrome in older adolescents: prevalence and correlates. J Adolesc 34: 391-395.

49. Ohayon MM, Roberts RE, Zulley J, Smirne S, Priest RG (2000) Prevalence and patterns of problematic sleep among older adolescents. J Am Acad Child Adolesc Psychiatry 39: 1549-1556.

50. Lack LC, Wright HR (2007) Clinical management of delayed sleep phase disorder. Behav Sleep Med 5: 57-76.

51. Dahl R: The regulation of sleep and arousal: Development and psychopathology. Dev Psychopathol 1996, 8:3-27.

52. Hasler B, Buysse D, Kupfer D, Germain A (2010) Phase relationships between core body temperature, melatonin, and sleep are associated with depression severity: further evidence for circadian misalignment in non-seasonal depression. Psychiatry Res 178: 205-207.

53. Horne JA, Ostberg O (1976) A self-assessment questionnaire to determine morningness-eveningness in human circadian rhythms. Int J Chronobiol 4: 97-110.

54. O'Brien LM, Mervis CB, Holbrook CR, Bruner JL, Klaus CJ, et al. (2004) Neurobehavioral implications of habitual snoring in children. Pediatrics 114: 44-49.

55. O'Brien LM (2009) The neurocognitive effects of sleep disruption in children and adolescents. Child Adolesc Psychiatr Clin N Am 18: 813-823.

56. Carotenuto M, Esposito M, Parisi L, Gallai B, Marotta R, et al. (2012) Depressive symptoms and childhood sleep apnea syndrome. Neuropsychiatr Dis Treat 8: 369-373.

57. Miller P, Iyer M, Gold AR (2012) Treatment resistant adolescent depression with upper airway resistance syndrome treated with rapid palatal expansion: a case report. J Med Case Rep 6: 415.

58. Chung F, Yegneswaran B, Liao P, Chung SA, Vairavanathan S, Islam S, Khajehdehi A, Shapiro CM: STOP questionnaire: a tool to screen patients for obstructive sleep apnea. Anesthesiology 2008, 108(5):812-821.

59. Knight JR, Sherritt L, Harris SK, Gates EC, Chang G (2003) Validity of brief alcohol screening tests among adolescents: a comparison of the AUDIT, POSIT, CAGE, and CRAFFT. Alcohol Clin Exp Res 27: 67-73.

60. Kennard B, Silva S, Vitiello B, Curry J, Kratochvil C, et al. (2006) Remission and residual symptoms after short-term treatment in the Treatment of Adolescents with Depression Study (TADS). J Am Acad Child Adolesc Psychiatry 45: 1404-1411.

61. Vitiello B, Emslie G, Clarke G, Wagner K, Asarnow J, et al. (2011) Long-term outcome of adolescent depression initially resistant to selective serotonin reuptake inhibitor treatment: A follow-up study of the TORDIA sample. J Clin Psychiatry 72: 388-396.

62. Morgenthaler T, Kramer M, Alessi C, Friedman L, Boehlecke B, et al. (2006) Practice parameters for the psychological and behavioral treatment of insomnia: an update. An american academy of sleep medicine report. Sleep 29: 1415-1419.

63. [No authors listed] (2005) NIH State-of-the-Science Conference Statement on manifestations and management of chronic insomnia in adults. NIH Consens State Sci Statements 22: 1-30.

64. Morin CM, Culbert JP, Schwartz SM (1994) Nonpharmacological interventions for insomnia: a meta-analysis of treatment efficacy. Am J Psychiatry 151: 1172-1180.

65. Murtagh DR, Greenwood KM (1995) Identifying effective psychological treatments for insomnia: a meta-analysis. J Consult Clin Psychol 63: 79-89.

66. Manber R, Edinger JD, Gress JL, San Pedro-Salcedo MG, Kuo TF, et al. (2008) Cognitive behavioral therapy for insomnia enhances depression outcome in patients with comorbid major depressive disorder and insomnia. Sleep 31: 489-495.

67. Fava M, McCall WV, Krystal A, Wessel T, Rubens R, et al. (2006) Eszopiclone co-administered with fluoxetine in patients with insomnia coexisting with major depressive disorder. Biol Psychiatry 59: 1052-1060.

68. Bootzin RR, Stevens SJ (2005) Adolescents, substance abuse, and the treatment of insomnia and daytime sleepiness. Clin Psychol Rev 25: 629-644.

69. Dimidjian S, Barrera M Jr, Martell C, Muñoz RF, Lewinsohn PM (2011) The origins and current status of behavioral activation treatments for depression. Annu Rev Clin Psychol 7: 1-38.

70. Kalak N, Gerber M, Kirov R, Mikoteit T, Yordanova J, et al. (2012) Daily morning running for 3 weeks improved sleep and psychological functioning in healthy adolescents compared with controls. J Adolesc Health 51: 615-622.

71. Dopp RR, Mooney AJ, Armitage R, King C (2012) Exercise for adolescents with depressive disorders: a feasibility study. Depress Res Treat 2012: 257472.

72. Swedo SE, Pleeter JD, Richter DM, Hoffman CL, Allen AJ, et al. (1995) Rates of seasonal affective disorder in children and adolescents. Am J Psychiatry 152: 1016-1019.

73. Terman M, Terman JS, Quitkin FM, McGrath PJ, Stewart JW, et al. (1989) Light therapy for seasonal affective disorder. A review of efficacy. Neuropsychopharmacology 2: 1-22.

74. Bogen S, Legenbauer T, Bogen T, Gest S, Jensch T, et al. (2013) Morning light therapy for juvenile depression and severe mood dysregulation: study protocol for a randomized controlled trial. Trials 14: 178.

75. Swedo SE, Allen AJ, Glod CA, Clark CH, Teicher MH, et al. (1997) A controlled trial of light therapy for the treatment of pediatric seasonal affective disorder. J Am Acad Child Adolesc Psychiatry 36: 816-821.

76. Niederhofer H, von Klitzing K (2012) Bright light treatment as mono-therapy of non-seasonal depression for 28 adolescents. Int J Psychiatry Clin Pract 16: 233-237.

77. The International Classification of Sleep Disorders, Diagnostic and Coding Manual. Second edition. Westchester, IL; 2005.

78. Gradisar M, Dohnt H, Gardner G, Paine S, Starkey K, et al. (2011) A randomized controlled trial of cognitive-behavioral therapy plus bright light therapy for adolescent delayed sleep phase disorder. Sleep 34: 1671-1680.

79. Emslie GJ, Kennard BD, Mayes TL, Nakonezny PA, Zhu L, et al. (2012) Insomnia moderates outcome of serotonin-selective reuptake inhibitor treatment in depressed youth. J Child Adolesc Psychopharmacol 22: 21-28.

80. Blumer JL, Findling RL, Shih WJ, Soubrane C, Reed MD (2009) Controlled clinical trial of zolpidem for the treatment of insomnia associated with attention-deficit/ hyperactivity disorder in children 6 to 17 years of age. Pediatrics 123: e770-776.

81. Ford JA, McCutcheon J (2012) The misuse of Ambien among adolescents: prevalence and correlates in a national sample. Addict Behav 37: 1389-1394.

82. Srinivasan V, Spence WD, Pandi-Perumal SR, Zakharia R, Bhatnagar KP, et al. (2009) Melatonin and human reproduction: shedding light on the darkness hormone. Gynecol Endocrinol 25: 779-785.

83. van Geijlswijk IM, Mol RH, Egberts TC, Smits MG (2011) Evaluation of sleep, puberty and mental health in children with long-term melatonin treatment for chronic idiopathic childhood sleep onset insomnia. Psychopharmacology (Berl) 216: 111-120.

84. Hartz I, Furu K, Bratlid T, Handal M, Skurtveit S (2012) Hypnotic drug use among 0-17 year olds during 2004-2011: a nationwide prescription database study. Scand J Public Health 40: 704-711.

85. Weiss SK, Garbutt A (2010) Pharmacotherapy in pediatric sleep disorders. Adolesc Med State Art Rev 21: 508-521, ix-x.

86. Eckerberg B, Lowden A, Nagai R, Akerstedt T (2012) Melatonin treatment

effects on adolescent students' sleep timing and sleepiness in a placebo-controlled crossover study. Chronobiol Int 29: 1239-1248.

87. Owens JA, Rosen CL, Mindell JA, Kirchner HL (2010) Use of pharmacotherapy for insomnia in child psychiatry practice: A national survey. Sleep Med 11: 692-700.

88. Brent D, Emslie G, Clarke G, Wagner K, Asarnow J, et al. (2008) Switching to another SSRI or to venlafaxine with or without cogntive behavioral therapy for adolescents with SSRI-resistant depression: the TORDIA randomized controlled trial. JAMA 8: 901-913.

89. Shamseddeen W, Clarke G, Keller M, Wagner K, Birmaher B, et al. (2012) Adjunctive sleep medications and depression outcome in the treatment of serotonin-selective reuptake inhibitor resistant depression in adolescents study. Journal of Child and Adolescent Psychopharmacology 22: 29-36.

90. Short M, Gradisar M, Lack L, Wright H, Chatburn A, et al. (2013) Estimating adolescent sleep patterns: parent reports versus adolescent self-report surveys, sleep diaries, and actigraphy. Nature and Science of Sleep 5: 23-26.

91. Beck A (Ed.): Beck Depression Inventory (BDI) Philadelphia, PA: Center for Cognitive Therapy; 1961.

92. Kovacs M: Children's Depression Inventory (CDI) North Tonawanda, N.Y: Multi-Health System; 1992.

93. Fendrich M, Weissman MM, Warner V (1990) Screening for depressive disorder in children and adolescents: validating the Center for Epidemiologic Studies Depression Scale for Children. Am J Epidemiol 131: 538-551.

94. Radloff L (1977) Center for Epidemiological Studies-Depression Scale (CES-D). The CES-D scale: a self-report depression scale for research in the general population. Applied Psychological Measurement 1: 385-401.

95. Reynolds W: Reynolds Adolescent Depression Scale Odessa, Fla: Psychological Assessment Resources; 1986.

13

Lifestyle Factors that Affect Youth's Sleep and Strategies for Guiding Patients and Families Toward Healthy Sleeping

Gruber Reut[1,2*] **and Bergmame Lana**[2]

[1]*McGill University, Montreal, Quebec, Canada*
[2]*Attention, Behavior and Sleep Lab, Douglas Mental Health University Institute, Quebec, Canada*

Abstract

Sleep is essential for optimal child and adolescent health, development, and academic performance. Lifestyle habits significantly influence child and adolescent sleep regulation, conferring either positive or negative effects on the attainment of sufficient and high-quality sleep. The primary objective of this paper is, thus, to review the lifestyle factors which may disrupt a child's sleep, on the one hand, and support healthy sleep, on the other. Lifestyle factors that have been found to negatively affect children and adolescents' sleep include: 1) exposure to modern technologies (e.g., television, computer and video games) leading to increased light exposure and night-time arousal; 2) consumption of wake-promoting substances, such as caffeine, that affect the physiological regulation of arousal and sleep; 3) consumption of late-evening meals; 4) aspects of the physical environment (e.g., air quality) that hinder sleep; and 4) cultural norms that place a low priority on sleep. Despite the negative impact of such factors on youths' sleep, such aspects are modifiable and can be easily targeted by simple and inexpensive interventions designed to promote healthy and sufficient sleep. This review offers several strategies to guide families in modifying unhealthy sleep habits and promoting refreshing, high-quality sleep.

Keywords: Lifestyle habits; Sleep; Health; Youth; Families

Abbreviations: SCN: Suprachiasmatic Nucleus

Introduction

Strong evidence indicates that sleep is extremely important to youth's health and success. Sleep deprivation has been empirically linked to obesity, diabetes, hypertension, metabolic syndrome, and cardiovascular problems [1-5]. In addition, poor sleep has been shown to impair academic performance, learning, memory and neurobehavioral functioning, especially in the context of activities that are essential for academic success, such as attention/response inhibition, memory, verbal creativity, problem solving, and general cognitive abilities (as reflected by IQ test scores) [6-10]. Poor sleep has also been linked to increased accidental injuries in younger children [11] and an increased risk of motor vehicle accidents, which is particularly relevant to adolescents of driving age [12-15]. Despite the very strong evidence indicating the importance of sleep, the sleep duration of children and adolescents has declined over time [16]. Recently, the Sleep in America Polls conducted by the National Sleep Foundation in 2004 showed that 34% of toddlers, 32% of preschoolers and 27% of school-aged children sleep fewer hours than their parents think they need. Although the optimal amount of sleep required in adolescence is reported to be at least 8.5 hours per night, as many as 70% of adolescent students get less than this amount of sleep [17] and more than half report feeling excessively tired or sleepy during the day [18]. Unfortunately, however, the significance of chronic sleep insufficiency is not adequately recognized in the current context of youth health.

Thus, we need to provide children and parents with tools to assist children in achieving sufficient sleep. For example, we could identify modifiable factors that influence the amount and quality of sleep among children and adolescents, and then target these factors as a means to optimize youth sleep.

Although sleep is a biological process, sleep habits are socially learned behaviors that are integrated with the natural rhythms of the body. Sleep physiology is regulated by two distinct physiological processes that interact to govern sleep timing and composition [19-21] The homeostatic sleep process (also known as process S) is a regulatory mechanism wherein sleep pressure accumulates as wake time lengthens and dissipates during a sleep episode. In contrast, circadian components (or process C) regulates the timing of sleep and awakening [22-24]. Process C is directly affected by environmental cues (see below for details), so the environment has a potent impact on sleep. This could be used to shape optimal sleep patterns, but if not cued properly, environmental factors can also create poor sleep patterns [25]. Because the rhythm of the circadian pacemaker (i.e., the "biological clock") is not precisely 24 hours, it must be realigned by an average of 0.2 hour each day through a process called "entrainment" [20]. The most powerful known synchronizer, or *zeitgeber* (from the German zeit, which means "time," and geben, which means "to give"), is the light-dark cycle [26,27]. Recent studies have shown that non-photic cues, such as food and activity levels, can also synchronize the Suprachiasmatic Nucleus (SCN) [28,29]. Thus, certain habits and environmental conditions, such as light exposure, meal times or engaging in stimulating activities, can affect the circadian and homeostatic sleep processes.

Lifestyle habits, which consist of repeated daily behavior, may positively or negatively affect a child's ability to obtain sufficient, high-quality sleep. Thus, we need to understand these elements in order to guide parents and children on optimizing sleep regulation and duration. The goals of the present paper are to: 1) review lifestyle factors that can affect youth sleep regulation, encourage later bedtimes and longer

***Corresponding author:** Reut Gruber, Department of Psychiatry, McGill University, Douglas Mental Health University Institute , 6875 LaSalle Blvd, Verdun (Quebec), Canada H4H 1R3 E-mail: reut.gruber@douglas.mcgill.ca

nighttime arousal, and disrupt and shorten sleep; and 2) review lifestyle habits that support healthy sleep and introduce strategies to modify the habits that negatively impact sleep.

Lifestyle Factors Affecting Sleep Regulation

The lifestyle factors that have been shown to affect the sleep regulation of children and adolescents include: modern technologies that cause light exposure and stimulate night-time arousal; consumption of wake-promoting substances (e.g., caffeine) that affect the physiological regulation of arousal and sleep; meal times; aspects of the physical environment (e.g., air quality) that hinder sleep; and cultural norms that place a low priority on sleep. Below, we will review each of these factors and their impacts on youth sleep.

Late-Night Use of Modern Technologies

A large percentage of children and adolescents have electronic media in their bedrooms and use these technologies late at night. A recent large study found that half of parents reported that their grade 5 children had a TV, DVD player and/or video game console in his or her bedroom, while 21% had computers and 17% had cellular phones [30]. Observational studies have consistently shown associations between media use and sleep problems among children [31-37]. These effects have been observed across cultures and in all media formats, including TV [36,38-40], video games [40-42], and computers [41,43,44]. The effects are also evident across the age spectrum, including preschoolers [32,37-39], school-aged children [31,33-36], adolescents and adults [43-45]. Access to and night-time use of electronic media has been associated with shortened sleep duration and excess body weight [30]. Children with increasingly more electronic media devices in their bedrooms reported shorter sleep durations, and students who used electronic devices on most or all nights reported sleeping less and more sleep problems [30]. The effect of night-time media use on sleep duration and quality is the result of: 1) the use of devices after bedtime at the expense of sleep; 2) the strong effect of light exposure [46], which suppresses melatonin and leads to circadian asynchrony, disrupted sleep and delayed sleep phase [47]; 3) the media content (exposure to violent media and games can lead to sleep problems); 4) sleep interruptions (cell phones and texting awakens children, and their content can increase arousal and make it difficult to disengage and fall asleep); and 5) poor parental control. In the latter context, Van den Bulck [41,48] has referred to electronic media exposure as an unstructured and boundless leisure activity that, unlike other hobbies or sports activities, has no clear endpoint. It has been suggested that the presence of a media device in the bedroom may indicate low parental control, contributing to increased exposure [48].

Caffeinated Beverages

Caffeine is a widely consumed psychoactive substance that activates dopaminergic reward circuits and produces behavioral effects similar to other dopaminergically mediated substances, such as cocaine and amphetamine [49]. Adenosine is a sleep-inducing neurochemical that decreases sensitivity to dopamine receptors and helps promote sleep. Caffeine blocks the adenosine receptor, increases the effect of dopamine on the D2 receptor and enhances the availability of dopamine, thus creating a stimulating effect [50]. As an adenosine antagonist, caffeine has been shown to attenuate electroencephalographic (EEG) markers associated with decreased homeostatic sleep pressure, thereby promoting wakefulness in humans [51]. Children may consume caffeine daily through caffeinated beverages. Energy drinks are particularly problematic, as they are treated as "dietary supplements" and are not subject to the same rules as soft drinks. In a recent study, 75% of children surveyed reported that they consumed caffeine on a daily basis, and the more caffeine the children consumed, the less they reported sleeping. In this study, children aged 5 to 7 years old consumed approximately 52 mg of caffeine per day, and children aged 8 to 12 years old consumed approximately 109 mg [52]. Habitual daily caffeine consumption has been related to sleep disruption, sleepiness [51,53,54], and impaired daytime functioning [55]. This is likely related to the long half-life of caffeine, which ranges from 3 to 7 hours [51]. Caffeine consumed during the afternoon or evening (e.g., dinnertime) is likely to last well into the night and affect the arousal system even at bedtime, hindering a child's ability to fall asleep.

Late-Evening Meals

Nutritional and hormonal cues are potent synchronizers of the circadian sleep process [56], and the feeding schedule can advance or delay the circadian phase. Under certain conditions of feeding, metabolic cues can alter both the master circadian clock and circadian responses to light [28,29,57,58]. Recent studies have shown that human mealtimes are important socio-environmental synchronizers of circadian rhythms, and late-evening meals have been associated with sleep onset delays, shortened sleep durations, and sleep deprivation [59]

Societal Values

A healthy diet, physical activity, and the proper amount of sleep are all interrelated and important for a child's health. Unfortunately, sleep is often neglected in this regard. Many perceive sleep time as lost time that could be spent more productively. In some ways, society's current view of sleep deprivation is similar to our past attitude toward smoking, which was characterized by ignorance, lack of concern regarding the serious consequences, and even humor. Our socio-cultural environment (long store hours, late-night sporting events, energy drinks, screen time, and artificial light exposure at night) does not promote healthy sleep habits, and people living in a 24/7 society place sleep low on their priority list. Parents' busy schedules and work hours may push dinner and family activities to later times. Children can also have busy schedules, as they are often enrolled in multiple extracurricular activities and attend late-ending social, sporting and school events that contribute to delayed bedtimes and short sleep durations. Sleep is often neglected as a crucial component of a healthy lifestyle, and sleep deprivation is not currently considered a public health concern. Thus, parents and children frequently push back bedtimes in order to accommodate other activities that are perceived as higher priority. Since school start times are fixed, children are unable to obtain sufficient sleep and become sleep deprived. Paradoxically, the effort to help children achieve more through late-night homework or extracurricular activities can have the opposite effect, as over-tired children will under-perform during the school day and may benefit far less from extracurricular opportunities.

Sleep is rarely integrated into programs and interventions designed to improve health. For example, weight regulation programs targeting childhood obesity typically focus on healthy eating and active living. Sleep is also not a typical focus of the government or pediatric practice, and the importance of sleep and its relevance to academic success is rarely addressed in educational programs aimed at optimizing academic performance. Thus, there is a general lack of awareness when it comes to the serious consequences of chronic sleep insufficiency on youth health and success.

In sum, certain lifestyle habits affect the physiological processes associated with sleep regulation and reflect cultural norms that prioritize busy schedules over sleep, contributing to the high prevalence of sleep deprivation in children and adolescents. Fortunately, however, these habits can be changed. Below, we review practical strategies that can help children and their families develop healthy sleeping patterns.

Lifestyle Choices that Support Healthy Sleep

The concrete strategies listed below may help guide children and families toward healthy sleeping. It is important to note that the quality of evidence for these recommendations is fairly low, as most of the information regarding potential harmful and beneficial factors come from observational studies, rather than rigorously designed intervention trials.

The creation of fixed bed- and wake-times is a recommended step in developing sleep patterns that allow a child to get enough sleep. The body "gets used" to falling asleep at a certain time, but only if this time is relatively consistent. It is important to set a bedtime that allows the child to get enough sleep. Although activities may occur at different times on weekends/holidays versus the school week, a child's bedtime should differ by no more than 1 hour.

To encourage the habit of falling asleep easily at the desired time, parents should create a consistent and calm bedtime routine that includes relaxing activities over about 20-30 min in the room where the child sleeps. In addition, they should create an optimal sleeping environment that is quiet, dark and cool in the evening, and well-lit in the morning. Importantly, the sleeping environment should be associated with positive experiences and emotions, and parents should not use banishment to the bedroom or an early bedtime as punishment [60, 61].

Young children who still nap should be encouraged to nap during the day; however, children older than 5 years (especially adolescents) should avoid napping during the day, as this interferes with the natural sleep homeostasis and creates difficulties with night-time sleeping. If an adolescent feels sleepy during the day, a nap should be limited to 15-20 minutes and should be scheduled for the early afternoon.

Parents should keep electronic devices (e.g., televisions, computers, cell phones, etc.) out of the bedroom and limit internet use in the evening.

Children who consume caffeinated substances, such as sodas, hot chocolate or solid chocolate, should avoid caffeine for at least 3 to 4 hours prior to bedtime. Coffee and energy drinks should be avoided, and this should be explained to adolescents who seek out these types of snacks or beverages.

Regular exercise, particularly in the afternoon, can help deepen sleep. However, strenuous exercise (e.g., intense hockey or soccer practice) within 2 hours prior to bedtime can compromise the ability to fall asleep.

Healthy sleep education that raises the awareness of the general public to the importance of sleep and offers age-specific sleep recommendations will be essential for preventing common sleep problems and sleep deprivation in our youth. Such education should emphasize the importance of developing a lifestyle that is conducive to healthy sleep behavior and prioritizing sleep over competing activities. The message and delivery method should be tailored to specific age groups, and both parents and children should be taught why and how to encourage healthy sleep [62].

In sum, parents can take simple steps to optimize their child's sleep and decrease negative habits that are detrimental to sleep. An understanding and awareness of the importance of sleep could help motivate them to reevaluate existing habits and make room for new habits that promote healthy sleep. One potential way to motivate parents to engage in such a process will be to educate them regarding the critical importance of sleep and the detrimental impact of sleep deprivation on their child's health and success.

Conclusion

Lifestyle habits, which are aspects of everyday life, can have significant impacts on sleep regulation. Because these habits are modifiable, they could be targeted by simple and inexpensive interventions aimed at helping families achieve healthy and sufficient sleep.

References

1. Cappuccio FP, Taggart FM, Kandala NB, Currie A, Peile E, et al. (2008) Meta-analysis of short sleep duration and obesity in children and adults. Sleep 31: 619-626.
2. Chaput JP, Lambert M, Gray-Donald K, McGrath JJ, Tremblay MS, et al. (2011) Short sleep duration is independently associated with overweight and obesity in Quebec children. Can J Public Health 102: 369-374.
3. Magee CA, Huang XF, Iverson DC, Caputi P (2010) Examining the pathways linking chronic sleep restriction to obesity. J Obes 2010.
4. George NM, Davis JE (2013) Assessing sleep in adolescents through a better understanding of sleep physiology. Am J Nurs 113: 26-31.
5. Geiger SD, Sabanayagam C, Shankar A (2012) The relationship between insufficient sleep and self-rated health in a nationally representative sample. J Environ Public Health 2012: 518263.
6. Buckhalt JA, El-Sheikh M, Keller PS, Kelly RJ (2009) Concurrent and longitudinal relations between children's sleep and cognitive functioning: the moderating role of parent education. Child Dev 80: 875-892.
7. El-Sheikh M, Buckhalt JA, Mark Cummings E, Keller P (2007) Sleep disruptions and emotional insecurity are pathways of risk for children. J Child Psychol Psychiatry 48: 88-96.
8. Meijer AM, Habekothé HT, Van Den Wittenboer GL (2000) Time in bed, quality of sleep and school functioning of children. J Sleep Res 9: 145-153.
9. Touchette E, Petit D, Séguin JR, Boivin M, Tremblay RE, et al. (2007) Associations between sleep duration patterns and behavioral/cognitive functioning at school entry. Sleep 30: 1213-1219.
10. Wolfson AR, Spaulding NL, Dandrow C, Baroni EM (2007) Middle school start times: the importance of a good night's sleep for young adolescents. Behav Sleep Med 5: 194-209.
11. Boto LR, Crispim JN, de Melo IS, Juvandes C, Rodrigues T, et al. (2012) Sleep deprivation and accidental fall risk in children. Sleep Med 13: 88-95.
12. Horne JA, Reyner LA (1995) Sleep related vehicle accidents. BMJ 310: 565-567.
13. Lyznicki JM, Doege TC, Davis RM, Williams MA (1998) Sleepiness, driving, and motor vehicle crashes. Council on Scientific Affairs, American Medical Association. JAMA 279: 1908-1913.
14. McConnell CF, Bretz KM, Dwyer WO (2003) Falling asleep at the wheel: aclose look at 1,269 fatal and serious injury-producing crashes. Behav Sleep Med 1: 171-183.
15. Pack AI, Pack AM, Rodgman E, Cucchiara A, Dinges DF, et al. (1995) Characteristics of crashes attributed to the driver having fallen asleep. Accid Anal Prev 27: 769-775.
16. Matricciani L, Olds T, Petkov J (2012) In search of lost sleep: secular trends in the sleep time of school-aged children and adolescents. Sleep Med Rev 16: 203-211.
17. Gibson ES, Powles AC, Thabane L, O'Brien S, Molnar DS, et al. (2006) "Sleepiness" is serious in adolescence: two surveys of 3235 Canadian students. BMC Public Health 6: 116.

18. Spilsbury JC, Storfer-Isser A, Drotar D, Rosen CL, Kirchner LH, et al. (2004) Sleep behavior in an urban US sample of school-aged children. Arch Pediatr Adolesc Med 158: 988-994.

19. Borbély AA (1982) A two process model of sleep regulation. Hum Neurobiol 1: 195-204.

20. Czeisler CA, Allan JS, Strogatz SH, Ronda JM, Sánchez R, et al. (1986) Bright light resets the human circadian pacemaker independent of the timing of the sleep-wake cycle. Science 233: 667-671.

21. Moore RY (1999) A clock for the ages. Science 284: 2102-2103.

22. Allada R, White NE, So WV, Hall JC, Rosbash M (1998) A mutant Drosophila homolog of mammalian Clock disrupts circadian rhythms and transcription of period and timeless. Cell 93: 791-804.

23. Blau J, Young MW (1999) Cycling vrille expression is required for a functional Drosophila clock. Cell 99: 661-671.

24. Ebadi M, Govitrapong P (1986) Neural pathways and neurotransmitters affecting melatonin synthesis. J Neural Transm Suppl 21: 125-155.

25. Carskadon MA, Acebo C, Jenni OG (2004) Regulation of adolescent sleep: implications for behavior. Ann N Y Acad Sci 1021: 276-291.

26. Czeisler CA, Duffy JF, Shanahan TL, Brown EN, Mitchell JF, et al. (1999) Stability, precision, and near-24-hour period of the human circadian pacemaker. Science 284: 2177-2181.

27. Mindell JA, Owens JA (2003) Sleep problems in pediatric practice: clinical issues for the pediatric nurse practitioner. J Pediatr Health Care 17: 324-331.

28. Challet E, Pévet P, Vivien-Roels B, Malan A (1997) Phase-advanced daily rhythms of melatonin, body temperature, and locomotor activity in food-restricted rats fed during daytime. J Biol Rhythms 12: 65-79.

29. Mendoza J, Graff C, Dardente H, Pevet P, Challet E (2005) Feeding cues alter clock gene oscillations and photic responses in the suprachiasmatic nuclei of mice exposed to a light/dark cycle. J Neurosci 25: 1514-1522.

30. Chahal H, Fung C, Kuhle S, Veugelers PJ (2013) Availability and night-time use of electronic entertainment and communication devices are associated with short sleep duration and obesity among Canadian children. Pediatr Obes 8: 42-51.

31. Owens J, Maxim R, McGuinn M, Nobile C, Msall M, et al. (1999) Television-viewing habits and sleep disturbance in school children. Pediatrics 104: e27.

32. Garrison MM, Liekweg K, Christakis DA (2011) Media use and child sleep: the impact of content, timing, and environment. Pediatrics 128: 29-35.

33. Li S, Jin X, Wu S, Jiang F, Yan C, et al. (2007) The impact of media use on sleep patterns and sleep disorders among school-aged children in China. Sleep 30: 361-367.

34. Nixon GM, Thompson JM, Han DY, Becroft DM, Clark PM, et al. (2008) Short sleep duration in middle childhood: risk factors and consequences. Sleep 31: 71-78.

35. Oka Y, Suzuki S, Inoue Y (2008) Bedtime activities, sleep environment, and sleep/wake patterns of Japanese elementary school children. Behav Sleep Med 6: 220-233.

36. Paavonen EJ, Pennonen M, Roine M, Valkonen S, Lahikainen AR (2006) TV exposure associated with sleep disturbances in 5- to 6-year-old children. J Sleep Res 15: 154-161.

37. Thompson DA, Christakis DA (2005) The association between television viewing and irregular sleep schedules among children less than 3 years of age. Pediatrics 116: 851-856.

38. Mistry KB, Minkovitz CS, Strobino DM, Borzekowski DL (2007) Children's television exposure and behavioral and social outcomes at 5.5 years: does timing of exposure matter? Pediatrics 120: 762-769.

39. Mindell JA, Meltzer LJ, Carskadon MA, Chervin RD (2009) Developmental aspects of sleep hygiene: findings from the 2004 National Sleep Foundation Sleep in America Poll. Sleep Med 10: 771-779.

40. Alexandru G, Michikazu S, Shimako H, Xiaoli C, Hitomi K, et al. (2006) Epidemiological aspects of self-reported sleep onset latency in Japanese junior high school children. J Sleep Res 15: 266-275.

41. Van den Bulck J (2004) Television viewing, computer game playing, and Internet use and self-reported time to bed and time out of bed in secondary-school children. Sleep 27: 101-104.

42. Dworak M, Schierl T, Bruns T, Strüder HK (2007) Impact of singular excessive computer game and television exposure on sleep patterns and memory performance of school-aged children. Pediatrics 120: 978-985.

43. Eggermont S, Van den Bulck J (2006) Nodding off or switching off? The use of popular media as a sleep aid in secondary-school children. J Paediatr Child Health 42: 428-433.

44. Mesquita G, Reimão R (2007) Nightly use of computer by adolescents: its effect on quality of sleep. Arq Neuropsiquiatr 65: 428-432.

45. Johnson JG, Cohen P, Kasen S, First MB, Brook JS (2004) Association between television viewing and sleep problems during adolescence and early adulthood. Arch Pediatr Adolesc Med 158: 562-568.

46. Higuchi S, Motohashi Y, Liu Y, Ahara M, Kaneko Y (2003) Effects of VDT tasks with a bright display at night on melatonin, core temperature, heart rate, and sleepiness. J Appl Physiol 94: 1773-1776.

47. Cajochen C, Frey S, Anders D, Späti J, Bues M, et al. (2011) Evening exposure to a light-emitting diodes (LED)-backlit computer screen affects circadian physiology and cognitive performance. J Appl Physiol 110: 1432-1438.

48. Van den Bulck J (2010) The effects of media on sleep. Adolesc Med State Art Rev 21: 418-429, vii.

49. Cauli O, Morelli M (2005) Caffeine and the dopaminergic system. Behav Pharmacol 16: 63-77.

50. Stahl SM (2008) Stahl's essential psychopharmacology : Neuroscientific basis and practical applications. (3rdedn), Cambridge University Press, Cambridge, New York.

51. Roehrs T, Roth T (2008) Caffeine: sleep and daytime sleepiness. Sleep Med Rev 12: 153-162.

52. Warzak WJ, Evans S, Floress MT, Gross AC, Stoolman S (2011) Caffeine consumption in young children. J Pediatr 158: 508-509.

53. Orbeta RL, Overpeck MD, Ramcharran D, Kogan MD, Ledsky R (2006) High caffeine intake in adolescents: associations with difficulty sleeping and feeling tired in the morning. J Adolesc Health 38: 451-453.

54. Pollak CP, Bright D (2003) Caffeine consumption and weekly sleep patterns in US seventh-, eighth-, and ninth-graders. Pediatrics 111: 42-46.

55. Calamaro CJ, Mason TB, Ratcliffe SJ (2009) Adolescents living the 24/7 lifestyle: effects of caffeine and technology on sleep duration and daytime functioning. Pediatrics 123: e1005-1010.

56. Tauman R (2012) Metabolic and Hormornal Regulation During Sleep, in Sleep Disordered Breathing in Children: A Comprehensive Clinical Guide to Evaluation and Treatment, L. Kheirandish-Gozal and D. Gozal, Editors. Humana Press.

57. Resuehr D, Olcese J (2005) Caloric restriction and melatonin substitution: effects on murine circadian parameters. Brain Res 1048: 146-152.

58. Mendoza J, Pévet P, Challet E (2007) Circadian and photic regulation of clock and clock-controlled proteins in the suprachiasmatic nuclei of calorie-restricted mice. Eur J Neurosci 25: 3691-3701.

59. Fleig D, Randler C (2009) Association between chronotype and diet in adolescents based on food logs. Eat Behav 10: 115-118.

60. Kuhn BR, Roane BM (2012) Pediatric insomnia and behavioral interventions, in therapy in sleep medicine, T.J. Barkoukis, et al., Editors. Elsevier Inc. (Saunders), Philadelphia.

61. Mindell JA, Kuhn B, Lewin DS, Meltzer LJ, Sadeh A; American Academy of Sleep Medicine (2006) Behavioral treatment of bedtime problems and night wakings in infants and young children. Sleep 29: 1263-1276.

62. Gruber R, Cassoff J, Knauper B (2011) Sleep health education in pediatric community settings: Rationale and practical suggestions for incorporating healthy sleep education into pediatric practice. Pediatr Clin North Am 58: 735-754.

Sleep Apnea in Traumatic Brain Injury: Understanding Its Impact on Executive Function

Tatyana Mollayeva[1]*, Tetyana Kendzerska[2], Shirin Mollayeva[3] and Angela Colantonio[4]

[1]Toronto Rehabilitation Institute, 550 University Avenue, Rm 11207, Toronto, Ontario M5G 2A2, Canada
[2]Institute of Health Policy, Management and Evaluation University of Toronto, 155 College Street, Suite 425 Toronto, Canada
[3]University of Toronto, Canada
[4]Saunderson Family Chair in Acquired Brain Injury Research, Toronto Rehabilitation Institute, University of Toronto, Canada

Abstract

Background: Persons who have sustained a traumatic brain injury are at a significantly increased risk for sleep disorders. One of the most commonly diagnosed sleep disorders after traumatic brain injury is sleep apnea, defined as a cessation of breathing accompanied by frequent arousals and hypoxia during sleep. The effects of untreated sleep apnea on a person's cognitive decline and the development of behavioral deficits have only recently been identified. It has been shown that axonal damage can occur because of sleep apnea and numerous neuropsychological studies of sleep apnea patients show deficits in cognitive domains, such as executive function and attention. However, there has been little published discussion regarding the interaction between sleep apnea and executive function among persons with traumatic brain injury.

Objectives: The objectives of this review were to 1) review/synthesize published work relevant to the discussion of sleep apnea influencing executive function; and 2) clarify the nature of the interface between executive function and sleep apnea in persons with traumatic brain injury.

Results: Until now, little attention has been directed to the neurobehavioral consequences of sleep apnea in persons with traumatic brain injury. There is an urgent need for more longitudinal research examining the effects of sleep apnea on executive function after traumatic brain injury and the effectiveness of sleep apnea treatment on executive function after injury.

Keywords: Traumatic brain injury; Executive function; Sleep apnea; Neurobehavior; Risk; Alzheimer's disease; Continuous positive airway pressure

Abbreviations: TBI: Traumatic Brain Injury; EF: Executive Function; SA: Sleep Apnea; CT: Computed Tomography; PET: Positron Emission Tomography; SDB: Sleep-Disordered Breathing; CSA: Central Sleep Apnea; OSA: Obstructive Sleep Apnea; RDI: Respiratory Disturbance Index; CNS: Central Nervous System; CPAP: Continuous Positive Airway Pressure; RCFT: Rey Complex Figure Test

Introduction

Traumatic brain injury (TBI) is a major global health problem. According to the World Health Organization, TBI will surpass many diseases as the major cause of death and disability by the year 2020 [1]. Although the prevalence of TBI, defined as chronic symptoms from an earlier TBI, is not widely studied, it is estimated that in the USA, around 5.3 million people experience long-lasting symptoms caused by TBI [2]. If this statistic is extrapolated to a global scale, an oft-quoted estimate is that approximately 140 million persons are living with a TBI-related disability; however there is a possibility that this number is overestimated or underestimated [3]. Of the various disabilities that are the result of TBI, cognitive and psychological deficits, particularly poor executive function (EF), prevent TBI survivors from reintegrating into the community, returning to school, and re-entering the workplace [4]. Executive function, the cognitive ability that underlies planning, problem-solving, self-monitoring, behavioral control and working memory [5], is therefore a major consideration in the cognitive rehabilitation of patients with brain injury [5]. While a discussion of neurocognitive impairment secondary to TBI would seem to be straightforward, the pathogenesis is likely to be a multifactorial process involving a diverse range of mechanisms. Consequently, it is essential that an examination of post-morbid executive function be done with reference to the other common disorders that can affect the brain. In the current review, we provide an overview of published work that is relevant to the discussion of sleep apnea's (SA) effects on EF and we examine different levels of evidence directed to clarifying the interface of executive function and SA in persons with TBI.

TBI and Cerebral Oxygenation as a Predictor of EF

When the brain is injured, normal pathways for EF performance are disturbed. The organic disruptions as well as cerebral ischemia resulting from post-traumatic hypotension and hypoxia together contribute to the poor cognitive outcomes that often follow TBI [6]. Decreased cerebral blood flow after TBI has been revealed using different diagnostic tools, such as computer tomography (CT) and positron emission tomography (PET) scans [7-8]. The mechanisms by which post-traumatic cerebral ischemia occurs include injury to the vessels as a result of mechanical displacement, hypotension in the presence of auto regulatory failure, inadequate availability of cholinergic neuro transmitters, and potentiation of prostaglandin-induced vasoconstriction. Because of an imbalance between cerebral oxygen consumption requirements and oxygen delivery, the brain

***Corresponding author:** Tatyana Mollayeva, Toronto Rehabilitation Institute, 550 University Avenue, Rm 11207, Toronto, Ontario M5G 2A2, Canada
E-mail: tatyana.mollayeva@utoronto.ca

tissue suffers from hypoxia [9]. It has been reported that the incidence, duration, and extent of tissue hypoxia is associated with poor neuropsychological outcomes post-TBI [10].

The phenomena of increased oxygen demand required for meta cognition and decreased oxygen delivery post-TBI are important concepts in understanding the underlying mechanism of EF decline after trauma to the brain. It is stipulated that persons with TBI who suffer from disorders causing decreased brain tissue oxygenation, constant or intermittent, due to other disorders (e.g.,SA), will demonstrate worse clinical outcomes post-TBI when compared to those who do not.

Defining SA

SA, an intermittent complete cessation of airflow during sleep, is the most frequently reported form of sleep-disordered breathing (SDB) after TBI. SA of at least 10 s is considered clinically important, but in many patients, apneas can last 20–30 s and in some cases as long as 3 min. SA can be central or obstructive in nature. In central sleep apnea (CSA), the neural drive to respiratory muscle is abolished. In obstructive sleep apnea (OSA), airflow ceases because of occlusion of the upper airway in sleep due to the specific anatomical structure of the upper airway or decreased muscle tonus resulting in muscle collapse during sleep. The resulting apnea leads to progression of asphyxia until there is an arousal from sleep, which restores the airway patency. The patient then returns to sleep and the sequence of the events repeats. In the most severe cases, SA occurs up to 500 times per night—resulting in sleep fragmentation and disturbances of sleep architecture. These nocturnal sleep disturbances result in vital exhaustion/daytime sleepiness/ impaired alertness and cognitive dysfunction, especially in the areas of attention and memory [11]. Furthermore, both OSA and CSA, highly prevalent after TBI, result in recurrent episodes of nocturnal asphyxia and decreased oxygenation (hypoxia) of brain tissue. Such brain tissue hypoxia is related to prefrontal lobe dysfunction [12]. Related respiratory events, hypopnea, and respiratory event-related arousals are characterized by a partial reduction in airflow in sleep, and consequent arousals from sleep with or without significant oxygen desaturation. The average number of all respiratory events per hour of sleep is termed the respiratory disturbance index (RDI). An RDI of 5 or greater is of clinical significance and can be an indication of SDB [13].

SA and Oxidative Stress

It is evident that SA may lead to a series of pathophysiologic events [14]. Xu et al. demonstrated that chronic intermittent hypoxia results in cortical neuronal cell apoptosis in mice [15]. Chronic intermittent hypoxia is also shown to be associated with inducible nitric oxide synthesis in the brain [16-17], which plays a role in nerve cell communication, and is associated with neuronal plasma membranes [18]. Other research has shown that free radicals formed as a result of oxidative stress in OSA lead to the up-regulation of transcription factors such as NF-κB [19]. Da Silva et al. reviewed the effects of OSA on homeostasis in the central nervous system (CNS) by examining the levels of biochemical markers of cerebral injury (neuron-specific enolase and the S100B protein derived from astrocytes) in OSA patients. The results of their study showed a significant increase in S100B markers, suggesting a CNS astrocyte reaction in response to cerebral hypoxemia in patients with OSA and supporting the view that OSA causes brain alterations, which can manifest as neuropsychological symptoms [20].

SA as a Predictor of Executive Function

Numerous studies have established a relationship between SA and cognitive deficits, including EF, attention/vigilance, language, memory, and psychomotor speed [21]. Of these various deficits, EF has been a research topic of particular interest. Several tasks, such as the Wisconsin Card Sorting Task, the Tower of Toronto, and the Stroop task, have been used to measure SA sufferers' deficits in EF [22].

Beebe and Gozal [12] studied the involvement of the frontal cortex in OSA patients and its link to EF. These authors reported decreased EF in their patients, which manifested as deficits in behavioral inhibition, self-regulation of affect and arousal, working and contextual memory, and analytical ability. They proposed a model in which sleep fragmentation, hypoxemia, and dysfunction of the frontal lobe cortex are interrelated through the disruption of homeostasis and altered glial viability within primarily frontal regions of the brain cortex. The authors stressed that executive dysfunction in OSA patients leads to reduced social relationships and job tasks; therefore, evaluation of social and work-related skills is crucial and should take precedence over other aspects of cognition (e.g., vocabulary, intelligence).

In one study, abnormal breathing and oxygen desaturation during sleep in heavy snorers were factors associated with obtaining fewer numbers of categories on the Wisconsin Card Sorting Task (i.e., domain of executive function: mental set shifting and abstract behavior). Using a modified version of the task, Naegele et al. [23] reported that poor performance on this task is predictive by the effect of severe hypoxemia in OSA patients. Behavioral manifestations in OSA patients also included difficulties with problem solving and initiation detected by the Tower of Toronto task (i.e., domain of executive function: problem solving). In addition, other researchers have found that persons with OSA require more time to complete EF tasks than do controls. When assessing planning abilities using the Maze task (i.e., domain of executive function: planning and foresight), Bedard et al. found that OSA participants had significant difficulties in completing the task [24].

Halbower et al. [25] studied links between OSA, cognitive deficits, and neuronal brain injury in children. Compared to controls, children with severe OSA had significant deficits in intelligence quotient (IQ) and EF (verbal working memory and verbal fluency), and demonstrated decreased neuronal metabolite ratios in the left hippocampus and the frontal cortex, as measured by proton magnetic resonance spectroscopic imaging. The authors speculated that untreated childhood OSA could permanently alter a developing child's cognitive potential.

Treatment of SA Executive Dysfunction

Several approaches to the treatment of SA have been advocated based on our current understanding of the mechanisms underlying the disorder. Milder OSA can often be managed effectively by weight reduction, avoidance of alcohol, improvement of nasal patency and avoidance of sleeping in a supine position. In more severe OSA cases, nasal continuous positive airway pressure (CPAP), a treatment which delivers positive pressure through a nasal/full-face mask to maintain opening of the upper airway during sleep, is widely used. Patients with CSA, whose apnea arises from instability of respiratory drive, have been shown to respond well to CPAP with or without adding nocturnal supplemental oxygen [26-27].

A current controversy regarding EF and treatment of SA revolves around an important issue: the efficacy of SA treatment in correcting executive dysfunction. Although newer research shows that cognitive deficits are resolved with treatment in the majority of cases, other research suggests some deficits in EF may remain unchanged [28-30]. This raises the possibility of permanent brain changes as a result of OSA.

In their review, Engleman et al. [31] indicated that most research to date has shown trends toward better cognitive performance after CPAP treatment compared to placebo. At least 3 studies comparing neuropsychological test scores of OSA patients before and after 6 months of CPAP treatment with test scores of healthy controls found notable cognitive improvement, including improvement in EF [23,32-33].

A recent randomized double-blind placebo-controlled trial by Ancoli-Israel et al. [34] examined the effect of CPAP on cognitive functioning in patients with Alzheimer's disease (AD). A comparison of pre-and post-treatment neuropsychological test scores (HVLT-R, Trail Making test) in Alzheimer's patients receiving 3 weeks of therapeutic CPAP showed a significant improvement in cognition, especially in episodic verbal learning and memory and in some aspects of EF such as cognitive flexibility and mental processing speed. These data, as well as the data of other researchers [35], seems promising and indicate that OSA may be a reversible cause of cognitive loss in this patient group; moreover, treatment of OSA, especially in the early stages of dementia when patients are still largely independent, may slow the progression of dementia. This reinforces the necessity of identifying and treating SA in individuals with TBI in the early stages post-injury.

Relationship Between TBI, SA, and Executive Dysfunction

Significant correlations have been reported between measures of EFs and regional cerebral glucose metabolism in medial and dorsolateral prefrontal cortical regions and the cingulate gyrus, despite the absence of detectable structural lesions on brain magnetic resonance imaging. These results suggest that impairments of EFs may be related not only to focal traumatic lesions of the prefrontal cortex, but also to lesions of the white matter tracts [36-37]. These effects appear to be non-specific to TBI, as similar results are reported in persons with Alzheimer's disease AD [38]. Interestingly, SA is a risk factor for AD and other neurological diseases [39]. Similarly, the implication of TBI as a contributing factor in the development of AD and dementia has been reported [40]. In some individuals, disruption of axonal transport following TBI can lead to the rapid accumulation of amyloid precursor proteins and other proteins associated with the neurodegenerative disease. The variation observed in the APOE E4 allele in persons with TBI prompted exploration of the role of genetic factors in modulating the risk for AD after TBI [41]. Coincidentally, O'Hara et al. [42] reported the relationship between sleep apnea and dementia through the APOE E4 allele, whose carriers may be at an increased risk for developing dementia. Numerous research studies also report a higher prevalence of SA in the TBI population, ranging from 25% to 35%, compared to 4–9% in the general world population [43].

Although the high numbers of SA in the TBI population can be partly attributed to pre-morbid undetected sleep disorders, which can be a proximate cause of the injury itself, some persons may develop the sleep disorder as a consequence of brain injury. A disturbed coordination of upper airway and diaphragmatic muscles due to damage to the brainstem might favor the appearance of SA. Aggregation of SA can occur with commonly prescribed medications after the injury, such as muscle relaxants, sedatives, or hypnotics. Furthermore, narcotics for pain can cause opioid-induced respiratory depression, defined as a combination of decreased respiratory drive, reduced level of consciousness, and upper-airway obstruction, manifesting as both central and obstructive respiratory events [44].

Theoretical links exist between levels of hypocretins, which play a part in the regulation of various functions, including arousal, muscle tone, locomotion, feeding behavior, and neuroendocrine/autonomic functions, and SA [45-46]. Baumann et al. reported low hypocretin-1 levels in the cerebrospinal fluid from over 90% of 27 patients in the early days post-TBI and in 19% of 21 patients at 6 months post-injury [47-48]. Hypocretin deficiency after TBI may cause the loss of control of respiratory-related activity of hypoglossal motoneurons during rapid eye movement (REM) sleep [49]. Similarly, the presence of motor activity disfacilitation during REM sleep in acute rat preparations, with experimentally induced hypoxia, hypercapnia, and/or reduced airway patency has been reported; many of these conditions are also present in OSA [50]. Therefore, it is possible that due to TBI, disfacilitation of respiratory-related inputs to hypoglossal motoneurons during REM sleep will result in aggravation of SA at the acute stages post-injury, but may resolve with time.

Another relationship relevant to the discussion of executive dysfunction in SA and post-TBI is comorbid psychopathology. Depression after TBI is common, ranging 27–61%, when structural diagnostic criteria are used [51-52]. A nearly twofold increase in the risk for developing major depressive disorders has been reported in persons suffering from SA [53]. Working with acute mild TBI patients, Chaput et al. found that depression and irritability were more frequent in those with sleep complaints [54]. Depression has been reported to be associated with poorer cognitive outcomes, and no published studies have shown that the cognitive effects of depression can be reliably differentiated from the cognitive effects of SA or TBI [55]. Moreover, depression can act as an amplifier of other neurobehavioral changes, including aggression and irritability, and modulate symptom overlap between the post-concussion syndrome and psychopathology [56]. Given the frequent co-occurrence of depression and SA in TBI, recognizing the cumulative evidence for the intertwined processes of mood, sleep, and neuroplasticity post-TBI may have important implications for cognitive rehabilitation.

One of the aims of this review was to determine whether current evidence suggests that SA is causally associated with executive dysfunction after TBI and whether there is any evidence that the treatment of SA is effective in improving EF of these persons. The intent was to shed light on the potential importance of SA screening and treatment post-TBI as a means of halting the progression of executive dysfunction after brain trauma. To directly examine this question, prospective longitudinal studies are required. However, this research design is expensive and demands sustained commitment from participants and investigators. Given the heterogeneity in TBI (e.g., sex, age, injury localization and severity, confounding factors, difference in medication regime, and genetic makeup), the main requirement of an effective prospective study—the recruitment and retention of a sufficiently large sample—is difficult to achieve. An alternative approach has been to focus on comparisons of outcome between groups of persons with TBI of similar age/gender/time since injury/injury localization/severity, but who differ in that some suffer SA and some do not.

Wilde et al. [57] performed such a study on 35 TBI patients, 18 years of age and older and at least 3 months post-TBI. Of these, 19 patients had OSA, as defined by polysomnography, with severity reported by the apnea–hypopnea index. Their EF performance was compared with 16 TBI participants without OSA. Both groups were comparable in terms of age, education, severity of injury, time post-injury, and Glasgow Coma Scale. The main outcome measures were: The Psychomotor Vigilance Test, Rey Complex Figure Test, Rey Auditory

Verbal Learning Test, Digit Span Test from the Wechsler Memory Scale, and finger-taping test. The Rey-Osterrieth Complex Figure Test (RCFT) [58] permits the evaluation of different cognitive functions believed to be EF measures, such as visuospatial abilities, attention, planning, organizational skills and analysis-synthesis. Persons with OSA performed significantly worse on RCFT delayed recall (t_{35}= -2.05, p=0.048), had greater numbers of lapses, and worse retention (i.e., deterioration of thinking ability and memory) compared to those without OSA. Interestingly, the researchers did not find significant differences in OSA vs. non-OSA patients on working memory tests such as the copy administration, total recall list, and the digit span test forward and backward (Table 1). These results are promising, suggesting the possibility of reversibility of executive deficits and the potential of recovery with treatment implementation.

The study has noted limitations. Some data were missing in 10 of 19 participants with OSA and in 8 of 16 non-OSA participants. The localization of brain damage was not reported, even though positive CT scan findings were found in 9 of 19 OSA and 8 non-OSA participants. The authors did not comment on the number of CSA events or whether any hypopneas that were included in the diagnoses were of central origin. Overall, this is valuable information because SA in TBI populations seems to differ from those being described in general. According to reports of Websters et al. [10], the majority of the events in their sample of 28 TBI participants were central in nature rather than obstructive, while in the general population, SA consists of 90% obstructive and only 10% central events [59]. Additional methodological concerns include the great number of variables and the small sample size consisted largely of male participants, which was not allowing definitive conclusions to be drawn.

In summary, executive dysfunction, encompassing impairments in cognitive, behavioral and emotional processes after TBI, presents significant challenges for recovery after injury. Similar process impairments are also found in persons with SA. This review suggests that undetected/untreated SA in persons with TBI may have profound effects on neurobehavioral processes, impacting both structure and function. Different lines of evidence are relevant to the mechanism of EF decline associated with TBI and untreated SA. These include, but are not limited to: 1) evidence from animal studies on hippocampal cell death and apoptosis of the forebrain regions as a result of recurrent SA resulting in secondary neuronal injury, 2) association between white-matter grade and severity of CSA reported, 3) results of CPAP treatment intervention studies showing improvement in EF test performance in SA sufferers, 4) studies on the prevalence of SA in TBI populations, placing affected individuals in a category of greater risk, 5) numerous studies showing the detrimental effects of SA on non-TBI persons' cognitive performance, especially EF, all of which advocate for an association between possible undiscovered and untreated SA and poor cognitive rehabilitation outcomes of TBI survivors. Finally, a recent study by researchers from the University of Pittsburgh School of Medicine retrospectively evaluated diffusion-tensor images from 64 consecutive patients with mild TBI who underwent magnetic resonance imaging. They found that more than half of the patients had sleep and wake disturbances. While researchers did not clarify the category of the sleep disorder, there was a significant reduction in fractional anisotropy in the parahippocampalgyri in patients with sleep and wake disturbances versus those without [36]. This region in the brain plays an important role in memory encoding and retrieval and in identifying social context as well, including paralinguistic elements of verbal communication [60].

Although we have presented a narrative review of published literature relevant to understanding the association between SA and executive function in TBI, a significant challenge in discussing these associations is disentangling the effect of brain injury from the effect of SA on executive function in TBI (Figure 1). It is possible that studies of executive function have been conducted often with TBI survivors who have suffered SA, where untreated pre-existing SA was

Author(s); year	Article Title, journal, pages; Study Objective	Research Design/ Sample Size; Inclusion/Exclusion	Participants	Data Collection Methods/Measures	Findings	Comments
Wilde M, Castriotta R, Lai J, Atanasov S, Masel B, Kuna S; 2007 [57]	Cognitive impairment in patients with traumatic brain injury and obstructive sleep apnea. Arch Phys Med Rehabil. 2007; 88(10):1284-8 ▪ To examine the impact of comorbid obstructive sleep apnea on the cognitive functioning of traumatic brain injury patients	Case-control study/35; subjects who were more than 18 years old and at least 3 months post-injury/ Subjects with other sleep disorders	Persons with traumatic brain injury (TBI) from 3 academic medical centers; 2 groups: obstructive sleep apnea (OSA) and non-OSA; n (OSA) =19, n (non-OSA) = 16 ▪ Age: mean for OSA, 47.25 y; non-OSA, 51.47 y ▪ Time since injury: OSA, 124 mo; non-OSA, 77 mo Male/Female: OSA, 17/2; non-OSA, 12/4 ▪ TBI severity (unknown/ moderate/moderate-severe/severe): OSA, 10/3/1/5; non-OSA, 8/2/3/3 ▪ Computed tomography (CT) findings (unknown/ negative/positive): OSA, 16/0/9; non-OSA, 8/1/7	Assessments: Clinical interview; Physical examination; Glasgow Coma Score (GSC); CT data; Neurological assessment; Polysomnography (PSG); Multiple Sleep Latency Test (MSLT)	Mean apnea–hypopnea index (AHI) for OSA group: 26.83/h; non-OSA: 4.49/h ▪ Mean MSLT score: OSA, 11.19; non-OSA, 5.06 ▪ Statistically significant difference in test performance for patients with and without OSA: • memory recall measures: worse in OSA • number of lapses: greater in OSA • retention: worse in OSA ▪ No statistically significant difference in performance between groups: • on the copy administration • total recall list • digit span test forward and backward	Definitions: Diagnosis of OSA: 5 or more apneas per hour and/or 10 or more apneas plus hypopneas per hour

Table 1: Literature review on association between traumatic brain injury and sleep apnea.

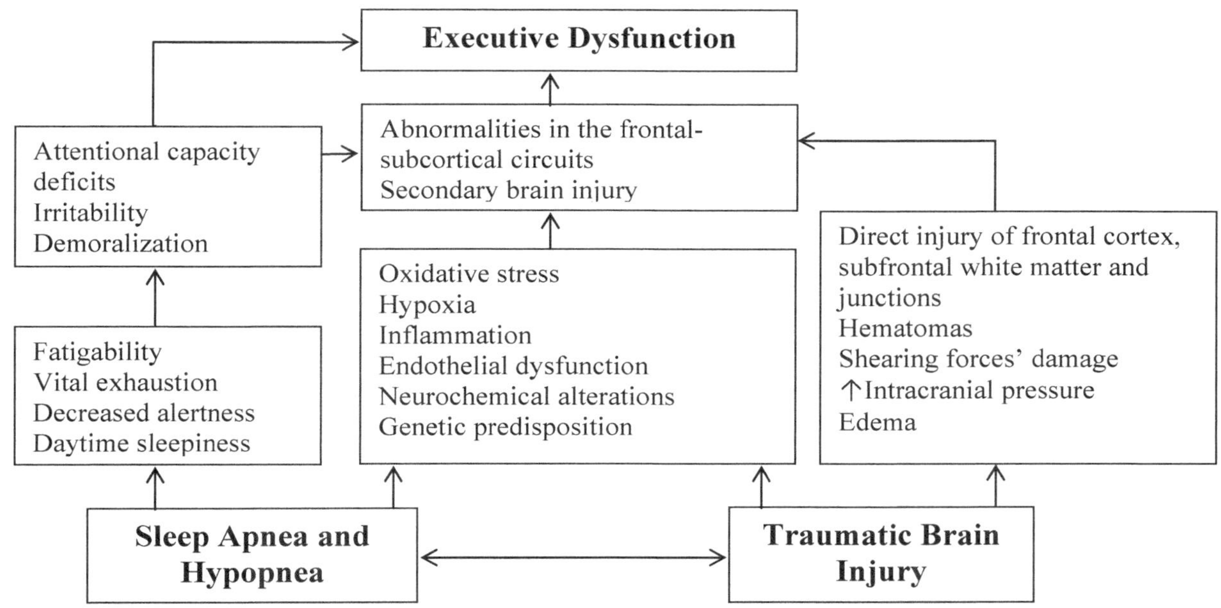

Figure 1: Pathogenesis of development of executive dysfunction among patients with Sleep Apnea and Traumatic Brain Injury.

a proximate cause of the brain injury itself. There is in fact growing evidence supporting an association between sleepiness and fatigue as a result of SA, and the probability of one's involvement in an incident involving injury [60]. As discussed above, non-specific alterations to white and grey matter integrity and aberrant prefrontal activity have been reported in both TBI and SA sufferers' studies. These provocative findings suggest a need for further study of brain connectivity among areas particularly relevant to executive function and vascular risk factors, taking into account the high likelihood of undetected/untreated SA in TBI persons. Given that there is no known cure for brain injury, addressing SA may provide benefits in terms of cognitive function which may be currently overlooked.

To conclude, the findings of this review suggest that limited research that has been done to identify EF outcomes in persons with TBI, and how these outcomes might be related to SA. Considering the impact of brain damage itself on cognitive functioning after TBI, it is still unknown whether executive dysfunction related to SA in the TBI population is a specific entity or whether the presence of SA exaggerates the TBI-related physiological changes in EF. The general processes slowing usually found in patients with brain injuries could explain, to a great extent, the decline in EF observed in persons with TBI, as well as persons with SA [14, 37-40]. More definitive evidence on SA as a cause of poor EF after TBI can be gathered through further research targeting TBI survivors. While it is premature to make strong conclusions regarding the nature of the synergy of SA and executive dysfunction in TBI, this literature review sheds light on the repercussions of SA, if left unrecognized and untreated, to cognitive dysfunction following brain damage. The prospect of improving impaired processes through the treatment of SA cannot be ignored. The current state of evidence indicating a hierarchy of post-morbid cognitive symptom clusters within similar injury severities, as well as sustained executive dysfunction after mild TBI years after injury, further strengthens the need to identify and treat people with TBI who experience SA at the early stages of cognitive rehabilitation.

Acknowledgment

This manuscript had no external funding source. The first author was supported by a 2012/13 Toronto Rehabilitation Institute Scholarship, 2012/13 Ontario Graduate Scholarship, and 2013/15 Frederick Banting and Charles Best Canada Graduate Scholarships-Doctoral Awards from the Canadian Institutes of Health Research. We also recognize the support of the Canadian Institute of Health Research - Institute of Gender and Health #CGW-126580.

References

1. Mathers CD, Loncar D (2006) Projections of global mortality and burden of disease from 2002 to 2030. PLoS Med 3: e442.
2. Langlois JA, Sattin RW (2005) Traumatic brain injury in the United States: research and programs of the Centers for Disease Control and Prevention (CDC). J Head Trauma Rehabil 20: 187-188.
3. Corrigan JD, Harrison-Felix C, Bogner J, Dijkers M, Terrill MS, et al. (2003) Systematic bias in traumatic brain injury outcome studies because of loss to follow-up. Arch Phys Med Rehabil 84: 153-160.
4. Mathias JL, Wheaton P (2007) Changes in attention and information-processing speed following severe traumatic brain injury: a meta-analytic review. Neuropsychology 21: 212-223.
5. Askenasy JJ, Rahmani L (1987) Neuropsycho-social rehabilitation of head injury. Am J Phys Med 66: 315-327.
6. Jellinger KA (2004) Traumatic brain injury as a risk factor for Alzheimer's disease. J Neurol Neurosurg Psychiatry 75: 511-512.
7. Dunham CM, Ransom KJ, Flowers LL, Siegal JD, Kohli CM (2004) Cerebral hypoxia in severely brain-injured patients is associated with admission Glasgow Coma Scale score, computed tomographic severity, cerebral perfusion pressure, and survival. J Trauma 56: 482-489.
8. Chang JJ, Youn TS, Benson D, Mattick H, Andrade N, et al. (2009) Physiologic and functional outcome correlates of brain tissue hypoxia in traumatic brain injury. Crit Care Med 37: 283-290.
9. Johnston AJ, Steiner LA, Coles JP, Chatfield DA, Fryer TD, et al. (2005) Effect of cerebral perfusion pressure augmentation on regional oxygenation and metabolism after head injury. Crit Care Med 33: 189-195.
10. Rose JC, Neill TA, Hemphill JC 3rd (2006) Continuous monitoring of the microcirculation in neurocritical care: an update on brain tissue oxygenation. Curr Opin Crit Care 12: 97-102.
11. Webster JB, Bell KR, Hussey JD, Natale TK, Lakshminarayan S (2001) Sleep

apnea in adults with traumatic brain injury: a preliminary investigation. Arch Phys Med Rehabil 82: 316-321.

12. Beebe DW, Gozal D (2002) Obstructive sleep apnea and the prefrontal cortex: towards a comprehensive model linking nocturnal upper airway obstruction to daytime cognitive and behavioral deficits. J Sleep Res 11: 1-16.

13. Young T, Palta M, Dempsey J, Skatrud J, Weber S, et al. (1993) The occurrence of sleep-disordered breathing among middle-aged adults. N Engl J Med 328 (17): 1230-5.

14. Finn L, Young T, Palta M, Fryback DG (1998) Sleep-disordered breathing and self-reported general health status in the Wisconsin Sleep Cohort Study. Sleep 21: 701-706.

15. Xu W, Chi L, Row BW, Xu R, Ke Y, et al. (2004) Increased oxidative stress is associated with chronic intermittent hypoxia-mediated brain cortical neuronal cell apoptosis in a mouse model of sleep apnea. Neuroscience 126: 313-323.

16. Schulz H, Wilde-Frenz J, Grabietz-Kurfürst U (1997) Cognitive deficits in patients with daytime sleepiness. Acta Neurol Belg 97: 108-112.

17. Schulz R, Seeger W, Grimminger F (2001) Serum nitrite/nitrate levels in obstructive sleep apnea. Am J Respir Crit Care Med 164: 1997-1998.

18. Southan GJ, Szabó C (1996) Selective pharmacological inhibition of distinct nitric oxide synthase isoforms. Biochem Pharmacol 51: 383-394.

19. Lavie L (2003) Obstructive sleep apnoea syndrome--an oxidative stress disorder. Sleep Med Rev 7: 35-51.

20. da Silva LG, Mottin CC, Souza DO, Portela LV, Braga CW, et al. (2008) Serum S100B but not NSE levels are increased in morbidly obese individuals affected by obstructive sleep apnea-hypopnea syndrome. Obes Surg 18: 993-999.

21. Naismith S, Winter V, Gotsopoulos H, Hickie I, Cistulli P (2004) Neurobehavioral functioning in obstructive sleep apnea: differential effects of sleep quality, hypoxemia and subjective sleepiness. J Clin Exp Neuropsychol 26: 43-54.

22. Harrison Y, Horne JA, Rothwell A (2000) Prefrontal neuropsychological effects of sleep deprivation in young adults--a model for healthy aging? Sleep 23: 1067-1073.

23. Halbower AC, Degaonkar M, Barker PB, Earley CJ, Marcus CL, et al. (2006) Childhood obstructive sleep apnea associates with neuropsychological deficits and neuronal brain injury. PLoS Med 3: e301.

24. [No authors listed] (1994) Indications and standards for use of nasal continuous positive airway pressure (CPAP) in sleep apnea syndromes. American Thoracic Society. Official statement adopted March 1944. Am J Respir Crit Care Med 150: 1738-1745.

25. Valencia-Flores M, Bliwise D, Guilleminault C, Cilveti R, Clerk A (1996) Cognitive function in patients with sleep apnea after acute nocturnal nasal continuous positive airway pressure (CPAP) treatment: sleepiness and hypoxemia effects. J ClinExpNeuropsychol 18(2): 197-210.

26. Bédard MA, Montplaisir J, Malo J, Richer F, Rouleau I (1993) Persistent neuropsychological deficits and vigilance impairment in sleep apnea syndrome after treatment with continuous positive airways pressure (CPAP). J Clin Exp Neuropsychol 15: 330-341.

27. Naegele B, Pepin JL, Levy P, Bonnet C, Pellat J, et al. (1998) Cognitive executive dysfunction in patients with obstructive sleep apnea syndrome (OSAS) after CPAP treatment. Sleep 21: 392-397.

28. Feuerstein C, Naegelé B, Pépin JL, Lévy P (1997) Frontal lobe-related cognitive functions in patients with sleep apnea syndrome before and after treatment. Acta Neurol Belg 97: 96-107.

29. Engleman HM, Kingshott RN, Martin SE, Douglas NJ (2000) Cognitive function in the sleep apnea/hypopnea syndrome (SAHS). Sleep 23 Suppl 4: S102-108.

30. Kotterba S, Rasche K, Widdig W, Duscha C, Blombach S, et al. (1998) Neuropsychological investigations and event-related potentials in obstructive sleep apnea syndrome before and during CPAP-therapy. J Neurol Sci 159: 45-50.

31. Naëgelé B, Thouvard V, Pépin JL, Lévy P, Bonnet C, et al. (1995) Deficits of cognitive executive functions in patients with sleep apnea syndrome. Sleep 18: 43-52.

32. Ancoli-Israel S, Gehrman P, Martin JL, Shochat T, Marler M, et al. (2003) Increased light exposure consolidates sleep and strengthens circadian rhythms in severe Alzheimer's disease patients. Behav Sleep Med 1: 22-36.

33. Bliwise DL (1996) Is sleep apnea a cause of reversible dementia in old age? J Am Geriatr Soc 44: 1407-1409.

34. Zappalà G, Thiebaut de Schotten M, Eslinger PJ (2012) Traumatic brain injury and the frontal lobes: what can we gain with diffusion tensor imaging? Cortex 48: 156-165.

35. Leclercq M, Couillet J, Azouvi P, Marlier N, Martin Y, et al. (2000) Dual task performance after severe diffuse traumatic brain injury or vascular prefrontal damage. J Clin Exp Neuropsychol 22: 339-350.

36. Fakhran S, Yaeger K, Alhilali L. Symptomatic white matter changes in mild traumatic brain injury resemble pathologic features of early Alzheimer dementia. (2013) Radiology. Published online before print.

37. Anderson KN, Bradley AJ (2013) Sleep disturbance in mental health problems and neurodegenerative disease. Nat Sci Sleep 5: 61-75.

38. Van Den Heuvel C, Thornton E, Vink R (2007) Traumatic brain injury and Alzheimer's disease: a review. Prog Brain Res 161: 303-316.

39. Jellinger KA, Paulus W, Wrocklage C, Litvan I (2001) Effects of closed traumatic brain injury and genetic factors on the development of Alzheimer's disease. Eur J Neurol 8: 707-710.

40. O'Hara R, Schröder CM, Kraemer HC, Kryla N, Cao C, et al. (2005) Nocturnal sleep apnea/hypopnea is associated with lower memory performance in APOE epsilon4 carriers. Neurology 65: 642-644.

41. Castriotta RJ, Wilde MC, Lai JM, Atanasov S, Masel BE, et al. (2007) Prevalence and consequences of sleep disorders in traumatic brain injury. J Clin Sleep Med 3: 349-356.

42. Mollayeva T, Shapiro CM. Medication Effects. In: Kushida CA (2013) The Encyclopedia of Sleep, Vol 2. Waltham: Academic Press 330-7.

43. Baumann CR, Bassetti CL (2005) Hypocretins (orexins) and sleep-wake disorders. Lancet Neurol 4: 673-682.

44. Saper CB (2006) Staying awake for dinner: hypothalamic integration of sleep, feeding, and circadian rhythms. Prog Brain Res 153: 243-252.

45. Baumann CR, Stocker R, Imhof HG, Trentz O, Hersberger M, et al. (2005) Hypocretin-1 (orexin A) deficiency in acute traumatic brain injury. Neurology 65: 147-149.

46. Baumann CR, Werth E, Stocker R, Ludwig S, Bassetti CL (2007) Sleep-wake disturbances 6 months after traumatic brain injury: a prospective study. Brain 130: 1873-1883.

47. Torterolo P, Yamuy J, Sampogna S, Morales FR, Chase MH (2003) Hypocretinergic neurons are primarily involved in activation of the somatomotor system. Sleep 26: 25-28.

48. Chase MH (2013) Motor control during sleep and wakefulness: clarifying controversies and resolving paradoxes. Sleep Med Rev 17: 299-312.

49. Jorge RE, Starkstein SE (2005) Pathophysiologic aspects of major depression following traumatic brain injury. J Head Trauma Rehabil 20: 475-487.

50. Bombardier CH, Fann JR, Temkin NR, Esselman PC, Barber J, et al. (2010) Rates of major depressive disorder and clinical outcomes following traumatic brain injury. JAMA 303: 1938-1945.

51. Peppard PE, Szklo-Coxe M, Hla KM, Young T (2006) Longitudinal association of sleep-related breathing disorder and depression. Arch Intern Med 166: 1709-1715.

52. Chaput G, Giguère JF, Chauny JM, Denis R, Lavigne G (2009) Relationship among subjective sleep complaints, headaches, and mood alterations following a mild traumatic brain injury. Sleep Med 10: 713-716.

53. Whelan-Goodinson R, Ponsford J, Schönberger M (2008) Association between psychiatric state and outcome following traumatic brain injury. J Rehabil Med 40: 850-857.

54. Fox DD, Lees-Haley PR, Ernest K, Dolezal-Wood S (1995) Post-concussive symptoms: base rates and etiology in psychiatric patients. ClinNeuropsychol 9: 89-92.

55. Wilde MC, Castriotta RJ, Lai JM, Atanasov S, Masel BE, et al. (2007) Cognitive impairment in patients with traumatic brain injury and obstructive sleep apnea. Arch Phys Med Rehabil 88: 1284-1288.

56. Lezak M (1995) Neuropsychological assessment. (3rdedn) New York: Oxford Univ Pr.

57. Hyafil A, Summerfield C, Koechlin E (2009) Two mechanisms for task switching in the prefrontal cortex. J Neurosci 29: 5135-5142.

58. Libby LA, Ekstrom AD, Ragland JD, Ranganath C (2012) Differential connectivity of perirhinal and parahippocampal cortices within human hippocampal subregions revealed by high-resolution functional imaging. J Neurosci 32: 6550-6560.

59. Lindberg E, Carter N, Gislason T, Janson C (2001) Role of snoring and daytime sleepiness in occupational accidents. Am J Respir Crit Care Med 164: 2031-2035.

60. Wittmann V, Rodenstein DO (2004) Health care costs and the sleep apnea syndrome. Sleep Med Rev 8: 269-279.

Frequency of Human Leukocyte Antigens, Plasminogen Activator Inhibitor-1 and Methylenetetrahydrofolate Reductase Gene Polymorphisms in Obstructive Sleep Apnea-Hypopnea Syndrome with or without Pulmonary Artery Hypertension

Domenico Maurizio Toraldo[1]*, Francesco De Nuccio[2], Salvatore Mauro[3], Francesco Spirito[4], Alessandro Distante[5] and Giuseppe Nicolardi[2]

[1]Department of Rehabilitation, Unit Care Respiratory, ASL/Lecce, Italy
[2]Laboratory of Human Anatomy and Neuroscience, Department of Biological and Environmental Sciences and Technologies, University of Salento, Italy
[3]Laboratory of Genetic, "Vito Fazzi", ASL Lecce, Italy
[4]Division of Cardiovascular disease, City of Lecce Hospital, Lecce, Italy
[5]ISBEM Research Institute, Medical School of University of Pisa, Pisa, Italy

Abstract

Background: The aim of this study was to investigate relationships between the genotypic frequencies of genes F5-coagulation factor V (proaccelerin, labile factor), F2-coagulation factor II (thrombin), MTHFR-methylenetetrahydrofolate reductase (NADPH), PAI-1 - plasminogen activator inhibitor-1, the frequencies of HLA haplotypes DQ2/DR3, DQ2/DR7, DQ8/DR4, **5,** DQ7/DR5 and clinical features and severity of OSAS in comparison to a control population of 163 patients without OSAS.

Methods and results: Eighty-two consecutive outpatients with OSAS were enrolled in the respiratory, cardio, and genetic study. By means of cluster analysis it was shown that 40% of patients with PAI-1 5G/5G polymorphism had pulmonary artery hypertension, with a mean value of 46 mm Hg, and also 40% of OSAS patients with pulmonary artery hypertension had PAI-1 5G/5G polymorphism, 50% had 4G/5G and 10% had 4G/4G; as regards OSAS patients without PH, 8.95% only had PAI-1 5G/5G polymorphism, 22.38% had PAI-1 4G/4G and 67.16% had PAI-1 4G/5G. PAI-1 polimorphisms were detected by RDB techniques**.** Moreover, these patients with OSAS showed HLA haplotypes polymorphism: DQ7 (40%), DQ2.5 (20%) and DQ2.2 (10%). Nevertheless, OSAS patients without PAH showed HLA polymorphism as follows: DQ7 (47, 76%); DQ2.5 (8.95%); DQ2.2 (16.41%). OSAS patients with pulmonary hypertension were 12.99 % of all OSAS patients. HLA polymorphism was analyzed by PCR amplification and gel electrophoresis.

Conclusions: Our results suggested a genotypic heterogeneity among OSAS patients PAI-1 5G/5G polymorphism with PAH possibly in relation with severity of the disease.

Keywords: PAI-1: Plasminogen activator inhibitor-1; HLA: Human leukocyte antigen; OSAS: Obstructive sleep apnoea syndrome; PAH: Pulmonary artery hypertension

Introduction

Obstructive Sleep Apnea Syndrome (OSAS) is affects 2-4% of the middle-aged population [1]. According to the American Sleep Disorder Association, OSAS is defined as an intrinsic sleep disturbance characterized by the appearance of repeated episodes of upper airways obstruction (apneas) occurring during sleep, usually associated with a reduction in oxygen blood saturation [2]. Several genetic factors, environmental influences as well as developmental factors are closely tied to OSAS. Redline and Tishler underline the genetic basis of several risk factors for obstructive sleep apnoea [3]. Earlier studies have examined the expression of various inflammatory factors in OSAS patients [4].

There is increasing evidence that OSAS is present with hypertension, myocardial ischemia, metabolic syndrome, including impaired glucose tolerance which increase the risk of stroke [5]. Existing research on the general population clearly indicate that an impaired fibrinolytic function is an important marker of cardiovascular risk [6,7].

For example, over-expression of the type 1 Plasminogen Activator Inhibitor (PAI-1), which is one of the primary regulators of the fibrinolytic system, enhances the pathological deposition of fibrin and facilitates the occurrence of thrombotic events [8]. An insertion/deletion polymorphism in the promoter region of this gene, where one allele sequence has four guanosines (4G) instead of five (5G), is collocated with a higher promoter activity [9] and increased PAI-1 levels in plasma [10]. A meta-analysis shows that this 4G allele is associated with an increased risk of myocardial infarct, particularly in high-risk populations [11]. In patients with OSAS, Range Mark et al. found increased PAI-1 levels and decreased fibrinolytic activity [12].

Moreover, several studies suggest that OSAS is strongly genetic, often found within families with progressively increasing risk which rises with the numbers of affected relatives [13,14]. The family pattern of OSAS is not only dependent on familial factors in increasing risk of the disorder but also by obesity, craniofacial malformations and ventilatory abnormalities [15,16]. The Human Leukocyte Antigen

***Corresponding author:** Domenico M Toraldo, Department of Rehabilitation, Unit Care Respiratory, ASL/Lecce, via a.c. Casetti n. 2 Zip Code 73100, Italy
E-mail: d.torald@tin.it

(HLA) is an objective genetic marker that may be implicated in the development of a disease through a genetic factor within the major histocompatibility complex [17].

Several studies have demonstrated an HLA DR2 and DQ1 gene polymorphism association with narcolepsy, suggesting a possible autoimmune connection [18-20]. Early research failed to demonstrate this hypothesis, finding that HLA-DR2 was only a linkage marker for another, unknown gene which causes narcolepsy. However, a Japanese study has shown an increased prevalence of HLA A2 in patients with OSAS as compared with the non OSAS population [21,22]. The frequency of HLA-A2 antigen was markedly increased in the patients with OSAS compared with control patients (81.3% vs. 40.6%) and compared with the general Japanese population. (40.7%)

The aim of this study was to investigate relationships between the genotypic frequencies of genes F5-coagulation factor V (proaccelerin, labile factor), F2-coagulation factor II (thrombin), MTHFR-methylenetetrahydrofolate reductase (NADPH), PAI-1 (plasminogen activator inhibitor-1), the frequencies of HLA haplotypes DQ2/DR3, DQ2/DR7, DQ8/DR4, 5, 10- DQ7/DR5 and clinical features and severity of OSAS in comparison to a control population of 163 patients without OSAS.

Methods

Patients and phenotypic parameters

Eighty-two consecutive outpatients with OSAS at the "A. Galateo" Department Rehabilitation, Respiratory Care Unit, San Cesario, Lecce, Italy, were enrolled in the respiratory study between June 2011 and January 2012. After enrolment in the study, all the patients were genetically evaluated at the laboratory of genetics of "Vito Fazzi" Hospital, ASL, Lecce, as well as at the Department of Cardiology at "City of Lecce Hospital" Lecce, Italy.

OSAS was diagnosed according to the American Academy of Sleep Medicine (AASM,) classification [23]. The following cardio-respiratory and morph metric parameters were also studied: BMI, Mallampati score as an independent predictor of obstructive sleep apnea [24], co morbidities, AHI (h/s), Mean $SatO_2$ (%), Nadir SaO_2 (%), T_{90} (%), PaO_2 (mmHg), $PaCO_2$ (mmHg); abdominal circumference and circumference of the neck (cm), Pulmonary Systolic Arterial Pressure (PAPs) (mmHg), Blood Pressure (mmHg), Epworth Sleepiness Scale (0-10), FEV_1 (%) , FEV_1/FVC (%), FCV (%). We studied the genotypic frequencies of genes haplotypes F5, F2, MTHFR, PAI-1 and the frequencies of HLA genes haplotype DQ2/DR3, DQ2/DR7, DQ8/DR4, and DQ7/DR5 in comparison to a control population of 163 patients without OSAS.

HLA genotyping of HLA DQ2-DQ8 genes

All patients included in the study were negative for tissue transglutaminase antibody typical of Celiac Disease. Blood was obtained with informed consent by vena puncture from patients.

Standard techniques for DNA extraction, PCR amplification and product detection have been used in the present work. A commercial reagent "DNA extraction from whole blood" ref AA1001 (Nuclear Laser Medicine, Settala, Mi, Italy) was used to purify genomic DNA from whole blood. HLA–DQ2 (DQA1*0501 and DQB1*02 alleles) and DQ8 (DQA1*0301 and DQB1*0302 alleles) genotyping was performed by PCR amplification using sequence specific primers (PCR-SSP) on a Gene Amp PCR 9700 System (Applied Bio system, Foster City, CA, USA). CELIAC DISEASE KIT 1 (Experteam, Venezia-Marghera, Italy), was used to determine HLA DQ2/DQ8 status in all patients. PCR products were detected by electrophoresis on 3% agarose gel and were visualized under UV light.

Coagulation factors and MTHFR genotyping

Assay for the identification of mutations associated with Cardiovascular Disease (CVD) based on Polymerase Chain Reaction (PCR) and reverse-hybridation was performed. Genomic DNA was extracted from whole blood samples using the "DNA extraction from whole blood" kit REF AA1001 (Nuclear Laser Medicine, Mi, Italy). The procedure includes three steps: 1) DNA isolation, 2) PCR amplification using biotinylated primers, 3) hybridization of amplification products to a test strip containing allele specific oligonucleotide probes (ASO) immobilized as an array of parallel lines. Bound biotinylated sequences are detected using streptavidin-alkaline phosphatase and colour substrates. "CVD Strip Assay"(Vienna Lab Diagnostics GmbH) contain all required material for the multiplex amplification on a Gene Amp PCR 9700 System (Applied Bio system, Foster City, CA, USA) of 12 mutations: Factor II G20210A; Factor V (Leiden) G1691A; Factor V H1299R; MTHFR A1298C and MTHFR C677T; Factor XIII V34L; β-Fibrinogen-455 G-A; PAI-1 4G/5G; GPIIIa L33P (HPA-1); ACE I/D; Apo B R3500Q; Apo E2/E3/E4.

Lung and heart function measurements

Static lung volumes were measured by body plethysmographs (6200 Auto box DL; Sensor Medics; Yorba Linda, CA) and dynamic lung volumes by mass flow sensors (V_{max}229; Sensor Medics) with the patients seated according to standard procedures [25].

Arterial blood gases were measured at the radial artery using microelectrodes (ABL 520; Radiometer; Copenhagen, Denmark), with the patient seated and spontaneously breathing air. Resting daytime PAPs was measured with a colour Doppler Echocardiograph (DE). Nocturnal desaturation was evaluated with polygraphic recording (Embletta *pds*, Recording System, Broomfield, CO, USA) of oxygen saturation, snoring, air flow, thoracic and abdominal respiratory movements, heart rate, including ECG in real-time mode, and body position. Polygraphic recordings were performed between 11:00 pm and 6:00 am. The signals, which were saved in a digital recorder, were computer-analyzed, and validated by a physician on the morning after the recording. Body mass index was calculated as the body weight/body weight ratio (in kilograms per square meter). Obesity was diagnosed when BMI > 29.9 kg/m^2.

Echocardiography analysis

Indirect noninvasive measurement of resting daytime PAPs was performed with a color Doppler Echocardiography (Acuson-Cypress-Siemens, Company by Business First of Louisville, 2005). Two-dimensional echocardiography was performed in apical views: four-chambers and two-chambers and parasternal views: long axis and short-axis. In all patients we excluded cardiac diseases that might determine arterial pulmonary hypertension. Tricuspid regurgitation was found in 86% of patients. The estimation of PAPs is based on simplified Bernoulli equation which describes the relationship of tricuspid regurgitation velocity and the peak pressure gradient of tricuspid regurgitation. This equation allows for estimation of PA systolic pressure taking into account right atrial pressure: PA systolic pressure=tricuspid regurgitation pressure gradient+estimated right atrial pressure. Right atrial pressure can be estimated based on the diameter and respiratory variation of the inferior vena cava although often a fixed value of 5 or 10 mmHg is assumed. Moreover Doppler-derived systolic PAP values are strongly correlated with pressure measured with catheterization [26].

Definition cardiac and respiratory parameters

The definition of apnoea and hypopnoea was based on standard criteria [27]. Nocturnal hypoxemia was defined as a $SatO_2$ of <90% for at least 5 min with an $NSatO_2$ of ≤ 85%. Time in bed was defined as the time from the start to the end of the recording. The percentage of Total Recording Time (TRT) spent in bed with a $SatO_2$ of 90% was defined as the T_{90}. The minimal TRT required for a satisfactory analysis of nocturnal recordings was 2 h [28]. Moreover, the subjective assessment of daytime sleepiness was carried out using the Epworth Sleepiness Scale (ESS) score of 10 [29]. According to ESC/ERS guidelines for echocardiographic diagnosis of pulmonary hypertension, pulmonary hypertension possible is defined as a systolic pulmonary artery pressure in the range of 37-50 mmHg with/without additional echocardiographic variables suggestive of pulmonary hypertension and with tricuspid regurgitation peak velocity of 2.9-3.4 m/s [30].

Statistical analysis

All variables first underwent descriptive statistical analysis to obtain the distribution fitting and to calculate average, variance, SD, range, standard skew ness and standard kurtosis. To evaluate whether the data variables were normally distributed, we calculated the _2 goodness-of-fit, the Shapiro-Wilk W test, the z-score for skewness, and the z-score for kurtosis. We also obtained a table of 95.0% Confidence Intervals (CI) with the mean of each variable to bind the sampling error in the estimates of these means. Patients were subdivided by gender and the variables of men and women in the N and ND groups were analyzed by *t* - test for unpaired data with comparison of means. The probability of type I error was minimized by the F-test of the Fisher-Snedecor test for comparison of variance, by the Mann-Whitney W test for comparison of medians, and with the Kolmogorov-Smirnov test, all of which were performed at a minimum 95% confidence level. The latter were carried out with the least-squares method so as to obtain linear prediction equations. Prediction accuracy referred to bias and precision, bias being the mean difference between predicted and measured values, and precision the 95% CI for the difference. Cluster analysis is used in such diverse fields as artificial intelligence, biology, medicine, psychology and business. It entails grouping similar objects into distinct, mutually exclusive subsets referred to as *clusters*. Elements within a cluster share a high degree of "natural association", whereas the clusters are relatively distinct from one another. We used the Fisher least significant differences method or the Bonferroni method, at 95% CI, to evaluate significant differences among the means with minimal probability of type I error, so as to assess significant differences between clusters.

Results

By means of cluster analysis it was shown that 40% of patients with PAI-1 5G/5G polymorphism had pulmonary artery hypertension, with a mean value of about 46 mm Hg, and also 40% of OSAS patients with pulmonary artery hypertension had PAI-1 5G/5G polymorphism, 50% are 4G/5G and 10% are 4G/4G; as regards OSAS patients without PH, 8.95% only had PAI-1 5G/5G polymorphism, 22.38% PAI-1 4G/4G and 67.16% PAI-1 4G/5G. Moreover, these OSAS patients showed HLA haplotypes polymorphism: DQ7 (40%), DQ2.5 (20%) and DQ2.2 (10%). Nevertheless, OSAS patients without PH showed HLA polymorphism as follows: DQ7 (47,76%); DQ2.5 (8.95%); DQ2.2 (16.41%). OSAS patients with pulmonary hypertension were 12.99 % of all OSAS patients (Table 1).

In the whole group of patients a relationship between FEV1 (%) and age was detected as follows: FEV1 (%)= 117,369 - 0,489893 Age (p-value=0,0004; R-squared=15,0023 %), outlining a worsening of pulmonary functions by age (Figures 1 and 2). Moreover, AHI (hs) was in relationship with neck circumference and FEV_1 (%) values, the model explaining 82,13% of AHI variability, as reported in the following equation: AHI=2,21 neck circumference-0,60 FEV_1 (%) (p-value=0,00001; R-squared (adj)=82,13 %). Nevertheless, FVC (%) alone was also in relation with AHI (hs) but only a 13,96 % of AHI (hs) variability was explained by this model: AHI=123,65 - 0,87 FVC (%) (p-value=0,0004; R-squared=15,06 %). PAP_S values correlates with AHI (%), neck and abdomen circumferences, FEV_1 (%) and Nadir $SatO_2$ (%) alone but not in a multiple regression model. Lastly, T_{90} (%) correlates with AHI (hs) as in the whole group of patients, as in OSAS not-PAH: T_{90}=-4,79804 + 0,747512 AHI (p-value=0,0000; R-squared (adjusted for d.f.)=65,736 %). As regards OSAS patients no-PAH only, we detected a relation between AHI values and both neck circumference and FEV_1 (%) predicted, the model explaining a 81,91% of AHI variability: AHI=2,37 neck circumference-0,69472 FEV_1 (%) (p-value=0,00001; R-squared (adjusted for d.f.)=81,91 %); PAPS is in relation only with neck circumference: PAP_S=0,64 neck circumference (p-value=0,00001; R-squared (adjusted for d.f.)=97,68 %).

As regarding the OSAS patients with pulmonary artery systolic hypertension, we detected the following relationship (Table 2):

1) Between AHI (hs) and abdominal circumference: AHI=-43,48+0,80 abdominal circumference (p-value=0,0453; R-squared (adjusted for d.f.)=33,90 %);

2) Between BMI and abdominal circumference: BMI=-20,12+0,46 abdominal circumference (p-value=0,0073; R-squared (adjusted for d.f.)=56,67 %);

	General (n=77) Mean ± SE	PAH (n=10) Mean ± SE	NoPAH (n=67) Mean ± SE	P
AHI/hs	41.39 ± 2.65	54.61 ± 6.52	39.45 ± 2.82	0.07NS
BMI(kg/m^2)	34.93 ± 0.89	36.29 ± 3.07	34.74 ± 0.92	0.56NS
Abdomen circumference/cm	116.03 ± 1.43	122.00 ± 5.21	115.18 ± 1.44	0.11NS
Neck circumference/ cm	43.43 ± 0.37	44.10 ± 1.33	43.33 ± 0.40	0.56NS
Age/years	56.24 ± 1.24	59.30 ± 4.36	55.80 ± 1.28	0.34NS
Ep worth Sleepiness Scale(0-10)	15.06 ± 0.49	14.3 ± 0.92	15.25 ± 0.54	0.52NS
FEV1 (%)	89.79 ± 1.57	80.80 ± 4.31	91.11 ± 1.63	0.025
FEV1/FVC (%)	93.74 ± 1.42	83.20 ± 3.89	95.29 ± 1.44	0.004
FVC (%)	94.45 ± 1.21	89.90 ± 3.22	95.12 ± 1.30	0.15NS
Mean SaO_2 (%)	90.57 ± 0.52	89.05 ± 1.22	90.80 ± 0.57	0.29NS
Nadir SaO_2 (%)	76.18 ± 1.10	73.20 ± 3.42	76.62 ± 1.16	0.34NS
Systolic Blood Pressure (mmHg)	141.60 ± 1.64	141.00 ± 4.58	141.69 ± 1.77	0.87NS
Diastolic Blood Pressure (mmHg)	86.35 ± 0.96	86.00 ± 1.63	86.40 ± 1.07	0.86NS
Pulmonary Artery Hypertension (systolic)(mmHg)	30.13 ± 0.79	44.70 ± 0.72	27.99 ± 0.52	0.00001
$PaCO_2$ (mmHg)	44.74 ± 1.22	46.50 ± 2.02	44.49 ± 1.37	0.58NS
PaO_2 (mmHg)	72.11 ± 1.48	66.95 ± 2.17	72.87 ± 1.65	0.18NS
T_{90} (%)	26.18 ± 2.49	38.40 ± 8.22	24.38 ± 2.54	0.08NS
pH	7.44 ± 0.025	7.40 ± 0.01	7.44 ± 0.03	0.57NS

Table 1: Clinical features of as patients with pulmonary artery systolic hypertension vs. as patients without pulmonary artery systolic hypertension.

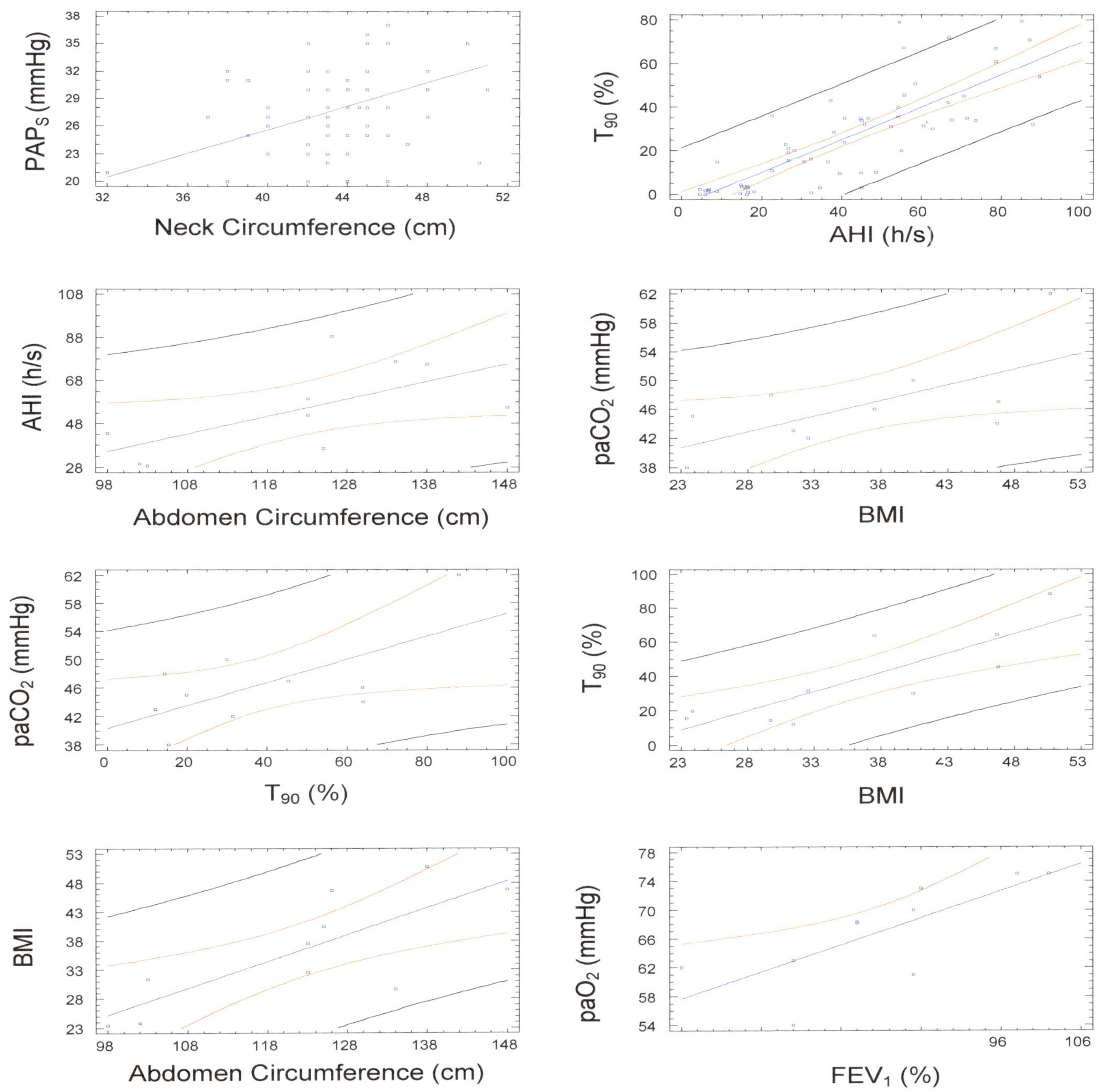

Figure 1: Changes of the variable in the study. In the whole group of patients was detected a relationship between FEV1 (%) and age, outlining a worsening of pulmonary functions by aging.

3) Between neck and abdominal circumference: neck circumference=24,35+0,16 abdominal circumference (p-value=0,0488; R-squared (adjusted for d.f.) =32,77 %).

4) Between $PaCO_2$ and BMI: $PaCO_2$=30,72+0,43 BMI (p-value=0,0380; R-squared (adjusted for d.f.) =36,444 %).

5) Between PaO_2 (mmHg) and abdominal circumference: PaO_2 (mmHg) =99,16-0,26 abdominal circumference (p-value=0,0487; R-squared (adjusted for d.f.) =32,83 %).

6) Between T_{90} and BMI: T_{90}=-42,50 + 2,23 BMI (p-value=0,0028; R-squared (adjusted for d.f.)=65,58 %).

7) Between T_{90} and AHI:T_{90} (%)=-5,48 + 0,80 AHI (hs) (p-value=0,0474; R-squared (adjusted for d.f.)=32,22 %).

8) Between PaO_2 mmHg and FEV_1 (%): PaO_2 mmHg=36,67 + 0,37 FEV_1 (%) (p-value=0,0133; R-squared (adjusted for d.f.)=50,0609 %).

9) Between PaCO2 (mmHg) and T_{90} (%): $PaCO_2$ (mmHg)=40,32

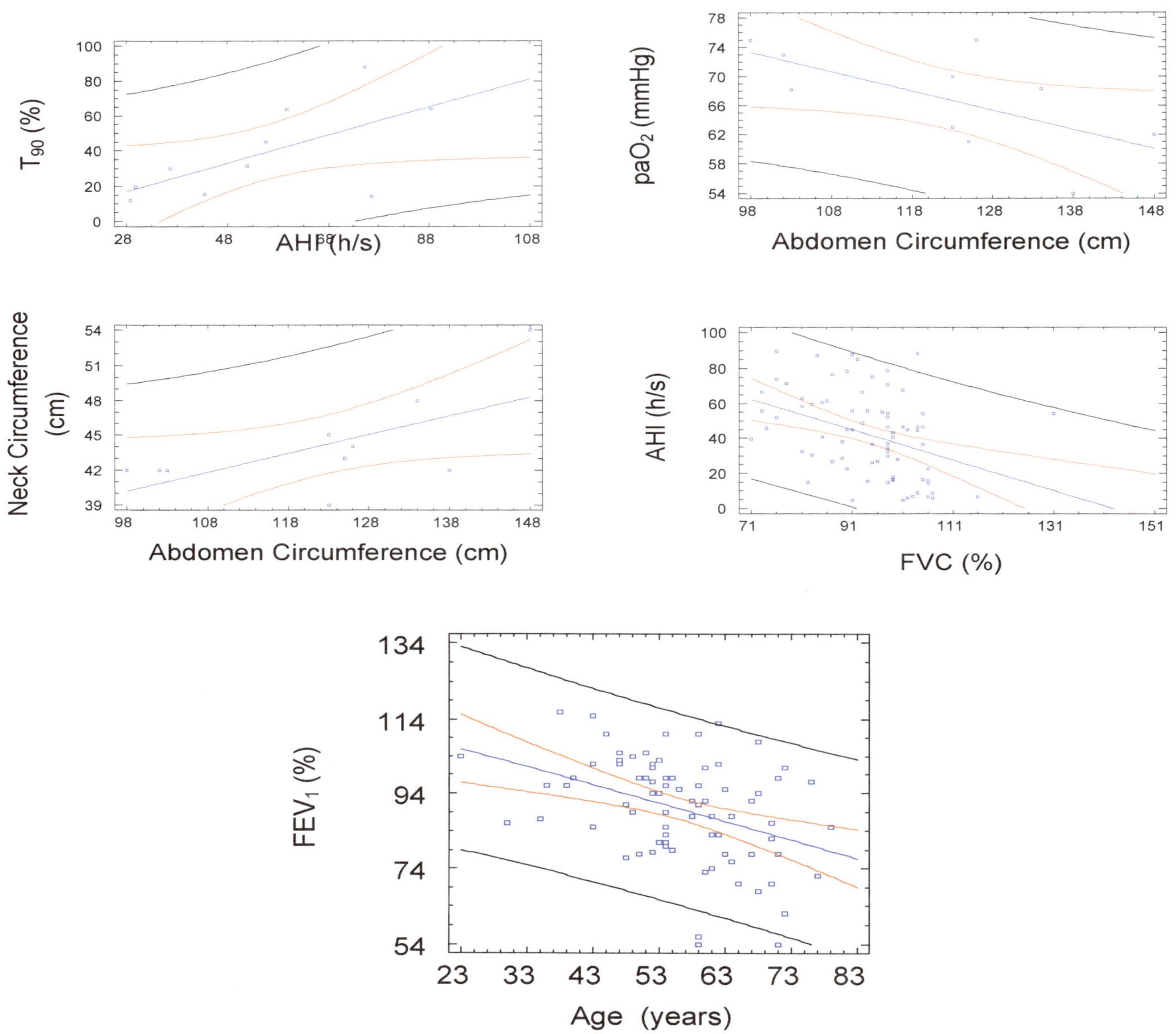

Figure 2: Changes of the variable in the study.

+ 0,16 T_{90} (%) (p-value=0,0405; R-squared (adjusted for d.f.)=35,5127 %)

Discussion

In our study, OSAS patients with pulmonary arterial hypertension were 12,99% of all OSAS patients. The reported prevalence of PAH in OSAS varies from 20% to 41% [31,32].

In this study, severity of OSAS did not always correlate with severity of pulmonary hypertension, but factors such as BMI and low daytime PaO_2 were more closely associated with mild degrees of pulmonary hypertension. Patients with OSAS and pulmonary hypertension have been shown to have increased pulmonary vascular press or responses to hypoxemia [33].

Two other studies showed a reduction in pulmonary artery pressure in patients treated with CPAP [34,35]. The research of Sajkov et al. showed a decrease in PAH as a response to hypoxemia with CPAP treatment [35]; in this study patients with baseline pulmonary hypertension showed the largest response; with CPAP treatment being key to this response. However, daytime pulmonary hypertension that occurs in patients with OSAS improves with CPAP and is more closely associated with BMI and daytime PaO_2 than with severity of OSAS. Nevertheless, there is no clear evidence linking OSAS to the aetiology of pulmonary hypertension [36]. Earlier data on pulmonary hypertension in patients with OSAS has been found to correlate more with a lower daytime PaO_2 and higher $PaCO_2$ than with severity of OSAS [37]. Our study has shown that the OSAS patients with PAH in comparison to the OSAS patients without PAH have an AHI and BMI greater and a lower mean SaO_2 and were more hypoxemic and mildly hypercapnic. It has been shown that intermittent hypoxia creates a chain of events involving oxidative stress and inflammatory response favourable to

	PAH (Mean ± SD)	NoPAH (Mean ± SD)	P	genpop
FEV1(%)	80,80	91.15	0.025	97.54
PAI15G/5G	40%	8.96%	0.006	14.12%
PAI14G/4G	10.0%	22.39		21.18%
PAI14G/5G	50%	67.16		63.53%
DQ2_2	10.0%	16.42%		16.47%
DQ2_5	20.0%	8.95%		9.41%
DQ7	40.0%	47.76%		47.06%
DQ8	0.0%	8.95%		7.06%
Et_F2	0.0%	1.49%		2.35%
Et_F5	0.0%	1.49%		1.18%
MTHFR_DEM	20.0%	28.36%		30.59%
MTHFR_EtAC	0.0%	13.43%		11.76%
MTHFR_EtCT	50%	19.40%	0.033	22.35%
MTHFR_OmAC	0.0%	10.45%		8.24%
MTHFR_OmCT	30%	25.37%		24.71%
MTHFR_wt	0.0%	4.48%		3.53%

Table 2: OSAS patients with pulmonary artery systolic hypertension vs. OSAS patients without pulmonary artery systolic hypertension. In the whole group of patients was detected a relationship between FEV1(%) and age as follows: FEV1(%)=117.369-0.489893, Age(P-value=0.0004); R-squared=15.0023%, suggesting a worsening of pulmonary functions by aging.

atherogenesis, which provides at least one pathway through which sleep apnoea affects the cardiovascular and metabolic systems [38]. However, most studies in this area were limited by the presence of co-morbidities which could have affected their pulmonary pressures [39,40].

Hypoxemia-induced endothelial cell dysfunction is a critical factor in pulmonary vascular remodelling [40]. Hypoxia induces up-regulation of vascular endothelial growth factor, which is a mediator of angiogenesis, resulting in vascular remodelling [41,42].

Conclusions and Outlook

Our results outlined no differences between OSAS patients with and without PAH, as regards HLA polymorphism; on the contrary a significant occurrence of PAI-1 5G/5G polymorphism in OSAS patients with PAH seems to be a relevant feature of these patients suggesting a role in the pathogenesis. According to these results, the occurrence of pulmonary artery hypertension in OSAS patients may be an associated pathology rather than a worsening of OSAS. Our results suggest a genotypic heterogeneity among OSAS patients with PAI-1 5G/5G polymorphism and with PAH, possibly in relation with the severity of illness.

Acknowledgements

We are grateful to Dr. Alexandru Cozma M.D., Internal Medicine Specialist, PhD, University PISA Italy, as to coordinate some study.

Conflict of Interest

The authors has declared that non conflict of interest exists

Ethical Conduct of Research

The local ethics committees approved the study. All patients gave their informed consent for participating in the study.

References

1. Young T, Palta M, Dempsey J, Skatrud J, Weber S, et al. (1993) The occurrence of sleep-disordered breathing among middle-aged adults. N Engl J Med 328: 1230-1235.
2. Chesson AL Jr, Ferber RA, Fry JM, Grigg-Damberger M, Hartse KM, et al. (1997) The indications for polysomnography and related procedures. Sleep 20: 423-487.
3. Redline S, Tishler PV (2000) The genetics of sleep apnea. Sleep Med Rev 4: 583-602.
4. Lévy P, Pépin JL, Arnaud C, Tamisier R, Borel JC, et al. (2008) Intermittent hypoxia and sleep-disordered breathing: current concepts and perspectives. Eur Respir J 32: 1082-1095.
5. Butt M, Dwivedi G, Khair O, Lip GY (2010) Obstructive sleep apnea and cardiovascular disease. Int J Cardiol 139: 7-16.
6. Valham F, Mooe T, Rabben T, Stenlund H, Wiklund U, et al. (2008) Increased risk of stroke in patients with coronary artery disease and sleep apnea: a 10-year follow-up. Circulation 118: 955-960.
7. van der Krabben MD, Rosendaal FR, van der Bom JG, Doggen CJ (2008) Polymorphisms in coagulation factors and the risk of recurrent cardiovascular events in men after a first myocardial infarction. J Thromb Haemost 6: 720-725.
8. Mohanty D, Ghosh K, Khare A, Kulkarni B (2004) Thrombophilia in coronary artery disease: a double jeopardy. Indian J Med Res 120: 13-23.
9. Dawson SJ, Wiman B, Hamsten A, Green F, Humphries S, et al. (1993) The two allele sequences of a common polymorphism in the promoter of the plasminogen activator inhibitor-1 (PAI-1) gene respond differently to interleukin-1 in HepG2 cells. J Biol Chem 268: 10739-10745.
10. Ye S, Green FR, Scarabin PY, Nicaud V, Bara L, et al. (1995) The 4G/5G genetic polymorphism in the promoter of the plasminogen activator inhibitor-1 (PAI-1) gene is associated with differences in plasma PAI-1 activity but not with risk of myocardial infarction in the ECTIM study. Etude CasTemoins de l'nfarctus du Mycocarde. Thromb Haemost 74: 837-841.
11. Iacoviello L, Burzotta F, Di Castelnuovo A, Zito F, Marchioli R, et al. (1998) The 4G/5G polymorphism of PAI-1 promoter gene and the risk of myocardial infarction: a meta-analysis. Thromb Haemost 80: 1029-1030.
12. Wolf J, Lewicka J, Narkiewicz K (2007) Obstructive sleep apnea: an update on mechanisms and cardiovascular consequences. Nutr Metab Cardiovasc Dis 17: 233-240.
13. Palmer LJ, Buxbaum SG, Larkin E, Patel SR, Elston RC, et al. (2003) A whole-genome scan for obstructive sleep apnea and obesity. Am J Hum Genet 72: 340-350.
14. Patel SR, Goodloe R, De G, Kowgier M, Weng J, et al. (2012) Association of genetic loci with sleep apnea in European Americans and African-Americans: the Candidate Gene Association Resource (CARe). PLoS One 7: e48836.
15. Manon-Espaillat R, Gothe B, Adams N, Newman C, Ruff R (1988) Familial 'sleep apnea plus' syndrome: report of a family. Neurology 38: 190-193.
16. Chay OM, Goh A, Abisheganaden J, Tang J, Lim WH, et al. (2000) Obstructive sleep apnea syndrome in obese Singapore children. Pediatr Pulmonol 29: 284-290.
17. Purcell S, Neale B, Todd-Brown K, Thomas L. Ferreira MA, et al. (2007) PLINK: a tool set for whole-genome association and population-based linkage analyses. Am J Hum Genet 81: 559-575.
18. Carmelli D, Colrain IM, Swan GE, Bliwise DL (2004) Genetic and environmental influences in sleep-disordered breathing in older male twins. Sleep 27: 917-922.
19. Lechler R, Warrens A. (2000) HLA in Health and Disease. 2rd ed. Academic Press.
20. Caylak E (2009) The genetics of sleep disorders in humans: narcolepsy, restless legs syndrome, and obstructive sleep apnea syndrome. Am J Med Genet A 149A: 2612-2626.
21. Lin L, Hungs M, Mignot E (2001) Narcolepsy and the HLA region. J Neuroimmunol 117: 9-20.
22. Brunetti L, Francavilla R, Leonardo Miniello V, Leone M, Rana M, et al. (2005) Influence of HLA antigens and OSAS in childhood: a preliminary report. J Sleep Res 14: 157-162.
23. [No authors listed] (1999) Sleep-related breathing disorders in adults: recommendations for syndrome definition and measurement techniques in clinical research. The Report of an American Academy of Sleep Medicine Task Force. Sleep 22: 667-689.
24. Nuckton TJ, Glidden DV, Browner WS, Claman DM (2006) Physical examination: Mallampati score as an independent predictor of obstructive sleep apnea. Sleep 29: 903-908.

25. Celli BR, MacNee W; ATS/ERS Task Force (2004) Standards for the diagnosis and treatment of patients with COPD: a summary of the ATS/ERS position paper. Eur Respir J 23: 932-946.

26. Abramson SV, Burke JB, Pauletto FJ, Kelly JJ Jr (1995) Use of multiple views in the echocardiographic assessment of pulmonary artery systolic pressure. J Am Soc Echocardiogr 8: 55-60.

27. Ferber R, Millman R, Coppola M, Fleetham J, Murray CF, et al. (1994) Portable recording in the assessment of obstructive sleep apnea. ASDA standards of practice. Sleep 17: 378-392.

28. Levi-Valensi P, Weitzenblum E, Rida Z, Aubry P, Braghiroli A, et al. (1992) Sleep-related oxygen desaturation and daytime pulmonary haemodynamics in COPD patients. Eur Respir J 5: 301-307.

29. Johns MW (1991) A new method for measuring daytime sleepiness: the Epworth sleepiness scale. Sleep 14: 540–45.

30. Galiè N, Hoeper MM, Humbert M, Torbicki A, Vachiery JL, et al. (2009) Guidelines for the diagnosis and treatment of pulmonary hypertension. The Task Force for the diagnosis and treatment of pulmonary hypertension of the European Society of Cardiology (ESC) and the European Respiratory Society (ERS), endorsed by the International Society of Heart and Lung Transplantation (ISHLT). Eur Respir J 34: 1219–63.

31. Adegunsoye A, Ramachandran S (2012) Etiopathogenetic mechanisms of pulmonary hypertension in sleep-related breathing disorders. Pulm Med 2012: 273591.

32. Garvey JF, Taylor CT, McNicholas WT (2009) Cardiovascular disease in obstructive sleep apnoea syndrome: the role of intermittent hypoxia and inflammation. Eur Respir J 33: 1195-1205.

33. Jilwan FN, Escourrou P, Garcia G, Jaïs X, Humbert M, et al. (2013) High occurrence of hypoxemic sleep respiratory disorders in precapillary pulmonary hypertension and mechanisms. Chest 143: 47-55.

34. Kario K (2009) Obstructive sleep apnea syndrome and hypertension: mechanism of the linkage and 24-h blood pressure control. Hypertens Res 32: 537-541.

35. Sajkov D, McEvoy RD (2009) Obstructive sleep apnea and pulmonary hypertension. Prog Cardiovasc Dis 51: 363-370.

36. Jones A, Vennelle M, Connell M, McKillop G, Newby DE, et al. (2013) Arterial stiffness and endothelial function in obstructive sleep apnoea/hypopnoea syndrome. Sleep Med 14: 428-432.

37. Arias MA, Garcia –Rio F, Alonso-Fernandez A, Martinez I, Villamor J (2006) Pulmonary hypertension in obstructive sleep apnoea:effects of continuous positive airway pressure A randomized, controlled cross-over study European Heart Journal 27: 1106–1113.

38. Lavie L (2012) Oxidative stress inflammation and endothelial dysfunction in obstructive sleep apnea. Front Biosci (Elite Ed) 4: 1391-1403.

39. Chaouat A, Weitzenblum E, Krieger J, Oswald M, Kessler R (1996) Pulmonary hemodynamics in the obstructive sleep apnea syndrome. Results in 220 consecutive patients. Chest 109: 380-386.

40. Atwood CW Jr, McCrory D, Garcia JG, Abman SH, Ahearn GS; American College of Chest Physicians (2004) Pulmonary artery hypertension and sleep-disordered breathing: ACCP evidence-based clinical practice guidelines. Chest 126: 72S-77S.

41. Arnardottir ES, Mackiewicz M, Gislason T, Teff KL, Pack AI (2009) Molecular signatures of obstructive sleep apnea in adults: a review and perspective. Sleep 32: 447-470.

42. Steiropoulos P, Kotsianidis I, Nena E, Tsara V, Gounari E, et al. (2009) Long-term effect of continuous positive airway pressure therapy on inflammation markers of patients with obstructive sleep apnea syndrome. Sleep 32: 537-543.

Hematic Cortisol and Craniofacial Morphology in Children with OSAS

Alberto Caprioglio[1]*, Alessandro Ollà[2], Franca Marino[3], Gian Marco Abbate[2], Federico Migliori[2], Carlo Mangano[4], Marco Cosentino[5] and Luana Nosetti[6]

[1]Associated Professor and Head, Department of Orthodontics, School of Dentistry, University of Insubria, Italy
[2]DDS, Department of Orthodontics, School of Dentistry, University of Insubria, Italy
[3]Assistant Professor, Centre of Research in Medical Pharmacology, School of Dentistry, University of Insubria, Italy
[4]Assistant Professor, Department of Oral Surgery, School of Dentistry, University of Insubria, Italy
[5]Associated Professor and Head, Centre of Research in Medical Pharmacology, School of Medicine, University of Insubria, Italy
[6]Assistant Professor, Department of Pediatrics, School of Medicine, University of Insubria, Italy

Abstract

Study objectives: This study wanted to evaluate the correlations between haematic cortisol levels and the craniofacial morphology in children with Obstructive Sleep Apnoea Syndrome (OSAS) in comparison with healthy children.

Design/setting/patients. This is a case-control study. Children referring to the Paediatric Department, University of Insubria, Varese, in the period between 1st and 31st October 2011 for a history of disturbed sleep were evaluated and 28 children, compliant to our criteria, were enrolled in the study.

Interventions: All patients underwent a full-night polysomnographic evaluation. Haematic cortisol levels were measured using a radioimmunoassay technique. An orthodontic evaluation and a cranial lateral cephalometric analysis were performed.

Measurements and results: Haematic cortisol concentration at 2.00 am was found higher in OSAS patients than in controls ($p<0.05$). An increase in craniomandibular ($p<0.05$) and intermaxillar ($p<0.01$) angles indicated a high angle tendency in OSAS with a posterior rotation of the mandible. A retro-position of the mandible ($p<0.05$), an increased overjet ($p<0.01$) and a reduction of overbite ($p<0.01$) were also found.

Conclusions: The altered hypothalamic-pituitary-adrenal activity and the craniofacial modification found are not enough to state if these conditions are causes rather than consequences of OSAS. Moreover cortisol and sleep fragmentation can cause a reduction of growth hormone secretion so it is possible that the alteration of facial morphology may also have a metabolic cause.

Keywords: Cephalometrics; Children; Growth; Orthodontics; Paediatric; Sleep apnoea

Introduction

Obstructive Sleep Apnoea Syndrome (OSAS) is a common problem in children [1]. The prevalence of OSAS in diagnostic studies ranges widely from 0.1 and 13%, even if great part of the literature converges on variations between 1 and 4% [1]. A difference in the prevalence based on age is not proven, even if several studies indicate a peak of incidence between 2 and 8 years, which is the age in which the tonsils and adenoids are the largest in relation to the underlying airway [2]. OSAS is defined by the American Academy of Pediatrics as "a disorder of breathing during sleep characterized by prolonged partial upper airway obstruction and/or intermittent complete obstruction (obstructive apnea) that disrupts normal ventilation during sleep and normal sleep patterns" [3].

Diagnosis of OSAS is based on medical history, physical examination and tests confirming the presence and severity of the upper airway obstruction, it is well known, however, that OSAS in children is not only associated with enlarged tonsils and adenoids, but also with the presence of abnormal airway collapsibility during sleep [4]. The gold standard for diagnosing OSAS is therefore the overnight polysomnography (PSG) [2,5]. Among the parameters measured with PSG, the Apnoea-Hypopnoea Index (AHI) is commonly used to evaluate the presence or absence of disease and to assess its severity; the AHI represents the number of obstructive apnoea and obstructive hypopne as observed per hour of Total Sleep Time (TST).

There is evidence suggesting that nocturnal awakenings in OSAS are associated with alterations in Hypothalamic-Pituitary-Adrenal (HPA) activity, specifically, increased pulsatile cortisol release [6]. Cortisol is the primary human glucocorticoid product of the HPA axis and major functions include metabolic (for example gluconeogenesis) and blood pressure regulation and immune suppression. Excess cortisol secretion is associated with numerous adverse systemic consequences, such as metabolic syndrome, diabetes, hypertension, depression and insomnia [7]. The circadian rhythm of secretion of cortisol is strongly related to sleep, an altered regulation of cortisol levels has been proposed as a mechanism through which sleep disorders manifest some of their pathologic effects [8]. In 1972, a study by Gillin et al. reported that glucocorticoids decreased REM sleep and increased time spent awake [9]. The human endogenous, SCN-controlled cortisol circadian rhythm is characterized by cortisol levels begin to rise about 2-3 h after sleep onset and a continuous arousal during the early waking hours. The peak, or acrophase, of the level of cortisol is indicated at about 09.00 h.

***Corresponding author:** Alberto Caprioglio, Department of Orthodontics, University of Insubria, Via Piatti, 10 – Varese, Italy
E-mail: alberto.caprioglio@uninsubria.it

As the day continues, there is a gradual decline in cortisol levels and as sleep ensues there is a continued decrease to the nadir [7].

In literature nocturnal awakenings has been associated with pulsatile cortisol release and autonomic activation leading to an increased release of catecholamine, Corticotropin-Releasing Hormone (CRH) and cortisol. OSAS seems to cause activation of the HPA axis through a similar mechanism of autonomic activation, awakening, and arousal [10,11]. HPA axis hyperactivity can have many negative effects on sleep. It can lead to sleep fragmentation, decreased Slow-Wave Sleep (SWS), and shortened sleep time. Likewise, OSAS can exacerbate HPA axis dysfunction, worsening the cycle [7].

In growing subjects, chronic obstructive airway disease is often associated with disorders of orthodontic interest [12-15]. In this field several studies has been conducted but the nature of the anatomical and functional relationships between respiratory and dental apparatuses makes it difficult to understand how the dysfunctions interact. It has been matter of discussion ascertain whether the craniofacial alterations are a cause or, rather, a consequence of increased resistance to oronasal airflow. Harvold et al. in 1981 showed the presence of cranial and muscle alteration in growing primates in which oral breathing was experimentally induced for an extended period of time [16].

Physiological breathing seems to play an active role in harmonious craniofacial development, therefore when external factors alter its mechanism functional and skeletal alterations can be observed. The most evident consequences of chronic nasal obstruction are represented by orofacial alterations related to an abnormal mandible displacement and a subsequent dysmorphism of the oral structures leading to a modified posture [13]. Under normal conditions tongue influence and regulate the upper jaw morphogenesis. Conversely, when breathing through the mouth, the tongue assumes a forward and downward position, moving its dorsum and the tonsillar tissue away from the posterior pharyngeal wall and does not perform its modelling function on the palate; for this reason the teeth and the maxilla are deprived of their natural support. The consequent "stretching" of the lips and the cheeks causes a centripetal force and inhibits a correct transverse maxillary growth predisposing lip incompetence [14]. It is interesting to note that, since the palate forms the basis of the nasal cavity, its contraction could represent a further cause to obstruction of the nasal flow, creating, also in this case, a vicious circle. The most frequent dysgnathia is represented by both dental and skeletal Class II, with reduction of the transverse diameter of the upper arch, ogival palate, mono- or bilateral posterior crossbite, and anterior open bite with buccally inclined upper incisors [13].

The aim of this preliminary study is to evaluate correlations between haematic cortisol levels and the craniofacial morphology in children diagnosed with OSAS, in comparison with a group of healthy children.

Materials and Method

Subjects

Children referring to the Paediatric Department, University of Insubria, Varese, in the period between 1st and 31st October 2011 for a history of disturbed sleep were evaluated. 28 children, compliant to our inclusion and exclusion criteria, showed Table 1, were enrolled in the study. The present study was conducted in accordance with the Helsinki Declaration and informed consent was obtained from all participants.

All 28 patients underwent a full-night polysomnographic evaluation and were divided in two groups. The group of paediatric OSAS included 18 patients (8 males, 10 female), with a mean age of 6.1 ± 0.9 (mean ± SD). The control group was represented by 10 children (4 males, 6 females) with a mean age of 5.9 ± 1.0 (Table 2).

Measurements

In the first phase of the study all patients underwent a overnight, 12 channels, polysomnographic evaluation (E-Series, Compumedics, Melbourne, Australia), performed in a sleep laboratory. The following parameters were analysed: nasal air flow, chest and abdominal movements, snoring, transcutaneous SaO_2 saturation, electroencephalogram, electrooculogram, electromyogram, body position and heart rate with electrocardiography.

All recordings were scored manually by the same operator. An obstructive apnoea was defined as the cessation of airflow for at least 10 seconds with continuing abdominal and thoracic movements according to the American Academy of Sleep Medicine [17]. An obstructive hypopnoea was defined as a 50% reduction in airflow for at least 10 seconds, compared with baseline, accompanied by abdominal and thoracic movements in combination with an arousal or an oxygen desaturation of 3% or more [17].

The obstructive apnoea-hypopnoea index was defined as the mean number of obstructive apnoea and hypopnoea per hour of sleep. According to the American Academy of Paediatrics' guidelines [3], we considered OSAS children showing AHI over 1.5.

Blood samples from the patients were collected and haematic parameters were evaluated.

Blood samples were collected at: 02.00 am and at 08.00 am with peripheral heparinized catheters and stored at 4°C.

Cortisol plasma levels were measured from each sample using a radioimmunoassay technique (Bridge Cortisol Kit, Adaltis, Roma, Italy) at the Section of Experimental and Clinical Pharmacology, Department of Clinical Medicine, University of Insubria, Varese.

In the second phase, the 18 patients of the OSAS group underwent also a specific clinical orthodontic evaluation and a cranial lateral cephalometry performed by the same specialist in orthodontics. The first phase's controls children were not taken as controls in the second phase, because, even if they were not diagnosed OSAS, they complained disturbed sleep that could be associated with several conditions, such as oral breathing, so they couldn't be considered representative of an healthy population. The mean cephalometric values in a 6 aged population of healthy children [18] were considered as controls.

Inclusion Criteria	Exclusion Criteria
Age in the range 5-7 years BMI in the range 13.5*-17** History of disturbed sleep	History of ENT surgery History of allergy Chronic illness Use of decongestant preparations Acute upper airway infections Acute otitis media Dysmorphic or craniofacial syndromes History of orthodontic treatment Primary adrenocortical hyperfunction

*5th percentile at 6 years; **85th percentile at 6 years

Table 1: Inclusion and Exclusion Criteria of the sample.

	Age (y)	Male	Female	Tot
OSAS	6.1 ± 0.9	8	10	18
Not OSAS	5.9 ± 1.0	4	6	10

Table 2: Age and gender of the sample.

All 18 cephalograms were digitally traced (NemoStudio 8.7.5 UV 10, Software Nemotec S.L., Madrid, Spain) by the same operator. For the cephalometric evaluation the Italian Board of Orthodontics' cephalometric analysis (IBO) was used [19]. The parameter considered were: angle sella - nasion - subspinale point (SNA), angle sella - nasion - pogonion point (SNPg), difference between SNA and SNPg (ANPg), inclination of the maxilla (SN-ANS.PNS), intermaxillar angle (ANS. PNS–GoMe), inclination of the mandible (SN-GoMe), upper incisor's inclination (1.1-ANS.PNS), lower incisor's inclination (4.1-GoMe), lower incisor's compensation (4.1-APg), overjet (OVJ), overbite (OVB), interincisal angle (1.1-4.1) (Figure 1).

Statistical analysis

Both cortisol data samples of OSAS and controls groups were found normally distributed by using Shapiro-Wilk test. Difference in haematic cortisol levels between the two groups was evaluated using Independent Samples t-test (MedCalc version 12.3.0.0, Mariakerke, Belgium).

For all OSAS subjects the cephalograms were traced twice by the same observer in two different moments to exclude method errors. No significant mean differences between the two series of records were found by employing paired t-tests. Dalhberg's formula was used to establish the method error [20]. Method error for the linear measurements was smaller than 0.5 mm while for the angular measurements it was smaller than 1 degree. Cephalometric data were found normally distributed by using Shapiro-Wilk test. The mean values of SNA, SNPg, ANPg, SN-ANS.PNS, ANS.PNS–GoMe, SN-GoMe, 1.1-ANS.PNS, 4.1-GoMe, 4.1-APg and 1.1-4.1 in a 6 aged population of healthy children [18] were taken as controls to evaluate the presence of significant differences in cephalometric parameters using One Sample t-test (MedCalc version 12.3.0.0, Mariakerke, Belgium). As the mean values of OVJ and OVB were not available in the control's source (18), we considered as control values the OVJ and OVB normal values indicated by the IBO [19].

Results

Among all the children recruited, 18 fulfilled the OSAS criteria according to the American Academy of Paediatrics [3]. There were no significant differences in age and gender between the groups (Table 2). Data obtained from polysomnographic monitoring underwent manual and instrumental reworking that allowed us to obtain the average percentage O_2 saturation (96.0 ± 2.8 in OSAS; 98.1 ± 0.6 in not OSAS), the minimum percentage of O_2 saturation (79.9 ± 14.3 in OSAS; 93.4 ± 2.2 in not OSAS) and the Apnoea-Hypopnoea Index (AHI=9.6 ± 5.0 in OSAS; AHI=0.8 ± 0.3 in not OSAS). The Sleep Efficiency and the Sleep Architecture were considered preserved in all subjects (Table 3).

Haematic cortisol concentration at 2.00 AM was found higher in OSAS patients (57 ± 50 ng/ml) than in controls (23 ± 11 ng/ml) ($p<0.05$). Conversely differences in concentrations at 8.00 AM were not found significant (176 ± 40 ng/ml in OSAS; 177 ± 56 ng/ml in controls) (Figure 2).

Cephalometric data are summarized in Table 4. A significant increase in craniomandibular (SN-GoMe, $p<0.05$) and intermaxillar (ANS.PNS-GoMe, $p<0.01$) angles indicated a high angle face in the OSAS group with a posterior rotation of the mandible. Retro-position of the mandible was detected by the reduction of SNPg angle ($p<0.05$) and the consequent enlargement of ANPg angle ($p<0.001$). Concerning the dentoalveolar parameters OVJ was found increased ($p<0.01$), according to the mandible's retro-position mentioned before, while 1.1-ANS.PNS and OVB were found reduced ($p<0.01$ for 1.1-ANS.PNS, $p<0.001$ for OVB).

Discussion

Few studies have been conducted to assess the craniofacial architecture of subjects with OSAS in young children with deciduous or mixed dentition. In the present study, according to Marino et al. [15], the OSAS children showed an orthognatic and harmonious maxilla in the sagittal (SNA) and vertical plane (SN-ANS.PNS). The cephalometric values that were disharmonious with the orthognatic facial pattern were observed in the mandible. The angles SNPg and SN-GoMe showed a retro-positioned mandible with a strong posterior inclination in clockwise direction, in relation to the anterior cranial base. This skeletal discrepancies lead to a hyperdivergent class II with an increased ANPg and anterior facial height. Inclinations of the upper incisors were found reduced and this result can be explained

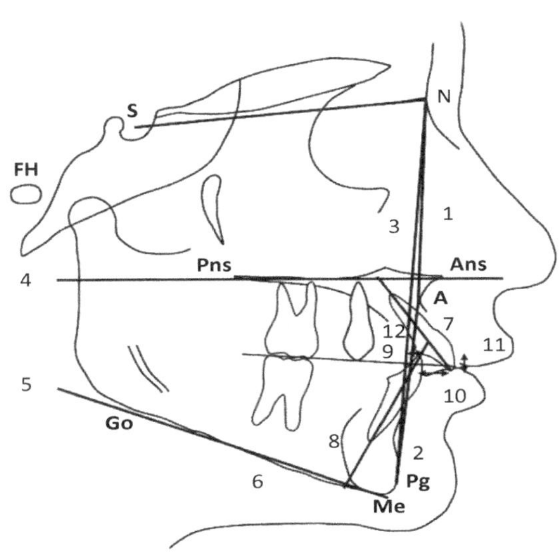

Figure 1: Cephalometric skeletal and dental measurements used in the study: (1) SNA; (2) SNPg; (3) ANPg; (4) SN-AnsPns; (5) SN-GoMe; (6) AnsPns-GoMe; (7) Maxillary incisors-AnsPns; (8) Mandibular incisors-GoMe; (9) Mandibolar incisors-APg; (10) Overjet; (11) Overbite; (12) Interincisal angle.

	OSAS	Not OSAS
AHI	9.6 ± 5.0	0.8 ± 0.3
SpO2 mean %	96.0 ± 2.8	98.1 ± 0.6
SpO2 min %	79.9 ± 14.3	93.4 ± 2.2
TST (min)	562 ± 30	517 ± 47

Table 3: Polysomnographic data.

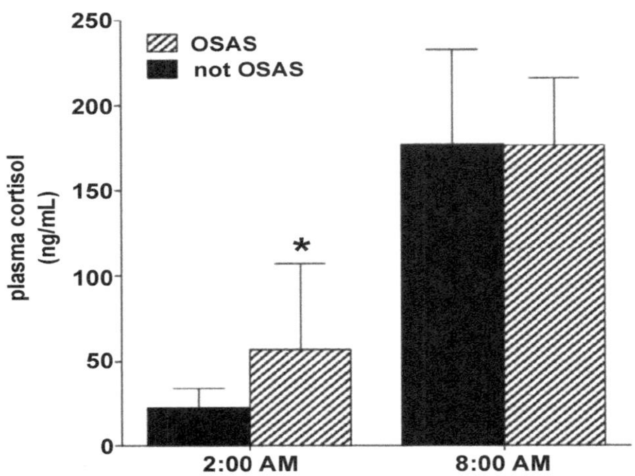

Figure 2: Mean cortisol dosage at 2.00 AM and 8.00 AM.

Variables[1]	OSAS subjects (mean ± sd)	Control values[2] (mean ± sd)	p-value
SNA	80.0 ± 3.7	80.1 ± 3.5	NS
SNPg	72.8 ± 3.8	76.2 ± 3.4	0.0168*
ANPg	7.1 ± 2.0	3.4 ± 2.0	0.0001***
SN-ANS.PNS	4.9 ± 1.2	6.8 ± 3.0	NS
ANS.PNS–GoMe	34.5 ± 3.8	30.2 ± 4.4	0.0029**
SN-GoMe	39.4 ± 3.4	37.0 ± 4.8	0.0491*
1.1-ANS.PNS	93.0 ± 10.6	105.2 ± 7.4	0.0039**
4.1-GoMe	87.5 ± 5.3	83.4 ± 7.3	NS
4.1-APg	0.4 ± 1.6	-1.8 ± 2.5	NS
OVJ	4.6 ± 1.8	3.5 ± 2.5	0.0032**
OVB	0.3 ± 1.0	2.5 ± 2.5	<0.0001***
Interincisal Angle	145.9 ± 12.1	140.9 ± 10.7	NS

1 all measures are expressed in degree, except 4.1-APg, OVJ and OVB that are reported in millimeters; 2 as reported in reference [18]; * p<0.05; ** p<0.01; *** p<0.001

Table 4: Mean cephalometric measures in OSAS subjects and respective control values.

by a dento-alveolar compensatory mechanism described by Solow in 1980 [21]. The increased OVJ is in line with the class II phenotype previously described, even if in literature OSAS and Class II skeletal pattern are not always correlated [12]. The decreased OVB is related to the increase of intermaxillary angle (ANS.PNS-GoMe). However, since the dentoalveolar parameters are evolving in preschool and school-age children, they are considered less indicative for the prediction of a future facial morphology. Many studies attest the correlation between upper airway obstruction and craniofacial modifications. Harvold in 1981 observed that when a growing primate is experimentally induced to be an oral breather it always develops muscle and cranial alterations [16]. It is important to note that this is a two-way problem: just as oral breathing can determine malocclusive patterns by affecting growth and craniofacial development, it is equally true that the various types of malocclusion can favour oral breathing [13]. Adenotonsillectomy generally resolves the upper airway obstruction, but the persistence or reappearance of snoring and OSAS later in life, after surgery at a prepubertal age, suggests that craniofacial modifications may be precocious and related to genetic or environmental factors [12,21].

The pathophysiology of OSAS has been associated with alterations of the Hypothalamic Pituitary Adrenal (HPA) axis; however a relationship between OSAS and altered cortisol levels has not been conclusively established [8]. Since nocturnal awakenings are associated with HPA axis activation and associated sympathetic activation it is expected that concentrations of cortisol could be higher in patients with OSAS [6]. However, many studies have failed to find differences in cortisol between OSAS subjects and normal controls [22]. Further, several studies have reported that Continuous Positive Airway Pressure (CPAP), the gold standard treatment for OSAS, does not reduce cortisol levels in patients with OSAS [23]. Finally, the removal of CPAP in OSAS patients has not been shown to result in immediate increases in cortisol levels [24]. Methodological concerns, such as infrequent sampling and inconsistent timing of sample collection, may have contributed to null findings for some studies. Recent studies using more extensive circadian sampling have reported differences in cortisol levels between OSAS patients and normal controls [10,11].

In our study we found an elevation in cortisol levels at night ($p<0.05$), while there were no significant differences in the morning, according to the results of Vgontzas et al. [11]. The absence of significant alterations in cortisol levels at 8.00 can be explained by the awakening response phenomena. The awakening response is the marked and rapid rise in cortisol and Adreno-Corticotropic Hormone (ACTH) that occurs after final morning awakening and continues for about a 60-min period, it is distinct from nocturnal awakenings and it is predictable and independent of the mode of awakening (naturally or with an alarm). It does not appear to be simply a continuation of the morning rise in cortisol or due to a wake-up stimulus. Spontaneous final awakening time is not linked to either a sleep stage or a specific cortisol level. Anticipation of awakening at a certain time can augment the early morning rise of cortisol that occurs before awakening. This effect is distinct from and has no impact on the subsequent cortisol awakening response [7].

The alteration of nocturnal cortisol levels might be important not only for the effects, mentioned above, that this hormone exerts on sleep, but also for the inhibitory activity that cortisol exerts on the secretion of the Growth Hormone (GH). It's known that elevated cortisol levels cause a reduction in the secretion of GH [25], moreover, since the peak of GH secretion occurs during SWS [25], OSAS itself, causing shortened SWS time, could cause an altered GH secretion. In fact, in literature it has been reported that children with obstruction of the upper airway show growth defects due to a reduced secretion of GH, which is restored after adenotonsillectomy [26]. In particular, in subjects with deficient GH secretion a reduced posterior facial height was found, when compared to healthy controls of the same age, due to a reduced growth of the ramus. Other studies report that the administration of GH in these patients lead to an acceleration in the growth of the mandibular ramus. Hence, if the obstruction of the upper airway can represent, through the modified tongue position and the consequent stretching of the soft tissues, a mechanical cause in the development of craniofacial alterations, it can be hypothized that an increased nocturnal secretion of cortisol in OSAS patients could provide a metabolic cause (Figure 3).

Altered HPA axis activity and craniofacial modification are often found in OSAS children. We are not able to state whether if these

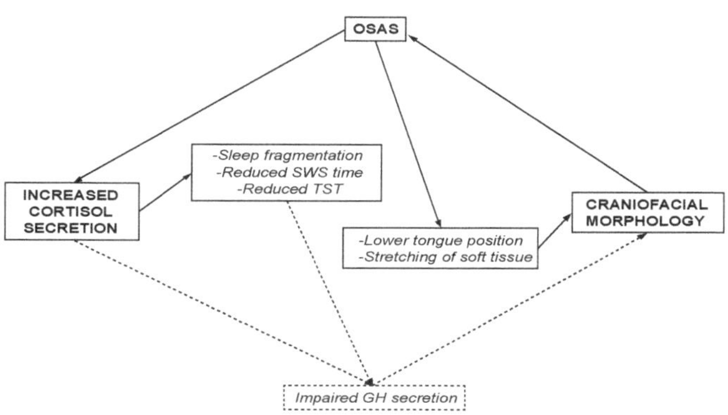

Figure 3: Simplified hypothetical model for developmental relationships between OSAS, cortisol, and craniofacial morphology.

conditions are causes rather than consequences of OSAS. It seems that they both present self-perpetuating vicious circles: in the former sleep fragmentation increase cortisol levels [6] and this increased HPA axis activity promotes sleep fragmentation itself [9], in the latter it is difficult to establish if the primary alteration is respiratory or maxillofacial [12,13]. Furthermore, due to the reduction of GH secretion caused by cortisol and sleep fragmentation, it can be assumed that, in OSAS subjects, the alteration of facial morphology may also have a metabolic cause. Independently of the primary cause of this vicious circle a multidisciplinary approach to OSAS children should be advisable.

Acknowledgement

The work was performed at the Department of Pediatrics and at the Department of Orthodontics, School of Medicine and Dentistry, University Of Insubria, Varese, Italy. All the authors declare the absence of any conflict of interest and financial support.

References

1. Lumeng JC, Chervin RD (2008) Epidemiology of pediatric obstructive sleep apnea. Proc Am Thorac Soc 5: 242-252.
2. Marcus CL (2001) Sleep-disordered breathing in children. Am J Respir Crit Care Med 164: 16-30.
3. Marcus CL, Brooks LJ, Draper KA, Gozal D, Halbower AC, et al. (2012) Diagnosis and management of childhood obstructive sleep apnea syndrome. Pediatrics 130: 714-755.
4. Marcus CL, McColley SA, Carroll JL, Loughlin GM, Smith PL, et al. (1994) Upper airway collapsibility in children with obstructive sleep apnea syndrome. J Appl Physiol 77: 918-924.
5. Li AM, Chan DF, Fok TF, Wing YK (2004) Childhood obstructive sleep apnoea: an update. Hong Kong Med J 10: 406-413.
6. Späth-Schwalbe E, Gofferje M, Kern W, Born J, Fehm HL (1991) Sleep disruption alters nocturnal ACTH and cortisol secretory patterns. Biol Psychiatry 29: 575-584.
7. Buckley TM, Schatzberg AF (2005) On the interactions of the hypothalamic-pituitary-adrenal (HPA) axis and sleep: normal HPA axis activity and circadian rhythm, exemplary sleep disorders. J Clin Endocrinol Metab 90: 3106-3114.
8. Tomfohr LM, Edwards KM, Dimsdale JE (2012) Is obstructive sleep apnea associated with cortisol levels? A systematic review of the research evidence. Sleep Med Rev 16: 243-249.
9. Gillin JC, Jacobs LS, Fram DH, Snyder F (1972) Acute effect of a glucocorticoid on normal human sleep. Nature 237: 398-399.
10. Henley DE, Russell GM, Douthwaite JA, Wood SA, Buchanan F, et al. (2009) Hypothalamic-pituitary-adrenal axis activation in obstructive sleep apnea: the effect of continuous positive airway pressure therapy. J Clin Endocrinol Metab 94: 4234-4242.
11. Vgontzas AN, Pejovic S, Zoumakis E, Lin HM, Bentley CM, et al. (2007) Hypothalamic-pituitary-adrenal axis activity in obese men with and without sleep apnea: effects of continuous positive airway pressure therapy. J Clin Endocrinol Metab 92: 4199-4207.
12. Zucconi M, Caprioglio A, Calori G, Ferini-Strambi L, Oldani A, et al. (1999) Craniofacial modifications in children with habitual snoring and obstructive sleep apnoea: a case-control study. Eur Respir J 13: 411-417.
13. Zicari AM, Albani F, Ntrekou P, Rugiano A, Duse M, et al. (2009) Oral breathing and dental malocclusions. Eur J Paediatr Dent 10: 59-64.
14. Caprioglio A, Levrini L, Nosetti L, Berini J, Macchi A, et al. (2011) Prevalence of malocclusion in preschool and primary school children with habitual snoring and sleep-disordered breathing. Eur J Paediatr Dent 12: 267-271.
15. Marino A, Malagnino I, Ranieri R, Villa MP, Malagola C (2009) Craniofacial morphology in preschool children with obstructive sleep apnoea syndrome. Eur J Paediatr Dent 10: 181-184.
16. Harvold EP, Tomer BS, Vargervik K, Chierici G (1981) Primate experiments on oral respiration. Am J Orthod 79: 359-372.
17. [No authors listed] (1999) Sleep-related breathing disorders in adults: recommendations for syndrome definition and measurement techniques in clinical research. The Report of an American Academy of Sleep Medicine Task Force. Sleep 22: 667-689.
18. Bhatia SN, Leighton BC (2003) A manual of facial growth - A Computer Analysis of Longitudinal Cephalometric Growth Data. Oxford Medical Publications.
19. http://www.sido.it/modules/ibo/Linee_Guida_IBO.pdf20.
20. Dahlberg G (1940) Statistical methods for medical and biological students. Interscience publication. New York.
21. Solow B (1980) The dentoalveolar compensatory mechanism: background and clinical implications. Br J Orthod 7: 145-161.
22. Entzian P, Linnemann K, Schlaak M, Zabel P (1996) Obstructive sleep apnea syndrome and circadian rhythms of hormones and cytokines. Am J Respir Crit Care Med 153: 1080-1086.
23. Nakamura T, Chin K, Shimizu K, Kita H, Mishima M, et al. (2001) Acute effect of nasal continuous positive airway pressure therapy on the systemic immunity of patients with obstructive sleep apnea syndrome. Sleep 24: 545-553.
24. Grunstein RR, Stewart DA, Lloyd H, Akinci M, Cheng N, et al. (1996) Acute withdrawal of nasal CPAP in obstructive sleep apnea does not cause a rise in stress hormones. Sleep 19: 774-782.
25. Giustina A, Veldhuis JD (1998) Pathophysiology of the neuroregulation of growth hormone secretion in experimental animals and the human. Endocr Rev 19: 717-797.
26. Peltomäki T (2007) The effect of mode of breathing on craniofacial growth--revisited. Eur J Orthod 29: 426-429.

17

Evaluation of Multiple Sleep-Related Parameters in Patients with Obstructive Sleep Apnea in Different Age Ranges

Gilbert Seda[1]*, Carolyn H Welsh[2], Massoud Daheshia[1], John Perri[1] and David Bradshaw[1]

[1]*Department of Pulmonary and Critical Care Medicine, Naval Medical Center San Diego, San Diego, CA 92134, USA*
[2]*Denver Veterans Affairs Medical Center, Denver, Colorado, USA*

Abstract

Purpose: No age-based comparative studies have investigated clinical and polysomnographic manifestations of adults with Obstructive Sleep Apnea (OSA).

Methods: Retrospective record review of 570 patients with OSA at Naval Medical Center San Diego. Patients were divided into one of four age cohorts: (1) ages 18-29 (n=209); (2) ages 30-39 (n=106); (3) ages 40-49 (n=102); and (4) ages > 50 (n=153). Group comparisons of demographics, Epworth Sleepiness Scale (ESS), Patient Sleep Questionnaire (PSQ), and polysomnography were analyzed.

Results: Patients, ages 18-29 reported more witnessed apneas, Excessive Daytime Sleepiness (EDS), and had higher respiratory related arousal indexes (p=0.018) compared to patients over 30 years old. Patients 50 years and older reported more nocturia (p=0.001), less snoring, and had higher Rapid Eye Movement (REM)-related apneas (p=0.008), and more severe oximetry desaturations than patients less than 50 years old (p=0.001 - 0.004). Age groups were similar with respect to Body Mass Index (BMI), self-reported sleep-related driving impairment, Apnea Hypopnea Index (AHI), non-REM (NREM) AHI, and total obstructive and central apneas.

Conclusions: Snoring, EDS, nocturia, arousal index, and lowest oxygen saturation most significantly differentiated OSA across different age groups of patients with OSA.

Keywords: Obstructive sleep apnea; Sleep-disordered breathing; Older adults; Young adults; Polysomnogram; Epworth sleepiness scale; Age; Apnea hypopnea index

Introduction

Obstructive sleep apnea is a common condition that is under recognized and under diagnosed. It is characterized by recurrent episodes of complete or partial collapse of the upper airway during sleep and is an important cause of medical morbidity and mortality. The Wisconsin-based cohort study of state employees less than 65 years of age found a prevalence of sleep-disordered breathing in 9% of women and 24% in men [1]. Risk factors for sleep-disordered breathing include obesity, male gender, menopause, alcohol consumption, craniofacial characteristics, and endocrine disorders such as hypothyroidism and acromegaly [2]. Symptoms of Obstructive Sleep Apnea (OSA) include excessive daytime sleepiness, insomnia, morning headaches, erectile dysfunction, snoring, witnessed apneas, and nocturia [2,3]. Polysomnographic features of OSA include increased wakefulness after sleep onset, reduced stage 3 and 4 sleep, reduced REM sleep, increased respiratory arousals, central and/or obstructive apneas, arterial oxygen desaturations, and cyclic variations in heart rate [2,3]. Potential consequences of sleep-disordered breathing include decreased survival [4], cognitive impairment [5], glucose intolerance [6], motor vehicle accidents [7], arterial hypertension [8], pulmonary hypertension [9], arrhythmias [10], stroke [11], sudden cardiac death [12], and diminished quality of life [13].

Age-related differences in sleep-disordered breathing are predominantly based on studies with middle-aged and older adults with minimal studies with young adults. Data from the community-based Sleep Heart Health Study have shown that disease prevalence increases steadily with age and reaches a plateau after the age of 60 years [14]. Similar trends with increasing age have also been noted in other cohorts in whom the prevalence of moderate to severe obstructive sleep apnea (AHI>15–20 events/h) remains relatively constant after the sixth decade of life [15]. Despite the increasing prevalence of OSA with age, this does not correlate with clinical symptoms or apnea severity [16]. In the Cardiovascular Health Study, the prevalence of reported snoring decreased with increasing age [17]. Snoring decreased from 41% in men ages 65 to 69 to 17% in those over 80. Furthermore, loud snoring, observed apneas, and daytime sleepiness in elderly subjects had no association with hypertension or cardiovascular disease prevalence. The negative correlation of snoring with advanced age and the lack of association between sleep apnea symptoms with cardiovascular disease raises the notion of whether sleep-disordered breathing in the elderly is a different disorder from that of middle age and younger adults.

In a recent study comparing the effects of age on the clinical features of OSA, elderly men had a higher percentage and duration of apneas and hypopneas [18]. It is possible there is an age-related spectrum of disease with obstructive sleep apnea with disease progression associated with advancing age. If this were the case, one would expect young adults to have more respiratory related arousals and REM related apneas and hypopneas while of this study was twofold: (1) to describe the age-related differences in clinical characteristics and polysomnographic findings of OSA in young adults, middle age adults, and the elderly and

***Corresponding author:** Gilbert Seda, Department of Pulmonary and Critical Care Medicine, Naval Medical Center San Diego, San Diego, CA 92134, USA, E-mail: gilbert.seda@gmail.com

(2) to determine whether there is an age related spectrum of disease that worsens with age.

Materials and Methods

Subjects

After approval by the Institutional Review Board, we selected the records of 570 patients evaluated by the Sleep Medicine Clinic, Naval Medical Center San Diego from 2006-2008. Patients had an overnight polysomnogram with sleep-disordered breathing defined by an apnea hypopnea index (AHI) ≥ 5 with clinical symptoms of sleep apnea. Patients with portable sleep studies were excluded. The study population had a mean age of 39 ± 13 (range 18-80), and a mean Body Mass Index (BMI) of 31 ± 6 kg/m^2 (range 17-62). There were 538 (94%) males and 32 (6%) females. The mean Epworth score was 12.71 ± 5.22 and mean Apnea-Hypopnea Index (AHI) was 32 ± 27.

Procedures

All subjects completed an Epworth Sleepiness Scale (ESS), Patient Sleep Questionnaire (PSQ), and an overnight polysomnogram (PSG). Demographic data included marital status, race, age, sex, and BMI. The ESS is a self-administered questionnaire to measure daytime sleepiness. A score ≥ 10 suggests significant daytime sleepiness. The Patient Sleep Questionnaire (PSQ) asks patients to rate various sleep behaviors and quantify other behaviors. Items from the PSQ include ratings about snoring, witnessed apneas, excessive daytime sleepiness, and use of alcohol to sleep. Furthermore, patients quantify nocturia frequency, driving impairment due to sleepiness, caffeine use, tobacco use, and alcohol consumption.

Experienced technicians visually scored polysomnographic records for sleep stage and apnea events using the Natus Sleep Works software. Obstructive apneas were defined as a drop in the peak thermal sensor excursion by > 90% of baseline and duration of the event for at least 10 seconds. Hypopneas required a greater than 50% decrease in airflow for at least 10 seconds with an accompanying ≥ 4% oxygen desaturation. The AHI was calculated for each patient based on the average number of events per hour. A physician with Sleep Medicine Certification reviewed the records and scoring. Polysomnographic data analyzed included the following: total sleep time, arousal index, AHI, AHI in REM sleep, AHI in NREM sleep, total number of obstructive and central apneas, lowest desaturation, time spent below 85% oxygen saturation, and whether the overnight polysomnogram was a split-night study. For split-night studies we used the data from the diagnostic portion of the study.

Statistical analysis

Patients were divided into one of four age cohorts: (1) group 1, ages 18-29 years old (n=209); (2) group 2, ages 30-39 (n=102); (3) group 3, ages 40-49 (n=106), and (4) group 4, ages 50 and older (n=153). Group demographics were evaluated using Fisher's exact test, and racial differences among age groups were evaluated with a chi-square test with pair-wise comparisons using the Fisher exact test with the Bonferroni critical value (significant if p ≤ 0.008). Since the data did not fit a normal distribution, age group differences were analyzed by the Kruskal-Wallis test. Significant differences between multiple age groups were analyzed by pair-wise "rank sum" tests with the Bonferroni critical value (significant if p ≤ 0.008).

Results

Demographics

The study age groups were predominantly male (94%). The ages ≥ 50 cohort had a greater proportion of females (13%, p<0.001) compared to other age cohorts (Table 1). There were no age group differences with respect to number of split-night studies (p=0.304). Ethnicity by age group showed p=0.002. Caucasians and African-Americans were the two most predominant ethnical groups, representing 49 & 15% of total patient populations, respectively, with an increasing prevalence of Caucasians and decreasing prevalence of African- Americans with increasing age (p<0.001). There were no other significant racial differences (Table 1). Number of non-married patients and the use of tobacco were significantly higher in the group 1. BMI was similar among all age groups (p=0.156).

ESS

Excessiveness daytime sleepiness is one of the most burdensome symptoms of sleep-disordered breathing and ESS is wildly used to assess patients' sleepiness. The questionnaire asks the patients to rate his or her probability of falling asleep on a scale of 0 to 3 on eight different parameters. Patients, ages 30-39 and 40-49, had higher Epworth scores than patients, ages ≥ 50 (median: 14 for groups 2 & 3 and 12 for group 4, p values: group 2 v. 4, p=0.008; group 3 v. 4, p=0.005). Patients, ages 18-29 had ESS scores similar to other age groups (Table 2 and 3).

PSQ

The sleep questionnaire contained a series of questions including sleep-related habits & complaints, and social behavior. Patients, ages 18-29, 30-39, and 40-49 endorsed more snoring in comparison to patients ages ≥ 50 (Group 1 v. 4, p=0.001; Group 2 v. 4, p<0.001; Group 3 v. 4, p<0.001). Patients, ages 18-29 reported more witnessed apneas and EDS than patients ages ≥ 50 (Group 1 v. 4 apneas, p=0.001, EDS p<0.001). Patients ages ≥ 50 endorsed more nocturia than other age groups (patients, ages 30-39, p<0.001; patients, ages 40-49, p<0.001;

	Total N=570	Group 1 N=209	Group 2 N=102	Group 3 N=106	Group 4 N=153	P value
Females	32 (6)	7 (3)	1 (1)	4 (4)	20 (13)*	p<0.001
Split night studies	194 (34)	76 (36)	32 (31)	29 (27)	57 (37)	p=0.304
Married	406 (75)	98 (55)*	75 (74)	95 (90)	138 (90)	p<0.001
Tobacco use	188 (33)	75 (36)	17 (17)	18 (17)	19 (13)	p=0.038
Race ^						p = 0.002**
White	168 (49)	44 (26)	27 (45)	27 (44)	70 (65)	
Black	55 (15)	25 (16)	14 (25)	9 (15)	7 (7)	
Asian/Pacific Islander	50 (15)	21 (16)	6 (16)	8 (13)	15 (14)	
Other	71 (21)	26 (42)	13 (13)	17 (28)	15 (14)	

*Values are given as number with % in ( ).
^ Because of the retrospective nature of analysis, we did not have access to ethnical data of 224 patients, and the reported data are based on total of 346 patients.
** P vale ethnicity by age group

Table 1: Demographics and Clinical Characteristics of Patients*.

	Group 1	Group 2	Group 3	Group 4
VARIABLE	Median	Median	Median	Median
BMI (kg/m^2)	29 (29-30)	31 (29-32)	29 (28-30)	30 (29-31)
Epworth	12 (11-13)	14 (12-15)	14 (12.4-16)	12 (10.9-12.1)
Sleep Questionnaire Items				
Snoring	5 (5)	5 (5)	5 (5)	4 (4-5)
Apneas	4 (4)	4 (4)	4 (4)	4 (3-4)
Excessive daytime sleepiness	4 (3-4)	3 (3-4)	3 (3-4)	3 (3)
Alcohol use to sleep	1 (1)	1 (1)	1 (1)	1 (1)
Nocturia	1 (1)	1 (1)	1 (1)	1.5 (1.5-2)
Sleep related MVA's	0 (0)	0 (0)	0 (0)	0 (0)
Sleep related near misses	0 (0)	0 (0-1)	0 (0-1)	0 (0)
Coffee consumption	0 (0)	0 (0-1)	1 (1-1.5)	1.5 (1-2)
Tea consumption (cup/day)	0 (0)	0 (0)	0 (0)	0 (0)
Cola consumption (can/day)	1 (0.9-1)	1 (1)	1 (1)	0.5 (0-1)
Cigarette use (pack/day)	0.26 (0.2-0.32)	0.12 (0.05-0.19)	0.14 (0.06-0.21)	0.12 (0.06-0.18)
Alcohol use (/week)				
Polysomnogram				
AHI (events/h^{-1})	21 (17-27)	21 (16-27.4)	21 (15-28.2)	25 (17-28)
Arousal index	22 (19-24)	16 (14-22.4)	16.5 (13-20)	20 (17-22)
Obstructive sleep apneas	34 (24-41)	22.5 (12-29.4)	21.5 (12.4-32.8)	29 (22.9-40.1)
Central sleep apneas	0 (0)	0 (0)	0 (0)	0 (0)
NREM AHI	20 (16-24)	20 (14.6-26.8)	18.5 (12-25.6)	19 (13.8-27)
REM AHI	12 (8.8-16)	17 (11.6-24)	22.5 (14.4-34.6)	25 (19.9-32.1)
Lowest oxygen saturation	83 (82-84)	82 (81-83.4)	81.5 (80-83)	81 (80-81)
Time less than 85%	0.1 (0-0.3)	0.4 (0.16-0.97)	0.4 (0.2-0.9)	0.9 (0.4-1.3)
ETOH	2 (1.5-3)	1.5 (1-2)	1 (0-1.5)	0.2 (0-1)

*Values are given as median with 95% confidence interval in ( )

Table 2: Age Group Rank Sum Medians*.

	Kruskal Wallis *p < 0.05	Pair-Wise Rank Sum Comparisons (Mann Whitney) *p < 0.008					
VARIABLE	1-4	1,2	1,3	1,4	2,3	2,4	3,4
BODY MASS INDEX	0.156	-	-	-	-	-	-
EPWORTH	0.002*	0.206	0.031	0.044	0.541	0.008*	0.005*
SLEEP QUESTIONNAIRE ITEMS							
Snoring	<0.001*	0.107	0.206	0.001*	0.770	<0.001*	<0.001*
Apneas	0.007*	0.117	0.615	0.001*	0.384	0.161	0.027
Excessive daytime sleepiness	0.001*	0.095	0.153	<0.001*	0.725	0.097	0.023
Alcohol use to sleep	0.051	-	-	-	-	-	-
Nocturia	<0.001*	0.175	0.001*	<0.001*	0.148	<0.001*	<0.001*
Sleep related motor vehicle accidents	0.528	-	-	-	-	-	-
Sleep related near misses	0.100	-	-	-	-	-	-
Coffee consumption	<0.001*	<0.001*	<0.001*	<0.001*	0.001*	<0.001*	0.124
Cola consumption	0.004*	0.151	0.982	0.014	0.200	<0.001*	0.022
Tea consumption	0.175	-	-	-	-	-	-
Cigarette use	<0.038*	0.841	0.783	0.003*	0.932	0.060	0.062
Alcohol use	<0.001*	0.050	0.004*	<0.001*	0.354	0.016	0.169
POLYSOMNOGRAM							
Apnea hypopnea index	0.802	-	-	-	-	-	-
Arousal Index	0.018*	0.021	0.006*	0.238	0.742	0.172	0.091
Obstructive sleep apneas	0.066	-	-	-	-	-	-
Central sleep apneas	0.553	-	-	-	-	-	-
NREM AHI	0.621	-	-	-	-	-	-
REM AHI	0.008*	0.171	0.009	0.003*	0.221	0.164	0.943
Lowest Oxygen Saturation	0.004*	0.272	0.051	<0.001*	0.525	0.054	0.208
Time less than 85%	0.001*	0.030	0.014	<0.001*	0.977	0.177	0.138

*Significant p value for Kruskal-Wallis is < 0.05. Significant p value for Mann Whitney is < 0.008.

Table 3: Age Group Differences*.

patients, ages 18-29, p<0.001). Patients, ages 40-49 also endorsed more nocturia than young adults (p=0.001). There were no age-related differences related to driving impairment due to excessive sleepiness.

Alcohol, caffeine, and tobacco

Patients, ages 18-29 reported more alcohol and tobacco use than patients, ages ≥ 50. Patients, ages 18-29 consumed the most alcohol compared to patients, ages 40-49 (p=0.004) and patients, ages ≥ 50 (p <0.001) with a trend toward use of alcohol to sleep (p=0.051). Although the majority of patients did not smoke (77%), there was a greater prevalence of smoking among patients, ages 18-29 compared to patients, ages ≥ 50 (p=0.003), but patients, ages ≥ 50 smokers used more tobacco than patients, ages 18-29. Patients, ages 30-39, 40-49 and ≥ 50 consumed more caffeinated beverages than patients, ages 18-29. Patients, ages 40-49 and ages ≥ 50 consumed more coffee than patients, ages 18-29 and 30-39. Patients, ages 30-39 consumed more coffee than patients, ages 18-29 (p<0.001). Patients, ages 30-39 reported more cola beverage consumption than patients, ages ≥ 50 (p<0.001).

Polysomnography

Arousal is an intrusion or disturbance in the patients' sleep pattern as measured by EEG brain wave activity. The arousal index is the average number of arousals per hour, regardless of the source of those arousals. In our study the arousal index was higher in patients, ages 18-29 compared to patients, ages 40-49 (p=0.006). Compared to patients, ages 18-29, patients, ages ≥ 50 had lower oxygen desaturations (p=0.003), more prolonged oxygen desaturations greater than 85% (p<0.001), and higher REM AHI's (p<0.001). There were no significant age-related differences with respect to AHI, total number of obstructive and central apneas, and NREM AHI.

Combined sleep-related parameters in function of age

A multiple linear regression analysis was conducted for different sleep-related parameters against OSA patients' ages. The plot of snoring, EDS, nocturia, arousal index, and lowest oxygen saturation against age had all individually significant p value (p<0.01). When these sleep-related parameters were used in combination (Combined Sleep-Related Parameters or CSRP) and a multiple linear regression statistic analysis was performed against patients' ages , an even stronger linear relationship was established, exhibiting a highly significant F-test of the overall fit p value < 0.00001, and a goodness of fit R-squared= 0.15 (Figure 1).

Discussion

Our study demonstrated an increased arousal index in patients, ages 18-29 compared to patients, ages ≥ 50, however, in the latter there was an increase in REM-related apneas and hypopneas as well as more severe desaturations despite similar AHI's. Our study suggests that the greatest differences in clinical symptoms and polysomnographic findings between patients, ages 18-29 and patients, ages ≥ 50 with OSA were not accounted for by BMI. Patients, ages 18-29 report many of the common symptoms associated with OSA such as snoring, witnessed apneas, and excessive daytime sleepiness. Patients, ages ≥ 50 report less snoring, less witnessed apneas, and less daytime sleepiness than patients, ages 18-29.Our study suggests that snoring, witnessed apneas, and obesity are insensitive indicators for identifying OSA in patients, ages ≥ 50. Data from the Sleep Heart Health Study on people ages 40 to 98 years demonstrated that male sex, BMI, neck size, snoring, and witnessed apneas were associated with OSA, but in older adults the magnitude of associations between OSA, body habitus, snoring and witnessed apneas decreased similar to our findings [19]. As a result, health care practitioners may not recognize CSA in older adults, and older adults may ascribe symptoms of OSA to aging, medications, or other medical problems. Maintaining a high index of suspicion and obtaining a complete medical history are valuable assets in assessing for OSA in the elderly.

Patients, ages ≥ 50 report more nocturia compared to the patients, ages 18-29. Nocturia has been previously reported as a common complaint in older adults and associated with increased falls and fractures [20,21]. A cross-sectional study investigating OSA in community-dwelling older adults demonstrated more nocturia with

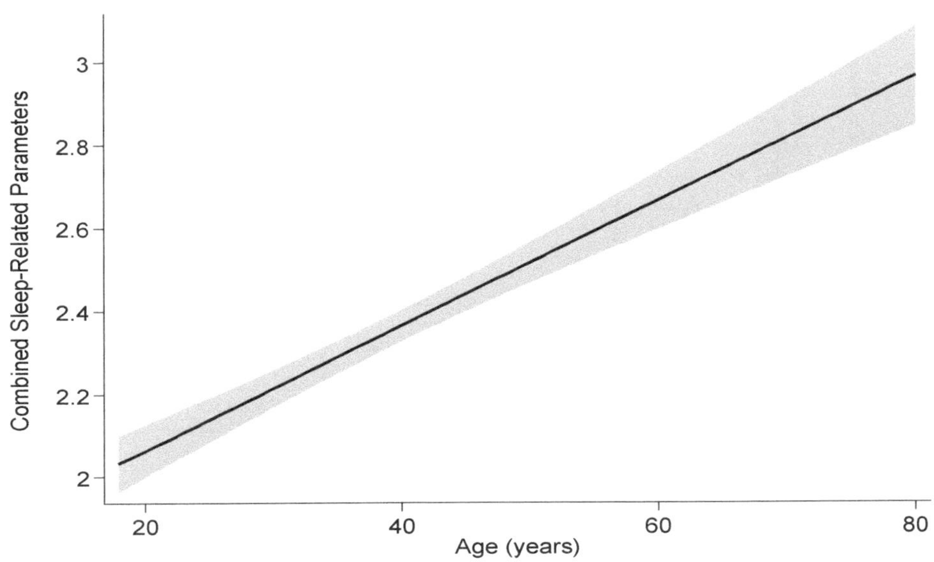

Figure 1: Multiple linear regression statistic analysis of the combined sleep-related parameters (CSRP), snoring, EDS, nocturia, arousal index and lowest oxygen saturation against patients' age. The significance at p<0.001 and R-squared=0.15 provide evidence of a linear relationship between the response (CSRP) and the explanatory variable (age). The higher the value of 'age' the more is the rate of CSRP. The shaded area represents 95% confidence interval

an AHI of 25 or greater [22]. The increased nocturia in the elderly and late middle age patients may be due to diuretic medications, increased intraabdominal pressure, confusion associated with arousals, and increased secretion of Atrial Natriuretic Peptide (ANP). Increased plasma and urine ANP result in increased natriuresis and dieresis [23]. The increased ANP levels in patients with severe sleep apnea are attributed to hemodynamic changes associated with sleep apnea to include atrial distension, acute hypoxemia, and pulmonary hypertension [24-26].

A greater proportion of patients, ages 18-29 reported alcohol and tobacco consumption compared to older age groups. The increased use of tobacco and alcohol consumption among patients, ages 18-29 may worsen sleep apnea severity in young adults. One epidemiologic study that focused on smoking found that current smokers were three times (95% CI, 1.4 to 6.4) more likely to have OSA than never-smokers [27]. There are several mechanisms to explain the link between smoking and OSA. Smoking can induce upper airway edema and increase sleep instability. Upper airway inflammation and edema may increase vulnerability to OSA. Sleep instability is associated with OSA and may be increased by reductions in blood nicotine levels. Nicotine may also cause a "rebound effect" where acutely nicotine increases upper airway tone that is reversed overnight with withdrawal of nicotine resulting in worsening OSA [27].

Many studies in which defined quantities of alcohol were administered to healthy subjects or patients with OSA before bedtime demonstrated increased number and duration of hypopnea and apnea events [28,29]. In one CPAP-titration experiment moderate alcohol consumption near bedtime increased the level of nasal pressure necessary to prevent apneas and hypopneas in patients with OSA [28]. Alcohol ingestion can inhibit the activity of upper airway muscles and increase airway collapsibility resulting in increased nasal and pharyngeal resistance. In addition, alcohol can diminish arousal responses resulting in prolonged apnea duration and worsening oxygen desaturation.

Although there was no difference in AHI between age cohorts, patients, ages ≥ 50 had more severe oxygen desaturations and an increased REM-related AHI while patients, ages 18-29 had an increased arousal index. The severe desaturation and high REM AHI in the elderly may be due to disease progression associated with age. The proposed mechanism may be increased deposition of parapharyngeal fat, lengthening of the soft palate, and changes in body structures surrounding the pharynx [27,28]. Respiratory related arousals are associated with Upper Airway Resistance Syndrome (UARS), and mild to severe OSA [29]. Frequent respiratory arousals disrupt sleep architecture and may account for the higher ratings of excessive daytime sleepiness on the PSQ.

Our study failed to demonstrate an increase in REM related apneas and hypopneas and a decrease in NREM-related apneas and hypopneas in patients, ages 18-29 compared to patients, ages ≥ 50. Our hypothesis was that sleep apnea has a continuum of disease severity that can be identified by examining age cohorts. Early manifestations of OSA in young patients would manifest with high arousals and REM predominant apneas and hypopneas while late manifestations of OSA would have predominantly NREM apneas and hypopneas. One explanation is that a number of patients, ages 18-29 already had moderate to severe apnea accounting for the REM and NREM apnea events. Another hypothesis is that apnea severity does not correlate with the proportion of REM vs. NREM apneas and hypopneas. A retrospective study examining the differences between patients with REM AHI vs. NREM AHI found that BMI, apnea severity, and severity of oxygen desaturation did not account for group differences. Only the duration of apnea was longer in the REM AHI group [30].

Our study has several limitations. First, the mean AHI was high which may have resulted in comparing age groups with severe OSA under representing adults with mild OSA, which may have better identified a spectrum of OSA. The study was also retrospective and patients were not randomized to the different age groups. Furthermore, investigators were not blinded when selecting patients for the different age cohorts and this could be perceived as a source of selection bias. A randomized double blind, prospective study with different age groups may have provided different data. Split-night studies compared to full-night diagnostic studies would potentially have shorter total sleep times that may alter sleep parameters; however, the number of split-night studies were similar between groups. There was also a significant proportion of male patients whose race was unknown as the information was either not available in the patient's electronic medical record or the patient's race was identified as "other." Finally, the findings may not apply to women as they were underrepresented in this study.

There were a greater percentage of women represented in the age ≥ 50 group which is consistent with epidemiological data which supports the higher prevalence of obstructive sleep apnea in postmenopausal women compared to premenopausal women [30]. The greater percentage of women in the older age group may have affected our results. With regards to the severity of sleep apnea among the younger age group, the main reasons young adults are referred for evaluation of sleep disordered breathing is due to occupational impairment due to daytime sleepiness or reports by roommates or spouses other of snoring and witnessed apneas. Young adults have similar risk factors for obstructive sleep apnea in comparison to older adults and therefore do not differ in apnea severity.

In conclusion, this study evaluated different sleep related parameters for patients with OSA at different age ranges. Patients, ages 18-29 had the largest differences in clinical and polysomnographic manifestations of OSA compared to patients, ages ≥ 50. Patients, ages 18-29 reported symptoms commonly associated with OSA and had higher arousal indexes. In contrast, patients, ages ≥ 50 reported more nocturia, less snoring, less witnessed apneas, and less daytime sleepiness and had an increased REM AHI with more severe oxygen desaturations.

References

1. Young T, Palta M, Dempsey J, Skatrud J, Weber S, et al. (1993) The occurrence of sleep-disordered breathing among middle-aged adults. N Engl J Med 328: 1230-1235.

2. Berry RB, Foster R. Obstructive sleep apnea hypopnea syndromes: definitions, epidemiology, diagnosis, and consequences. In Carney PR, Berry RB, Geyer JD, eds. Clinical Sleep Disorders. New York, NY: Lippincott; 254-277.

3. Patil SP, Schneider H, Schwartz AR, Smith PL (2007) Adult obstructive sleep apnea: pathophysiology and diagnosis. Chest 132: 325-337.

4. He J, Kryger MH, Zorick FJ, Conway W, Roth T (1988) Mortality and apnea index in obstructive sleep apnea. Experience in 385 male patients. Chest 94: 9-14.

5. Findley LJ, Barth JT, Powers DC, Wilhoit SC, Boyd DG, et al. (1986) Cognitive impairment in patients with obstructive sleep apnea and associated hypoxemia. Chest 90: 686-690.

6. Reichmuth KJ, Austin D, Skatrud JB, Young T (2005) Association of sleep apnea and type II diabetes: a population-based study. Am J Respir Crit Care Med 172: 1590-1595.

7. Hartenbaum N, Collop N, Rosen IM (2006) Sleep Apnea and Commercial

Motor Vehicle Operators: Statement From the Joint Task Force of the American College of Chest Physicians, the American College of Occupational and Environmental Medicine, and the National Sleep Foundation Chest 130: 902-905.

8. Peppard PE, Young T, Palta M, Skatrud J (2000) Prospective study of the association between sleep-disordered breathing and hypertension. N Engl J Med 342: 1378-1384.
9. Sajkov D, Cowie RJ, Thornton AT, Espinoza HA, McEvoy RD (1994) Pulmonary hypertension and hypoxemia in obstructive sleep apnea syndrome. Am J Respir Crit Care Med 149: 416-422.
10. Guilleminault C, Connolly SJ, Winkle RA (1983) Cardiac arrhythmia and conduction disturbances during sleep in 400 patients with sleep apnea syndrome. Am J Cardiol 52: 490-494.
11. Shahar E, Whitney CW, Redline S, Lee ET, Newman AB, et al. (2001) Sleep-disordered breathing and cardiovascular disease: cross-sectional results of the Sleep Heart Health Study. Am J Respir Crit Care Med 163: 19-25.
12. Gami AS, Howard DE, Olson EJ, Somers VK (2005) Day-night pattern of sudden death in obstructive sleep apnea. N Engl J Med 352: 1206-1214.
13. D'Ambrosio C, Bowman T, Mohsenin V (1999) Quality of life in patients with obstructive sleep apnea: effect of nasal continuous positive airway pressure--a prospective study. Chest 115: 123-129.
14. Young T, Peppard PE, Gottlieb DJ (2002) Epidemiology of obstructive sleep apnea: a population health perspective. Am J Respir Crit Care Med 165: 1217-1239.
15. Durán J, Esnaola S, Rubio R, Iztueta A (2001) Obstructive sleep apnea-hypopnea and related clinical features in a population-based sample of subjects aged 30 to 70 yr. Am J Respir Crit Care Med 163: 685-689.
16. Bixler EO, Vgontzas AN, Ten Have T, Tyson K, Kales A (1998) Effects of age on sleep apnea in men: I. Prevalence and severity. Am J Respir Crit Care Med 157: 144-148.
17. Enright PL, Newman AB, Wahl PW, Manolio TA, Haponik EF, et al. (1996) Prevalence and correlates of snoring and observed apneas in 5,201 older adults. Sleep 19: 531-538.
18. Chung S, Yoon IY, Lee CH, Kim JW (2009) Effects of age on the clinical features of men with obstructive sleep apnea syndrome. Respiration 78: 23-29.
19. Young T, Shahar E, Nieto FJ, Redline S, Newman AB, et al. (2002) Predictors of sleep-disordered breathing in community-dwelling adults: the Sleep Heart Health Study. Arch Intern Med 162: 893-900.
20. Brown JS, Vittinghoff E, Wyman JF, Stone KL, Nevitt MC, et al. (2000) Urinary incontinence: does it increase risk for falls and fractures? Study of Osteoporotic Fractures Research Group. J Am Geriatr Soc 48: 721-725.
21. Stewart RB, Moore MT, May FE, Marks RG, Hale WE (1992) Nocturia: a risk factor for falls in the elderly. J Am Geriatr Soc 40: 1217-1220.
22. Endeshaw YW, Johnson TM, Kutner MH, Ouslander JG, Bliwise DL (2004) Sleep-disordered breathing and nocturia in older adults. J Am Geriatr Soc 52: 957-960.
23. Ichioka M, Hirata Y, Inase N, Tojo N, Yoshizawa M, et al. (1992) Changes of circulating atrial natriuretic peptide and antidiuretic hormone in obstructive sleep apnea syndrome. Respiration 59: 164-168.
24. Rubattu S, Volpe M (2001) The atrial natriuretic peptide: a changing view. J Hypertens 19: 1923-1931.
25. Wetter DW, Young TB, Bidwell TR, Badr MS, Palta M (1994) Smoking as a risk factor for sleep-disordered breathing. Arch Intern Med 154: 2219-2224.
26. Malhotra A, Huang Y, Fogel R, Lazic S, Pillar G, et al. (2006) Aging influences on pharyngeal anatomy and physiology: the predisposition to pharyngeal collapse. Am J Med 119: 72.
27. Eikermann M, Jordan AS, Chamberlin NL, Gautam S, Wellman A, et al. (2007) The influence of aging on pharyngeal collapsibility during sleep. Chest 131: 1702-1709.
28. Guilleminault C, Stoohs R, Clerk A, Simmons J, Labanowski M (1992) From obstructive sleep apnea syndrome to upper airway resistance syndrome: consistency of daytime sleepiness. Sleep 15: S13-16.
29. Siddiqui F, Walters AS, Goldstein D, Lahey M, Desai H (2006) Half of patients with obstructive sleep apnea have a higher NREM AHI than REM AHI. Sleep Med 7: 281-285.
30. Lee W, Nagubadi S, Kryger MH, Mokhlesi B (2008) Epidemiology of Obstructive Sleep Apnea: a Population-based Perspective. Expert Rev Respir Med 2: 349-364.

18

Media, Sleep and Memory in Children and Adolescents

Markus Dworak[1]* and Alfred Wiater[2]

[1]Harvard Medical School, West Roxbury, MA, USA
[2]Department of Pediatrics, Hospital Cologne Porz/Rhine, Cologne, Germany

Abstract

Media usage across children and adolescents is steadily increasing and captures a significant amount of their usual waking time. Excessive media use affects sleep quality and quantity including increased sleep onset latency, night awakenings and overall reduced sleep duration. Healthy sleep is important for overall health, as well as physical and mental performance and disrupted sleep during early childhood and adolescent results in emotional and behavioral consequences including impaired school performance, attention problems and a higher risk for ADHD and obesity. The present review summarizes recent findings related to the effects of media on sleep and memory in children and adolescent and provides practical recommendations for children's' and adolescent's media and sleep behavior.

Keywords: Sleep; Memory; Adolescents; REM sleep

Introduction

Media are one of the most powerful forces in young people's lives today. In western society average media consumption in children and adolescents is steadily increasing and accounts for over 7.5 hours a day, seven days a week [1]. Within the last decade the impact of media on children's health and wellbeing is increasingly recognized and considered as a serious problem in modern society. Excessive television and videogame usage has been associated with somatic problems, obesity and multiple psychiatric symptoms such as aggressive behavior, attention problems and hyperactivity [2-7]. Within the last years there is also accumulating evidence that excessive media consumption can significantly impair sleep behavior and memory performance [8,9]. This topical review gives an overview of the recent key findings that addressed the relationship between media, sleep and memory in children and adolescents.

Media Exposure and Sleep Behavior in Children and Adolescents

Clinical experience with adults and children with sleep problems strongly implicates television-viewing habits as a potentially significant influence on sleep behavior [8]. Media exposure is associated with sleeping difficulties, bedtime resistance, sleep-onset delay, sleep anxiety, night awakenings, and shortened sleep duration [8-10]. A study by Johnson et al. showed that watching television three or more hours per day during adolescence elevated significantly the risk for frequent sleep problems by early adulthood [10,11]. The reasons how media exposure affects sleep behavior seems to be multiple: Especially late evening television viewing can contribute to heightened alertness and increased physiological arousal, which are associated with difficulty falling asleep [8,12,13]. Second, extended exposure to the bright light of a television screen may contribute to delayed or reduced melatonin secretion, adversely affecting the sleep-waking cycle [12-14]. Third, both news media and entertainment fiction may lead to short-term and enduring fright reactions. Even TV programs, movies and news made for children may trigger fear [15] therefore selectively supporting to the development of sleep problems [16-18]. Also, physical inactivity, which seems to be associated with extensive television viewing, may contribute to increased restlessness and difficulty falling or staying asleep [5,19]. Indeed, an inverse relationship between time spent using video games and daily physical activity has been observed [20-22]. Positive effects of physical activity on children's overall health, sleep quality, sleep latency and deep NREM sleep have been observed in different studies [19-24]. Beside the reduced physical activity, excessive media use appears to be clearly associated with elements of a less healthy diet including lower fruit and vegetable consumption; higher consumption of energy-dense snacks, drinks, and fast foods; and higher total energy intake [25-27], therefore increasing the risk for overweight and obesity. Indeed, recent results from a 30-year study indicate that increased daily hours of TV consumption on weekends predicted a higher BMI at the age of 30 and that each additional hour of TV watched on weekends at age 5, increased the risk of adult obesity by 7% [28].

But what is the most powerful predictor for sleep problems among children and adolescent? Multiple independent studies identified the occurrence of a TV in children's bedroom as major predictor for sleep problems [29]. A bedroom television increases the opportunity for young children to watch frightening or violent content as well as adult-targeted television content which has been linked to an increased for sleep problems [30]. In general, regular bedroom television usage was associated with delayed bedtimes, difficulty falling asleep, and less overall sleep, and thus seems to be the most powerful predictor of overall sleep disturbance and bedtime resistance [9,29]. These data are supported by recent observations from real life daily practice whereby 20% to 43% of US preschool-aged children have a television in their bedroom, and increasing numbers of families report sleep problems as one of the primary reasons [29]. Since sleep problems itself can clearly influence daytime physical and mental performance, special care is needed to prevent potential negative effects of poor sleep on children's health and cognitive development.

Sleep and Memory in Children and Adolescents

It is widely known that the newborn brain continues to develop

***Corresponding author:** Markus Dworak, Harvard Medical School, West Roxbury, MA, USA, E-mail: Markus_Dworak@hms.harvard.edu

rapidly through the first few years of life and that considerable plasticity exists during this time period [31,32]. In the last decades, extensive research has been accumulated demonstrating that sleep is essential for important processes of brain development, neuronal plasticity and memory consolidation in children and adolescents [33-37].

Sleep seems to be particularly important during early brain development up to the age of two years when a child still spends more time asleep than awake. Even when starting school, sleep accounts for up to 50 percent of the 24-h day. Often, total sleep duration in children and adolescents is also below general recommendations and despite cultural differences, many studies have shown that adolescents world-wide sleep significantly less than the recommended 9-10 h [38]. Compared to adulthood, childhood is characterized by longer sleep duration and higher amounts of deep and restorative non-rapid-eye-movement (NREM) sleep and active (rapid-eye-movement) REM sleep which is characterized by a high-frequent brain activity as measured in the electroencephalogram (EEG) [38,39]. Results from longitudinal EEG sleep studies suggest that sleep regulation undergoes a period of maturation during infancy and a lower frontal predominance of NREM slow wave activity has been observed in children and adolescents compared to adults, possibly reflecting the late maturation of the frontal cortex [40].

Presumably, both REM and NREM sleep are involved in the consolidation process, in which NREM sleep is particularly favorable to explicit memory, whereas REM sleep favors implicit memory processes [41,42].

Various studies have investigated the impact of sleep on learning and memory in children and adolescents and evidence is condensing that disrupted sleep negatively affects these processes. Steenari et al. showed that longer sleep latency and lower sleep efficiency were associated with poorer auditory and visual working memory, whereas shorter sleep duration was associated with lower working memory performance. The authors concluded that sleep quality rather than sleep duration appeared to be strongly associated with working memory performance [42]. Sadeh et al. examined the association between sleep and neurobehavioral functioning, including the encoding of declarative memory content in school-age children. "Good" and "Poor" sleepers were identified and the "Poor" sleepers showed more fragmented sleep and reduced sleep efficiency. Overall, good sleepers showed better results learning digits compared to the poor sleepers. Interestingly, this difference only showed up in a morning but not in the noon hours. The authors hypothesized that the findings are in line with theories of general cognitive performance emphasizing the contribution of both chronobiological and homeostatic factors on cognitive performance [43,44].

One night of total sleep deprivation in young adolescents (12-15 years) resulted in a significant decline of correctly recalled words in the Williams Word Memory Test. In a further study, Sadeh et al. [43] examined the effects of prolonged modest sleep restriction or extension in children. After two regular nights with normal sleep duration, children (9-12 year old) were asked to extend or restrict their sleep time by 1 h for three consecutive nights. Children, who extended their sleep time, improved their memory task performance significantly compared to baseline and compared to the sleep-restriction group. Other studies compared the effects of nocturnal sleep versus daytime wakefulness on declarative memory consolidation and procedural memory consolidation in 6-8 year old children and adults [33,42]. Declarative memory performance was enhanced when sleep followed learning. Interestingly, in contrast to the hypothesis and to findings in adults, in children procedural performance was impaired after periods of nocturnal sleep in comparison to periods of daytime wakefulness. The authors concluded that the sleep-related consolidation process of distinct memory systems might depend on developmental stage. Together these and other studies provide evidence that sleep is critically involved in memory encoding and working memory in children and adolescents.

Effects of Excessive Media Consumption on Sleep-Dependent Memory Performance

Poor sleep quality may result in mental health problems, impaired school performance, and somatic complaints. Sleep difficulties are significantly associated with both behavioral problems, such as school attendance problems, and higher levels of tiredness [9]. Most studies examined long-term effects of media exposure on sleep timing, whereas only a few studied the effects of television and computer exposure on children's and adolescence sleep quality and associated health problems.

In one of our previous studies, we examined the effects of intense media use on sleep and cognitive performance in school-aged children. Children were exposed to voluntary television use (TV-movie for 90 minutes) and video game consumption for 90 minutes or no media at all a few hours before their usual bedtime. Sleep behavior was measured in all participants in the following night by using polysomnographic measurements to determine sleep-architecture and sleep-continuity parameters. Furthermore, a visual and verbal memory test was used before media stimulation and on the following day after one night of sleep to determine visuo spatial and verbal memory performance [45]. Playing an exciting video prolonged sleep-onset latency and increased the percentage of stage 2 sleep, which reflects a lighter and more interference-prone sleep stage, whereas NREM slow-wave sleep (stage 3 and 4) was significantly reduced. Playing the video game was also associated with a decline in verbal memory performance in the participating children. Television viewing reduced sleep efficiency but did not affect sleep patterns. Overall, no effects on REM-sleep were observed.

Previous studies showed different effects of television viewing and video game playing on several physiologic parameters [46]. Unlike television viewing, which expends the same energy as sitting quietly, interactive video game consumption resulted in significant increases in various physiologic and metabolic variables in young children, including heart rate, blood pressure, respiratory rate, energy expenditure, and ventilation, and thus a higher arousal state of the central nervous system [46]. The magnitude of these changes was below standard physical exercise and national health recommendations and did not affect metabolic, cardiovascular, pulmonary, hemodynamic, and endocrine systems in the whole body and the brain as physical activity does [47]. A higher arousal state within the hours before sleeping might be a strong factor that influences subsequent sleep. Further different effects of television viewing and video game playing could influence emotional factors. TV viewers are in a receptive state, whereas video game users are playing an interactive role. Children might identify themselves with the role they take within the game and aggressive or violent contents could be encoded [48].

The observation that playing a heart-pounding video game can impair verbal memory performance is in line with several studies showing that strong emotional experiences, such as computer games and thrilling films, could influence learning processes decisively. Since recently acquired knowledge is very sensitive in the following

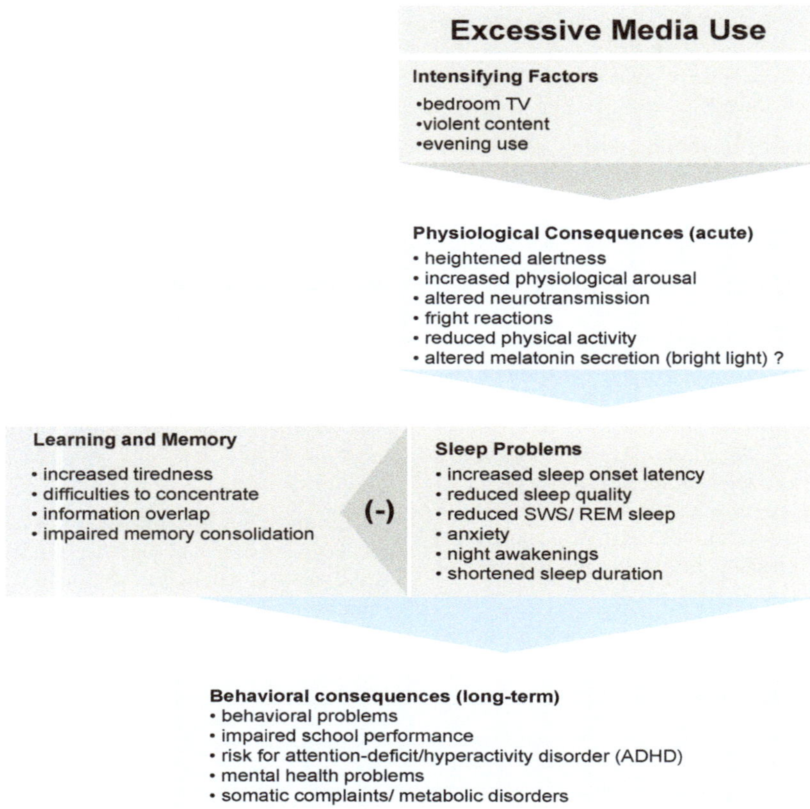

Figure 1: Theoretical relationship between excessive media use, sleep problems, memory processing and behavioral consequences in children and adolescent.

consolidation period, emotional experiences within the hours after learning could strongly influence processes related to memory consolidation [49-51]. Often, interactive video games are challenging, sometimes frustrating, exciting, and often surprising for children and adolescents, and during playing, individuals may experience a range of emotions accompanied by neurophysiological changes.

Exposure to adult media potentially has a stronger impact than media exposure time [52,53]. Especially adult (violent/sexual) media content and associated individual excitement can affect sleep and learning in children [54], but only 13% have parental control with rules about the content of their consumed media [1].

Movie, television, and video game use during the middle school years was uniformly associated with a negative impact on school performance [53]. Children with lowest grades spend more time playing video games and less time reading than those with the best grades [1]. Limiting young children's exposure to television as a medium during formative years of brain development may reduce children's subsequent risk for developing ADHD and social and scholastic problems [53-55].

Conclusion and Recommendations

Media use is steadily increasing and captures a significant amount of children's and adolescents waking time. Excessive media use can affect sleep quality and quantity including increased sleep onset latency, night awakenings and shortened sleep duration. Healthy sleep is important for overall health and development and disrupted sleep during early childhood and adolescent can result in neuro-developmental implications and emotional and behavioral consequences including impaired school performance, attention problems and a higher risk for ADHD and obesity (Figure 1).

Parents and educator should be aware of their children`s media use. Children`s and adolescents bedroom is no place for a TV. Parents and teachers should provide directions about total media use including the time spent with television and computer as well as the contents of TV and video games. Restriction of media time should be associated with alternative challenging activities. Insofar, physical activity and team sport can absolutely be recommended. Physical activity is an important component in the development of self-esteem in children. It has a preventive function concerning obesity and an improving influence on sleep quality. However, further research is needed to examine the long-term consequences of excessive media use in children and adolescents on overall health and behavior.

References

1. Rideout V, Roberts DF, Foehr UG (2007) Generation M: media in the lives of 8–18 year-olds.
2. Johnson JG, Cohen P, Smailes EM, Kasen S, Brook JS (2002) Television viewing and aggressive behavior during adolescence and adulthood. Science 295: 2468-2471.
3. Christakis DA, Zimmerman FJ, DiGiuseppe DL, McCarty CA (2004) Early television exposure and subsequent attentional problems in children. Pediatrics 113: 708-713.
4. Toyran M, Ozmert E, Yurdakök K (2002) Television viewing and its effect on physical health of schoolage children. Turk J Pediatr 44: 194-203.
5. Robinson TN, Wilde ML, Navracruz LC, Haydel KF, Varady A (2001) Effects of reducing children's television and video game use on aggressive behavior: a randomized controlled trial. Arch Pediatr Adolesc Med 155: 17-23.

6. Oginska H, Pokorski J (2006) Fatigue and mood correlates of sleep length in three age-social groups: School children, students, and employees. Chronobiol Int 23: 1317-1328.

7. Owens J, Maxim R, McGuinn M, Nobile C, Msall M, et al. (1999) Television-viewing habits and sleep disturbance in school children. Pediatrics 104: e27.

8. Van den Bulck J (2004) Television viewing, computer game playing, and Internet use and self-reported time to bed and time out of bed in secondary-school children. Sleep 27: 101-104.

9. Tazawa Y, Okada K (2001) Physical signs associated with excessive television-game playing and sleep deprivation. Pediatr Int 43: 647-650.

10. Johnson JG, Cohen P, Kasen S, First MB, Brook JS (2004) Association between television viewing and sleep problems during adolescence and early adulthood. Arch Pediatr Adolesc Med 158: 562-568.

11. Kubota T, Uchiyama M, Suzuki H, Shibui K, Kim K, et al. (2002) Effects of nocturnal bright light on saliva melatonin, core body temperature and sleep propensity rhythms in human subjects. Neurosci Res 42: 115-122.

12. Higuchi S, Motohashi Y, Liu Y, Maeda A (2005) Effects of playing a computer game using a bright display on presleep physiological variables, sleep latency, slow wave sleep and REM sleep. J Sleep Res 14: 267-273.

13. Higuchi S, Motohashi Y, Liu Y, Ahara M, Kaneko Y (2003) Effects of VDT tasks with a bright display at night on melatonin, core temperature, heart rate, and sleepiness. J Appl Physiol 94: 1773-1776.

14. Custers K, Van den Bulck J (2012) Fear effects by the media. Eur J Pediatr 171: 613-616.

15. Harrison K, Cantor J (1999) Tales from the screen: enduring fright reactions to scary media. Media Psychol 1: 97-116.

16. Singer MI, Slovak K, Frierson T, York P (1998) Viewing preferences, symptoms of psychological trauma, and violent behaviors among children who watch television. J Am Acad Child Adolesc Psychiatry 37: 1041-1048.

17. Cantor J (1994) Fright reactions to mass media. In: Bryant J, Zillmann D, eds. Media Effects: Advances in Theory and Research. (2ndedn). Mahwah, NJ: Lawrence Erlbaum Associates Inc: 287-306.

18. Dworak M, Wiater A, Alfer D, Stephan E, Hollmann W, et al. (2008) Increased slow wave sleep and reduced stage 2 sleep in children depending on exercise intensity. Sleep Med 9: 266-272.

19. Robinson TN (2001) Television viewing and childhood obesity. Pediatr Clin North Am 48: 1017-1025.

20. Strauss RS, Rodzilsky D, Burack G, Colin M (2001) Psychosocial correlates of physical activity in healthy children. Arch Pediatr Adolesc Med 155: 897-902.

21. Janz KF, Golden JC, Hansen JR, Mahoney LT (1992) Heart rate monitoring of physical activity in children and adolescents: the Muscatine Study. Pediatrics 89: 256-261.

22. Janz KF, Burns TL, Torner JC, Levy SM, Paulos R, et al. (2001) Physical activity and bone measures in young children: the Iowa bone development study. Pediatrics 107: 1387-1393.

23. Strong WB, Malina RM, Blimkie CJ, Daniels SR, Dishman RK, et al. (2005) Evidence based physical activity for school-age youth. J Pediatr 146: 732-737.

24. Pearson N, Biddle SJ (2011) Sedentary behavior and dietary intake in children, adolescents, and adults. A systematic review. Am J Prev Med 41: 178-188.

25. DuRant RH, Baranowski T, Johnson M, Thompson WO (1994) The relationship among television watching, physical activity, and body composition of young children. Pediatrics 94: 449-455.

26. Matheson DM, Killen JD, Wang Y, Varady A, Robinson TN (2004) Children's food consumption during television viewing. Am J Clin Nutr 79: 1088-1094.

27. Skelton JA, Cook SR, Auinger P, Klein JD, Barlow SE (2009) Prevalence and trends of severe obesity among US children and adolescents. Acad Pediatr 9: 322-329.

28. Garrison MM, Liekweg K, Christakis DA (2011) Media use and child sleep: the impact of content, timing, and environment. Pediatrics 128: 29-35.

29. Paavonen EJ, Pennonen M, Roine M, Valkonen S, Lahikainen AR (2006) TV exposure associated with sleep disturbances in 5- to 6-year-old children. J Sleep Res 15: 154-161.

30. Barkovich AJ, Kjos BO, Jackson DE Jr, Norman D (1988) Normal maturation of the neonatal and infant brain: MR imaging at 1.5 T. Radiology 166: 173-180.

31. Yamada H, Sadato N, Konishi Y, Muramoto S, Kimura K, et al. (2000) A milestone for normal development of the infantile brain detected by functional MRI. Neurology 55: 218-223.

32. Backhaus J, Hoeckesfeld R, Born J, Hohagen F, Junghanns K (2008) Immediate as well as delayed post learning sleep but not wakefulness enhances declarative memory consolidation in children. Neurobiol Learn Mem 89: 76-80.

33. Buckhalt JA, El-Sheikh M, Keller P (2007) Children's sleep and cognitive functioning: race and socioeconomic status as moderators of effects. Child Dev 78: 213-231.

34. Diekelmann S, Born J (2010) The memory function of sleep. Nat Rev Neurosci 11: 114-126.

35. Jan JE, Reiter RJ, Bax MC, Ribary U, Freeman RD, et al. (2010) Long-term sleep disturbances in children: a cause of neurona loss. Eur J Paediatr Neurol 14: 380-390.

36. Fischer S, Wilhelm I, Born J (2007) Developmental differences in sleep's role for implicit off-line learning: comparing children with adults. J Cogn Neurosci 19: 214-227.

37. Ohayon MM, Carskadon MA, Guilleminault C, Vitiello MV (2004) Meta-analysis of quantitative sleep parameters from childhood to old age in healthy individuals: developing normative sleep values across the human lifespan. Sleep 27: 1255-1273.

38. Anders TF (1994) Infant sleep, nighttime relationships, and attachment. Psychiatry 57: 11-21.

39. Giedd JN (2004) Structural magnetic resonance imaging of the adolescent brain. Ann N Y Acad Sci 1021: 77-85.

40. Gais S, Born J (2004) Declarative memory consolidation: mechanisms acting during human sleep. Learn Mem 11: 679-685.

41. Wilhelm I, Diekelmann S, Born J (2008) Sleep in children improves memory performance on declarative but not procedural tasks. Learn Mem 15: 373-377.

42. Steenari MR, Vuontela V, Paavonen EJ, Carlson S, Fjallberg M, et al. (2003) Working memory and sleep in 6- to 13-year-old schoolchildren. J Am Acad Child Adolesc Psychiatry 42: 85-92.

43. Sadeh A, Gruber R, Raviv A (2002) Sleep, neurobehavioral functioning, and behavior problems in school-age children. Child Dev 73: 405-417.

44. Dworak M, Schierl T, Bruns T, Strüder HK (2007) Impact of singular excessive computer game and television exposure on sleep patterns and memory performance of school-aged children. Pediatrics 120: 978-985.

45. Wang X, Perry AC (2006) Metabolic and physiologic responses to video game play in 7- to 10-year-old boys. Arch Pediatr Adolesc Med 160: 411-415.

46. Cotman CW, Berchtold NC (2002) Exercise: a behavioral intervention to enhance brain health and plasticity. Trends Neurosci 25: 295-301.

47. Frölich J, Lehmkuhl G: Computer and Internet erobern die Kindheit. Schattauer, Stuttgart/Germany 2012.

48. Maquet P (2001) The role of sleep in learning and memory. Science 294: 1048-1052.

49. Stickgold R, Hobson JA, Fosse R, Fosse M (2001) Sleep, learning, and dreams: off-line memory reprocessing. Science 294: 1052-1057.

50. Dolan RJ (2002) Emotion, cognition, and behavior. Science 298: 1191-1194.

51. Bernard-Bonnin AC, Gilbert S, Rousseau E, Masson P, Maheux B (1991) Television and the 3- to 10-year-old child. Pediatrics 88: 48-54.

52. Sharif I, Sargent JD (2006) Association between television, movie, and video game exposure and school performance. Pediatrics 118: e1061-1070.

53. Brady SS, Matthews KA (2006) Effects of media violence on health-related outcomes among young men. Arch Pediatr Adolesc Med 160: 341-347.

54. Christakis DA, Ebel BE, Rivara FP, Zimmerman FJ (2004) Television, video, and computer game usage in children under 11 years of age. J Pediatr 145: 652-656.

55. Subrahmanyam K, Greenfield P, Kraut R, Gross E (2001) The impact of computer use on children's and adolescents' development. J Appl Dev Psychol 22: 7-30.

The Development of Posttraumatic Stress Disorder after Mild Traumatic Brain Injury in Civilian Populations

Xi Han[1], Ping Sheng[2,3]*, Chengguang Huang[2], Mingkun Yu[2], Lijun Hou[2] and Yan Dong[2,3]*

[1]*Department of Neurosurgery, Huashan Hospital, Fudan University, China*
[2]*Department of Neurosurgery, Second Military Medical University, China*
[3]*Neuroscience center, Second Military Medical University, China*

Abstract

Background: Posttraumatic stress disorder (PTSD) is an anxiety disorder following exposure to a traumatic event. Recent studies demonstrate that mild traumatic brain injury (mTBI) is strongly associated with PTSD among soldiers returning from Iraq. However, the effect of mTBI on development of PTSD in civilian populations is quite controversial. The study is aimed at identifying whether mTBI contributes to an increased risk of PTSD in civilian populations as it happens in the service members.

Methods: A comprehensive search of literature was undertaken in order to identify published studies on PTSD associated with mTBI. mTBI was defined according to the American Congress of Rehabilitation Medicine (ACRM). PTSD was operationalized as the presence of symptoms consistent with those defined by the *Diagnostic and Statistical Manual of Mental Disorders.* The effect of mTBI on the development of PTSD was assessed with odds ratio (OR) with 95% confidence intervals (CIs).

Results: The pooled data consisted of 1222 mTBI patients and 1468 general trauma participants. 14% of mTBI patients reported PTSD, and 9% of general trauma patients developed PTSD. Or of the pooled studies indicates a 61% increase in the prevalence of PTSD, suggesting that mTBI might increase the risk of development of PTSD in civilian settings (or 1.61, 95% CI 1.25-2.06. p=0.0002, I^2=0%). The occurrence of PTSD was not significantly different among 3-months, 6-months and 12-months follow up subgroups (p=0.28). A sensitivity analysis shows the results are affected by sequential exclusion of study reported by Bryant et al. (2010). When Bryant et al. data were removed, OR of the other six studies demonstrates that the prevalence of PTSD in mTBI and general trauma groups doesn't significantly differ (OR 1.30, 95% CI 0.88-1.93. p=0.19, I^2=0%). The study from Bryant et al contributed 57% of patients to overall data, which was derived from four levels I trauma centers across three states in Australia.

Conclusion: Our data indicate that mTBI patients are more prone to develop PTSD than general trauma patients without mTBI in civilian settings.

Keywords: Mild traumatic brain injury; Minor brain injury; Posttraumatic stress disorder; Anxiety.

Introduction

Traumatic brain injury (TBI) is a major public health problem. In the United States, more than 1.5 million individuals sustain TBI every year [1]. It is estimated that almost 320,000 deployed American personnel may have suffered varying degrees of TBI [2]. Mild TBI (mTBI) is the most frequent type of TBI among both veteran and civilian populations. In the civilian sector, the majority of cases with mTBI are associated with early symptoms that typically resolve within a few days to a few months post injury [3-6]. However, a minority of individuals continue to complain of ongoing post concussive somatic, cognitive, and/or behavioral symptoms that may lead to long-term functional limitation [7-10].

Posttraumatic stress disorder (PTSD) is an anxiety disorder characterized by reexperiencing, avoidance, and hyper arousal symptoms following exposure to a traumatic event. Historically, it was argued that trauma survivors with mTBI have no painful traumatic memories and, therefore cannot develop core PTSD symptoms characterized by intrusive re-experiencing of the event. However, evidence has accrued showing that PTSD symptoms can develop after mTBI [11-16]. Recent studies demonstrate that mTBI are strongly associated with PTSD among soldiers returning from Iraq [17]. On examination of multiple potential predictors of PTSD including non-TBI-related injuries, only combat intensity and mTBI with loss of consciousness (LOC) were significantly associated with PTSD once other variables were controlled. These findings suggest that mTBI might increase the likelihood of developing PTSD in service members. There has been extensive debate in the literature regarding whether mTBI has a strong effect on the development of PTSD in civilian populations [18-28]. So far, the published data investigating the incidence of PTSD after mTBI in civilian populations are difficult to interpret due to variations in the methodology and conflicting results. As indicated in a recent study by the World Health Organization Collaborating Centre Task Force on mTBI, different criteria used to define mTBI and lack of control groups or comparison of inappropriate control groups have been often found in the existing literature [29].

The current study employed meta-analysis to integrate the available literature on the incidence of PTSD associated with mTBI and bring

***Corresponding author:** Yan Dong, Department of Neurosurgery, Shanghai Institute of Neurosurgery, Military Institute of Neurosurgery, Changzheng Hospital, Second Military Medical University, 415 Fengyang Road, Shanghai 200003, China, E-mail: smmudongyan@163.com or li_hou@hotmail.com

a more clear evidence for the question whether PTSD can confer the risk of PTSD development after mTBI in civilian populations with a rigorous methodological quality assessment.

Materials and Methods

Selection of studies

A comprehensive search of Pubmed and PSYCHInfo databases was undertaken in order to identify published studies on PTSD associated with mTBI. Key search terms included "mild traumatic brain injury", "minor traumatic brain injury", "mild brain injury", "minor brain injury", "mild head injury", "minor head injury", "mild closed head injury", "minor closed head injury", "mild head trauma" and "minor head trauma". These search terms were paired with "posttraumatic stress", "posttraumatic stress disorder" and "anxiety disorder". The search was limited to English language published in peer-reviewed journals from January 1980 to December 2013 that involved human subjects and presented primary data. Reference lists from the relevant studies were searched for additional references.

Inclusion criteria

Original studies were considered for inclusion in the meta-analysis if they met with the following criteria: (1) adult civilians were studied; (2) mTBI was defined according to the American Congress of Rehabilitation Medicine (ACRM) [30]; (3) PTSD was operationalized as the presence of symptoms consistent with those defined by the *Diagnostic and Statistical Manual of Mental Disorders (DSM-III, SDM-III-R, DSM IV, or DSM-IV-TR)* [31-33], which were assessed through clinical diagnoses or interviews or "probable PTSD" based on indicated cutoff scores using self-report inventories or screening measures in not less than 3 months after injury. (4) Results were sufficient to allow calculation of effect sizes. (5) Results were not reported elsewhere.

Data collection

Titles and abstracts from all references identified in the literature search process were reviewed by two independent study investigators. For each study included in the meta-analysis, the author, date of publication, country and assessment tools for PTSD were summarized in Table 1. Several sample characteristics were also noted, including sample size, mean age, mean education, sex, CT examination, and severity of injury as measured by Injury Severity Score (ISS) for patients and control samples when available. Results were reviewed with another member of the research team. Studies included in the meta-analysis were assessed for risk of bias using Newcastle-Ottawa score (NOS) [34]. The score assigns a study a maximum of 9 points, with higher scores indicating a lower risk of bias.

Statistical analysis

The effect of mTBI on the development of PTSD was assessed with odds ratio (or) with 95% confidence intervals (CIs). A subgroup analysis was carried out based on education, mean age, NOS, follow-up, ISS and country. Egger's test was applied to check the potential publication bias. The statistical estimates of effect were derived using a random-effects model with Mantel-Haenszel statistics. Heterogeneity of mTBI effect on the development of PTSD between studies was investigated visually by scatter plot analysis and statistically by the heterogeneity I^2 statistic. I^2 statistic of 0%-40% indicates unimportant heterogeneity, 30%-60% indicates moderate heterogeneity, 50-90% indicates substantial heterogeneity, and 75%-100% indicates considerable heterogeneity. P values were calculated by χ^2 tests. All the reported P values are two-sided and value of P less than 0.05 was regarded as statistically significant for all included studies. All analyses were calculated using STATA (version 10.0).

Results

We identified 853 potentially relevant studies from our combined database, of which 734 were excluded after a preliminary review. The remaining 75 studies were retrieved for detailed assessment. Ultimately, 7 prospective cohort studies met the inclusion criteria (Figure 1). For the study from Bryant et al. [26], outcomes at 3-months and 12-months follow up were both included for analyses. A total of 1222 mTBI patients and 1468 general trauma participants were included. There was no evidence of publication bias for the development of PTSD after mild traumatic brain injury (P value for Egger's test, 0.38). Five high quality studies were judged by a NOS score of 7 or above. The baseline characteristics of the participants and the design of the studies were summarized in the Table 1.

The pooled data consisted of 2690 individuals with 304 PTSD patients. 14 % of mTBI patients reported PTSD, and 9% of general trauma patients developed PTSD. As shown in Figure 2, OR of the pooled studies indicates a 61% increase in the prevalence of PTSD in mTBI patients when compared with general trauma participants, suggesting that mTBI might increase the risk of development of PTSD in civilian settings (OR 1.61, 95% CI 1.25-2.06, p=0.0002, I^2=0%) (Figure 2). In order to evaluate the effect of time after injury on development of PTSD in mTBI populations, the pooled data were classified into 3 subgroups (3-months, 6-months and 12-months follow up groups). There was no significant difference among subgroups (p=0.28) (Figure 2). A sensitivity analysis shows the results are affected by sequential exclusion of study reported by Bryant et al. [26] When Bryant's research was removed, OR of the other six studies demonstrates that

Source	mTBI group		control group		follow up (month)	sex (male)	mean age (year)	ISS	education (year)	CT examination	Newcastle-Ottawa score	country	diagnosis of TBI	screening tools for PTSD
	PTSD	total	PTSD	total										
Levin HS [21] (2001)	8	60	6	52	3	71%	36	5.13	10.84	-/+	6	USA	ACRM	SCID
Jones C [23] (2005)	10	58	11	61	3	40%	37	3.22	N/A	N/A	4	UK	ACRM	PSS
Bryant RA [24] (2010)	48	377	43	555	3	73%	38	10.42	N/A	N/A	7	Australia	ACRM	CAPS
Ponford J [26] (2011)	7	90	3	80	3	70%	35	ND	13.87	-	7	Australia	ACRM	PCL-C
Bryant RA[19] (1999)	15	63	18	71	6	68%	32	6.82	N/A	N/A	7	Australia	ACRM	CIDI
Friedland JF [20] (2001)	17	64	7	35	7	64%	33	20.06	N/A	N/A	7	Canada	ACRM	IES+GHQ
Creamer M [22] (2005)	24	189	8	118	12	76%	37	13.67	N/A	N/A	7	Australia	ACRM	CAPS
Bryant RA [24] (2010)	43	321	36	496	12	73%	38	10.42	N/A	N/A	7	Australia	ACRM	CAPS

N/A, not available; ACRM, American Congress of Rehabilitation Medicine; CIDI, Composite International Diagnostic Interview; PCL-C, PTSD Checklist-civilian version; CAPS, Clinician-Administered PTSD Scale; SCID, structured clinical interview for DSM-IV; PSS, PTSD symptom scale; -/+, negative/positive; IES, Impact of Event Scale; GHQ, General Health Questionaire; CT, computed tomography.

Table 1: Design and patient characteristics for studies included in the meta analysis.

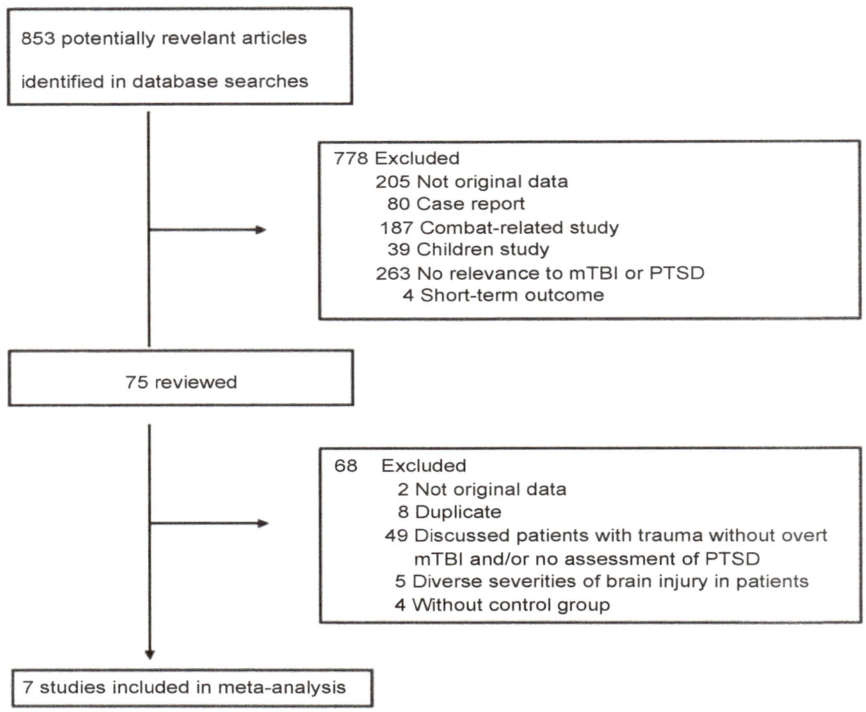

Figure 1: Flow diagram of the literature search and studies selection process.

Study or Subgroup	mTBI Events	mTBI Total	Control Events	Control Total	Weight	Odds Ratio M-H, Random, 95% CI
4.1.1 3 months follow up						
Bryant RA 2010	48	337	43	555	32.4%	1.74 [1.13, 2.68]
Jones C 2005	10	58	11	61	6.9%	0.95 [0.37, 2.43]
Levin HS 2001	8	60	6	52	4.8%	1.18 [0.38, 3.65]
Ponford J 2011	7	90	3	80	3.2%	2.16 [0.54, 8.67]
Subtotal (95% CI)		585		748	47.3%	1.55 [1.08, 2.22]
Total events	73		63			
Heterogeneity: Tau² = 0.00: Chi² = 1.76, df = 3 (P = 0.62); I² = 0%						
Test for overall effect: Z = 2.40 (P = 0.02)						
4.1.2 6 months follow up						
Bryant RA 1999	15	63	18	71	9.8%	0.92 [0.42, 2.02]
Friedland JF 2001	17	64	7	35	6.2%	1.45 [0.53, 3.92]
Subtotal (95% CI)		127		106	16.0%	1.10 [0.59, 2.03]
Total events	32		25			
Heterogeneity: Tau² = 0.00: Chi² = 0.49, df = 1 (P = 0.49); I² = 0%						
Test for overall effect: Z = 0.29 (P = 0.77)						
4.1.3 12 months follow up						
Bryant RA* 2010	43	321	36	496	28.0%	1.98 [1.24, 3.15]
Creamer M 2005	24	189	8	118	8.8%	2.00 [0.87, 4.61]
Subtotal (95% CI)		510		614	36.8%	1.98 [1.32, 2.98]
Total events	67		44			
Heterogeneity: Tau² = 0.00: Chi² = 0.00, df = 1 (P = 0.98); I² = 0%						
Test for overall effect: Z = 3.29 (P = 0.001)						
Total (95% CI)		1222		1468	100.0%	1.61 [1.25, 2.06]
Total events	172		132			
Heterogeneity: Tau² = 0.00: Chi² = 4.77, df = 7 (P = 0.69); I² = 0%						
Test for overall effect: Z = 3.76 (P = 0.0002)						
Test for subgroup differences: Chi² = 2.53. df = 2 (P = 0.28). I² = 20.9%						

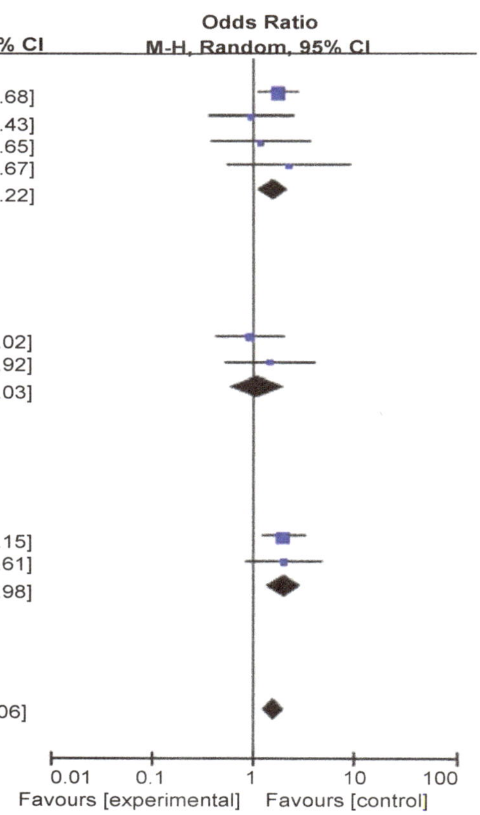

Figure 2: Effect of mTBI on the risk of development of PTSD in civilian populations. * Outcomes at 3-months and 12-months follow up were both included for analyses.

the prevalence of PTSD in mTBI and general trauma groups doesn't significantly differ (OR 1.30, 95% CI 0.88-1.93, p=0.19, I^2=0%). The study from Bryant et al. [26] contributed 57% of patients to overall data, which was derived from four levels I trauma centers across three states in Australia.

Subgroup analyses were carried out based on education, mean age, NOS, follow-up, ISS and country (Table 2). Outcomes at 12-months follow up were included for subgroup analyses in the study from Bryant et al. [26], with the exception of education, mTBI attributed to an increase in the prevalence of PTSD in the other five subgroup analyses, where Bryant's study contributed an overwhelming portion to overall data due to its huge sample size. It is possible that statistical significant difference might come out of contribution of specific study rather than subset factors.

Discussion

Our study is aimed at identifying whether mTBI contributes to a increased risk of PTSD in civilian populations as it happens in the service members. In this review, we surveyed 804 publications related to mTBI and PTSD and 7 studies were finally included in our meta-analysis. The overall incidence of PTSD is 14% in the mTBI patients in a civilian sample. The military or veteran studies reported probable PTSD in 33% to 39% of respondents who endorsed having experienced a probable mTBI [17,35,36]. Since a substantial number of mTBI survivors in the military is the result of non-combat-related injuries (i.e., sports injuries, assaults, motor vehicle accidents), comparison between civilian studies and military studies helps assess how often PTSD is due to the stress of combat/military life. The meta-analysis demonstrates that patients suffering mTBI are at higher risk of PTSD development compared to general trauma patients in the civilian populations. Some literature on PTSD following TBI has shown that PTSD symptoms decrease significantly over time within a year post injury [37-38]. However, quite a quantity of studies disputes the opinion because of the fact that the rates of PTSD don't drop over a year after TBI [26,39,40] Our stratified analyses showed that the prevalence of PTSD at 3-months, 6-months and 12-months follow up didn't differ, supporting the idea that the occurrence of PTSD may be maintained or even increase over time after injury.

Hesdorffer *et al.* [20] reported their systematic review on the long-term psychiatric outcomes following traumatic brain injury in 2009. They concluded, on the basis of their evaluation, that there is inadequate/insufficient evidence to determine whether an association exists between mTBI and PTSD in civilian populations [20]. Of note, they drew their conclusion mainly depending on the study reported by Creame, which was derived from one trauma center in Australia including 189 mTBI patients and 118 general trauma patients. In the present review, we included 2690 individuals in 7 studies with a broad range of baseline characteristics. We argue that the insufficient data might lead to the uncertainty about the relationship between PTSD and mTBI in Hesdorffer *et al.* [20] research.

There are several important limitations in the review. The major limitation is the quality of studies involved. Of the 7 studies, 71% (n=5) were from centers in Australia. Although all the studies are prospective investigation, only the study reported by Bryant, *et al.* [26] is a multisite design with a big sample size of more than 300 mTBI participants. The numbers of mTBI patients vary across the other six studies from 58 to 189. The meta-analysis demonstrates that patients suffering mTBI are at higher risk of PTSD development compared to general trauma patients in the civilian populations, which is in accordance with findings from Bryant *et al.* [26]. However, when the data were removed, a meta-analysis of the other six small studies does not predict the effect of mTBI on the development of PTSD. In some cases, a meta-analysis of several small studies may fail to predict the results of a single large study although it is now widely used to provide evidence to support clinical strategies [41]. The heterogeneity of sample sizes may partially account for the divergence in our study. When divergences are seen between meta-analysis and a large study, few will disagree that the value of the large and well designed studies is of more guidance to clinical practice than meta-analyses. Thus, more large researches of high quality will help us come to a consistent conclusion in the future.

Another limitation is the inconsistent assessment tools of PTSD applied in the studies, consisting of clinical interview and self-reported

Group	PTSD event/total patients		Odds Ratios (OR) and 95%CI	P value	heterogeneity	P value for heterogeneity
	mTBI	GT				
Education (years)						
≥ 12	7/90	3/80	2.16 [0.54, 8.67]	0.28	-	-
<12	8/60	6/52	1.18 [0.38, 3.65]	0.77	-	-
Mean age						
≥ 35	92/718	64/807	1.72 [1.22, 2.43]	0.002	0	0.64
<35	32/127	25/106	1.10 [0.59, 2.03]	0.77	0	0.49
NOS						
≥ 7	106/727	72/800	1.68 [1.21, 2.34]	0.002	0	0.54
<7	18/118	17/113	1.04 [0.50, 2.14]	0.92	0	0.77
Follow-up						
≥ 6	99/637	69/720	1.66 [1.18, 2.33]	0.004	0	0.40
<6	28/208	20/193	1.21 [0.64, 2.31]	0.55	0	0.63
ISS						
>10	60/385	43/531	1.87 [1.22, 2.85]	0.004	0	0.58
<10	33/181	35/184	0.98 [0.58, 1.67]	0.95	0	0.94
Country						
Australia	89/663	65/765	1.71 [1.21, 2.43]	0.003	0	0.39
Other	35/182	24/148	1.16 [0.65, 2.09]	0.61	0	0.83
Overall	124/845	89/913	1.55 [1.15, 2.09]	0.004	0	0.60

Table 2: Subgroup analyses based on education, mean age, NOS, follow-up, ISS and country.

questionnaires. Clinician-Administered PTSD Scale-IV (CAPS), a structured clinical interview with good sensitivity and specificity relative to the Structured Clinical Interview for DSM-IV (SCID), as well as sound test-retest reliability, was utilized to assess PTSD in the studies of Bryant and Creamer Compared to CAPS, self-reported questionnaires could interfere with the ascertainment of PTSD in the studies. Three of the studies used self-reported questionnaires to diagnose probable PTSD. The inclusion of such articles could elevate the estimated incidence of PTSD in the participants.

An additional limitation of the review is the classification of mTBI. All the studies categorized TBI patients according to Glasgow Coma Scale (GCS), widely used to assess the level of consciousness after TBI. GCS score ranges from 3 (most severely impaired) to 15 (no neurologic impairment). GCS 13-15 is often employed as one of criteria to define mTBI. However, GCS score doesn't accord with severity of brain damage all the time. Mild traumatic brain injury can be classified into two categories-complicated and uncomplicated mTBI, in which complicated mTBI means presence of an intracranial abnormality on neuroimaging. Almost all the studies included in our meta-analysis didn't discriminate complicated mTBI from uncomplicated mTBI. Data by Smits *et al.* [42] indicated that complicated mTBI was significantly associated with worse outcome [42]. Grouping all mTBI participants into a single category may oversimplify the complex characteristics of brain injury and obscure important differences related to mTBI severity [43]. In future study, it is necessary to clarify whether injury in the specific sites of brain tissue might confer the risk of development of PTSD following mTBI.

mTBI patients develop post concussion symptoms (PCS), a constellation of physical, cognitive and emotional symptoms. The presence of persistent PCS complicates the diagnosis of PTSD after mTBI because many of the complaints are similar, including irritability, depressive symptoms, sleep disturbance and cognitive difficulties. The issue that PCS are a result of organic or psychological factors, or an interaction between the two has been long debated. The facts that PCS is frequently encountered among healthy adults [44-45] and clinical groups without a history of mTBI [46] indicate that PCS might be nonspecific to mTBI. Recent studies show that PCS complaints after mTBI are more likely to be ascribed to psychological factors, such as anxiety, depression or PTSD rather than mTBI [47-50]. Apart from PTSD, mTBI could be associated with other psychiatric disorders, such as depression, generalized anxiety disorder, obsessive-compulsive disorder and substance abuse. It is a well-studied fact that PTSD patients have high rates of psychiatric comorbidity. Apparently, public health concerns are needed to address the huge health burden caused by the psychiatric effects of mTBI. New approaches that ease early identification of psychiatric disorders and prompt early interventions to prevent psychiatric condition might facilitate optimal recovery from mTBI.

Conclusion

This meta-analysis represents synthesis of the available data on the development of PTSD after mTBI in civilian populations. The overall incidence of PTSD is 14% in mTBI patients and 9% in general trauma patients among the civilian populations. Our data indicate that mTBI patients are more prone to develop PTSD than general trauma patients without mTBI in civilian settings.

References

1. Beauchamp K, Mutlak H, Smith WR, Shohami E, Stahel PF (2008) Pharmacology of traumatic brain injury: where is the "golden bullet"? Mol Med 14: 731-740.
2. Ling G, Bandak F, Armonda R, Grant G, Ecklund J (2009) Explosive blast neurotrauma. J Neurotrauma 26: 815-825.
3. Dikmen S, Machamer J, Temkin N (2001) Mild head injury: facts and artifacts. J Clin Exp Neuropsychol 23: 729-738.
4. Ryan LM, Warden DL (2003) Post concussion syndrome. Int Rev Psychiatry 15: 310-316.
5. Powell TJ, Collin C, Sutton K (1996) A follow-up study of patients hospitalized after minor head injury. Disabil Rehabil 18: 231-237.
6. Carroll LJ, Cassidy JD, Peloso PM, Borg J, von Holst H, et al. (2004) Prognosis for mild traumatic brain injury: results of the WHO Collaborating Centre Task Force on Mild Traumatic Brain Injury. J Rehabil Med 43: 84-105.
7. Hartlage LC, Durant-Wilson D, Patch PC (2001) Persistent neurobehavioral problems following mild traumatic brain injury. Arch Clin Neuropsychol 16: 561-570.
8. Vanderploeg RD, Curtiss G, Luis CA, Salazar AM (2007) Long-term morbidities following self-reported mild traumatic brain injury. J Clin Exp Neuropsychol 29: 585-598.
9. Deb S, Lyons I, Koutzoukis C (1999) Neurobehavioural symptoms one year after a head injury. Br J Psychiatry 174: 360-365.
10. van der Naalt J, van Zomeren AH, Sluiter WJ, Minderhoud JM (1999) One year outcome in mild to moderate head injury: the predictive value of acute injury characteristics related to complaints and return to work. J Neurol Neurosurg Psychiatry 66: 207-213.
11. Harvey AG, Bryant RA (1999) The relationship between acute stress disorder and posttraumatic stress disorder: a 2-year prospective evaluation. J Consult Clin Psychol 67: 985-988.
12. Hickling EJ, Gillen R, Blanchard EB, Buckley T, Taylor A (1998) Traumatic brain injury and posttraumatic stress disorder: a preliminary investigation of neuropsychological test results in PTSD secondary to motor vehicle accidents. Brain Inj 12: 265-274.
13. Mayou RA, Black J, Bryant B (2000) Unconsciousness, amnesia and psychiatric symptoms following road traffic accident injury. Br J Psychiatry 177: 540-545.
14. Gil S, Caspi Y, Ben-Ari IZ, Koren D, Klein E (2005) Does memory of a traumatic event increase the risk for posttraumatic stress disorder in patients with traumatic brain injury? A prospective study. Am J Psychiatry 162: 963-969.
15. Bombardier CH, Fann JR, Temkin N, Esselman PC, Pelzer E, et al. (2006) Posttraumatic stress disorder symptoms during the first six months after traumatic brain injury. J Neuropsychiatry Clin Neurosci 18: 501-508.
16. Yurgil KA, Barkauskas DA2, Vasterling JJ3, Nievergelt CM4, Larson GE5, et al. (2014) Association between traumatic brain injury and risk of posttraumatic stress disorder in active-duty Marines. JAMA Psychiatry 71: 149-157.
17. Hoge CW, McGurk D, Thomas JL, Cox AL, Engel CC, et al. (2008) Mild traumatic brain injury in U.S. Soldiers returning from Iraq. N Engl J Med 358: 453-463.
18. Bryant RA, O'Donnell ML, Creamer M, McFarlane AC, Silove D (2013) A multisite analysis of the fluctuating course of posttraumatic stress disorder. JAMA Psychiatry 70: 839-846.
19. Sbordone RJ, Liter JC (1995) Mild traumatic brain injury does not produce post-traumatic stress disorder. Brain Inj 9: 405-412.
20. Hesdorffer DC, Rauch SL, Tamminga CA (2009) Long-term psychiatric outcomes following traumatic brain injury: a review of the literature. J Head Trauma Rehabil 24: 452-459.
21. Bryant RA, Harvey AG (1999) The influence of traumatic brain injury on acute stress disorder and post-traumatic stress disorder following motor vehicle accidents. Brain Inj 13: 15-22.
22. Friedland JF, Dawson DR (2001) Function after motor vehicle accidents: a prospective study of mild head injury and posttraumatic stress. J Nerv Ment Dis 189: 426-434.
23. Levin HS, Brown SA, Song JX, McCauley SR, Boake C, et al. (2001) Depression and posttraumatic stress disorder at three months after mild to moderate traumatic brain injury. J Clin Exp Neuropsychol 23: 754-769.
24. Creamer M, O'Donnell ML, Pattison P (2005) Amnesia, traumatic brain injury, and posttraumatic stress disorder: a methodological inquiry. Behav Res Ther 43: 1383-1389.

25. Jones C, Harvey AG, Brewin CR (2005) Traumatic brain injury, dissociation, and posttraumatic stress disorder in road traffic accident survivors. J Trauma Stress 18: 181-191.

26. Bryant RA, O'Donnell ML, Creamer M, McFarlane AC, Clark CR, et al. (2010) The psychiatric sequelae of traumatic injury. Am J Psychiatry 167: 312-320.

27. Zatzick DF, Rivara FP, Jurkovich GJ, Hoge CW, Wang J, et al. (2010) Multisite investigation of traumatic brain injuries, posttraumatic stress disorder, and self-reported health and cognitive impairments. Arch Gen Psychiatry 67: 1291-1300.

28. Ponsford J, Cameron P, Fitzgerald M, Grant M, Mikocka-Walus A (2011) Long-term outcomes after uncomplicated mild traumatic brain injury: a comparison with trauma controls. J Neurotrauma 28: 937-946.

29. Carroll LJ, Cassidy JD, Holm L, Kraus J, Coronado VG, et al. (2004) Methodological issues and research recommendations for mild traumatic brain injury: J Rehabil Med 43: 113-125.

30. The Mild Traumatic Brain Injury Committee of the Head Injury Interdisciplinary Special Interest Group of the American Congress of Rehabilitation Medicine (1993) Definition of mild traumatic brain injury. J Head Trauma Rehabil 8: 86-87.

31. Arntz A (1999) Do personality disorders exist? On the validity of the concept and its cognitive-behavioral formulation and treatment. Behav Res Ther 37 Suppl 1: S97-134.

32. Diagnostic and Statistical Manual of Mental Disorders. 3rd ed. Washington, DC, American Psychiatric Association.

33. Diagnostic and Statistical Manual of Mental Disorders. 4th ed. Washington, DC,American Psychiatric Association.

34. Wells GA, Shea B, O'Connell D, Peterson J, Welch V, et al. The Newcastle-Ottawa Scale (NOS) for assessing the quality of nonrandomised studies in meta-analyses.

35. Schneiderman AI, Braver ER, Kang HK (2008) Understanding sequelae of injury mechanisms and mild traumatic brain injury incurred during the conflicts in Iraq and Afghanistan: persistent postconcussive symptoms and posttraumatic stress disorder. Am J Epidemiol 167: 1446-1452.

36. Center for Military Health Policy Research (2008) Invisible Wounds of War: Psychological and Cognitive Injuries, Their Consequences, and Services to Assist Recovery. Rand Corporation.

37. Blanchard EB1, Hickling EJ, Barton KA, Taylor AE, Loos WR, et al. (1996) One-year prospective follow-up of motor vehicle accident victims. Behav Res Ther 34: 775-786.

38. Shalev AY1, Freedman S, Peri T, Brandes D, Sahar T, et al. (1998) Prospective study of posttraumatic stress disorder and depression following trauma. Am J Psychiatry 155: 630-637.

39. Mayou R1, Bryant B, Duthie R (1993) Psychiatric consequences of road traffic accidents. BMJ 307: 647-651.

40. O'Donnell ML1, Creamer M, Pattison P, Atkin C (2004) Psychiatric morbidity following injury. Am J Psychiatry 161: 507-514.

41. LeLorier J1, Grégoire G, Benhaddad A, Lapierre J, Derderian F (1997) Discrepancies between meta-analyses and subsequent large randomized, controlled trials. N Engl J Med 337: 536-542.

42. Smits M1, Hunink MG, van Rijssel DA, Dekker HM, Vos PE, et al. (2008) Outcome after complicated minor head injury. AJNR Am J Neuroradiol 29: 506-513.

43. Pertab JL1, James KM, Bigler ED (2009) Limitations of mild traumatic brain injury meta-analyses. Brain Inj 23: 498-508.

44. Paniak C1, Reynolds S, Phillips K, Toller-Lobe G, Melnyk A, et al. (2002) Patient complaints within 1 month of mild traumatic brain injury: a controlled study. Arch Clin Neuropsychol 17: 319-334.

45. Iverson GL1, Lange RT (2003) Examination of "postconcussion-like" symptoms in a healthy sample. Appl Neuropsychol 10: 137-144.

46. Meares S1, Shores EA, Taylor AJ, Batchelor J, Bryant RA, et al. (2011) The prospective course of postconcussion syndrome: the role of mild traumatic brain injury. Neuropsychology 25: 454-465.

47. Lippa SM1, Pastorek NJ, Benge JF, Thornton GM (2010) Postconcussive symptoms after blast and nonblast-related mild traumatic brain injuries in Afghanistan and Iraq war veterans. J Int Neuropsychol Soc 16: 856-866.

48. Meares S1, Shores EA, Taylor AJ, Batchelor J, Bryant RA, et al. (2011) The prospective course of postconcussion syndrome: the role of mild traumatic brain injury. Neuropsychology 25: 454-465.

49. Ponsford J1, Cameron P, Fitzgerald M, Grant M, Mikocka-Walus A, et al. (2012) Predictors of postconcussive symptoms 3 months after mild traumatic brain injury. Neuropsychology 26: 304-313.

50. Wilk JE1, Thomas JL, McGurk DM, Riviere LA, Castro CA, et al. (2010) Mild traumatic brain injury (concussion) during combat: lack of association of blast mechanism with persistent postconcussive symptoms. J Head Trauma Rehabil 25: 9-14.

CPAP for Obstructive Sleep Apnea in the Post-Operative Setting: An Oximetry Evaluation Study

Inderjeet S Brar[1], Ramakant Sharma[2], Gaurav Khanna[3] and Dennis Auckley[4*]

[1]*Affinity Medical Center, Massillon, OH, USA*
[2]*Louis Stokes Cleveland VA Medical Center, Cleveland, OH, USA*
[3]*University of Cincinnati, Cincinnati, OH, USA*
[4]*MetroHealth Medical Center, Case Western Reserve University, Cleveland, OH, USA*

Abstract

Objective: To study the prevalence and associations of nocturnal hypoxia following surgery in PAP-treated (CPAP or bilevel pressure support) OSA patients.

Patients and Methods: PAP-treated OSA patients presenting for elective surgery (n=38) between August 2007 and October 2008 underwent overnight oximetry monitoring on their prescribed PAP therapy on postoperative night one. The lowest oxygen (O_2) saturation (SpO_2), time spent with SpO_2 <89% and the presence of sleep disordered breathing (saw-tooth oscillations) were determined from the oximetry tracings. Need for supplemental O_2, nursing/ respiratory interventions, and complications were recorded. Records were reviewed for the type and duration of surgery and anesthesia, net fluid balance, narcotic / sedative use, demographics and co-morbidities.

Results: Seven of 38 subjects (18.4%) spent at least 30 minutes with SpO_2 <90% during the night (hypoxic group=HG) on their prescribed PAP therapy. The severity of baseline OSA (total and supine apnea-hypopnea index), pre-CPAP SpO_2 (asleep on diagnostic PSG and awake evening after surgery), net fluid balance, and total IV narcotic dose were associated with the HG. Nursing interventions and addition of O_2 were more common in the HG, though other adverse events were not. Review of the oximetry tracings suggested 71% of the HG, and 42% of the non-hypoxic group, had findings of uncontrolled sleep apnea.

Conclusions: Despite the use of prescribed PAP therapy the night following surgery, some OSA patients become hypoxic. Postoperative oximetry monitoring may be indicated in PAP-treated OSA patients undergoing surgery.

Keywords: Obstructive sleep apnea; CPAP; Perioperative care; Postoperative complications

Abbreviations: AHI: Apnea Hypopnea Index; BPAP: Bilevel Positive Airway Pressure; CPAP: Continuous Positive Airway Pressure; ODI: Oxygen Desaturation Index; OSA: Obstructive Sleep Apnea; O_2: Oxygen; PAP: Positive Airway Pressure; CPAP: Continuous Positive Airway Pressure; BPAP: Bilevel Positive Airway Pressure; PSG: Polysomnogram; REM: Rapid Eye Movement; SpO_2: Oxygen Saturation Ibrar

Introduction

The estimated prevalence of Obstructive Sleep Apnea (OSA) is 5% in adults in western countries [1]. The prevalence of OSA in the surgical population is likely similar to that of the general population [2-4]. The majority of these patients are not diagnosed at the time of their presentation [2,3].

Patients with OSA are at increased risk for postoperative adverse events. Both surgery and general anesthesia alter pulmonary function, resulting in hypoxemia that could deteriorate during sleep [5,6]. Residual effects of general anesthesia and neuromuscular relaxants, as well as effects of narcotics and sedatives, may relax the pharyngeal muscles and depress the arousal response, leading to more frequent and prolonged apneas with ensuing hypoxia and hypercapnia [7-9]. Supine positioning, often required following surgery, and REM sleep rebound after the first postoperative night can both worsen sleep apnea [10,11]. All of these factors can translate into worsened postoperative outcomes, often catastrophic, for OSA patients undergoing surgery [12].

Retrospective case control studies have suggested higher rates of myocardial ischemia, arrhythmias, need for respiratory interventions, postoperative atrial fibrillation, encephalopathy / delirium, infections and a longer ICU length of stay in patients with OSA [13-15]. A recent retrospective review of over 6 million orthopedic and general surgeries from the National Inpatient Sample found OSA to be an independent risk factor for perioperative pulmonary complications [16].

The first line treatment of OSA remains CPAP therapy [17]. Limited data suggests that CPAP may be protective in the perioperative setting for patients with OSA. A case series of 14 OSA patients undergoing a variety of surgeries reported no postoperative complications following institution of a policy to use CPAP postoperatively [18]. In a retrospective orthopedic case control study, preoperative CPAP use was suggested to reduce postoperative complications, though the data set was too small for analysis [13]. However, there are concerns that a pressure setting established in a stable outpatient state may not be effective in perioperative environment.

***Corresponding author:** Dennis Auckley, 2500 MetroHealth, MetroHealth Medical Center, Cleveland, OH 44109, USA, E-mail: dauckley@metrohealth.org

We hypothesized that in OSA patients undergoing elective surgery, PAP (CPAP or bilevel pressure support=BPAP) set at prescribed home settings would not effectively eliminate hypoxia on the first night following surgery.

Methods

Subjects and design

This was an observational cohort study conducted at MetroHealth Medical Center (MHMC, Case Western Reserve University), an urban academic tertiary care hospital. Consecutive OSA patients undergoing elective surgery were recruited from the pre-surgical clinic between August 2007 and October 2008. All patients provided informed consent and the study was approved by the MHMC's Institution Review Board (IRB #07-00732).

Subjects enrolled were required to have polysomnogram (PSG) diagnosed OSA, (an apnea-hypopnea index (AHI) of $\geq$ 5 events per hour with OSA symptoms), and have been successfully manually titrated on CPAP or BPAP. A successful titration consisted of an AHI <10 (or a 50% or greater reduction in the AHI if the baseline AHI was <15) and oxygen saturation (SpO_2) $\geq$ 89% on the best pressure setting. Subjective compliance with CPAP or BPAP prior to surgery was required. Subjects were excluded if they were unable to use their PAP postoperatively (i.e. remained intubated), if they were on supplemental oxygen preoperatively (daytime or nocturnal), if they required >40% FiO_2 following surgery, if they were pregnant or if they were unwilling/unable to consent to the study.

Subjects (n=38) enrolled in the study brought their own PAP units (certified by the hospital engineering department) and interface to the hospital. Following surgery, patients were recovered in the Post Anesthesia Care Unit (PACU) and then transferred to a general surgical floor under the care of the primary surgical service. Subjects were placed on their PAP when ready for sleep and a pulse-oximeter with recording capability (Nellcor N-595®) was placed on the patient's index finger. Respiratory therapy and nursing personnel verified successful PAP placement and an adequate oximetry recording. Oximetry recordings were obtained between the hours of 2100 and 0615. A minimum of 5 hours of recording time was required (63% had more than 6 hours of recording).

Subjects were monitored throughout the night by nursing under the hospital's sleep apnea protocol (vitals at 2 hour intervals or more frequently as clinically indicated, monitoring oxygenation). Respiratory therapy and nursing personnel documented if (and what time) the subjects removed their PAP therapy and, if so, they helped to replace the PAP therapy. Unsuccessful attempts were documented (3 subjects spent part of the night off of PAP therapy). The use of supplemental oxygen was also documented (occurred in 5 subjects).

Data collection

Upon completion of the oximetry recording, data was downloaded from the oximeter. Automated analysis included the oxygen desaturation index (4% or >desaturation from baseline events per hour=ODI) and time spent with SpO_2 <89% (time off PAP therapy was excluded from analysis). The lowest SpO_2 and mean SpO_2 were also noted. Manual inspection of the oximetry tracings was performed and low SpO_2 readings resulting from artifacts were removed from the analysis.

Waveform tracings were downloaded for review and independently evaluated by 2 Sleep-Boarded Sleep Specialists in a blinded fashion (clinical oximetries were mixed in). Each tracing was categorized as either normal, consistent with cardiopulmonary disease (steady low hypoxic pattern), consistent with sleep apnea (saw-tooth pattern waveforms) or consistent with both cardiopulmonary disease and sleep apnea (elements of both). If disagreements arose, a 3rd Sleep-Boarded Sleep Specialist reviewed the tracing and a consensus was obtained.

Data was abstracted from the electronic medical record for patient demographics, comorbidities, past polysomnography details, anesthesia type, surgery type and duration, postoperative fluid balance, postoperative narcotic and benzodiazepine use, any postoperative complications, and length of stay. Postoperative complications recorded included respiratory complications (new addition of oxygen, intubation, new hypercapnia [pCO_2 >45 mm Hg], atelectasis [independent Radiologist report], pneumonia, pulmonary embolism), cardiovascular complications (hypotension, uncontrolled hypertension requiring urgent intervention, chest pain, myocardial infarction, new arrhythmia), transfer to a higher level of care, and general complications (delirium, fever, hypoglycemia, ileus, new anemia).

Statistical analysis

The cohort was divided into 2 groups based on the result of their oximetry recording. The groups included the Hypoxic Group (HG, n=7, 18.4% of the total cohort) and the NonHypoxic Group (NHG, n=31, 81.6% of the total cohort). To be part of the HG, subjects had to spend $\geq$ 30 minutes of the oximetry recording time, while on PAP therapy, with SpO_2 <89%. All subsequent data is presented with subjects categorized into one of these groups. For the purposes of analysis, the 2 subjects on BPAP (one in each group) had their PAP pressure recorded as the expiratory pressure setting.

Data is expressed as mean ± SD or, median with 25th and 75th percentiles or percentages. Comparisons of continuous data were made by Wilcoxon rank sum test or Welch two sample t-test for two group comparisons, Analysis of variance (ANOVA) or Kruskal-Wallis test for multiple group comparisons; and of the proportions by Fisher's exact test. Statistical analysis was done using statistical software R version 2.5.1 (2007-06-27) (Copyright (C) 2007 The R Foundation for Statistical Computing ISBN 3-900051-07-0). P values <0.05 were considered significant.

Results

Thirty eight subjects completed the study and 7 (18.4%) of these met the criteria for the Hypoxic Group (HG). Baseline data for the HG and the NonHypoxic Group (NHG) are presented in Table 1. In general, the cohort as a whole was predominantly female, middle-aged and obese with significant rates of co-morbid cardiopulmonary disease. There were no significant differences between the oximetry categorized groups in baseline demographics or co-morbidities.

Baseline PSG data for the 2 groups is displayed in Table 2. Compared to the NHG, the HG had more severe OSA (AHI 36 vs. 22, p=0.03) and supine OSA (AHI 37 vs. 22, p<0.01), as well as a lower average SpO_2 during sleep (93% vs. 95%, p<0.01). Despite this, the CPAP settings and control of OSA by CPAP were similar in the 2 groups. Baseline PAP titration studies were performed further out from the date of surgery in the HG compared to the NHG, though this was not statistically significant.

Data related to the specifics of anesthesia and surgery, as well as sedative and narcotic medication use on the first postoperative night are shown in Table 3. There were no significant differences between the 2 groups in the anesthesia delivery method, type of surgery, duration

	Hypoxic Group (N = 7)		NonHypoxic Group (N = 31)		
	Median or Percent	25th, 75th percentile	Median or Percent	25th, 75th percentile	P-value
Gender					
Males	14%		26%		1
Females	86%		74%		
Ethnicity					
African American	29%		61%		0.35
Caucasian	71%		36%		
Hispanic	0%		3%		
Age (years old)	50	46, 55	50	46, 59	0.87
BMI (kg/m^2)					
At PSG	39	36, 42	39	34, 44	0.90
At Surgery	43	37, 44	40	33, 45	0.58
Past Medical History					
Arrhythmias	0%		10%		1
CAD	0%		7%		1
CHF	0%		3%		1
Stroke	0%		3%		1
Diabetes Mellitus	57%		36%		0.40
Hypertension	71%		61%		1
Lung Disease	71%		39%		0.21

Abbreviations: PSG=Polysomnogram, BMI=Body Mass Index, CAD=Coronary Artery Disease, CHF=Congestion Heart Failure

Table 1: Baseline Demographic Data.

	Hypoxic Group (N = 7)		NonHypoxic Group (N = 31)		
	Median	25th, 75th percentile	Median	25th, 75th percentile	P-value
Diagnostic PSG					
AHI	36	33, 52	22	14, 29	0.03
Supine AHI	37	35, 57	22	13, 32	<0.01
REM AHI	43	33, 51	40	15, 67	0.97
Average SpO_2 (%)	93	92, 94	95	95, 97	<0.01
Lowest SpO_2 (%)	79	73, 86	84	79, 88	0.27
CPAP titration PSG*					
Prescribed CPAP ($cm\ H_20$)	10	9, 13	10	8, 12	0.94
AHI on best PAP setting	2	1, 3	1	0, 4	0.61
Average SpO_2 (%)	94	94, 97	97	96, 98	0.21
Lowest SpO2 (%)	91	90, 92	93	91, 95	0.07
Time from titration PSG to surgery (days)	627	398, 856	343	74, 812	0.24

*Two subjects were titrated on bilevel pressure support. Both were in the NonHypoxic Group. The expiratory pressure (EPAP) was used for statistical analysis for these 2 subjects.

Abbreviations: PSG=Polysomnogram, AHI=Apnea-Hypopnea Index, Spo_2=Oxygen Saturation, CPAP=Continuous Positive Airway Pressure

Table 2: Baseline PSG Data.

	Hypoxic Group (N = 7)		NonHypoxic Group (N = 31)		
	Median or Percent	25th, 75th percentile	Median or Percent	25th, 75th percentile	P-value
Preoperative SpO_2 (%)	97	96, 98	98	96, 99	0.14
Anesthesia					
Type of anesthesia					
General	86%		87%		
Conscious sedation	0%		10%		0.40
Spinal	14%		3%		
Benzodiazepine dose					
(Midazolam IV mg)	2	2, 3.5	2	2, 2	0.40
Anesthesia finish time					
Morning	43%		39%		
Afternoon	57%		55%		1
Evening	0%		6%		
Surgery					
Type of surgery					
Head & Neck	0%		7%		
Upper Abdomen	57%		29%		
Lower Abdomen	14%		29%		0.54
Limb	14%		29%		
Lumbar Spine	14%		3%		
Skin	0%		3%		
Length of Surgery					
< 2 hours	14%		42%		
2 – 6 hours	86%		55%		0.32
> 6 hours	0%		3%		

Net Fluid Balance (liters) (From OR till midnight on the general ward)	2.9	2.6, 3.85	2.2	1.55, 2.65	0.03
Morphine Equivalent Dose (MEQ) (From OR till oximetry completion) Total IV MEQ dose (mg) Total PO MEQ dose (mg)	63 0	52, 67 0,10	41 4.5	31 54 0,35	0.03 0.21
Benzodiazepine Use (General ward post-operative night 1) IV Benzodiazepine (%) PO Benzodiazepine (%)	14% 0%		0% 10%		0.18 1

Abbreviations: Spo_2=Oxygen Saturation, OR=Operating Room

Table 3: Anesthesia, Surgery and Postoperative Night 1 Data.

	Hypoxic Group (N = 7)		NonHypoxic Group (N = 31)		
	Median or Percent	**25th, 75th percentile**	**Median or Percent**	**25th, 75th percentile**	**P-value**
Pre-CPAP Average SpO_2 (%) (On ward, prior to CPAP)	95	94, 96	97	95, 99	0.02
Oximetry Results (On CPAP Ist post-operative night) Time below SpO_2 of 89% (minutes) Average SpO_2 (%) Lowest SpO_2 (%) *Oxygen Desaturation Index (ODI)	172 89 77 19	118, 240 88, 90 75, 80 7, 23	0 95 89 1	0, 1 93, 97 86, 91 1, 3	< 0.01 <0.01 <0.01 <0.01
Postoperative Complications Nursing intervention (adding O_2 bleed to CPAP or changing to high-flow O_2 mask)	43%		10%		0.03
O_2 added to CPAP (liters per min)	0		0	0, 0	0.01
Atelectasis **Non-cardiovascular complications ***Cardiovascular complications	29% 57% 0%	0, 2	0% 29% 16%		<0.01 0.20 0.56
Post-operative Day 1 Lowest SpO_2 recorded (%)	92	86, 93	94	86, 95	<0.05

*ODI – defined as number of desaturation events (4% or more drop in SpO_2) per hour.
**Non-cardiovascular complications: delirium, fever, hypoglycemia, ileus, new anemia.
***Cardiovascular complications: hypotension, uncontrolled hypertension requiring urgent intervention, chest pain, myocardial infarction, new arrhythmia.
Abbreviations: Spo_2=Oxygen Saturation, CPAP=Continuous Positive Airway Pressure

Table 4: Postoperative Night 1 Oximetry Data.

of surgery, or time of day of the surgery. Subjects in the HG had a more positive net fluid balance on the day of surgery (2.9 liters vs. 2.2 liters, p=0.03) and received more narcotics on the day of surgery / first postoperative night (morphine equivalent dose of 63 mg vs. 41 mg, p=0.04) compared to the NHG.

Table 4 displays the data from the first night following surgery for both groups. The baseline pre-PAP SpO_2 was lower in the HG group, though still in the normal range (95% vs. 97%, p=0.02). From the oximetry, the HG had a lower average SpO_2 (89% vs. 95%, p<0.01), lower average nadir SpO_2 (77% vs. 89%, p< 0.01) and higher ODI (19 vs. 1, p< 0.01). Figure 1 shows the lowest SpO_2 encountered for each subject on their diagnostic PSG, on their titration PSG on the chosen CPAP setting, and on the oximetry postoperative night 1 on that same CPAP setting. While the HG required more nursing intervention/use of supplemental oxygen than the NHG, the rates of other complications was similar with the exception of more atelectasis noted in the HG.

Results of the oximetry interpretations are shown in Figure 2. Those in the HG had more studies interpreted as being consistent with sleep disordered breathing, as well as cardiopulmonary disease, than the NHG. Of note, 42% of the NHG oximetries were interpreted as consistent with uncontrolled sleep apnea. An example of a patient's oximetry tracings on their diagnostic PSG, on their chosen CPAP setting, and then on postoperative night 1 on the same CPAP setting is displayed in Figure 3. The postoperative oximetry was interpreted as consistent with sleep apnea.

Discussion

Use of positive airway pressure therapy has been advocated as a protective therapy for use in patients with OSA during the postoperative time [18,19] and recent guidelines agree with this approach [20-24]. However, current data are limited to case series and PAP use in OSA patients postoperatively has not been systematically studied. The results of the present study call into question the efficacy of previously determined PAP pressure settings in the postoperative setting and suggest that postoperative nocturnal oximetry monitoring may be indicated even in PAP-treated OSA patients.

While the majority of the subjects in this study were not hypoxic on the night after surgery, the duration and severity of hypoxia in a subset of subjects was significant. In some cases, the degree of nocturnal hypoxia mirrored that of untreated OSA (Figure 1) and, in the postoperative setting, could place them at risk for cardiopulmonary

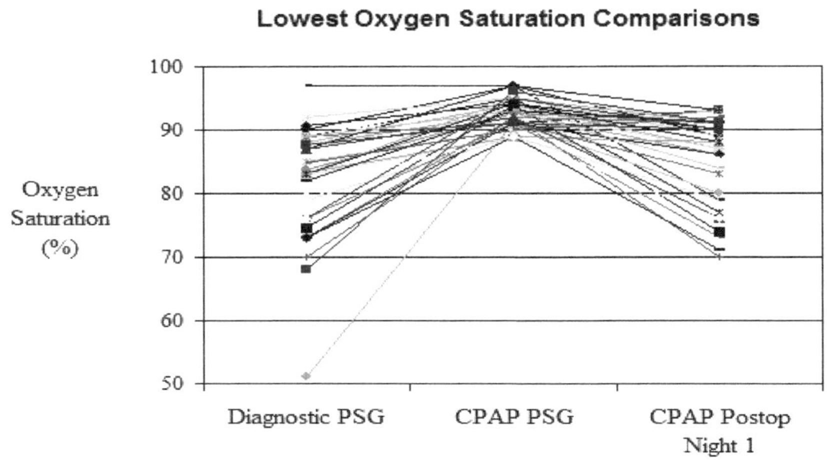

Abbreviations: PSG=polysomnogram, CPAP=continuous positive airway pressure, Postop=postoperative

Figure 1: Lowest Oxygen Saturation on Diagnostic PSG, CPAP PSG and Postoperative Night 1 Oximetry on CPAP.

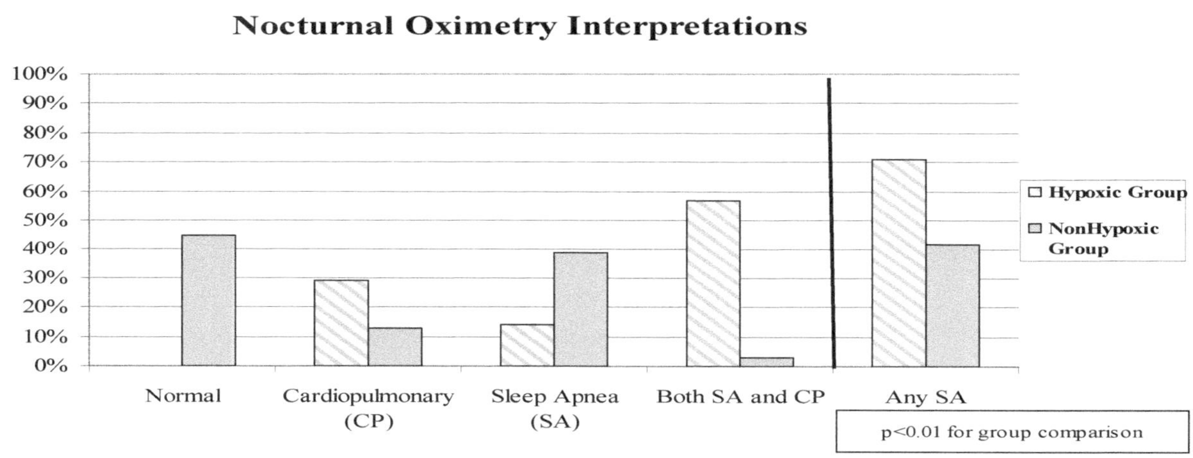

Abbreviations: CP=cardiopulmonary, SA=sleep apnea, Any SA=combined total of oximetries with elements of uncontrolled sleep apnea (sleep apnea and both sleep apnea and cardiopulmonary categories)

Figure 2: Nocturnal Oximetry on CPAP on Postoperative Night 1.

complications [13,22]. In this study, nursing interventions in the HG may have prevented the development of some adverse events that might otherwise be seen.

The American Academy of Sleep Medicine's most recent (2003) clinical practice review on the perioperative care of individuals with OSA recommended PAP use postoperatively in those with known OSA on PAP prior to surgery, and that "patients should be monitored for evidence of impaired gas exchange and upper airway obstruction (following surgery)." [20]. The duration of this monitoring was not specified. The current study suggests that oximetry monitoring for at least the first postoperative night may be indicated. The American Society of Anesthesiologists Task Force recommendations (2006) also advocated the use of PAP therapy postoperatively for patients with PAP-treated OSA, and felt that continuous pulse oximetry monitoring was warranted in patients who are "at increased perioperative risk from OSA" [21]. Details regarding who is at "increased perioperative risk" were not stated.

More recently, a postoperative management algorithm recommended continuous oximetry monitoring in OSA patients using PAP therapy postoperatively, though only in those noncompliant with PAP therapy preoperatively, those with severe OSA (defined as an AHI >30), and those with "recurrent respiratory events" in the PACU (recurrent hypoxia, episodes of bradypnea, a witnessed apnea or pain-sedation mismatch) [23]. These recommendations do not take into account the baseline supine AHI, postoperative fluid balance, and narcotic dose, factors associated with the development of nocturnal hypoxia in the present study.

The etiology for the hypoxia noted in some of the subjects could not be fully determined in this study. Based on the oximetry waveforms, uncontrolled sleep apnea appears to play a role, though it is unclear if it is due to uncontrolled obstructive apneas or the development of central apneas, which could result from the use of narcotics. It is noteworthy that 42% of the nonhypoxic group had evidence of uncontrolled sleep apnea on their oximetry tracings (Figure 2). It is possible that either the

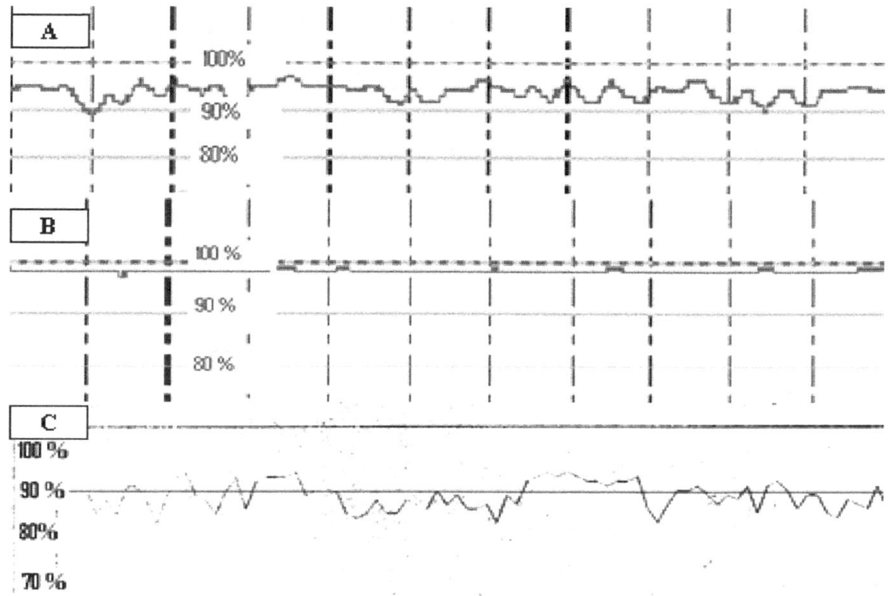

Panel A: oximetry sample from diagnostic PSG showing typical sawtooth pattern of uncontrolled OSA
Panel B: oximetry sample from CPAP titration PSG showing good control of OSA on CPAP at 9 cm H2O
Panel C: oximetry sample from 1st postoperative night on CPAP at 9 cm H2O showing recurrence of sawtooth pattern suggesting uncontrolled OSA

Figure 3: Oximetry Example of Uncontrolled Sleep Apnea on 1st Postoperative Night.

residual effects of anesthesia (especially in those undergoing afternoon surgeries) and/or the use of narcotic analgesics postoperatively may have resulted in worsening of the baseline sleep apnea and thus a lack of control on the subject's home PAP setting. Another consideration is that the subject's sleep apnea is no longer controlled on their home PAP settings as the titration studies were performed, on average, 1-2 years prior to their surgery. Weight did increase in both groups, though not significantly and thus this possibility cannot be excluded. However, it should be noted that there are no current guidelines recommending a repeat PAP titration prior to elective surgery in OSA patients on PAP therapy at home. Significant PAP mask leak, while not noted by the nursing or respiratory personnel, could also contribute to the appearance of uncontrolled sleep apnea. Further study with formal PSG testing will be required to determine the nature of the respiratory events and the potential role of air leaks. Alternative PAP therapies, such as autoadjusting CPAP (for OSA) or adaptive servo ventilation (for central apnea), may be useful in postoperative OSA management.

Some of the nocturnal hypoxia seen may also have been related to anesthetic / narcotic-induced hypoventilation. Arterial blood gas analysis and CO_2 monitoring were not performed in this study, and thus this possibility cannot be excluded. Future studies should include CO_2 monitoring as hypoventilation may influence the choice of PAP therapy. The increased positive net fluid balance and rates of clinically determined atelectasis in the hypoxic group could have also contributed to hypoxia postoperatively by a mechanism unrelated to the upper airway.

Use of CPAP postoperatively appears feasible. A 2009 study noted that 63% of patients using CPAP preoperatively were placed on CPAP the night after surgery [24]. In the present study, subjects were required to use CPAP following surgery and over 90% tolerated it without significant difficulty. This suggests that CPAP use should be encouraged postoperatively in patients accustomed to using PAP therapy at home.

There are some limitations to this study. Oximetry recording does not reveal the cause of hypoxemia and thus studies with PSG and CO_2 monitoring are needed. Oximetry recordings also do not allow for sleep-wake differentiation and some of the hypoxia noted may represent wake-time hypoxia. On the other hand, the ODI is determined by the number of desaturations divided by the recording time, not sleep time, and thus the ODI is likely underestimated. Another limitation is the lack of objective pre and postoperative CPAP compliance data. Subjective compliance was required to enroll in the study, though subjective reporting typically overestimates use. Postoperatively, CPAP use was documented by nursing and respiratory personnel, but objective time-on-pressure data was not available. Likewise, objective leak data was not obtained, which could be an important factor in poorly controlled sleep apnea. And finally, the number of subjects in the study was small and larger studies with more advanced monitoring are needed.

In summary, this study provides evidence supporting the use of routine oximetry monitoring in OSA patients following surgery, even in those treated with PAP therapy. It is hoped that by doing so, adverse events may be avoided, though larger studies are needed to confirm this. The mechanism(s) for the hypoxia noted, and how best to manage it, warrant further investigation.

Acknowledgments

Dr. Brar: contributed to the study design, data collection, analysis and manuscript preparation. Dr. Sharma: contributed to the study design, data collection and manuscript preparation. Dr. Khanna: contributed to data collection and manuscript preparation. Dr. Auckley: contributed to study design, analysis and manuscript preparation. Dr. Auckley takes responsibility for the integrity of the work as a whole.

References

1. Young T, Peppard PE, Gottlieb DJ (2002) Epidemiology of obstructive sleep apnea: a population health perspective. Am J Respir Crit Care Med 165: 1217-1239.

2. Chung F, Ward B, Ho J, Yuan H, Kayumov L, et al. (2007) Preoperative identification of sleep apnea risk in elective surgical patients, using the Berlin questionnaire. J Clin Anesth 19: 130-134.

3. Finkel KJ, Searleman AC, Tymkew H, Tanaka CY, Saager L, et al. (2009) Prevalence of undiagnosed obstructive sleep apnea among adult surgical patients in an academic medical center. Sleep Med 10: 753-758.

4. Stierer TL, Wright C, George A, Thompson RE, Wu CL, et al. (2010) Risk assessment of obstructive sleep apnea in a population of patients undergoing ambulatory surgery. J Clin Sleep Med 6: 467-472.

5. Craig DB (1981) Postoperative recovery of pulmonary function. Anesth Analg 60: 46-52.

6. Marshall BE, Wyche MQ Jr (1972) Hypoxemia during and after anesthesia. Anesthesiology 37: 178-209.

7. Esclamado RM, Glenn MG, McCulloch TM, Cummings CW (1989) Perioperative complications and risk factors in the surgical treatment of obstructive sleep apnea syndrome. Laryngoscope 99: 1125-1129.

8. Catley DM, Thornton C, Jordan C, Lehane JR, Royston D, et al. (1985) Pronounced, episodic oxygen desaturation in the postoperative period: its association with ventilatory pattern and analgesic regimen. Anesthesiology 63: 20-28.

9. Sollevi A, Lindahl SG (1995) Hypoxic and hypercapnic ventilatory responses during isoflurane sedation and anaesthesia in women. Acta Anaesthesiol Scand 39: 931-938.

10. Richard W, Kox D, den Herder C, Laman M, van Tinteren H, et al. (2006) The role of sleep position in obstructive sleep apnea syndrome. Eur Arch Otorhinolaryngol 263: 946-950.

11. Charbonneau M, Marin JM, Olha A, Kimoff RJ, Levy RD, et al. (1994) Changes in obstructive sleep apnea characteristics through the night. Chest 106: 1695-1701.

12. Ostermeier AM, Roizen MF, Hautkappe M, Klock PA, Klafta JM (1997) Three sudden postoperative respiratory arrests associated with epidural opioids in patients with sleep apnea. Anesth Analg 85: 452-460.

13. Gupta RM, Parvizi J, Hanssen AD, Gay PC (2001) Postoperative complications in patients with obstructive sleep apnea syndrome undergoing hip or knee replacement: a case-control study. Mayo Clin Proc 76: 897-905.

14. Mooe T, Gullsby S, Rabben T, Eriksson P (1996) Sleep-disordered breathing: a novel predictor of atrial fibrillation after coronary artery bypass surgery. Coron Artery Dis 7: 475-478.

15. Kaw R, Golish J, Ghamande S, Burgess R, Foldvary N, et al. (2006) Incremental risk of obstructive sleep apnea on cardiac surgical outcomes. J Cardiovasc Surg (Torino) 47: 683-689.

16. Memtsoudis S, Liu SS, Ma Y, Chiu YL, Walz JM, et al. (2011) Perioperative pulmonary outcomes in patients with sleep apnea after noncardiac surgery. Anesth Analg 112: 113-121.

17. Epstein LJ, Kristo D, Strollo PJ Jr, Friedman N, Malhotra A, et al. (2009) Clinical guideline for the evaluation, management and long-term care of obstructive sleep apnea in adults. J Clin Sleep Med 5: 263-276.

18. Rennotte MT, Baele P, Aubert G, Rodenstein DO (1995) Nasal continuous positive airway pressure in the perioperative management of patients with obstructive sleep apnea submitted to surgery. Chest 107: 367-374.

19. Arisaka H, Sakuraba S, Kobayashi R, Kitahama H, Nishida N, et al. (2008) Perioperative management of obstructive sleep apnea with nasal continuous positive airway pressure. Anesth Prog 55: 121-123.

20. Meoli AL, Rosen CL, Kristo D, Kohrman M, Gooneratne N, et al. (2003) Upper airway management of the adult patient with obstructive sleep apnea in the perioperative period--avoiding complications. Sleep 26: 1060-1065.

21. Gross JB, Bachenberg KL, Benumof JL, Caplan RA, Connis RT, et al. (2006) Practice guidelines for the perioperative management of patients with obstructive sleep apnea: a report by the American Society of Anesthesiologists Task Force on Perioperative Management of patients with obstructive sleep apnea. Anesthesiology 104: 1081-1093.

22. Hwang D, Shakir N, Limann B, Sison C, Kalra S, et al. (2008) Association of sleep-disordered breathing with postoperative complications. Chest 133: 1128-1134.

23. Seet E, Chung F (2010) Management of sleep apnea in adults - functional algorithms for the perioperative period: Continuing Professional Development. Can J Anaesth 57: 849-864.

24. Liao P, Yegneswaran B, Vairavanathan S, Zilberman P, Chung F (2009) Postoperative complications in patients with obstructive sleep apnea: a retrospective matched cohort study. Can J Anaesth 56: 819-828.

The Correlation of Physical Parameters and Apnea-Hypopnea Index in OSA Suspected Thai Patients

Nuntigar Sonsuwan[1], Sutida Ameiam[2] and Kittisak Sawanyawisuth[3]*

[1]*Department of Otolaryngology, Chiang Mai University, Chiang Mai, 50200, Thailand*
[2]*Uttaradit Hospital, Uttaradit, Thailand*
[3]*Department of Medicine, Faculty of Medicine, Khon Kaen University, Khon Kaen, 40002, Thailand*

Abstract

Most Asian countries have limited resources for polysomnography. Risk factors for Obstructive Sleep Apnea (OSA) in Asian populations may be different from the Western countries. Knowing the physical risk factors for OSA may be a helpful tool for clinicians to select suitable patients to be tested for OSA. We enrolled consecutive OSA-suspected patients between October 1st, 2006 and September 30th, 2007. Physical factors including Body Mass Index (BMI), Neck Circumference (NC), and Waist Circumference (WC) were recorded. The correlations of BMI, NC, WC and Apnea-Hypopnea Index (AHI) were executed. Various cut points of BMI, NC, and WC were calculated for sensitivity and specificity of severity of OSA. During the study period, there were 66 patients enrolled. All three parameters (BMI, NC, and WC) were significantly correlated with AHI. The highest correlation index was between BMI and AHI (0.604), whereas the correlation index of AHI-WC and AHI-NC were 0.571 and 0.440, respectively. Only BMI and WC, but not NC, were significantly related to severity of OSA. The BMI of more than 25 kg/m^2 had the highest sensitivity (93.8%) for severe OSA, whereas WC more than 101.8 cm had the highest specificity (92%). In conclusion, BMI, WC, and NC are correlated with AHI in OSA suspected Thai patients. BMI and WC, but not NC, were associated with severity of OSA. In resource-limited facilities, these parameters may be helpful for clinicians to evaluate the risk of OSA more appropriately.

Keywords: Body mass index; Waist circumference; Neck circumference; Association; Obstructive sleep apnea; Severity

Introduction

Obstructive Sleep Apnea (OSA) is defined as Apnea-Hypopnea Index (AHI) more than 5 times/hour by polysomnography. The prevalence of OSA is 4% in males and 2% in females of general population [1-3]. It is a strong risk factor for hypertension, coronary artery disease, and stroke [4-6]. However, OSA is under diagnosed and neglected in clinical practice [7] particularly in Southeast Asian countries where healthcare resources are limited.

Common risk factors of OSA include older age, male gender, obesity, craniofacial anomalies, and particular diseases such as hypothyroidism. Among those risk factors, obesity is the major risk factor in the Western countries. Neck Circumference (NC) more than 43 cm is related with severity of OSA in American patients. The sensitivity and specificity of this cut point are 67% and 83%, respectively [3]. Data for these physical factors and OSA is still limited in Southeast Asian populations. We evaluated the correlation of various physical factors and OSA in Thai patients that would be clinically helpful for selecting patients to perform polysomnography in a resource-limited setting.

Materials and Methods

We enrolled consecutive patients (age 25-60 years) with history of snoring or suspected of OSA at Department of Otolaryngology, Faculty of Medicine, Chiang Mai University between October 1st, 2006 and September 30th, 2007. The exclusion criteria were patients with craniofacial anomalies or one of the following diseases: hypothyroidism, acromegaly, vocal cord paralysis, post-polio syndrome, neuromuscular disorders, Marfan's syndrome, Down syndrome, Pierre-Robin syndrome, and amyloidosis.

All eligible patients were tested with Somnocheck® V2.04 and recorded for baseline characteristics, Body Mass Index (BMI), NC, and Waist Circumference (WC). OSA was defined if the AHI was more than 5 times/hour. The severity of OSA was classified by AHI as mild (AHI 5-14.9 times/hour), moderate (AHI 15-29.9 times/hour), and severe (AHI>30 times/hour), respectively. The Somnocheck® device has been shown to be highly correlated with polysomnography (r = 0.98) [8].

NC and WC were measured by the same physician and tape throughout the study period. The landmark for NC and WC were upper border of cricothyroid membrane of each patient in sitting position and umbilical line, respectively. The study protocol was approved by the institute review board of Chiang Mai University and all patients signed informed consent prior to the study participation.

Statistical analysis

The correlation of BMI, NC, WC and AHI were executed by Pearson correlation coefficient and Fisher Exact test. Various cut points of BMI, NC, and WC were calculated for sensitivity and specificity of severity of OSA.

Results

During the study period, there were 66 patients met the study criteria. The mean (S.D.) age of all patients was 51.4 (8.2) years. Of those,

***Corresponding author:** Kittisak Sawanyawisuth, Faculty of Medicine, Department of Medicine, Khon Kaen University, Khon Kaen, 40002, Thailand
E-mail: kittisak@kku.ac.th

48 patients (72.7%) were male and had at least one underlying diseases. The most three common underlying diseases were hypertension (23 patients, 34.9%), dyslipidemia (21 patients, 31.4%), and allergic rhinitis (10 patients, 15.1%), respectively. Abnormal physical signs were found in 55 patients (83.7%). The most three common anatomical findings were redundant soft palate (46 patients, 69.8%), long uvula (27 patients, 40.7%), and enlarged tonsils (12 patients, 18.6%), respectively.

According to the Asian classification of obesity, 9 patients (13.6%), 11 patients (16.7%), 32 patients (48.5%), and 14 patients (21.2%) were classified as normal, overweight, obesity class 1, and obesity class 2, respectively. The mean (S.D.) of NC and WC were 38.8 (3.2) cm and 91.6 (11.6) cm, respectively.

There were 58 patients (87.9%) with AHI more than 5 times/hour. Of those, 25 patients (37.9%) had mild OSA, while 17 patients (25.8%) and 16 patients (24.2%) had moderate and severe OSA, respectively.

All three parameters (BMI, NC, and WC) were significantly correlated with AHI by Pearson correlation method. The highest correlation index was between BMI and AHI (0.604), whereas the correlation index of AHI-WC and AHI-NC were 0.571 and 0.440, respectively.

We categorized all patients and severity of OSA by level of BMI, WC, and NC (Tables 1-3). Only level of BMI and WC were statistically correlated with severity of OSA (p value < 0.05). All patients with BMI more than 30 kg/m^2 had AHI more than 5 times/hour (Table 1). Patients with WC less than 75.5 cm were not severe OSA, while patients with WC more than 101.8 cm were moderate or severe OSA (Table 2). Level of NC was not statistically related with level of AHI (Table 3).

The BMI of more than 25 kg/m^2 had the highest sensitivity for severe OSA, whereas WC more than 101.8 cm had the highest specificity (Table 4).

Discussion

This study showed that BMI, WC, and NC were all statistically correlated with AHI but only BMI and WC were statistically related with severity of OSA in the Thai population.

BMI, WC, and NC are parameters that associated with obesity. From the analysis, BMI was the factor that mostly correlated with AHI (correlation coefficient 0.604). Only nine patients (13.6%) had normal BMI. Of those, only one patient had severe OSA. This patient had enlarged tonsils (grade 3) that may enhance severity of OSA. For those patients with BMI more than 30 kg/m^2 with snoring or symptoms of OSA, all of them had OSA. The BMI cut point of 25 kg/m^2 had sensitivity of 93.8% for severe OSA. Therefore, Thai patients with snoring or symptoms of OSA had BMI more than 25 kg/m^2, the likelihood of having severe OSA is 93.8%. Previous report also showed that BMI was negatively related with night time desaturation in OSA patients [9].

BMI	AHI<5	AHI 5-14.9	AHI 15-29.9	AHI ≥ 30	Total
18.5-22.9	2	4	2	1	9
23.0-24.9	1	8	2	0	11
25.0-29.9	5	12	9	6	32
≥ 30	0	1	4	9	14
Total	8	25	17	16	66

Note. AHI: apnea-hypopnea index

Table 1: The correlation between Body Mass Index (BMI) and severity of obstructive sleep apnea (p value < 0.05).

AHI (Events / Hr.) / WC (cm)	AHI<5	AHI 5-14.9	AHI 15-29.9	AHI ≥ 30	Total
62.5-75.5	3	4	1	0	8
75.6-88.6	2	7	4	2	15
88.7-101.7	3	14	8	7	32
≥ 101.8	0	0	4	7	11
Total	8	25	17	16	66

Note. AHI: Apnea-Hypopnea Index

Table 2: The correlation between Waist Circumference (WC) and severity of obstructive sleep apnea (p value < 0.05).

AHI (Events/Hr.) / NC (cm.)	AHI<5	AHI 5-14.9	AHI 15-29.9	AHI ≥ 30	Total
32.0 - 36.0	2	8	2	1	13
36.1 - 40.1	4	14	7	6	31
≥ 40.2	2	3	8	9	22
Total	8	25	17	16	66

Note. AHI: apnea-hypopnea index

Table 3: The correlation between Neck Circumference (NC) and severity of obstructive sleep apnea (p value>0.05).

Parameters	Sensitivity	Specificity
BMI>25 kg/m^2	93.8	38.0
WC>101.8 cm	43.8	92.0
NC>40.2 cm	56.3	74.0

Note. BMI: Body Mass Index; WC: Waist Circumference; NC: Neck Circumference

Table 4: Sensitivity and specificity of various parameters for severe OSA.

WC was also correlated with AHI and severity of OSA in OSA suspected Thai patients. All patients with WC more than 101.8 cm had moderate or severe OSA. This cut point had lower sensitivity but higher specificity for severe OSA compared to BMI. If one had WC more than 101.8 cm with snoring, the specificity for severe OSA is 92%.

Neck circumference more than 43 cm is related with severity of OSA in American patients. The sensitivity and specificity of this cut point are 67% and 83%, respectively [3]. Unlike a study from the Western country, NC was not significantly associated with severity of OSA in Thai patients. It also had the lowest correlation coefficient (0.440) compared to BMI and WC [3]. Previous studies showed that NC was the most significant factor correlated with severity of OSA and survival factor of stroke [10,11]. However, a study from Asia [12] did not find the correlation of NC and the severity of OSA similar to the present study. NC therefore may not be correlated with OSA severity in Asian population.

Even though BMI and WC were strongly correlated with severe OSA, the diagnosis of OSA is still needed to be confirmed by polysomnography. These results will be helpful for clinicians in facilities without polysomnography devices. Currently, there are very few hospitals that sleep study is available. It would be worthy to refer patients with snoring or symptoms of OSA who have BMI more than 25 kg/m^2 or WC more than 101.8 cm to sleep specialists. Another caution for our study is that we excluded patients with craniofacial anomalies and the diseases mentioned in the exclusion criteria. In other words, this study may not apply to OSA patients from anatomical abnormalities.

There are some limitations in the present study. Study variables were only physical parameters. Other factors such as symptoms of

OSA or complications of OSA were not included in the analysis as risk factors for OSA. Some factors however may not be valid such as daytime sleepiness symptoms, or unexplained nocturia. In contrast, physical parameters were measurable and can be used universally. Secondly, the statistical analyses showed only the correlation of physical factors and AHI but not as the independent factor for OSA. Further studies should be conducted in larger sample size and analyzed by advanced statistical method such as multiple logistic regression analysis.

Conclusion

BMI, WC, and NC are correlated with AHI in OSA suspected Thai patients. BMI and WC, but not NC, were predictors for severity of OSA. BMI is the most valuable parameter for the prediction of severe OSA. In resource limited facilities, these parameters may be helpful for clinicians to evaluate the risk of OSA more appropriately.

References

1. Young T, Palta M, Dempsey J, Skatrud J, Weber S, et al. (1993) The occurrence of sleep-disordered breathing among middle-aged adults. N Engl J Med 328: 1230-1235.
2. Kyzer S, Charuzi I (1998) Obstructive sleep apnea in the obese. World J Surg 22: 998-1001.
3. Dixon JB, Schachter LM, O'Brien PE (2003) Predicting sleep apnea and excessive day sleepiness in the severely obese: indicators for polysomnography. Chest 123: 1134-1141.
4. Peppard PE, Young T, Palta M, Skatrud J (2000) Prospective study of the association between sleep-disordered breathing and hypertension. N Engl J Med 342: 1378-1384.
5. Shahar E, Whitney CW, Redline S, Lee ET, Newman AB, et al. (2001) Sleep-disordered breathing and cardiovascular disease: cross-sectional results of the Sleep Heart Health Study. Am J Respir Crit Care Med 163: 19-25.
6. Drager LF, Polotsky VY, Lorenzi-Filho G (2011) Obstructive sleep apnea: an emerging risk factor for atherosclerosis. Chest 140: 534-542.
7. Silverberg DS, Oksenberg A, Iaina A (1997) Sleep related breathing disorders are common contributing factors to the production of essential hypertension but are neglected, underdiagnosed, and undertreated. Am J Hypertens 10: 1319-1325.
8. Ficker JH, Wiest GH, Wilpert J, Fuchs FS, Hahn EG (2001) Evaluation of a portable recording device (Somnocheck) for use in patients with suspected obstructive sleep apnoea. Respiration 68: 307-312.
9. Hannon TS, Rofey DL, Ryan CM, Clapper DA, Chakravorty S, et al. (2012) Relationships among obstructive sleep apnea, anthropometric measures, and neurocognitive functioning in adolescents with severe obesity. J Pediatr 160: 732-735.
10. Medeiros CA, Bruin VM, Castro-Silva Cd, Araújo SM, Chaves Junior CM, et al. (2011) Neck circumference, a bedside clinical feature related to mortality of acute ischemic stroke. Rev Assoc Med Bras 57: 559-564.
11. Pinto JA, Godoy LB, Marquis VW, Sonego TB, Leal Cde F, et al. (2011) Anthropometric data as predictors of Obstructive Sleep Apnea Severity. Braz J Otorhinolaryngol 77: 516-521.
12. Ugur KS, Ark N, Kurtaran H, Kizilbulut G, Cakir B, et al. (2011) Subcutaneous fat tissue thickness of the anterior neck and umbilicus in patients with obstructive sleep apnea. Otolaryngol Head Neck Surg 145: 505-510.

22

Solution to the Humanity's Age-old Problem "Sore Waist and Aching Back": Using NON-Conventional Sleeping Positions and Bedding to Alleviate Back Pain and Regain Energy

Jinhui Chiang* **and Ryan Chiang**

Chinese Medicine Clinic, I-I-Tang (IIT), Taiwan

Abstract

For eons, human beings walked using their four limbs. It was not until relatively recently that human beings started to walk on their two feet. By standing on two feet, the waist takes the weight from the upper part of the body, which accounts for three-fifths of their total weight. If people stand, sit or walk too long, they will have a sore waist and an aching back. The frequency of the symptoms is similar to that of a cold. The back pain problem particularly occurs to laborers, athletes, those who physically challenge themselves, or those who have to stand and sit for a long time due to the requirements of their work, such as teachers, barbers or hairdressers, store sales clerks, dentists, nurses, long-distance drivers, or some assembly line operators. Those people easily get a sore waist and aching back. Thus, calling this problem "humanity's age-old problem" is not an exaggeration. Numerous methods were developed to solve the problem. Much research has also been conducted to find out the factors of the problem. However, one crucial problem has been overlooked. It derives from existing kinds of beds that are made by misusing the ergonomic spines movement curve. So, when people lie on a bed, they still feel tension from moving or working. Therefore, NON-conventional sleeping positions and bedding are needed based on human's natural smiling curve. In other words, to get a real relaxation, the spine needs to be in the shape of a smiling curve, like the shape of a bow, crescent moon, so that people can lie down and sleep with relaxation from head to toe, from inside to outside, from internal to external organs, and the ten body systems (integument system, skeletal system, muscular System, circulatory system, lymphatic system, nervous system, digestive system, respiratory system, urinary system, endocrine system, reproductive system). The compression in lumbar spine can also be alleviated. Then the body can be physically and mentally relaxed and get enough rest.

Keywords: Back pain; Sleeping disorder; Nonconventional sleeping position; Bedding; S –curve; Smiling curve

Incorrect Sleeping Positions and Bedding Exhaust Your Physical Strength Every night

It is very common for people to get bone spurs, sciatica, sore neck and thigh bone, tingling pain in knees and feet. The advice that they commonly receive from doctors is to avoid incorrect sitting and standing postures or inappropriate postures especially when bending over to lift heavy objects. However, doctors seldom mention the problem of sleeping postures. Specialty physicians have also avoided talking about the importance of sleeping postures. At most, they show their concern by asking whether the mattress is too hard or soft, or whether the waist is being supported in bed. It seems that the matter is not that serious, so it is often postponed until a later time to deal with it.

Speaking of sleeping postures, the choices are usually limited to lying on one's back, sleeping on one's side, and sleeping on one's stomach. People tend to toss and turn restlessly without a fixed posture. It perhaps does not make sense if one is told to have a particular sleeping posture. Nevertheless, people are supposed to be vigorous, energetic, and high-spirited after a good night sleep. Surprisingly, it often turns out to be the other way around after they get up in the morning. For example, most people have the symptoms such as a sore waist, aching back, stiff tendons and tight muscles. It may seem strange and most people might wonder whether they were sleeping or working during the night. Without quality sleep to help people regain energy, how can they deal with work during the day time? It is a small everyday issue but turns out to be a big problem that has bothered people for thousands of years without any solution having been found. According to the researcher's experimental research study, it was found that the inability of people to sleep well, be relaxed, and get good rest certainly has something to do with their sleeping postures and bedding. If sleeping is not helping people to regain their energy and restore their vitality but instead causes fatigue, they may fall sick from exhaustion and overwork.

State of Incomplete Sleep

Sleeping disorder is a condition or disease that interferes with sleep. It can be caused by various factors, including stress, substance abuse, body weight, BMI (Body Mass Index), maxillofacial and craniofacial deformities, and bedding. Sleeping disorders can also be considered as life style diseases, which is associated with the way a person or a group of people lives, including atherosclerosis, heart disease, and stroke. A variety of factors that contribute to sleeping disorder have been identified through numerous studies; however, little research has been done to detect the problem— the body posture during sleep. Koninck et al. [1] also pointed out that despite the fact that many aspects of sleep and dreaming have been studied extensively, the bodily positions during sleep have not received very much attention.

***Corresponding author:** Jinhui Chiang, Chinese Medicine Clinic, I-I-Tang (IIT), Taiwan, E-mail: lisung@yahoo.com

During sleep, people commonly move or change sleeping positions. In Koninck et al. [1] study, the data results show that the average of good sleepers' position changes per night is 22.3. In general, people can change their sleeping positions as few as 30 to 40 times and as many as50 to 60 times. We can count the times within six hours (i.e. 360 minutes) per night. If people change their sleeping positions 30 times, the frequency is once every 12 minutes. If people toss and turn 60 times, the frequency is once every 6 minutes. In other words, people change their sleeping positions one time within 6 to 12 minutes. The change of their sleeping positions is due to uncomfortable sleeping postures, which puts pressure on skin, muscles, blood vessels and results in soreness and tingling pain. The brain gets the message of the tingling pain, makes an internal inductive analysis, and then sends out a message to turn over. That is to say, part of the brain is not resting; it is busy receiving and sending messages to change their sleeping positions the entire night. This kind of sleep is called "state of incomplete sleep" People who do not change their sleeping postures or bedding will have this problem to some extent.

In summary, sleeping disorder has causal relationship with sleeping positions. As Koninck et al. [1] indicate, "sleep positions constitute an interesting dimension of sleep and that further study may reveal causal links between the quality of sleep and the amount of time spent in particular positions. Certain sleep disorders may indeed be related to sleep positions." Their research provides good evidence showing the causal relationship between the bodily positions and sleeping disorder.

The Syndrome Derived from Incomplete Sleep

Sleeping is crucial because it directly influences life span. For example, hibernating animals, such as turtles and snakes, have a long life. On the contrary, incomplete sleep or sleeping deficiency may cause brain fatigue, brain degradation or premature aging, and immune system problems. Those who have long-term insomnia have a problem with their immune system. The diseases involved in the immune system include cancer, tumors, infectious diseases, and many other inflammation diseases, which can be described as all-encompassing and are too numerous to mention. Most of them are related to the immune system. On the other hand, if people's immunity is balanced, they will not be infected with any diseases and will live a long life.

As known, getting a cold has a correlation with incomplete sleep. For instance, people usually catch a cold during the night time, but the cold is not discovered until the next morning. The symptoms of a cold include a pharyngeal nose, feeling dry and pain between the nose and pharynx, nasal congestion, sneezing, a runny nose, dizziness, muscle aches, fatigue, and migraine. It is not until people get up in the morning, they may find they get a cold with the symptoms stated above. As a matter of fact, the cold is usually caused by the constant change of bodily position during sleep, which actually results from incomplete sleep. Without a good night's sleep, people can easily get a cold, which is the root cause of all diseases. Therefore, we can conclude that all of the ailments and diseases mentioned above can be classified as "the syndrome derived from incomplete sleep."

"Seeking it my whole life; Looking back all of a sudden; It has not been far from my side" (from a poem by Chi-Ji Xin in Chinese Song Dynasty)

To unlock the eternal suspenseful mystery of back pain, it was found that specialists, scholars, and physicians did spend a huge amount of effort in this area, such as injections and medicine, titanium implant surgery, perfusion of bone cement, neck supporter (or neck supporting collar), frame brace, waist frame protection belt, spinal scoliosis braces, electric massage chairs, ice packs, hot packs, traction, tai-chi, yoga, abdominal movement exercise, waist power exercise, acupuncture, massage therapy, chiropractic [1], cupping therapy [1], stretching, qigong, low-frequency electrical stimulation therapy, thermal treatment, aqua therapy, steam therapy, medicated wash, or medicated plaster. Numerous methods were developed, but the most crucial solution for back pain was ignored. Back pain can actually be repaired through sleeping naturally during the night time. It is as one western proverb says, "Time, nature, and patience are three great physicians", which are sent by God to treat people's diseases every night." If we really understand the proverb, we should take advantage of the night time lying in the "appropriate" bed naturally rest patiently to recover peacefully, and relax thoroughly. After we sleep soundly for five or six hours with the help of the three physicians, our body will feel soft and comfortable. This is the most comfortable state that can avoid a sore waist and an aching back. Consequently, all of our diseases can be cured and our good health can be maintained. In other others, this is the real remedy for back pain. It is a natural repair actually working at night while people sleep.

The Bed Industry has Made a Serious Mistake

It is time to seriously discuss what kind of sleeping positions and bedding are needed in order to achieve a deep and sound sleep without tossing and turning at night. Spring beds have been manufactured for 130 years. While they have really brought unprecedented comfort, they unfortunately cannot reduce back pain. Some physicians even advocate the use of a hard wooden bed and convince patients to sleep on it. In fact, sleeping on a hard wooden bed is not as comfortable as sleeping on the spring bed, nor is it helpful for alleviating back pain. After a careful examination of all the beds sold on the market, it was discovered that bed manufacturers made a fatal mistake. They mistook the S sports curvature (Figure 1) of a person's spine as the rest curvature. Consequently, beds made for people to sleep on have unexpectedly led to more fatigue. That's why most people are dissatisfied with their bed. This is reflected in a poll in which60% of people stated that they do not

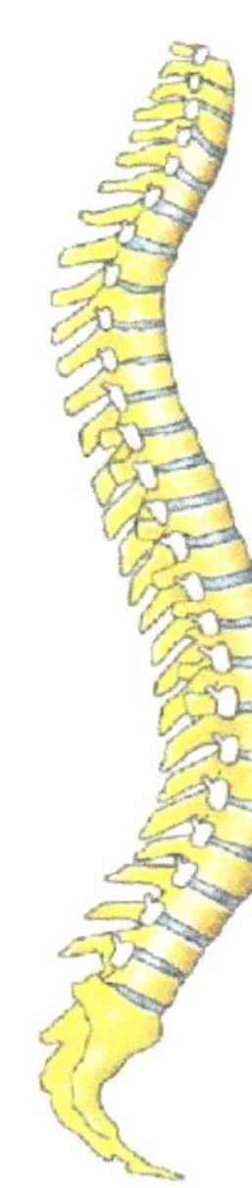

Figure 1: S curvature of the spine.

feel sleep well and do not get enough sleep, and 90% of people stated their sleeping was disturbed.

Sleeping Position Changing from the S-Curve to Smiling Curve Will Double People's Life-Span

Spinal physiological curvature has more than one pattern. The curvature can be divided into at least two states: the state of motion and the state of rest. When a person is in the state of motion, such as standing, walking, running and jumping, or working, his or her spinal curvature turns into S-curve. The cervical spine turns forward convex; the thoracics acral concave back. If we look at a person from the side, an S-curve is observed. On the other hand, if a person is in the state of rest, the curvature of a person's spine is in a relaxed state, which appears as "a smiling curve" (Figure 2). Thus, if a bed is made according to this relaxed smiling curve, it can really allow a person to take a good rest. In contrast, if a bed is made according to the S-curve, it does not provide a person with any rest at all. What's worse, it forces a person to continue to be in the state of motion.

However, most people choose to sleep on the beds leaving them in the state of movement, tension, and exhaustion instead of resting, because they have typically believed that a bed should be flat. Experts in the field of preventive medicine also believe that the best sleeping position should be the same as the standing position, which has become a slogan in the bed industry. Therefore, the bed industry has only concerned about making flat bedsteads based on the S-curve of the human body. In fact, without further investigation or research conducted, there is a problem with the logic. For a healthy person, lying down and standing up make no difference because their back can keep in the shape of S-curve. But, for those who are injured or ill and have no physical strength, it will be difficult for them to maintain the shape of S-curve. Thus, a bed that is flat is not possible to support, hold, and pad a person's body to get sufficient rest.

One bed manufacturer who calls himself "doctor" claimed that the former U.S. President, George W Bush, and his family members all sleep on the beds he made. He also affirmed that for decades he changed the concept of "misunderstanding of the bed, misusing of the bed." One of the sentences in his article puzzled many readers. He said that the function of his bed is to reach the goal of "the best posture of standing at attention with relaxation –straight waist, upright chest, narrow abdomen." This is definitely a posture that will exhaust a person's energy. Those who have received military training courses know that being "at ease" is slightly more relaxing than being "at attention." When one is "at attention", one is in a NON-relaxing state: having chin up and chest out, shrinking the lower abdomen, eyes looking straight ahead, high spirits, full of energy, combat readiness, straight and impressive looking. So, standing "at attention" is the most uneasy position. If a bed is made by reflecting such a ridiculous understanding and misconception, how can people expect to have a bed that can offer them a good night's sleep? Not only this bed manufacturer but also other manufacturers have madesuch a big mistake. This manufacturer "doctor" simply put his bed-making concept into words. As a matter of fact, over the past 130 years, all beds made by the bed industry are pretty much the same. They are not made to keep people in the state of motion, tension, combat readiness, and exhaustion instead of having them rest, recuperate and regain energy.

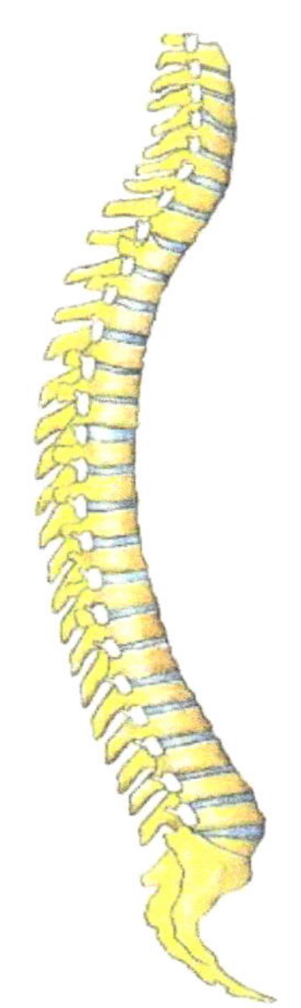

Figure 2: Smiling curvature of the spine.

Sleeping on the Back and on One Side in a Smiling Curve Can Help One Sleep Without Changing Positions All Night

Ancient Chinese Buddhist practitioners were required to "sit like bells, walk like wind, stand like a pine tree, sleep like a bow" because these postures were perceived as the best postures for Buddhist practice. Similarly, the smiling-curve sleeping position is perceived as the most comfortable position, which can be divided into two: one is sleeping on the back; the other is sleeping on the side.

The first one is sleeping on one side. Sleeping on one's side retracts one's spine into the shape of a bow, which is also called the shape of crescent moon. The School of Medicine at Oklahoma State University published a paper on sleeping quality. It mentioned that sleeping on one side the whole night can better help the spine to relax. This type of sleeping position is certainly good for the spine, but it presses hard on the area between the shoulders to the ribs and to the flank, and from the armpit to the waist. The press often makes people to feel uncomfortable and has them constantly their sleeping positions while sleeping.

The other position is sleeping on the back. If a person who is sleeping on the back is watched from the side of the body, the shape of the person's body appears as a smiling curve. The head and knees move to the same height and the waist moves to the lower position. The angle between the body and legs of the person is around 140 degrees. The position of sleeping on the side is formed by means of a bed with a smiling curve. If people sleep on the bed like that, it certainly makes them feel comfortable. When people sleep on the back on the bed with a smiling curve, their chest and shoulders are relaxed without being moved upwards, their lower part of abdomen sinks down naturally, and their belly and lower part of abdomen are soft and loose. This is similar to the movement of *T'aichi*– having the chest and back relieved and the neck pulled up, breathing from the abdomen, and having long and gentle breathing, which do not make people feel like moving their body. People's back pain can be totally alleviated.

In regard of this issue, Jacobson et al. [2] research also discusses back pain, sleep quality, and bedding by comparing "personal and new bedding systems between subjects with reported high and low base line sleep quality." The findings of their research show that new, medium- firm bedding systems can yield significant differences for good and poor sleep quality. They also found that the variables, such as age, weight, height, and body mass index, are independent of such improvements.

Three Examples About Posturing With a Spine that is Hunched in the Shape of a Smiling Curve Like a Bow

As mentioned earlier, from the traditional perspective, the two examples—standing at attention and lying flat on the bed—may seem to be the easiest positions. However, if a person has the two positions, his or her spine is in the shape of the S sports curvature, which often leads to some sort of pain, soreness and fatigue. In contrast, from some common facts in our daily life, we can easily find out that the spine in the resting state is in the shape of a smiling curve, which is the most comfortable curve. This concept will be illustrated by the three examples: the fetus, the animal, and the biker.

The fetus in the womb has its feet crossed and its body hunched in the resting state.

After it is born, it begins to learn to walk with a vertical backbone. When in the walking state, the baby's spine resembles an S-curve, but when in the resting state, its spine often appears in the shape of a smiling curve (Figure 3).

Another example is the animal.

The spine of all four-legged animals, including cats, dogs, cattle, sheep, pigs, tigers, leopards, lions, and deer, appears as an S-curve when they are in the state of standing, running, jumping and walking. However, when they are in the resting state, their spines naturally turn into the shape of a smiling curve, like a crescent.

The third example is bicyclists.

We often see most bicyclists riding a bike with their back hunched (Figure 4). The position of sitting on a bike makes a person lean forward or squat with two feet bent in the same level, so that the bicyclist's spine will feel more comfortable. According to Dr. Wen-Ji Tsai [3], the dean of Bone Care orthopaedics Center in Taiwan, the degree of a person's spine curve in the state of standing is 1.145 and bike-riding position is 1.031. He concludes that bike-riding can help alleviate the compression particularly between the fourth lumbar and fifth lumbar of a person's spine.

Evidence in Literature of Physiology and Anatomy Confirmed that the Spine Stretches to its Extent When Sleeping in the Shape of a Smiling curve, Matching the Measurement of X-Ray

There is plenty of evidence in the literature of physiology and anatomy in regard to the smiling curve of the spine. For example, if the spine of a donated dead body is bent forwards and backwards, the forward-bent smiling curve stretches the body to its fullest. That is to say, the position of smiling curve is the most beneficial to the circulation of the spinal marrow, blood, nerves, and the air in the governing vessel. In addition, people's back muscles are longer than their abdominal muscles; their governing vessel is longer than their Conception Vessel. Having a position with a slight smiling curve is actually the most comfortable position though many children and the elderly are often reminded to have their chins up, chests out, and shrink the lower abdomen. As a matter of fact, people stoop and hunch their back unconsciously because it is the most comfortable position. If it weren't for the desire to create positive impression, such as elegance

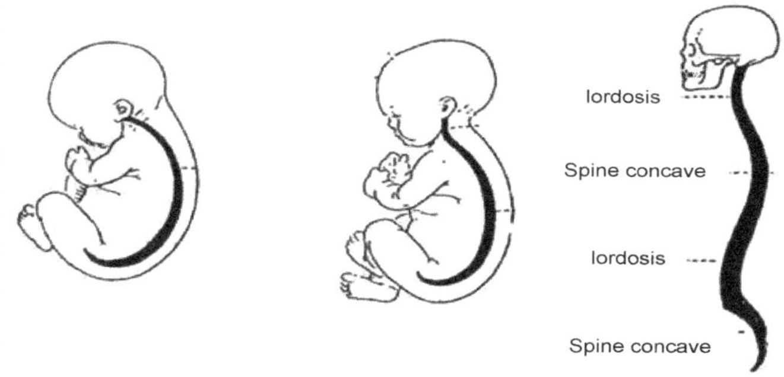

Figure 3: Human Spine Development.

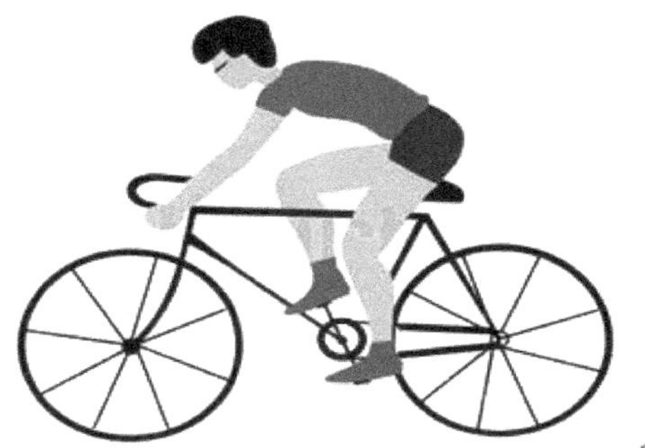

Figure 4: The spine curve of a bicyclist.

and dignity, people would feel most comfortable with the position of a smiling curve.

In addition, according to a measurement done by X-ray, the length ratio of the anterior and posterior spinal longitudinal ligament should be less than1. Only with this ratio can the space of the lumbar spinal cord canal be expanded to its extent. When a person is in the standing state, the ratio is 1.145. If the body slightly leans forward for approximately 0.95, like a bike-riding position, the lumbar posterior longitudinal ligament can be stretched open by the position of leaning forward, which can effectively increase spinal cavity space, lower the pressure in the lower lumbar backside, and reduce nerve compression.

In conclusion, there are many ways that can help people keep in good health, including various kinds of foods, equipment, and exercises. All of them can strengthen a human body to a certain degree. However, the most important thing is to solve the age-old problem—sore waist and aching back. The best solution found so far is using the NON-conventional sleeping positions and bedding in the shape of a smiling curve in order to regain people's energy and alleviate their waist soreness and back pain. Once people's waist soreness and back pain are alleviated, they can really get a good rest and can eventually maintain good health.

References

1. Koninck, JD, Gagnon P, Lallier S (1983) Sleep positions in the young adult and their relationship with the subjective quality of sleep. Sleep 6: 52-59.
2. Jacobson BH, Wallace T, Gemmell H (2006) Subjective rating of perceived back pain, stiffness and sleep quality following introduction of medium-firm bedding systems. Journal of Chiropractic Medicine 5: 128-134.
3. Tsai W (2012) Bike riding can alleviate the compression in lumbar spine. Apple Daily, August 28, 2012.

The Association of Troponin I Levels with Severity of Obstructive Sleep Apnea Syndrome

Nalan Demir[1],Oğuz Köktürk[2], Tansu Ulukavak Ciftçi[2], Ozlem Gülbahar[3], Neslihan Celik Bukan[3] and Kenan Köse[4]

[1]*Department of Chest Diseases, School of Medicine, Ankara University, Ankara, Turkey*
[2]*Department of Chest Diseases, School of Medicine, Gazi University, Sleep Medicine Unit, Ankara, Turkey*
[3]*Department of Biochemistry, School of Medicine, Gazi University, Ankara, Turkey*
[4]*Department of Statistics, School of Medicine, Ankara University, Ankara, Turkey*

Abstract

Background: As a result of repeated nocturnal hypoxemia, pulmonary arterial vasoconstriction, acute right ventricular dilatation and hypokinesia and myocardial injury may occur in patients with Obstructive Sleep Apnea Syndrome (OSAS). As it is known, Cardiac Troponin I (cTnI) is an important marker of myocardial injury.

Objectives: The aim of this study is to investigate the degree of myocardial injury which is created with nocturnal hypoxemia by measuring cTnI levels in patients with OSAS and to evaluate the association between cTnI levels and severity of OSAS.

Methods: Seventy-six subjects who had OSAS symptoms were examined with standard polysomnography (PSG) and classified according to their Apnea-Hypopnea Index (AHI). Forty-seven patients with AHI ≥ 5 were considered as OSAS and 29 subjects with AHI<5 were included into control group. OSAS patients were divided into three groups according to their AHI values as mild (AHI=5-15) (n:13), moderate (AHI=15-30) (n:14) and severe (AHI>30) OSAS (n:20). Serum cTnI levels were measured twice in all subjects after the PSG.

Results: When the levels of cTnI were compared, there was no significant difference between patients and controls (OSAS=3.6 ± 2.7 ng/ml and controls=3.1 ± 1.8 ng/ml, p=0.3). Also no significant difference was detected between mild-moderate OSAS (2.93 ± 1.67 ng/ml), severe OSAS (4.57 ± 3.47 ng/ml) and controls comparing with their cTnI levels (p=0.053). But cTnI levels in severe OSAS patients were significantly higher than controls (p=0.01). According to the logarithmic transformation, log-cTnI was 0.49 ± 0.21 ng/ml and 0.47 ± 0.21 ng/ml in OSAS subjects and controls, respectively (p=0.74). Severe OSAS patients had higher log-cTnI levels (0.59 ± 0.22 ng/ml) than mild-moderate OSAS subjects and controls (p=0.018, f=4.26). There was a positive correlation between AHI and cTnI levels in patients with OSAS (r=0.276, p=0.019, R^2=0.076).

Conclusion: Cardiac troponin I measurements may be useful to show the degree of myocardial injury in severe OSAS.

Keywords: Cardiac troponin I; Obstructive sleep apnea syndrome; Polysomnography; Apnea-hypopnea index; Myocardial injury

Introduction

Obstructive sleep apnea syndrome (OSAS), characterized by repeated upper airway obstruction episodes and nocturnal desaturation is a common disorder that occurs at least 2% to 4% of the adult population. The severity of OSAS is described according to the apnea-hypopnea index (AHI) [1].

The relationship of OSAS with cardiovascular diseases including hypertension, congestive heart failure, arrhythmias, and Coronary Artery Disease (CAD) is well known [2,3]. The acute hemodynamic changes of OSAS include systemic and pulmonary hypertension, increased right and left ventricle after load, and increased cardiac output [4]. Recent studies have shown that at the end of the repeated nocturnal hypoxemia, pulmonary arterial vasoconstriction may be observed in OSAS. In addition, Right Ventricle (RV) dilatation and hypokinesia due to repetitive hypoxemia may lead to myocardial injury and ischemia without CAD [5-8].

Cardiac troponins are high sensitive biochemical markers of acute myocardial infarction [9]. Serum troponins are also increased in a number of clinical settings such as acute and chronic heart failure, cardioversion, ablation, cardiac arrest, sepsis/septic shock and SIRS, end stage renal failure, acute pulmonary embolism, cardiac trauma and acute stroke in addition to acute coronary syndrome [10-16]. Recently, cardiac troponin testing is increasingly used in non-coronary diseases to indicate cardiac injury [17,18]. Cardiac troponin I (cTnI) levels may also be elevated in patients with OSAS who occurred myocardial injury due to repeated nocturnal hypoxemia [19].

The aim of this study is to evaluate the degree of myocardial injury in patients with OSAS and to determinate association between AHI values and cTnI levels.

Material and Methods

Study subjects

A total number of 76 patients admitted to Gazi University Sleep Medicine Unit were included in this study, prospectively. The study

***Corresponding author:** Nalan Demir, MD, Department of Pulmonary Medicine, School of Medicine, Ankara University 06100 Cebeci-Ankara, Turkey
E-mail: dr.ndemir@gmail.com

was approved by the local ethics review board. Inclusion criteria were as follows: being older than 18 years, having OSAS symptoms (snoring, witnessed apneas, excessive daytime sleepiness) on admission, to give informed consent for the study, performing full-night polysomnography. Exclusion criteria were accepted as: having acute coronary syndrome, renal and heart failure, sepsis, chronic obstructive pulmonary diseases, recent cardiac trauma or intervention.

Sleep study

Overnight Polysomnography (PSG) was performed in all patients by a computerized system (Somnostar alpha; Sensormedics, USA) and included the following variables: electrooculogram (2 channels), electroencephalogram (4 channels), electromyogram of submental muscles (2 channels), electromyogram of the anterior tibialis muscle of both legs (2 channels); electrocardiogram and airflow (with a nasal cannule). Chest and abdominal efforts (2 channels) were recorded using inductive plethysmography, arterial oxyhemoglobin saturation (SaO_2: 1 channel) by pulse oximetry with a finger probe. The recordings were conducted at a paper speed of 10 mm/s, and sleep stage were scored according to the standard criteria of Rechtschaffen and Kales [20]. Arousals were scored according to accepted definitions [21]. The AHI was obtained by dividing the total number of apneas and hypopneas by the Total Sleep Time (TST). Apneas were defined as complete cessation of airflow ≥ 10 s. Hypopneas were defined as reduction of >50% in one of three respiratory signals, airflow signal or either respiratory or abdominal signals of respiratory inductance plethysmography, with an associated fell of ≥ 3% in oxygen saturation or an arousal [22]. According to the recently updated International Classification of Sleep Disorders published by the American Academy of Sleep Medicine, a diagnosis of OSAS was made if the AHI is ≥ 15, independent of occurrence of symptoms, or whenever an AHI>5 is associated with any of the following: 1) sleep attacks excessive daytime sleepiness (EDS), 2) unrefreshing sleep, fatigue or insomnia, or 3) witnessed heavy snoring and/or breathing pauses referred by the partner [23]. Patients with sleep disorders, except OSAS, such as Upper Airway Resistance Syndrome (UARS), Periodic Legs Movements' Syndrome (PLMs) or narcolepsy were excluded.

Study design

Totally 76 patients who had performed PSG due to OSAS symptoms (snoring, witnessed apneas, excessive daytime sleepiness) without acute coronary syndrome were included to this study, prospectively. In 47 cases of all OSAS diagnoses were confirmed by PSG. The remaining 29 patients without OSAS were evaluated as control group (AHI<5). The cases with OSAS were also divided in 3 groups according to severity of disease: Mild OSAS (AHI: 5-15), moderate OSAS (AHI: 15-30) and severe OSAS (AHI>30).

For all patients, clinical data (symptoms, physical examination findings, body mass index, X-ray, electrocardiography, lung function tests, complete blood count, routine biochemical analysis and thyroid hormone levels) were obtained on admission. According to the body mass index, the patients classified as normal, overweight (BMI ≥ 25), obese (BMI ≥ 30), and morbid obese (BMI ≥ 40). After the sleep study, the findings of PSG, AHI values, and cTnI levels were recorded.

Laboratory analyses

In all patients, the venous blood samples were obtained after the PSG for cTnI measurements. Blood samples were centrifuged at 3000 rpm for 15 minutes and saved at -80°C. All samples were analyzed with cTnI ELISA test (solid phase enzyme-linked immunosorbent assay) (specificity: 87.5%, sensitivity: 100%, CI: 95%). The lower limit of cTnI ELISA=0.48 ng/ml; upper limit=1.0 ng/ml.

Statistical analysis

Data were analyzed by using SPSS for Windows release 10.0.1 (SPSS, Chicago, IL). Values were expressed as mean ± SD. The chi-square test was used to compare categorical variables. The *t*-test was used to compare the mean differences in independent samples. In addition, case summary reports and frequency charts were used to analyze the group variables. Kruskal wallis one way analysis was used for comparison of mild, moderate, severe OSAS subjects and controls. The comparison of groups was performed by ANOVA test. Pearson correlation was used to evaluate an association between AHI and cTnI values. All p values were two-tailed and a p value<0.05 was considered statistically significant.

Results

In the analysis of all cases (n: 76, female/male: 28/48), the mean age was 50.2 ± 10.9 (27-76) years. Mean body mass index (BMI) was 30.5 ± 6.1 kg/m^2. According to the BMI, 14 (18.4%) cases were normal. Thirty (39.5%) of them was overweight. Obesity and morbid obesity were seen in 23 (30.3%) and 9 (11.8%) of all cases. Thirty-three patients (43.4%) were active smoker on admission. Existing co-morbidities were hypercholosterolemia (n:29, 38.2%), hypertension (n:17, 22.4%), diabetes mellitus (n:10, 13.2%), artymia (n:5, 6.6%), coronary artery disease (n:5, 6.6%), and chronic heart failure (n: 2, 2.6%).

OSAS was detected in 47 (61.8%) (M/F:27/20) of all cases, and these cases were subdivided to the three groups as mild (n:13), moderate (n:14) and severe OSAS (n:20), according to the their AHI values. The remaining 29 (38.2%) patients of all who had normal PSG were accepted as controls (Figure 1).

When demographic data of subjects and controls were analyzed; sex, mean body mass index (BMI-kg/m^2), smoking history, existing co-morbidities, first SaO_2 levels and electrocardiographic changes (left and right bundle block, arytmia) on PSG were similar between subjects and controls (p>0.05). Nonetheless, OSAS subjects were older than controls (p=0.01), and obesity was more frequent in cases with OSAS (p=0.03). At the sleep study, mean AHI values and minimum SaO_2 were different for each group as expected (p=0.00). First SaO_2, mean was 94.9 ± 1.5

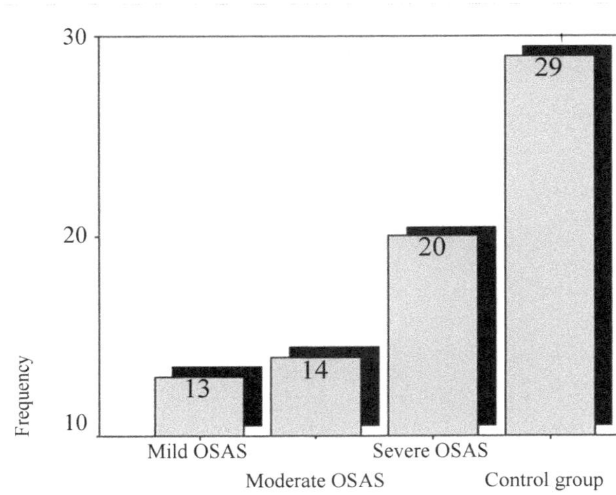

Figure 1: The frequency of OSAS subjects and controls that had normal polysomnography.

and 94.8 ± 5.4 in subjects and controls, respectively (p=0.8 and 0.0). Whereas mean AHI values in cases with OSAS were 38.5 ± 36.7, it was 2.1 ± 1.3 in controls. The levels of cTnI were similar in both groups (OSAS=3.6 ± 2.7 ng/ml and controls=3.1 ± 1.8 ng/ml, p=0.3) (Table 1).

At the comparison of mild-moderate and severe OSAS and controls, females were predominant in controls than mild-moderate and severe OSAS (p=0.04). In OSAS subjects min SaO_2 levels were gradually decreased according to the severity of OSAS during the PSG (p=0.00). When cTnI levels were compared between mild-moderate OSAS (2.93 ± 1.67 ng/ml), severe OSAS (4.57 ± 3.47 ng/ml) and controls (3.13 ± 1.83 ng/ml), there was no significant difference (p=0.053). But levels of cTnI in patients with severe OSAS were significantly higher than controls (p=0.01) (Table 2).

In present study, logaritmic transformation was used for normalization of cTnI levels. According to this analysis, log-cTnI was 0.49 ± 0.21 ng/ml and 0.47 ± 0.21 ng/ml in OSAS subjects and controls, respectively (p=0.74) (Table 3). When mild and moderate OSAS were compared with severe OSAS and controls, the patients with severe OSAS had higher log-cTnI levels (0.59 ± 0.22 ng/ml) than mild-moderate OSAS subjects and controls (p=0.018, f=4.26, Kruskal wallis one way analysis) (Table 4).

At the analysis of demographic features according to the log-cTnI; smoker patients had higher log-cTnI levels (0.52 ± 0.25 ng/ml) than non-smokers (0.44 ± 0.16 ng/ml), statistically (p=0.01) (Table 5), there was no relation between smoking and AHI values (p=0.8). Age, BMI, and min SaO_2 during the sleep study were no associated with log-cTnI as given in table 6 (p>0.05, Pearson correlation). When the presence of comorbidity was compared with AHI and cTnI values, there was no statistically significance (p>0.05).

There was a positive correlation between AHI and cTnI levels in patients with OSAS (r=0.276, p=0.019, R^2=0.076, Pearson correlation) (Table 7; Figure 2).

Discussion

This study showed that cardiac troponin I is a detectable marker in OSAS patients and high levels of cTnI might be observed in severe OSAS.

	OSAS subjects	Controls	p
Sex (F/M)	20/27	8/21	0.2
Mean age (year)	52.5 ± 10.5	46.3 ± 10.6	0.01
Body mass index (BMI-kg/m²), mean	31.3 ± 6.4	29.1 ± 5.5	0.1
According to BMI			
Normal	9	5	
Overweight	13	17	
Obesity	19	4	0.03
Morbid obesity	6	3	
Smoking history	19	14	0.6
Co-morbidities			
Hypercholesterolemia	18	11	1.0
Hypertension	12	5	0.5
Diabetes mellitus	7	3	0.7
Arytmia	4	1	0.6
Coronary artery disease	4	1	0.6
Chronic heart failure	1	1	1.0
Polisomnography			
AHI, mean	38.5 ± 36.7	2.1 ± 1.3	0.0
First SaO_2, mean	94.9 ± 1.5	94.8 ± 5.4	0.8
Min SaO_2, mean	74.9 ± 12.2	85.8 ± 6.0	0.0
ECG changes	15	8	0.7
cTnI, mean	3.6 ± 2.7	3.1 ± 1.8	0.3

Table 1: The comparison of OSAS subjects and controls according to the clinical characteristics, polysomnographic findings and mean troponin (cTnI) values.

	Controls	Mild+Moderate OSAS	Severe OSAS	F	p
Age, mean	46.25 ± 10.62	50.30 ± 9.53	55.55 ± 11.15	4.67	**0.012**
Sex					
Female	21	8	12		**0.04**
Male	8	19	8		
Smoking history					
Smokers	14	12	7		0.64
Non-smokers	15	15	13		
BMI, mean	29.06 ± 5.48	29.95 ± 6.19	33.19 ± 6.29	2.98	0.057
ECG changes					
+	8	7	8		0.53
-	21	20	12		
Min SaO_2 on PSG	85.85 ± 6.04	79.37 ± 9.22	68.90 ± 13.32	18.39	0.00
$cTnI_{mean}$ (ng/ml)	3.13 ± 1.83	2.93 ± 1.67	4.57 ± 3.47	3.06	0.053

Table 2: The clinical and laboratory findings in patients with mild-moderate and severe OSAS, and controls (ANOVA test).

	Log-cTnI, mean ± SD	p
OSAS subjects	0.49 ± 0.21	
Controls	0.44 ± 0.19	0.74
Total	0.47 ± 0.21	

Table 3: The comparison of OSAS subjects and controls according to the log-cTnI levels.

	Log-cTnI, mean ± SD	F	p
Mild+Moderate OSAS	0.44 ± 0.19		
Severe OSAS	**0.59 ± 0.22**	4.26	0.018
Controls	0.44 ± 0.19		
Total	0.47 ± 0.21		

Table 4: The evaluation of the OSAS subjects and controls according to the log-cTnI levels.

	Log-cTnI	p
Female	0.42 ± 0.16	0.18
Male	0.50 ± 0.22	
Smokers	0.52 ± 0.25	0.01
Non-smokers	0.44 ± 0.16	
Hypertension		
+	0.53 ± 0.24	0.91
-	0.46 ± 0.20	
ECG changes		
+	0.47 ± 0.17	0.92
-	0.47 ± 0.22	

Table 5: The demographic features according to the Log-cTnI levels in all subjects.

	r	p
Age and Log-cTnI	-0.033	0.78
BMI and Log-cTnI	0.014	0.90
SaO_2 min and Log-cTnI	-0.141	0.24

Table 6: The comparison of age, BMI, min SaO_2 and Log-cTnI in study subjects.

Obstructive sleep apnea syndrome is an important risk factor for cardiovascular diseases [2,3,24-28]. In literature, angina-like symptoms and ischemic changes on electrocardiogram have been detected in patients without CAD previously [1,5,29]. Whether nocturnal ischemic events in patients with OSAS has not been clear adequately, previous studies have suggested that OSAS is associated with myocardial injury without CAD due to possible mechanisms such as repeated hypoxemia and related sympathetic activation [24,30]. Acute hemodynamic changes involving the pulmonary artery and RV during apneic episodes are well

	Log-AHI
Log-cTnI	r=0.28 p=0.019 R^2=0.076

Table 7: The correlation of Log-AHI and Log-cTnI in patients.

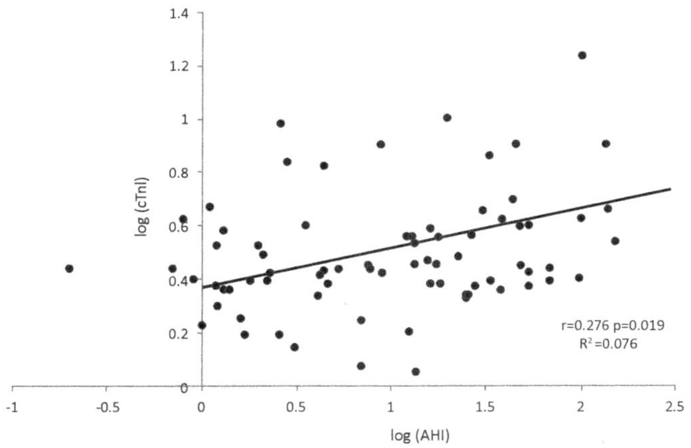

Figure 2: The association of log-AHI and log-cTnI in OSAS subjects.

recognized so far. It is known that pulmonary hypertension and RV dysfunction may occur in OSAS patients due to nocturnal hypoxemia. Hypoxemia-induced endothelial cell dysfunction is a critical factor in pulmonary artery remodeling because of the repeated apnea-related hypoxic events may induce oxidative stress of vascular endothelium [6,8,31-33]. Chronic Intermittent Hypoxia (CIH) is considered to be one of the most important causes of cardiovascular diseases in OSAS patients. The repeated hypoxia and reoxygenation cycle in sleep is similar to hypoxia-reperfusion injury, which initiates oxidative stress. In animal OSA models, there have been shown that CIH induced to myocardial injury, and cardiac troponin I levels was significantly higher in the CIH [34,35]. Thus cTnI levels might be elevated in OSAS patients due to possible factors such as RV dysfunction and repeated nocturnal hypoxemia as reported earlier studies.

The Sleep Heart Health Study showed a modest increase in the odds ratio of coronary artery disease in patients with severe OSAS compared with controls and the other studies showed that patients with OSAS have nocturnal ST segment changes that correlate with oxyhemoglobin desaturation and severity of OSA [5,29,30,36]. In our study, cTnI levels were detected higher in severe OSAS than mild, moderate OSAS and controls, too. This result was compatible with the results of previous studies which ischemic changes were found to be associated with severity of disease. The significant difference in cTnI between mild, moderate and severe OSAS groups considered that myocardial injury induced by repeated nocturnal hypoxemia and apnea-hypopnea. However, there was no statistically significance between nocturnal desaturation during the PSG and cTnI values in our study. In a study which cardiac troponin T levels were studied of 15 OSAS patients without CAD, there was observed that cardiac troponin T levels was not detectable marker in OSAS [37]. In another study performing to establish cardiac damage related to nocturnal ischemia in fifty OSAS patients, cTnI levels were found similar to the controls [38]. However, recently published a study has been shown that high sensitivity cardiac troponin T levels were associated with severity of OSAS [39]. As compatible with this, although cTnI levels were detected similar between OSAS patients and controls, cTnI levels were increased with severity of diseases in our study.

As emphasized in previous studies, myocardial injury without CAD can be detected in OSAS by cardiac troponins or another biomarker [30,33,40]. The presence of any possible contribution of cardiac troponins to the pathophysiology of OSAS because of cardiac troponins might be useful in detection of myocardial injury in patients with OSAS and CAD could be prevented by CPAP therapy in early stage. Considering the cardiovascular morbidity and mortality rates, myocardial injury in OSAS should be diagnosed immediately and the decision of CPAP therapy should be made as early as possible [29,30].

In a recent study which was evaluated the association between severity of OSAS and coronary vasoconstriction there was significant correlation between AHI values and endothelial function of coronary arteries [41]. The results of our study were confirmed to this opinion.

One of the limitations of our study is that histopathologic diagnosis could not be performed for subclinical coronary artery disease in patients. But the patients included to the study had no symptoms suggesting acute coronary syndrome and there was no relation found between troponin I values and existing cardiovascular diseases, statistically. However, further imaging techniques are needed to determine underlying coronary artery disease. Another limitation of our study is that control group consisted of patients who admitted to sleep clinic, therefore may not reflect healthy controls.

In conclusion, high levels of cTnI were observed in severe OSAS. This study has been thought that cardiac troponin I measurements may be may be useful to show the degree of myocardial injury in severe OSAS.

References

1. Epstein LJ, Kristo D, Strollo PJ Jr, Friedman N, Malhotra A, et al. (2009) Clinical guideline for the evaluation, management and long-term care of obstructive sleep apnea in adults. J Clin Sleep Med 5: 263-276.
2. Bradley TD, Floras JS (2009) Obstructive sleep apnoea and its cardiovascular consequences. Lancet 373: 82-93.
3. Bhadriraju S, Kemp CR Jr, Cheruvu M, Badhriraju S (2008) Sleep apnea syndrome: implications on cardiovascular diseases. Crit Pathw Cardiol 7: 248-253.
4. Bananian S, Lehrman SG, Maguire GP (2002) Cardiovascular consequences of sleep-related breathing disorders. Heart Dis 4: 296-305.
5. Koehler U, Dübler H, Glaremin T, Junkermann H, Lubbers C, et al. (1991) Nocturnal myocardial ischemia and cardiac arrhythmia in patients with sleep apnea with and without coronary heart disease. Klin Wochenschr 69: 474-482.
6. Niijima M, Kimura H, Edo H, Shinozaki T, Kang J, et al. (1999) Manifestation of pulmonary hypertension during REM sleep in obstructive sleep apnea syndrome. Am J Respir Crit Care Med 159: 1766-1772.
7. Sanner BM, Konermann M, Sturm A, Müller HJ, Zidek W (1997) Right ventricular dysfunction in patients with obstructive sleep apnoea syndrome. Eur Respir J 10: 2079-2083.
8. Sajkov D, McEvoy RD (2009) Obstructive sleep apnea and pulmonary hypertension. Prog Cardiovasc Dis 51: 363-370.
9. Falahati A, Sharkey SW, Christensen D, McCoy M, Miller EA, et al. (1999) Implementation of serum cardiac troponin I as marker for detection of acute myocardial infarction. Am Heart J 137: 332-337.
10. Nunes JP (2001) Cardiac troponin I in systemic disease. A possible role for myocardial strain. Rev Port Cardiol 20: 785-788.
11. Meyer T, Binder L, Hruska N, Luthe H, Buchwald A (2000) Cardiac troponin I elevation in acute pulmonary embolism is associated with right ventricular dysfunction. J Am Coll Cardiol 36: 1632-1636.
12. Adams JE 3rd, Bodor GS, Davila-Roman VG, Delmez JA, Apple FS, et al. (1993) Cardiac troponin I. A marker with high specificity for cardiac injury. Circulation 88: 101-106.

13. Higgins JP, Higgins JA (2003) Elevation of cardiac troponin I indicates more than myocardial ischemia. Clin Invest Med 26: 133-147.

14. Guest TM, Ramanathan AV, Tuteur PG, Schechtman KB, Ladenson JH, et al. (1995) Myocardial injury in critically ill patients. A frequently unrecognized complication. JAMA 27: 1945-1949.

15. Agzew Y (2009) Elevated serum cardiac troponin in non-acute coronary syndrome. Clin Cardiol 32: 15-20.

16. Roongsritong C, Warraich I, Bradley C (2004) Common causes of troponin elevations in the absence of acute myocardial infarction: incidence and clinical significance. Chest 125: 1877-1884.

17. Giannitsis E, Katus HA (2004) Comparison of cardiac troponin T and troponin I assays--implications of analytical and biochemical differences on clinical performance. Clin Lab 50: 521-528.

18. Berroëta C, Provenchère S, Mongredien A, Lasocki S, Benessiano J, et al. (2006) The use of cardiac troponins (T or I) measurement in cardiology and various clinical settings. Ann Fr Anesth Reanim 25: 1053-1063.

19. Lorenzi-Fillho G, Drager LF (2010) Sleep apnea: why should we look for cardiac biomarkers? J Clin Sleep Med 6: 420-421.

20. Rechtschaffen A, Kales A (1968) A manual of standardized terminology, techniques, and scoring system for sleep stages in human subjects. CA: Brain Information Service, VCLA, Los Angeles.

21. American Sleep Disorders Association (1992) EEG arousals, scoring rules and examples: a preliminary report from the Sleep Disorders Atlas Task Force of the American Sleep Disorders Association. Sleep 15: 173-184.

22. (1999) Sleep-related breathing disorders in adults: Recommendations for syndrome definition and measurement techniques in clinical research. The report of an American Academy of Sleep Medicine Task Force. Sleep 22: 667-689.

23. American Academy of Sleep Medicine (AASM) International Classification of Sleep Disorders. (2ndedn). Westchester IL, AASM, 2005.

24. Khayat R, Patt B, Hayes D Jr (2009) Obstructive sleep apnea: the new cardiovascular disease. Part I: obstructive sleep apnea and the pathogenesis of vascular disease. Heart Fail Rev 14: 143-153.

25. Devulapally K, Pongonis R Jr, Khayat R (2009) OSA: the new cardiovascular disease: part II: Overview of cardiovascular diseases associated with obstructive sleep apnea. Heart Fail Rev 14: 155-164.

26. Parish JM, Somers VK (2004) Obstructive sleep apnea and cardiovascular disease. Mayo Clin Proc 79: 1036-1046.

27. Kato M, Adachi T, Koshino Y, Somers VK (2009) Obstructive sleep apnea and cardiovascular disease. Circ J 73: 1363-1370.

28. Lüthje L, Andreas S (2008) Obstructive sleep apnea and coronary artery disease. Sleep Med Rev 12: 19-31.

29. Hanly P, Sasson Z, Zuberi N, Lunn K (1993) ST-segment depression during sleep in obstructive sleep apnea. Am J Cardiol 71: 1341-1345.

30. Peled N, Abinader EG, Pillar G, Sharif D, Lavie P (1999) Nocturnal ischemic events in patients with obstructive sleep apnea syndrome and ischemic heart disease: effects of continuous positive air pressure treatment. J Am Coll Cardiol 34: 1744-1749.

31. Marrone O, Bonsignore MR (2002) Pulmonary haemodynamics in obstructive sleep apnoea. Sleep Med Rev 6: 175-193.

32. McLaughlin VV, Archer SL, Badesch DB, Barst RJ, Farber HW, et al. (2009) ACCF/AHA 2009 expert consensus document on pulmonary hypertension. A report of the American College of Cardiology Foundation Task Force on Expert Consensus Documents and the American Heart Association developed in collaboration with the American College of Chest Physicians; American Thoracic Society, Inc.; and the Pulmonary Hypertension Association. J Am Coll Cardiol. 53: 1573-1619.

33. Kasasbeh E, Chi DS, Krishnaswamy G (2006) Inflammatory aspects of sleep apnea and their cardiovascular consequences. South Med J 99: 58-67.

34. Liu JN, Zhang JX, Lu G, Qiu Y, Yang D, et al. (2010) The effect of oxidative stress in myocardial cell injury in mice exposed to chronic intermittent hypoxia. Chin Med J (Engl) 123: 74-78.

35. Fletcher EC (2000) Cardiovascular consequences of obstructive sleep apnea: experimental hypoxia and sympathetic activity. Sleep 23: 127–131.

36. Shahar E, Whitney CW, Redline S, Lee ET, Newman AB, et al. (2001) Sleep-disordered breathing and cardiovascular disease: cross-sectional results of the Sleep Heart Health Study. Am J Respir Crit Care Med 163: 19-25.

37. Gami AS, Svatikova A, Wolk R, Olson EJ, Duenwald CJ, et al. (2004) Cardiac troponin T in obstructive sleep apnea. Chest 125: 2097-2100.

38. Oktay B, Akbal E, Firat H, Ardic S, Akdemir R, et al. (2008) Evaluation of the relationship between heart type fatty acid binding protein levels and the risk of cardiac damage in patients with obstructive sleep apnea syndrome. Sleep Breath 12: 223-228.

39. Randby A, Namtvedt SK, Einvik G, Hrubos-Strøm H, Hagve TA, et al. (2012) Obstructive Sleep Apnea is Associated with Increased High-Sensitivity Cardiac Troponin T Levels. Chest 142: 639-646.

40. Kokturk O, Ciftci TU, Mollarecep E, Ciftci B (2005) Elevated C-reactive protein levels and increased cardiovascular risk in patients with obstructive sleep apnea syndrome. Int Heart J 46: 801-809.

41. Kadohira T, Kobayashi Y, Iwata Y, Kitahara H, Komuro I (2011) Coronary Artery Endothelial Dysfunction Associated With Sleep Apnea. Angiology 62: 397-400.

Does CPAP Use in the First 15 Days Predict its Use after 4 Months? A Prospective French Cohort Study

Thibaut Gentina[1], Elodie Gentina[2,*], Catherine Lamblin[1], François Jouniaux[1], François Codron[1] and Aiman Tulaimat[3]

[1]*Hôpital Privé La Louvière, Générale de Santé, Lille, France*

[2]*Skema Business School – Université de Lille, MERCUR Research, France*

[3]*Cook County Health and Hospital Systems, Division of Pulmonary, Critial Care, and Sleep Medicine, USA*

Abstract

Objective: Early prediction of which patients with obstructive sleep apnea will not adhere with CPAP can trigger physicians to correct possible causes or offer alternative therapies. This study aims to determine the ability of early CPAP use to predict long-term adherence with CPAP independent from its definition and to test previously described predictors of adherence.

Method: This is a prospective, observational cohort study that was performed in nine sleep disorder centers in France. Patients were newly diagnosed with obstructive sleep apnea and a CPAP was prescribed for the first time. We collected socioeconomic, medical, sleep, and psychological variables to be associated with adherence with CPAP. The patients were evaluated 15 days after CPAP set up and monthly for 4 months until they were adherent. We assessed potential predictors of CPAP adherence at 4 months with emphasis on CPAP use at 15 days. CPAP adherence was defined as an average daily use of at least 3, 4, 5, and 6 hours.

Results: We enrolled 420 patients. Early CPAP use and CPAP use at 4 months were similar. At 4 months, 94% of patients used a CPAP ≥3 hours and 49% of patients used it ≥6 hours. The area under the ROC curve for early CPAP use predicting adherence at 4 months was ≥0.85 for all adherence definitions. The optimal threshold for early CPAP use to predict adherence increased from 3.2 to 6.4 hours as the definition of CPAP adherence increased from 3 to 6 hours. CPAP use at 4 months was higher in older patients.

Conclusions: Early CPAP use was the single best predictor of CPAP adherence and was independent of how adherence was defined. Physicians must assess CPAP use no later than 2 weeks to address its causes or prescribe an alternative therapy.

Keywords: Obstructive sleep apnea (OSA); Continuous positive airway pressure (CPAP); Adherence; predictors

Introduction

Treatment of obstructive sleep apnea (OSA) with continuous positive airway pressure (CPAP) improves sleep quality, reduces sleepiness, enhances quality of life and reduces cardiovascular morbidities [1-3]. As in most medical conditions, the benefits of therapy are reaped only by adherent patients. Unfortunately, and as in other conditions, adherence to the use of a CPAP is suboptimal. In one study which defined adherence arbitrarily as using a CPAP ≥3 hours on 70% of nights, found that 54% of patients were non-adherent [4]. Understanding the barriers to and predictors of CPAP treatment uptake and long-term adherence is therefore critical for successfully establishing and maintaining patients on effective CPAP treatment [5]. It allows physicians to apply interventions that improve adherence early because waiting until patients declare themselves after few months of treatment to be non-adherent might be too late. It also allows physicians to select the patients that need these interventions instead of applying these interventions to all patients at a much higher cost. Knowing which patients are unlikely to adhere to the use of CPAP also prompts physicians to discuss alternative treatments early [6,7].

Socio-economic factors, disease severity, health problems, psychological variables, social variables, testing methods, side effects, and behavioural traits have been associated with adherence to the use of a CPAP. This large number of variables suggests that adherence is a complex process (Appendix 1).

This complexity underscores some of the limitations of published reports. First, the reports focus on one variable or a limited number of variables to predict CPAP adherence. Second, the samples of many of these studies are small. This not only reduces the generalizability of the findings, but also reduces the number of variables that can be reliably tested. Lastly, the sometimes vaguely described follow-up process of the patients reduces the reproducibility of the findings.

Furthermore, the definitions of adherence are arbitrary. The most frequently used definition is 4 hours per night and it is based on the improvement in consequences of OSA in patients that use CPAP for at least 4 hours. There is, however, growing interest in setting CPAP targets based on a patient needs [8-10].

Therefore, we conducted this study to validate a large number of variables as predictors of the adherence to CPAP use in a large sample of patients that were followed meticulously for 4 months. We focused on early use of CPAP and we defined adherence at 4 months in various ways.

***Corresponding author:** Elodie Gentina, 2SKEMA Business School – Université de Lille, MERCUR Research, France E-mail: elodie.gentina@skema.edu

Materials and Methods

Study design

This prospective cohort study was performed in nine medical centers in the north of France. The protocol was approved by the French Research Ethics Board of The Patient Protection Committee. All patients provided written informed consent before participation.

Study sample

Adult patients (18-75 years old) were recruited from nine centers in France. Each center utilized the same method to recruit and follow their patients in order to avoid any differences between centers (Table 1).

All consecutive patients for whom CPAP had been prescribed for the first time for the treatment of OSA between March 2013 and June 2013 were eligible for the present study. We excluded patients that were cognitively deficient and unable to fill in the questionnaires, patients unable (or refused) to give their informed consent, patients unable to read and/or speak French, and patients with neuromuscular diseases.

Diagnosis of obstructive sleep apnea

The diagnosis was based on a full in-laboratory polysomnogram (PSG) or home sleep test (HST). The PSG was performed with the Alice 5 (Philips, Eindhoven, Netherlands) that included 6 EEG channels, 2 EOG channels, chin EMG, bilateral anterior tibialis EMG, nasal/oral thermister, nasal pressure transducer, chest and abdominal wall movements, EKG, and pulse oximetry. The PSG scoring was standardized across centers. HST was performed with Embletta polygraph (Resmed, San Diego, CA) that included nasal/oral thermister, nasal pressure transducer, chest and abdominal wall movements, heart rate, and pulse oximetry.

Sleep was scored with the Rechtschaffen and Kales criteria. Apneas, hypopneas, and arousals were scored according to the American Academy of Sleep Medicine 2007. The apnea hypopnea index that was calculated by dividing the number of apneas and hypopnea by the total sleep time (recording time for HST) in hours.

Prescription of CPAP

CPAP was prescribed if a patient met 1 of 2 conditions: 1) the apnea-hypopnea index (AHI) ≥30 events per hour, or 2) the AHI index was between 15 and 30 events per hour with respiratory arousal >10 per hour and at least 2 symptoms of OSA symptoms (snoring, choking or gasping during sleep, unrefreshing sleep, daytime fatigue, impaired concentration, or nocturia).

CPAP initiation and monitoring

Patients were seen by sleep physicians in consultation and then referred for a sleep study [11-13]. Because knowledge is a pre-condition for health behavior or a change in health behavior, patient were subjected to a specific educational intervention [14]. Before starting CPAP, each patient was educated by a physician and a technician about the health risk of OSA and about the use of the CPAP machine. Patients also watched a 10-min video about the definition of OSA, symptoms of OSA, CPAP machine, the sensation of wearing CPAP, and benefits of using CPAP [15]. The delay between seeing the physician and the sleep study was 15 days and between the sleep study and starting CPAP was less than 48 hours.

The CPAP devices include counters that measure machine-on time using a microprocessor. Patient adherence data was obtained on day 15 and at the end of the first month. Patients with CPAP use ≥3 hours at the end of the first month were evaluated at the end of fourth months. Patients with CPAP use <3 hours at the end of the first month were visited monthly until they became adherent. During each visit, the average nightly use CPAP hours over the last month was recorded (Table 1).

Data collected

Independent variables: The socio-economic variables were age, gender, marital status (married or living as a couple versus living alone), employment status (fulltime, part-time, or unemployed), type of health insurance (government or government insurance with private health insurance). The health variables were infarction, or arrhythmia. The psychological variables were assessed with two scales: The Pichot scale16 and the Epworth Sleepiness Scale (ESS17). The Pichot scale is divided in 2 subscales: depression (13 items) and fatigue (8 items). The ESS measures the level of sleepiness (8 items). OSA related variables were method of diagnosing OSA (PSG or HST), the apnea-hypopnea index (AHI), average nightly use of CPAP in the first 15 days (early CPAP use).

Dependent variable: Adherence was monitored using the smart card technology embedded in the CPAP machines and was defined as the average nightly use of CPAP at the set pressure.

Statistical analysis

To determine the ability of early CPAP use in predicting adherence with CPAP at 4 months, we calculated the area under the receiver operator characteristic curve (AU-ROC) for 4 adherence definitions (3, 4, 5, 6 hours).We determined the optimal thresholds of early CPAP use to predict adherence based on the Youden Index and calculated the sensitivity (Sn) and specificity (Sp) for these thresholds. We also determined, at each definition of adherence, the thresholds of early CPAP use that had a sensitivity of 90% (Sn90) or a specificity of 90% (Sp90). Bias-corrected bootstrapping of 1000 iterations was used to determine these thresholds and their confidence intervals.

The French government reimburses patients for CPAP if they use it for more than 3 hours per night. Therefore, we used the 3-hour definition for the rest of the analysis, with patients using CPAP ≥ 3 hours per day considered as adherent, patients using CPAP <3 hours considered as non-adherent.

We compared between adherent and non-adherent patients all other variables available for the physician before initiating CPAP (pre-CPAP predictors). We used the t-test or chi-squared as indicated by the data type. Differences were significant if the p value is ≤0.05. We tested the significant pre-CPAP predictors with early CPAP use in a multiple regression analysis to determine the smallest number of independent predictors of adherence.

Results

Patients

We give the study questionnaire to 465 patients: 429 patients responded, 9 were lost during the follow-up, and 420 patients were included in the final analysis (useable response rate of 92%). Most patients were men, obese, and had severe sleep apnea. The majority of patients had private insurance in addition to government insurance (Table 2).

Adherence CPAP use: early CPAP use (5.6 ± 2.0 hours) and CPAP use at 4 months (5.7 ± 1.7 hours) were similar, p=0.09. The correlation

Visit	Patients	Where	Personnel	What was done	Education
CPAP set up	All patients	Clinic	Physician	Questionnaire	A 15-min video about the definition of OSA, symptoms of OSA, CPAP machine, the sensation of wearing CPAP, and benefits of using CPAP. Discussion and demonstration
Visit 15 days	All patients	Home	Technician	Early CPAP use	Individualized and face to face education and specific information about OSA, performance, treatment relevance, symptom change with CPAP, troubleshooting advice... A written document on CPAP was provided Demonstration of the Website "Elia Medical Education http://eliamedical-education.com/
First month	All patients	Clinic	Physician	CPAP use	Discussion, demonstration and support
Second month	Non-adherent first month	Home	Technician	CPAP use	Discussion, demonstration and support
Third month	Non-adherent second month	Home	Technician	CPAP use	Discussion, demonstration and support
Fourth month	All patients	Clinic	Physician	CPAP use	Discussion, demonstration and support

Table 1: Visit types during the 1-4 month study.

between early CPAP use and CPAP use at 4 months was high (r=0.71, p<0.001). The linear regression equation for CPAP was use at 4 months (hours)=2.2 + 0.6 × early use of CPAP (hours).

Early CPAP use was equally predictive of use of CPAP at 4 months no matter what the threshold was (Table 3 and Figure 1). The accuracy of early CPAP in predicting adherence changed with the type of insurance. The AU-ROC was higher when patients had only government insurance than when they had additional private insurance (4-hours: 0.95 ± 0.04 versus 0.86 ± 0.02, p=0.04; 5-hours: 0.92 ± 0.06 versus 0.85 ± 0.02, p=0.2; 6-hours: 0.96 ± 0.03 versus 0.83 ± 0.02, p=0.002). We did not evaluate the 3 hours adherence because the sample was two small. The accuracy of early CPAP use in predicting adherence at 4 months was not affected by ESS, age, gender, employment, or marital status.

As the threshold to define CPAP adherence increased from 3 hours to 4 hours, the optimal threshold of early CPAP use increased, then was stable for adherence defined as 4 or 5 hours, and then increased again for adherence define as 6 hours. The ranges of thresholds for Sn90 (3.3-4.6 hours) and for Sp90 (5.5-6.5 hours) were narrow.

When the definition of adherence changes, the distribution of adherence status (remained adherent, became non-adherent, remained non-adherent, became adherent) at 4 months changes. When we used the same threshold to define adherence at 15 days and at 4 months, increasing the threshold for adherence from 3 to 6 hours increased the percentage of patients that remain non-adherent at 4 months and decreased the percentage remained adherent over the 4 month (Figure 2).

Pre-CPAP predictors of adherence at 4 months

Adherent patients were older than non-adherent patients (57 ± 12 versus 49 ± 11, p=0.002). The AU-ROC curve for age as a predictor of adherence was 0.67 and the optimal threshold was 53 years with a sensitivity of 0.62 and a specificity of 0.67. The threshold for a specificity of 90% was 67.

We divided patients into 2 groups: older patients>53 years (252 patients), and younger patients ≤ 53 years (168 patients). In comparison to the older patients, the younger patients had a higher BMI (34 ± 7 versus 31 ± 6), had a higher Pichot fatigue score (15 ± 8 versus 14 ± 8, p=0.01), and a higher ESS score (11, IQR 8-15 versus 10, IQR 6-14, p=0.03), and they used CPAP slightly less in the first 15 days (0.5 ± 0.2 hours). There was also a weak but significant correlation between the Pichot fatigue score and the drop in CPAP use from 15 days to 4 months (r=0.1, p=0.036).

When age and early use of CPAP were entered in a logistic regression, age became non-significant and early use of CPAP was the only predictor of adherence at 4 months. The odds ratio associated with every hour of early CPAP use for predicting CPAP adherence at 4 months was 2.1 (95% CI: 1.6-2.7, p<0.001). On the other hand, in a linear regression model with the hours of CPAP use as the dependent variable, age and early CPAP use were significant and the regression equation was CPAP use at 4 months=1.5+ [early CPAP use in hours × 0.62] + [age in years×0.01].

There was no correlation between CPAP use at 4 months and ESS (r=-0.05, p=0.3) or between CPAP use and AHI (r=0.09, p=0.06). Similarly, none of the other pre-CPAP variables (including the methods of diagnosing OSA) was associated with CPAP use at 4 months.

Discussion

In this relatively large sample of patient with OSA that was followed closely for 4 months, we found that early CPAP use was the strongest predictor of adherence at 4 months independent of its definition. Of the variables available for the physician before starting CPAP, age was the only variable associated, though weakly, with CPAP adherence at 4 months.

Our results complement the results reported by others that long-term CPAP adherence patterns are often established within the first weeks of therapy [15-18]. Budhiraj et al. [12] reported that CPAP use by the third day was predictive of CPAP use at 30 days. Popescu et al. [13] reported that CPAP use in the first 2 weeks predicts CPAP adherence at 1 year. Chai-Coetzer et al. [19] reported that adherence at one month predicted CPAP adherence at 1 year. McArdle et al. [5] reported that CPAP use at 3 months predicts adherence after 2 years. This composite of evidence suggests that adherence to CPAP use must be evaluated early and continuously after initiating therapy.

A novel and interesting finding of our study was the relationship between the area under the ROC curve for early CPAP use and the insurance type. It has been shown in the past that socioeconomic status (especially poverty) is associated with CPAP use (see appendix). In our study, early CPAP use was more predictive of long-term use in patients with government only (suggestive lower income). The type of insurance was not, however, associated the adherence itself. This finding deserves

Socio-economic variables	
Men, %	70
Age, years	56 ± 12
Married, %	78
Fully employed, %	59
Government insurance with private health insurance,%	94
Health variables	
Body mass index, kg/m^2	32 ± 6
Treated Hypertension, %	49
Heart disease (arrhythmia or congestive heart failure),%	12
Stroke,%	12
Myocardial infarction, %	11
Loss of libido, %	32
OSA related variables	
AHI	46 ± 19
Diagnosis made with HST, %	38
Daily CPAP use in the first 15 days	5.6±2
Psychological Variables	
Epworth Sleepiness Scale	10.7 ± 5
Pichot Fatigue Scale	14.2 ± 7
Pichot Depression Scale	4.7 ± 4

Table 2: Baseline characteristics of the patients at the onset of CPAP therapy (n=420).

Definition of adherence at 4 months	Adherence at 4 month based on definition	Threshold at 15 days	Sn	Sp	Sn_{90}	Sp_{90}
3 hours	94%	3.2 (2.2-3.9)	91%	70%	3.3	6.0
4 hours	81%	5.4 (3.3-5.6)	72%	86%	3.8	5.5
5 hours	69%	5.5 (5.1-5.5)	77%	83%	4.2	6.2
6 hours	49%	6.4 (5.7-6.8)	66%	89%	4.6	6.5

Table 3: The percentage of adherent patients at various definitions at four months, the optimal threshold of early use (15 days) to predict adherence based on bootstrap analysis, its sensitivity and specificity, and the threshold of early CPAP use with sensitivity of 90% (Sn_{90}) and specificity of 90% (Sp_{90}).

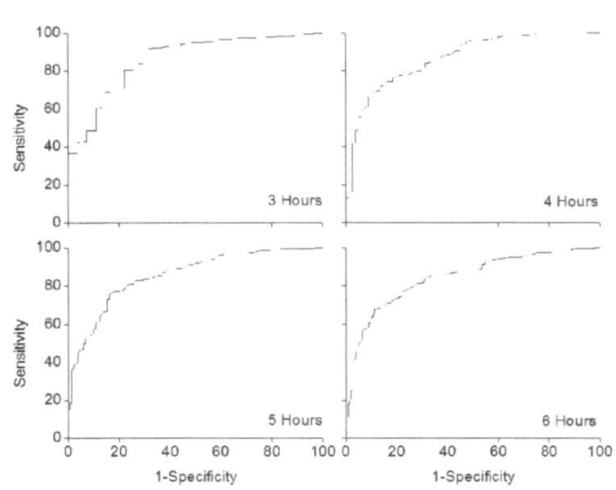

Figure 1: ROC curves for early CPAP use predicting adherence at the 4 thresholds at 4 months. The area was 0.86 (0.82-0.89) for 3 hours, 0.87 (0.83-0.89) for 4 hours, 0.86 (0.82-0.88) for 5 hours, and 0.85 (0.81-0.88) for 6 hours.

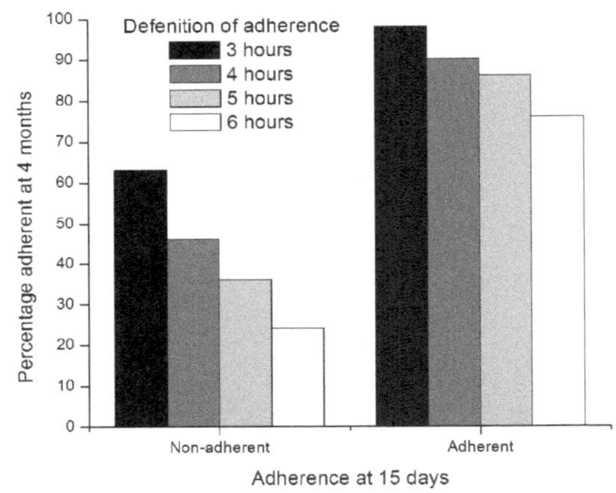

Figure 2: The relation between adherence on day 15 (x-axis) and adherence at 4 months defined with the same hours of CPAP use. When patients were non-adherent at 15 days, they are unlikely to be adherent at 4 months with a decreasing chance of adherence as the threshold for adherence increases. When patients were adherent at 15 days, the were likely to be adherent at 4 month but with a decreasing likelihood as the threshold for adherence increased; but, the lowest adherence rate, which was with a threshold of 6 hours, was still >70%.

further evaluation because it might reflect a motive behind the use of CPAP such as employment for drivers or just to avoid monetary penalty for not using CPAP.

Because the definition of CPAP adherence is arbitrary and studies have used definitions varying between 2 and 6 hours, we tested 3, 4, 5, and 6 hour thresholds. The AU- ROC curve for early CPAP use predicting later adherence was similar between all definitions of adherence. Therefore, our conclusions can be extended to settings where the criterion of adherence is different from that used in France, especially since Chai-Coetzer and colleagues have shown that the relation between early use and long-term adherence is independent from country [19].

Currently most clinicians rely on a single definition to identify patients not adherent to CPAP use. In the United States, patients are considered adherent if they use a CPAP for more than 4 hours most night of the week. This definition of adherence is required by Medicare to pay for CPAP. Nevertheless, to achieve maximal alertness and cognitive functioning, a reduction in carbon dioxide in patients with obesity hypoventilation syndrome, or a reduction in blood pressure, a patient must use a CPAP for more than 6 hours a day [20-22]. The thresholds we identified can help physicians predict if a patient will meet the required CPAP use. Therefore, for example, if a patient was a commercial driver that required maximal cognitive functioning, early CPAP use of less than 6.5 hours would be concerning and less than 4.5 hours would be very concerning.

Predicting non-adherent patients early helps physicians select patients that need attention and intensive follow-up. Of the patients that were using CPAP ≥3 hours in the first two weeks, 98% were using it ≥3 hours at 4 months. On the other hand, 37% of the patients that were using CPAP < 3 hours at 15 days were still using it <3 hours at 4 months. Thus, when the desired dose of CPAP use is low, only patients with very low early use should probably be followed closely for the first few months.

Variable	This study
Socio-economic variables	
Age [12,13]	Confirmed
Gender [30]	Not confirmed
Marital status [26,30]	Not confirmed
Employment status [26,31]	Not confirmed
Type of health insurance [32]	Not confirmed
Race [33]	Not tested
Life events [34]	Not tested
Health variables	
Treated Hypertension [35]	Not confirmed
Heart disorders [4]	Not confirmed
BMI [13,36]	Not confirmed
Stroke [37]	Not confirmed
Myocardial infarction [38]	Not confirmed
Nasal anatomy [39]	Not tested
Psychological or behavioural variables	
Epworth Sleepiness [17]	Not confirmed
Pichot Fatigue Scale [40]	Not confirmed
Pichot Depression scale [16]	Not confirmed
Self-efficacy [27,28]	Not tested
Coping-styles [41]	Not tested
Locus of control [29]	Not tested
Initial CPAP exposure variables	
CPAP use in the first 15 days [4,13]	Confirmed
Diagnosed with HST [42]	Not confirmed
AHI [43]	Not confirmed
Social variables	
Spousal involvement [27,44]	Not tested
Bed partner sleep quality [45,46]	Not tested
Technical variable	
Mask-interface [47]	Not tested
Heated vs. cold pass-over humidity [48]	Not tested
Flexible pressure on CPAP (C-Flex vs continuous positive airway pressure) [49]	Not tested
Claustrophobia [50]	Not tested
Side effect [19]	Not tested

Table 4: Summary of variables from prior studies on significant predictors of CPAP.

In contrast, 76% of patients using a CPAP more than 6 hours at 15 days were still doing so at 4 months and only 24% of patients using a CPAP less than 6 hours increased above this threshold. Therefore, when the desired dose of CPAP is high, as in drivers and patients with obesity hypoventilation, all patient should be followed closely.

Age was the only pre-CPAP variable predictor of adherence: older patients were more likely to use a CPAP than younger patients. Sin et al. [23] reported a similar relation between age and CPAP adherence. In fact they reported that CPAP use increased by 0.24 hours per decade, while in our study it was 0.34 hours in a univariate regression and 0.1 hours after adjustment for early CPAP use. Similarly, Budhiraja et al. [12] showed that adherent (defined as >4 hours) patients were on average 3 years older than non-adherent patients. If we use the 4 hour definition, adherent patients were 8 years older.

Although they were more fatigued and sleepy, younger patients used a CPAP less than older ones. This profile is similar to that report by Pepin et al. [24] as a predictor of residual sleepiness after treatment with a CPAP. Because of the correlation between the Pichot fatigue score and the drop in CPAP use from 15 days to 4 months, it is plausible that these young, fatigued patients gradually reduced their CPAP use because they did not feel better with it. This observation is also concerning because younger patients will live longer than older ones, and if they remain non-adherent, they are likely to suffer cardiovascular complications at a younger age, further leading to a larger societal impact of OSA.

Many investigators have reported that AHI [4,13] and the ESS4, [25] predicted adherence. We did not find such a relationship. This is not due to spectrum bias because the distribution of both AHI and ESS were wide. A larger sample size might have resulted in a weak correlation between AHI and adherence, but it would have been too weak to be useful predictor. Yet, patients with high AHI and ESS should receive special attention from physicians because they are more likely to benefit when they adhere to CPAP use than patients with lower AHI or ESS.

This study has two particular strengths. First, the sample is relatively large (only 5 other studies included more than 500 patients) and the patients were recruited from multiple centers. This allowed us to simultaneously test a large number of variables previously tested by other investigators (Table 4). Second, the patients were followed monthly if they remained non-adherent and at 4 months. In comparison, the study by Gagnadoux et al. [26] included more than 1000 patients that were followed at the end of the first week, and then at the end of the third month. The follow-up was not regular or based on adherence. Another study from Sin et al. [23] provided a very detailed follow-up of the patients but the sample was small.

Follow-up and adherence in this study was higher than what is reported by others. Two reasons might explain this observation. First, the study had a dedicated physician who was specifically involved in the coordination of data collection to monitor the quality of the collection processing. Second, the French government reimbursed patients for CPAP use if they used it for more than 3 hours per night, which encouraged the patients to use the CPAP. This is slightly different from reimbursement in the United States where Medicare purchases the CPAP machine once the patients is deemed adherent. In fact, the relationship between the accuracy of early CPAP use in predicting adherence and the type of insurance suggests that the reimbursement mechanism might play a role in the change in adherence between the first 15 days and 4 months.

There are several limitations in this study. The first limitation is that we did not test side effects. Early complaints of side effects have previously been associated with long-term non-adherence with CPAP [19]. We assume that they were addressed with the patients during the frequent visits and should have been resolved by the fourth months of follow-up. The second limitation is that we did not test coping, locus of control, and self-efficacy, which have previously been shown to predict adherence [19,20,21,26-29]. They are probably mechanisms that lead to early non-adherence that ultimately continues long-term. Once a patient is identified early on to be at risk of non-adherence, the clinician must evaluate that patient's coping and self-efficacy. Lastly, our follow-up was 4 months only. The longer the follow-up, the more events that can affect adherence: seasonal allergy, mask failure, change work hours, etc. The 4 four month follow-up is probably optimal to reduce external events that can affect adherence.

In conclusion, CPAP use in the first 15 days is the best predictor of adherence to the use of a CPAP at 4 months and it was more accurate in patients than in government only insured patients. The threshold of early CPAP use should be adjusted based on the desired long term adherence. These observations might assist physicians identify early the patients that will not meets their target of CPAP use and these patients will be suitable for intensive follow-up or alternative therapy.

Contributions

Study conception and design: Thibaut Gentina. Thibaut Gentina designed the research plan and organized the study.

Acquisition of data: François Jounieaux, Catherine Lamblin and François Codron developed the methodology, participated in the collection of data and coordinated the data-analysis.

Analysis and interpretation of data: Elodie Dancoine and Aiman Tulaimat performed the analyses.

Drafting of manuscript: Thibaut Gentina, Elodie Dancoine and Aiman Tulaimat contributed to the writing of the manuscript.

Critical revision: Elodie Dancoine and Aiman Tulaimat.

Acknowledgment

1. Elia Medical (Manufacture and Installation of Medical-Surgical EquipmentaAnd Instruments) by supporting financially this research.

Elia Medical, 11 Avenue Léon Blum, 59370 Mons-en-Barœul, France.

2. Bernard DOUAY by supporting his help in the coordination of the mouse work.

3. Doctors by supporting their help in collecting data: François FORTIN, Lille (59), Jean Marc DERNIS, Lille (59), Marc BURE, Lille (59), Arnaud PRIGENT, Rennes (35), Christophe VERKINDRE, Béthune (62), Pierre Marie BROUSSIER, Bois Guillaume (76), Jean-Jacques GRES, Havre (76), Dominique GUFFROY, Maubeuge (59), Jamal KABBANI, Chelles (77), Laurent KEDZIORA, Denain (59).

Conflict of Interest

There is not conflict of interest in this research.

References

1. Meslier N, Lebrun T, Grillier-Lanoir V, Rolland C, Henderick JC, et al. (1998) A French survey of 3225 patients treated with CPAP for obstructive sleep apnoea: benefits, tolerance, compliance and quality of life. European Respiratory Journal 12: 185-92.
2. Bazzano LA, Khan Z, Reynolds K, He J (2007) Effect of nocturnal nasal continuous positive airway pressure on blood pressure in obstructive sleep apnea. Hypertension 50: 417-423.
3. Marin JM, Carrizo SJ, Vicente E, Agusti AG (2005) Long-term cardiovascular outcomes in men with obstructive sleep apnoea-hypopnoea with or without treatment with continuous positive airway pressure: an observational study. Lancet 365: 1046-1053.
4. McArdle N, Devereux G, Heidarnejad H, Engleman HM, Mackay T, et al. (1999) Long-term use of CPAP therapy for sleep apnoea-hypopnoea syndrome. American Journal of Respiratory and Critical Care Medicine 159: 1108-1114.
5. Bouloukaki I, Giannądaki K, Mermigkis C, Tzanakis N, Mauroudi E, et al. (2014) Intensive versus standard follow-up to improve continuous positive airway pressure compliance. Eur Respir J 44: 1262-1274.
6. Chan AS, Lee RW, Cistulli PA (2008) Non positive airway pressure modalities: mandibular advancement devices/ positional therapy. Proceedings of the American Thoracic Society 5: 179-184.
7. Won CH, Li KK, Guilleminault C (2008) Surgical treatment of obstructive sleep apnea upper airway and maxillomandibular surgery. Proceedings of the American Thoracic Society 5: 193-199.
8. Rosenthal L, Gerhardstein R, Lumley A, Guido P, Day R, et al. (2000) CPAP therapy in patients with mild OSA: implementation and treatment outcome. Sleep Med 1: 215-220.
9. Mortimore IL, Kochlar P, Douglas NJ (1996) Effect of chronic continuous positive airway pressure (CPAP) therapy on upper airway size in patients with sleep apnoea/ hypopnoea syndrome. Thorax 51: 190-192.
10. Weaver TE, Maislin G, Dinges DF, Bloxham T, George CF, et al. (2007) Relationship between hours of CPAP use and achieving normal levels of sleepininess and daily functioning. Sleep 30: 711-719.
11. Boquillon A (2013) L'apnée du sommeil: les patients en colère. L'Express. http://www.lexpress.fr/actualite/societe/sante/l-apnee-du-sommeil-les-patients-en-colere_1215626.html#JM8ikBekF08wBU7y.99.
12. Budhiraja R, Parthasarathy S, Drake CL, Roth T, Sharief I, et al. (2007) Early CPAP use identifies subsequent adherence to CPAP therapy. Sleep 30: 320-324.
13. Popescu G, Latham M, Allhar V, Elliott MW (2001) Continuous positive airway pressure for sleep apnoea/hypopnoea syndrome: usefulness of a 2 week trial to identify factors associated with long term use. Thorax 56: 727-733.
14. Bandura A (1977) Self-efficacy: Toward a unifying theory of behavioral change. Psychological Review 84: 191-215.
15. Wiese HJ, Boethel C, Phillips B, Wilson JF, Peters J, et al. (2005) CPAP compliance: Video education may help! Sleep Medicine 6: 171-174.
16. Pichot P, Boyer P, Pull CB, Rein W, Simon M, et al. (1984) Un questionnaire d'auto-évaluation de la symptomatologie dépressive: le QD2. Construction, structure factorielle, propriétés métrologiques. Revue de Psychologie Appliquée 3: 229-250.
17. Johns MW. The Epworth Sleepiness Scale: The official website of the Epworth Sleepiness
18. Aloia MS, Arnedt JT, Stanchina M, Millman RP, (2007) How early in treatment is PAP adherence established? Revisiting night-to-night variability. Behavioral Sleep Medicine 5: 229–240.
19. Chai-Coetzer CL, Luo YM, Antic NA, Zhang XL, Chen BY, et al. (2013) Predictors of long-term adherence to continuous positive airway pressure therapy in patients with obstructive sleep apnea and cardiovascular disease in the SAVE study. Sleep 36: 1929-1937.
20. Martínez-García MA, Campos-Rodríguez F, Soler-Cataluña JJ, Catalán-Serra P, Román-Sánchez P, et al. (2012) Increased incidence of nonfatal cardiovascular events in stroke patients with sleep apnoea: effect of CPAP treatment. Eur Respir J 39: 906-912.
21. Babak M, Tulaimat, Evans AT, Wang Y, Itania AA, et al. (2006) Impact of adherence with positive airway pressure therapy on hypercapnia in obstructive sleep apnea. Journal of Clinical Sleep Medicine 2: 57-62.
22. Antic NA, Catcheside P, Buchan C, Hensley M, Naughton MT, et al. (2011) The effect of CPAP in normalizing daytime sleepiness, quality of life, and neurocognitive function in patients with moderate to severe OSA. Sleep 34: 111-119.
23. Sin DD, Mayers I, Man GC, Pawluk L (2002) Long-term compliance rates to continuous positive airway pressure in obstructive sleep apnea: A population-based study. Chest 121: 430–435.
24. Pepin JL, Viot-Blanc V, Escourrou P, Racineux JL, Sapene M, et al. (2009) Prevalence of residual excessive sleepiness in CPAP-treated sleep apnoea patients: the French multicentre study. European Respiratory Journal 33: 1062-1067.
25. Krieger J, Kurtz D, Petiau C, Sforza E, Trautmann D (1996) Long-term compliance with CPAP therapy in obstructive sleep apnea patients and in snorers. Sleep 19: S136-143.
26. Gagnadoux F, Le Vaillant M, Goupil F, Chollet S, Masson P, et al. (2011) Influence of marital status and employment status on long-term adherence with continuous positive airway pressure in sleep apnea patients. Plos One 6: 225-303.
27. Baron KG, Berg CA, Czajkowski LA, Smith TW, Gunn H, et al. (2011) Self-efficacy contributes to individual differences in subjective improvements using CPAP. Sleep & Breathing 15: 599-606.
28. Sawyer AM, Canamucio A, Moriarty H, Weaver TE, Richards KC, et al. (2011) Do cognitive perceptions influence CPAP use? Patient Educ Couns 85: 85-91.
29. de Zeeuw J, Baberg HT, Duchna HW, Kempkens DJ, Walther JW, et al. (2007) [Locus of control belief is a predictor of CPAP-compliance in patients with obstructive sleep apnea syndrome]. Pneumologie 61: 283-290.
30. Ye L, Pien GW, Ratcliffe SJ, Weaver TE (2009) Gender differences in obstructive sleep apnea and treatment response to continuous positive airway pressure. Journal of Clinincal Sleep Medicine 5: 512–518.

31. Platt AB, Field SH, Asch DA, Chen Z, Patel NP, et al. (2009) Neighborhood of residence is associated with daily adherence to CPAP therapy. Sleep 32: 799–806.

32. Hoffstein V, V iner S, Mateika S, Conway J (1992) Treatment of obstructive sleep apnea with nasal continuous positive air way pressure. Patient compliance, perception of benefits, and side effects. American Review of Respiratory Disease 145: 745-841.

33. Scharf S, Seiden L, DeMore J, Carter-Pokras O (2004) Racial differences in clinical presentation of patients with sleep-disordered breathing. Sleep & Breathing 8: 173–183.

34. Lewis KE, Seale L, Bartle IE, Watkins AJ, Ebden P (2004) Early predictors of CPAP use for the treatment of obstructive sleep apnea. Sleep 27: 134-138.

35. Phillips B, Shafazand S (2013) CPAP and hypertension in nonsleepy patients. J Clin Sleep Med 9: 181-182.

36. Redenius R, Murphy C, O'Neill E, Al-Hamwi M, Zallek SN (2008) Does CPAP lead to change in BMI? J Clin Sleep Med 4: 205-209.

37. Palombini L, Guilleminault C (2006) Stroke and treatment with nasal CPAP. Eur J Neurol 13: 198-200.

38. Hung J, Whitford EG, Parsons RW, Hillman DR (1990) Association of sleep apnea with myocardial infarction. Lancet 336: 261-264.

39. Sugiura T, Noda A, Nakata S, Yasuda Y, Soga T, et al. (2007) Influence of nasal resistance on initial acceptance of continuous positive airway pressure in treatment for obstructive sleep apnea syndrome. Respiration 74: 56–60.

40. Low Y Preud'homme X, Goforth HW, Omonuwa T, Krystal AD (2011) The association of fatigue with depression and insomnia in HIV-seropositive patients: a pilot study. Sleep 34: 1723-1726.

41. Stepnowsky CJ Jr, Bardwell WA, Moore PJ, Ancoli-Israel S, Dimsdale JE (2002) Psychologic correlates of compliance with continuous positive airway pressure. Sleep 25: 758-762.

42. Lettieri CF, Lettieri CJ, Carter K (2011) Does home sleep testing impair continuous positive airway pressure adherence in patients with obstructive sleep apnea? Chest 139: 849-854.

43. Meurice J, Dore P, Paquereau J, Neau JP, Ingrand P, et al. (1994) Predictive factors of long-term compliance with nasal continuous positive airway pressure treatment in sleep apnea syndrome. Chest 105: 429–433.

44. Ye L, Malhotra A, Kayser K, Willis DG, Horowitz JA, et al. (2015) Spousal involvement and CPAP adherence: A dyadic perspective. Sleep Medicine Reviews 19: 67-74.

45. McArdle N, Kingshott R, Engleman HM, Mackay TW, Douglas NJ (2001) Partners of patients with sleep apnoea/hypopnoea syndrome: effect of CPAP treatment on sleep quality and quality of life. Thorax 56: 513-518.

46. Parish JM, Lyng PJ (2003) Quality of life in bed partners of patients with obstructive sleep apnea or hypopnea after treatment with continuous positive airway pressure. Chest 124: 942-947.

47. Mortimore IL, Whittle AT, Douglas NJ (1998) Comparison of nose and face mask CPAP therapy for sleep apnoea. Thorax 53: 290-292.

48. Massie C, Hart R, Peralez K, Richards G (1999) Effects of humidification on nasal symptoms and compliance in sleep apnea patients using continuous positive airway pressure. Chest 116: 403-408.

49. Aloia MS, Stanchina M, Arnedt JT, Malhotra A, Millman RP (2005) Treatment adherence and outcomes in flexible vs standard continuous positive airway pressure therapy. Chest 127: 2085-2093.

50. Chasens ER, Pack AI, Maislin G, Dinges DF, Weaver TE (2005) Claustrophobia and adherence to CPAP treatment. West J Nurs Res 27: 307-321.

Appendix 1

Reference	Factors associated with compliance	Country	Sample (n)	threshold value to be adherent (/ night)
	Socio-economic variables			
Mc Ardle et al. (1999)[1]	Age	U.K.	1211	2 hours
Krieger et al. (1996)[2]	Age	France	728	4 hours
Budhiraja et al. (2007)[3]	Age, race	U.S.	100	4 hours
Olsen et al. (2008)[4]	Age	Australia	77	2 hours
Popescu et al. (2001)[5]	Age, gender	England	209	
Sin et al. (2002)[6]	Age, gender	Canada	296	4 hours
Simon-Tuval et al. (2009)[7]	Age, monthly income	Israel	162	Not indicated
Young et al. (1993)[8]	Gender	U.S.	602	4 hours
Pelletier et al. (2001)[9]	Gender	France	163	3 hours
Lewis et al. (2004)[10]	Gender, marital status, life event	United Kingdom	82	4 hours
Ye et al. (2009)[11]	Gender	7 sleep centers in the U.S. and Canada	176	4 hours
Bakker et al.[12]	Age, gender, ethnicity, education, employment, annual income, type of health insurance, health literacy	New Zealand	126	4 hours
Ye et al. (2012)[13]	Marital status, race	U.S.	91	4 hours
Gagnadoux et al. (2011)[14]	Marital status, employment status	France	1141	4 hours
Scharf et al. (2004)[15]	Race	U.S.	128	Not indicated
Billings et al. (2011)[16]	Race	U.S.	191	2 hours
Platt et al. (2009)[17]	Race, employment status, Neighborhood of residence	U.S.	266	4hours
Hoffstein et al. (1992)[18]	Type of health insurance	U.S.	96	4 hours

Reference	Factors associated with compliance	Country	Sample (n)	threshold value to be adherent (/ night)
		health variables		
Popescu et al. (2001)[5]	BMI	England	209	2 hours
Krieger et al. (1996)[2]	BMI	France	728	4 hours
Young et al. (1993)[8]	BMI	U.S.	602	4 hours
Pelletier et al. (2001)[9]	BMI	France	163	3 hours
Gagnadoux et al. (2011)[14]	BMI	France	1141	4 hours
Loredo et al. (2007)[19]	BMI, heart disorder	U.S.	76	6 hours
Wild et al. (2004)[20]	BMI	United Kingdom	119	3 hours
Olsen et al. (2008)[4]	BMI	Australia	77	4 hours
Redenius et al. (2008)[21]	BMI	U.S.	309	4 hours
Sugiera et al. (2007)[22]	BMI	Japan	77	5 hours
Reishten et al. (2010)[23]	Erectile dysfunction	U.S. and Canada	123	Not indicated
Margel et al. (2005)[24]	Erectile dysfunction	Israel	60	Not indicated
Mc Ardle et al. (1999)[1]	Treated Hypertension, heart disorder	U.K.	1211	2 hours
Hung et al. (1990)[25]	Treated Hypertension, myocardial infarction	Australia	101	Not indicated
Philips et al. (2013)[26]	Treated Hypertension	Spain	725	4 hours
Palombini et al. (2006)[27]	Stroke	Italy	50	4 hours
Martínez-García et al. (2012)[28]	Stroke, myocardial infarction	Italy	223	4 hours

Reference	Factors associated with compliance	Country	Sample (n)	threshold value to be adherent (/night)
		osa related variables		
Mc Ardle et al. (1999)[1]	AHI	U.K.	1211	2 hours
Popescu et al. (2001)[5]	AHI	England	209	2 hours
Krieger et al. (1996)[2]	AHI	France	728	4 hours
Pelletier et al. (2001)[9]	AHI	France	163	3 hours
Gagnadoux et al. (2011)[14]	AHI	France	1141	4 hours
Wild et al. (2004)[20]	AHI	United Kingdom	119	3 hours
Palombini et al. (2006)[27]	AHI	Italy	50	4 hours
Hui et al. (2001)[29]	AHI	China	112	4 hours
Krieger (1992)[30]	AHI	France	233	Not indicated
Meurice et al. (1994)[31]	AHI	France	44	5 hours
Bollig (2010)[32]	AHI	Synthetical article		
Baron et al. (2011)[33]	AHI	U.S.	31	Not indicated
Hoffstein et al. (1992)[18]	Minimum nasal cross-sectional area + reduced volume	U.S.	96	4 hours
Sugiera et al. (2007)[22]	AHI, Minimum nasal cross-sectional area + reduced volume	Japan	77	5 hours
Morris et al. (2006)[34]	Minimum nasal cross-sectional area + reduced volume	U.S.	34	Not indicated
Fletcher et al. (1991)[35]	Minimum nasal cross-sectional area + reduced volume	U.S.	Not indicated	Not indicated
Bakker et al. (2011)[12]	AHI	USA	126	4 hours
Simon-Tuval et al. (2009)[7]	AHI	Israel	162	Not indicated

Reference	Factors associated with compliance	Country	Sample (n)	threshold value to be adherent (/ night)
		psychological/ behavioral variables		
Mc Ardle et al. (1999)[1]	Epworth Sleepiness, Pichot Fatigue Scale	U.K.	1211	2 hours
Krieger et al. (1996)[2]	Epworth Sleepiness	France	728	4 hours
Pelletier et al. (2001)[9]	Epworth Sleepiness	France	163	3 hours
Lewis et al. (2004)[10]	Epworth Sleepiness	United Kingdom	82	4 hours
Ye et al. (2012)[11]	Epworth Sleepiness	U.S.	91	4 hours
Sin et al. (2002)[6]	Epworth Sleepiness, self-efficacy	Canada	296	4 hours

Loredo et al. (2007)[19]	Epworth Sleepiness	U.S.	76	6 hours
Wild et al. (2004)[20]	Epworth Sleepiness, self-efficacy	United Kingdom	119	3 hours
Meurice et al. (1994)[31]	Epworth Sleepiness	France	44	5 hours
Engleman et al. (1994)[36]	Epworth Sleepiness	U.K.	16	3.2 hours
Waldhorn et al. (1990)[37]	Epworth Sleepiness	U.S.	125	2 hours
Olsen et al. (2008)[4]	Pichot Fatigue Scale, Pichot Depression scale	Australia	77	4 hours
Yinghui et al. (2011)[38]	Pichot Fatigue Scale, Pichot Depression scale	U.S.	57	Not indicated
Bakker et al. (2011)[12]	Epworth Sleepiness, self-efficacy	USA	126	4 hours
Baron et al. (2011)[33]	Self-efficacy	U.S.	31	Not indicated
Sawyer et al. (2011)[39]	Self-efficacy	U.S.	66	20 minutes at effective pressure
Stepnowsky et al. (2002)[40]	Coping-styles	U.S.	23	Not indicated
de Zeeuw et al. (2007)[41]	Locus of control	Germany	85	Not indicated
Tyrrell et al. (2006)[42]	Locus of control	France	9	Not indicated

Reference	Factors associated with compliance	Country	Sample (n)	Minimum threshold value to be adherent (/night)
	initial cpap exposure variables			
Mc Ardle et al. (1999)[1]	CPAP use (in the first 15 days stage <3 hours)	U.K.	1211	2 hours
Popescu et al. (2001)[5]	CPAP use (in the first 15 days stage <3 hours)	England	209	2 hours
Lewis et al. (2001)[10]	Initial problems with CPAP use (in the first night)	United Kingdom	82	4 hours
Balachandran et al.(2013)[43]	CPAP perception questionnaire over the first 30 days of therapy	U.S.	1226	4 hours
Rosen et al. (2012)[44]	Diagnosed with HST	U.S.	373	4 hours
Lettieri et al. (2011)[45]	Diagnosed with HST	U.S.	210	4 hours

Reference	Factors associated with compliance	Country	Sample (n)	Minimum threshold value to be adherent (/night)
	social variables			
Baron et al. (2011)[33]	Spousal involvement	U.S.	31	Not indicated
Mc Ardle et al. (1999)[1]	Bed partner's sleep quality and overall quality of life	U.K.	1211	2 hours
Parish et al. (2003)[46]	Bed partner's sleep quality and overall quality of life	U.S.	51	6 hours (mean)
McArdle et al. (2001)[47]	Bed partner's sleep quality and overall quality of life	U.K.	49	Not indicated
Simon-Tuval et al. (2009)[7]	Partners sleeps separately and family and/or friends with positive experience of CPAP	Israel	162	Not indicated
Cartwright. (2008)[48]	Shared sleeping		20	
Ye et al. (2009)[49]	Spousal involvement	Synthetical article		

Reference	Factors associated with compliance	Country	Sample (n)	Minimum threshold value to be adherent (/night)
	technical variables			
Anderson et al. (2003)[50]	Mask-interface (types of nasal vs face mask innovations)	New Zealand	11	Not indicated
Khanna et al. (2003)[51]	Mask-interface (types of nasal vs face mask innovations)	U.S.	38	4 hours

Massie et al. (2003)[52]	Mask-interface (types of nasal vs face mask innovations)	U.S.	39	4 hours
Mortimore et al. (1998)[53]	Mask-interface (types of nasal vs face mask innovations)	U.K.	30	Not indicated
Massie et al. (1999)[54]	Heated vs cold pass-over humidity	U.S.	38	1 hour
Aloia et al. (2005)[55]	Flexible pressure on CPAP adherence	U.S.	89	Not indicated
Pepin et al. (2009)[56]	Flexible pressure on CPAP adherence	France	218	4 hours
Chasen et al. (2005)[57]	Claustrophobia	U.S.	153	2 and 5 hours
Chai et al. (2013)[58]	Side effect	China, Australia, and New Zealand	275	3 hours

Appendix References

1. McArdle N, Devereux G, Heidarnejad H, Engleman HM, Mackay TW, et al. (1999) Long-term use of CPAP therapy for sleep apnea/hypopnea syndrome. Am J Respir Crit Care Med 159: 1108-1114.
2. Krieger J, Kurtz D, Petiau C, Sforza E, Trautmann D (1996) Long-term compliance with CPAP therapy in obstructive sleep apnea patients and in snorers. Sleep 19: S136-143.
3. Budhiraja R, Parthasarathy S, Drake CL, Roth T, Sharief I, et al. (2007) Early CPAP use identifies subsequent adherence to CPAP therapy. Sleep 30: 320-324.
4. Olsen S, Smith S, Oei T, Douglas J (2008) Health belief model predicts adherence to CPAP before experience with CPAP. Eur Respir J 32: 710-717.
5. Popescu G, Latham M, Allgar V, Elliott MW (2001) Continuous positive airway pressure for sleep apnoea/hypopnoea syndrome: usefulness of a 2 week trial to identify factors associated with long term use. Thorax 56: 727-733.
6. Sin DD, Mayers I, Man GC, Pawluk L (2002) Long-term compliance rates to continuous positive airway pressure in obstructive sleep apnea: a population-based study. Chest 121: 430-435.
7. Simon-Tuval T, Reuveni H, Greenberg-Dotan S, Oksenberg A, Tal A, et al. (2009) Low socioeconomic status is a risk factor for CPAP acceptance among adult OSAS patients requiring treatment. Sleep 32: 545-552.
8. Young T, Palta M, Dempsey J, Skatrud J, Weber S, et al. (1993) The occurrence of sleep-disordered breathing among middle-aged adults. N Engl J Med 328: 1230-1235.
9. Pelletier-Fleury N, Rakatonanahary D, Fleury B (2001) The age and other factors in the evaluation of compliance with nasal continuous positive airway pressure for obstructive sleep apnoea syndrome. Acox proportional hazars analysis. Sleep Medicine 2: 225-232.
10. Lewis KE, Seale L, Bartle IE, Watkins AJ, Ebden P (2004) Early predictors of CPAP use for the treatment of obstructive sleep apnea. Sleep 27: 134-138.
11. Ye L, Pien GW, Ratcliffe SJ, Weaver TE (2009) Gender differences in obstructive sleep apnea and treatment response to continuous positive airway pressure. J Clin Sleep Med 5: 512-518.
12. Bakker JP, O'Keeffe KM, Neill AM, Campbell AJ (2011) Ethnic disparities in CPAP adherence in New Zealand: Effects of socioeconomic status, health literacy and self-efficacy. Sleep 1: 1595-1603.
13. Ye L, Pack A, Maislin G, Dinges D, Hurley S, et al. (2012) Predictors of continuous positive airway pressure use during the first week of treatment. J Sleep Res 21: 419-426.
14. Gagnadoux F, Le Vaillant M, Goupil F, Pigeanne T, Chollet S, et al. (2011) Influence of marital status and employment status on long-term adherence with continuous positive airway pressure in sleep apnea patients. PLoS One 6: e22503.
15. Scharf SM, Seiden L, DeMore J, Carter-Pokras O (2004) Racial differences in clinical presentation of patients with sleep-disordered breathing. Sleep Breath 8: 173-183.
16. Billings ME, Auckley D, Benca R, Foldvary-Schaefer N, Iber C, et al. (2011) Race and residential socioeconomics as predictors of CPAP adherence. Sleep 34: 1653-1658.
17. Platt AB, Field SH, Asch DA, Chen Z, Patel NP, et al. (2009) Neighborhood of residence is associated with daily adherence to CPAP therapy. Sleep 32: 799-806.
18. Hoffstein V, Viner S, Mateika S, Conway J (1992). Treatment of obstructive sleep apnea with nasal continuous positive airway pressure. Patient compliance, perception of benefits, and side effects. American Review of Respiratory Disease 145: 841-745.
19. Loredo JS, Berry C, Nelesen RA, Dimsdale JE (2007) Prediction of continuous positive airway pressure in obstructive sleep apnea. Sleep Breath 11: 45-51.
20. Wild MR, Engleman HM, Douglas NJ, Espie CA (2004) Can psychological factors help us to determine adherence to CPAP? A prospective study. Eur Respir J 24: 461-465.
21. Redenius R, Murphy C, O'Neill E, Al-Hamwi M, Zallek SN (2008) Does CPAP lead to change in BMI? J Clin Sleep Med 4: 205-209.
22. Sugiura T, Noda A, Nakata S, Yasuda Y, Soga T, et al. (2007) Influence of nasal resistance on initial acceptance of continuous positive airway pressure in treatment for obstructive sleep apnea syndrome. Respiration 74(1): 56–60.
23. Reishtein JL, Maislin G, Weaver TE; Multisite Study group (2010) Outcome of CPAP treatment on intimate and sexual relationships in men with obstructive sleep apnea. J Clin Sleep Med 6: 221-226.
24. Margel D, Tal R, Livne PM, Pillar G (2005) Predictors of erectile function improvement in obstructive sleep apnea patients with long-term CPAP treatment. Int J Impot Res 17: 186-190.
25. Hung J, Whitford EG, Parsons RW, Hillman DR (1990) Association of sleep apnoea with myocardial infarction in men. Lancet 336: 261-264.
26. Phillips B, Shafazand S (2013) CPAP and hypertension in nonsleepy patients. J Clin Sleep Med 9: 181-182.
27. Palombini L, Guilleminault C (2006) Stroke and treatment with nasal CPAP. Eur J Neurol 13: 198-200.
28. Martínez-García MA, Campos-Rodríguez F, Soler-Cataluña JJ, Catalán-Serra P, Román-Sánchez P, et al. (2012) Increased incidence of nonfatal cardiovascular events in stroke patients with sleep apnoea: effect of CPAP treatment. Eur Respir J 39: 906-912.
29. Hui DS, Choy DK, Li TS, Ko FW, Wong KK, et al. (2001) Determinants of continuous positive airway pressure compliance in a group of Chinese patients with obstructive sleep apnea. Chest 120: 170-176.
30. Krieger J (1992) Long-term compliance with nasal continuous positive airway pressure (CPAP) in obstructive sleep apnea patients and nonapneic snorers. Sleep 15: S42-46.
31. Meurice JC, Dore P, Paquereau J, Neau JP, Ingrand P, et al. (1994) Predictive factors of long-term compliance with nasal continuous positive airway pressure treatment in sleep apnea syndrome. Chest 105: 429-433.
32. Bollig SM (2010) Encouraging CPAP adherence: it is everyone's job. Respir Care 55: 1230-1239.
33. Baron KG, Berg CA, Czajkowski LA, Smith TW, Gunn HE, et al. (2011) Self-efficacy contributes to individual differences in subjective improvements using CPAP. Sleep Breath 15: 599-606.
34. Morris LG, Setlur J, Burschtin OE, Steward DL, Jacobs JB, et al. (2006) Acoustic rhinometry predicts tolerance of nasal continuous positive airway pressure: a pilot study. Am J Rhinol 20: 133-137.
35. Fletcher E, Luckett R (1991) The effect of positive reinforcement on hourly

compliance in nasal continuous positive airway pressure users with obstructive sleep apnea. American Review of Respiratory Disease 143(5): 936-41.

36. Engleman HM, Martin SE, Deary IJ, Douglas NJ (1993) Effect of continuous positive airway pressure treatment on daytime function in sleep apnoea/ hypopnoea syndrome. Lancet 343(8897): 572–575.

37. Waldhorn RE1, Herrick TW, Nguyen MC, O'Donnell AE, Sodero J, et al. (1990) Long-term compliance with nasal continuous positive airway pressure therapy of obstructive sleep apnea. Chest 97: 33-38.

38. Yinghui L, Preud'homme X, Harold W, Goforth MD, Omonua T, et al. (2011) The association of fatigue with depression and insomnia in HIV-seropositive patients: A pilot study. Sleep 34(12): 1723-1726.

39. Sawyer AM, Canamucio A, Moriarty H, Weaver TE, Richards KC, et al. (2011) Do cognitive perceptions influence CPAP use? Patient Educ Couns 85: 85-91.

40. Stepnowsky CJ Jr, Bardwell WA, Moore PJ, Ancoli-Israel S, Dimsdale JE (2002) Psychologic correlates of compliance with continuous positive airway pressure. Sleep 25: 758-762.

41. de Zeeuw J, Baberg HT, Duchna HW, Kempkens DJ, Walther JW, et al. (2007) Locus of control belief is a predictor of CPAP-compliance in patients with obstructive sleep apnea syndrome. Pneumologie 61(5): 283-290.

42. Tyrrell J, Poulet C, Pe Pin JL, Veale D (2006) A preliminary study of psychological factors affecting patients' acceptance of CPAP therapy for sleep apnoea syndrome. Sleep medicine 7(4): 375-379.

43. Balachandran JS, Yu X, Wroblewski K, Mokhlesi B (2013) A brief survey of patients' first impression after CPAP titration predicts future CPAP adherence: a pilot study. Journal of Clinical Sleep Medicine 9(3): 199-205.

44. Rosen CL , Auckley D , Benca R., Foldvary-Schaefer N, Iber C, et al (2012) A multisite randomized trial of portable sleep studies and positive airway pressure autotitration versus laboratory-based polysomnography for the diagnosis and treatment of obstructive sleep apnea: the HomePAP study . Sleep 35(6): 757-767.

45. Lettieri CF, Lettieri CJ, Carter K (2011) Does home sleep testing impair continuous positive airway pressure adherence in patients with obstructive sleep apnea? Chest 139: 849-854.

46. Parish JM, Lyng PJ (2003) Quality of life in bed partners of patients with obstructive sleep apnea or hypopnea after treatment with continuous positive airway pressure. Chest 124: 942-947.

47. McArdle N, Kingshott R, Engleman HM, Mackay TW, Douglas NJ (2001) Partners of patients with sleep apnoea/hypopnoea syndrome: effect of CPAP treatment on sleep quality and quality of life. Thorax 56: 513-518.

48. Cartwright R (2008) Sleeping together: a pilot study of the effects of shared sleeping on adherence to CPAP treatment in obstructive sleep apnea. J Clin Sleep Med 4: 123-127.

49. Ye L, Malhotra A, Kayser K, Willis DG, Horowitz JA, et al. (2015) Spousal involvement and CPAP adherence: a dyadic perspective. Sleep Med Rev 19: 67-74.

50. Anderson FE, Kingshott RN, Taylor DR, Jones DR, Kline LR, et al. (2003) A randomized crossover efficacy trial of oral CPAP (Oracle) compared with nasal CPAP in the management of obstructive sleep apnea. Sleep 26: 721-726.

51. Khanna R, Kline LR (2003) A prospective 8 week trial of nasal interfaces vs. a novel oral interface (Oracle) for treatment of obstructive sleep apnea hypopnea syndrome. Sleep Med 4: 333-338.

52. Massie C, Hart R (2003) Clinical outcomes related to interface type in patients with obstructive sleep apnea/hypopnea syndrome who are using continuous positive airway pressure. Chest 123(4): 1112–1118.

53. Mortimore IL, Whittle AT, Douglas NJ (1998) Comparison of nose and face mask CPAP therapy for sleep apnoea. Thorax 53: 290-292.

54. Massie CA1, Hart RW, Peralez K, Richards GN (1999) Effects of humidification on nasal symptoms and compliance in sleep apnea patients using continuous positive airway pressure. Chest 116: 403-408.

55. Aloia MS, Stanchina M, Arnedt JT, Malhotra A, Millman RP (2005) Treatment adherence and outcomes in flexible vs standard continuous positive airway pressure therapy. Chest 127: 2085-2093.

56. Pepin JL, Muir JF, Gentina T, Dauvilliers Y, Tamisier R, et al (2009) Pressure reduction during exhalation in sleep apnea patients treated by continuous positive airway pressure. Chest 136(2):490-497.

57. Chasens ER, Pack AI, Maislin G, Dinges DF, Weaver TE (2005) Claustrophobia and adherence to CPAP treatment. West J Nurs Res 27: 307-321.

58. Chai-Coetzer CL, Luo YM, Antic NA, Zhang XL, Chen BY, et al. (2013) Predictors of long-term adherence to continuous positive airway pressure therapy in patients with obstructive sleep apnea and cardiovascular disease in the SAVE study. Sleep 36: 1929-1937.

Sleep Apnea and Other Sleep Disorders: Survey in Individuals with Idiopathic Pulmonary Fibrosis (IPF)

Swathy Puthalapattu[1]*, Jesse Roman-Rodriguez[2,3], Rafael L Perez[2,3], Srinivas Bhadriraju[4] and Octavian C Ioachimescu[1,5]

[1]Division of Pulmonary and Critical Care Medicine, Emory University School of Medicine, Atlanta, Georgia, USA
[2]University of Louisville, Louisville, Kentucky, USA
[3]Louisville Veterans Affairs Medical Center, Louisville, Kentucky, USA
[4]Baylor College of Medicine, Houston, Texas, USA
[5]Atlanta Veterans Affairs Medical Center, Atlanta, Georgia, USA

Abstract

Purpose: The aim of this survey was to gather data about the incidence of various sleep disorders, particularly sleep apnea, in subjects with IPF who participated in a regional patient-oriented seminar on this condition. We hypothesized that the frequency of Obstructive Sleep Apnea (OSA) and psychiatric sleep disorders would be disproportionately high in the IPF population.

Methods: The project was a one-time survey administered to stable patients with IPF and their family members from the South eastern USA who participated in the "Living with IPF" public seminar at the Emory University campus. The survey used a validated questionnaire, i.e., Sleep Disorders Questionnaire (SDQ), to detect presence of Sleep Apnea (SA) and selected sleep disorders - Restless Legs Syndrome (RLS), Psychiatric Sleep Disorders (PSY) and narcolepsy (NAR). The questionnaire was administered to all participants (with and without IPF), in a confidential manner. The findings were used to determine if there were differences in the incidence of SA and other sleep disorders between individuals with IPF and those without the disease.

Results: A total of 52 people agreed to participate in the study. One subject was excluded due to unclear IPF status. The median SDQ raw scores in IPF patients for SA, RLS, PSY and NAR were 28.7, 27.1, 26.2 and 26.5, respectively; overall, they were not statistically different in IPF patients versus control subjects. However, as validated in other studies, patients with history of OSA had significantly higher SDQ-SA scores.

Conclusions: The present study aimed to investigate cross-sectionally the incidence of self-reported sleep conditions in patients with IPF versus healthy family member controls. Overall, we did not find a disproportionately higher incidence of sleep disorders in the IPF population. This may be explained by inherent methodological limitations and the small sample size.

Keywords: Idiopathic pulmonary fibrosis; Obstructive sleep apnea; Restless legs syndrome; Narcolepsy; Psychiatric sleep disorders

Introduction

Obstructive Sleep Apnea (OSA) associated with excessive daytime sleepiness, or OSA syndrome, is estimated to occur in 1 of 20 adults or about 5% of the general population in the United States [1]. An epidemiological review by Young et al. estimates that about 1 in 5 adults have at least mild OSA and 1 in 15 adults have at least moderate OSA [2]. OSA is becoming increasingly prevalent. Nevertheless, mainly due to lack of awareness by the public and healthcare professionals, the vast majority remain undiagnosed and untreated. Data from the Wisconsin Sleep Cohort study estimated that 93% of women and 82% of men with moderate-to-severe sleep apnea were undiagnosed [3]. A follow-up publication from the Wisconsin Cohort Study five years later indicated that the prevalence of OSA in people aged 30-60 years was 9-24% for men and 4-9% for women [2].

Idiopathic Pulmonary Fibrosis (IPF) is a progressive fibrosing lung disease of unknown etiology that affects an estimated 160,000 Americans, and accounts for over 15,000 deaths a year [4]. The median survival from the time of diagnosis is 2 to 3 years [5]. To date, most of the pharmacologic agents evaluated in clinical trials in IPF have failed to demonstrate improvement in clinically meaningful outcomes (e.g. symptoms, functional status or survival) [6]. The absence of any effective treatment for IPF suggests that the recognition and treatment of comorbid sleep conditions in IPF patients should become a priority in their management [7,8].

The aim of this survey was to gather data about the incidence of restless legs syndrome, psychiatric sleep disorders, narcolepsy and OSA in subjects with IPF, who participated in a regional patient-oriented seminar on this condition. Recently published studies report an increased incidence of OSA in patients with IPF [7,9,10]. Prior studies have demonstrated interdependence between upper airway size in OSA and lung volumes. Snorers with OSA were found to have a more dramatic fall in measured pharyngeal cross-sectional area as lung volume decreased [11,12]. In spite of overall lack of effectiveness in IPF, until recent years Gluco Cortico Steroids (GCS) were often used in treatment regimens for IPF. The well known corticosteroid-related central fat deposition in the neck region may be a reason for the deterioration of underlying OSA during the course of IPF.

To the best of our knowledge, there are no published English

***Corresponding author:** Swathy Puthalapattu, Fellow, Pulmonary and Critical Care Medicine, Division of Pulmonary, Allergy and Critical Care Medicine, Emory University School of Medicine, 615 Michael Street - Suite 211, Atlanta, GA 30322, USA
E-mail: swathy.puthalapattu@emory.edu

studies investigating the frequency of insomnia, narcolepsy and restless legs syndrome in patients with IPF. The main goal of the present study was to investigate cross-sectionally the frequency of common sleep disorders in patients with IPF. We hypothesized that the frequency of sleep apnea and psychiatric sleep disorders is disproportionately increased in the IPF population.

Methodology

Aims

This survey was designed to serve as a pilot investigation on the types and incidence of comorbid sleep disorders, particularly sleep apnea, in subjects with IPF participating in a regional patient-oriented awareness day. Unaffected participants (family members attending the event) were also surveyed and analyzed as controls. This project was a one-time survey of participants in the "Living with IPF" seminar, using a validated questionnaire to detect the presence of sleep apnea and selected sleep disorders. The questionnaire was administered to all participants with and without IPF in a confidential manner. The findings are used to determine if there are differences in the incidence of sleep apnea and other sleep disorders between individuals with IPF and those without the disease.

Study population and study site

The survey was administered to stable patients with IPF from the South eastern USA who participated in the "Living with IPF" public seminar on November 12, 2005 at the Emory University campus. Unaffected participants were also surveyed and represented the control group. The "Living with IPF" public seminars typically had up to 50 subjects with IPF in addition to family members, leading to about 200 participants in total. Institutional Review Board (IRB) at Emory University approved the protocol prior to the survey. The diagnosis of IPF was generally made according to the standard of clinical care at that time, i.e., in approximately 60% of the patients by lung biopsy and in 40% by correlating the clinical and tomographic features of their presenting condition.

Survey instrument - Sleep disorders questionnaire (SDQ)

The SDQ was designed and validated by Sleep Lab Software Ltd., (Ann Arbor, MI). SDQ is a 175-item questionnaire which ascertains the risk of having or developing a sleep disorder. The SDQ was derived from Sleep Questionnaire and Assessment of Wakefulness (SQAW), used since the 1970s at Stanford University. Four sleep domains are assessed: Sleep Apnea (SA), narcolepsy (NAR), Psychiatric Sleeps Disorders (PSY), and Restless Legs Syndrome (RLS). For each category, total score ranges from 0 to 60. In validative cohorts, SA and NAR scales proved to be the most discriminating and to have the highest sensitivity, specificity, positive and negative predictive values compared to PSY and RLS scales. Typically, the survey takes 60–90 minutes to complete, though individuals with a high school reading level may finish as quickly as 25 minutes [13].

The questionnaire was offered to all participants along with a demographic sheet with queries about age, gender, height, weight, history of OSA, other sleep problems, Positive Airway Pressure (PAP) use, oxygen use, lung problems, heart problems and smoking status. The sheet clearly states that no identifying information is to be added to any part of the survey. Self-addressed stamped envelopes were provided to all participants to return the completed envelope to the Emory Center for Interstitial Lung Diseases. A Center coordinator not involved in the survey received the questionnaires, assured that no identifying information was present and destroyed the envelopes. The questionnaires were then given to the investigators for analysis.

Analysis

Each question of the SDQ was rated by the subject nominally as "never," "rarely," "sometimes," "usually," or "always." The responses are converted to an ordinal scale of 1 to 5, respectively. Higher numerical scores reflect greater clinical severity of symptom. The sum of individual responses previously validated to predict the presence of each of the four categories of sleep disorders - sleep apnea, narcolepsy, psychiatric sleep disorder, and restless leg syndrome, generate a raw score for each category. The raw scores of subjects with IPF were compared to individuals without the disease in each category using nonparametric methods (Wilcoxon test). The Chi-square test (with Fisher correction, where needed) was used to test for differences between the control group and subjects with IPF, among the four categories of sleep disorders. JMP 9.0 (SAS Inc., Cary, NC) was used for the statistical analysis.

Results

A total of 52 people agreed to participate in the study. One subject was excluded due to unclear IPF status. The participant characteristics for IPF patients (n = 27) and control subjects (n = 24) are shown in table 1. The subjects in the IPF group were generally older than the control group. The age distribution of the cohort is shown in Figure 1 (median age of 62). As expected, more males were present in the IPF group. The Body Mass Indes (BMI) was slightly lower in the control group, although not statistically significant (p = 0.24).

The median raw scores for sleep apnea, restless legs syndrome, psychiatric sleep disorders and narcolepsy were not statistically different in the IPF patients vs control subjects. The median score and 25th-75th interquartile ranges are shown in table 2. Of note, the median raw scores did not differ between males and females of the IPF and the control groups (data not shown). Patients with history of sleep apnea had on average a higher SDQ-SA score, which was statistically

Demographic Variable	IPF Median (25th, 75th percentiles*)	Control Median (25th, 75th percentiles*)
Age	65 (59, 71)	56 (48.5, 64)
Gender (M/F)	16/11	6/18
BMI**	28.1 (24.5, 1.8)	26.9 (22.3, 29)
Smoking status 0/27		3/24

*Non-normally distributed data shown as median (25th, 75th percentiles).
**BMI, Body Mass Index

Table 1: Demographic data.

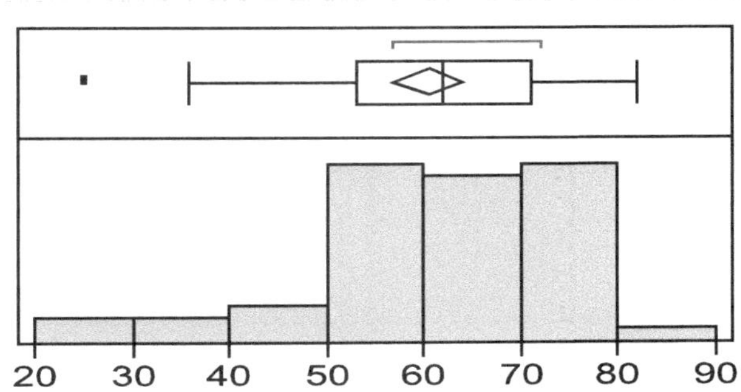

Figure 1: Age distribution of the cohort. Median age – 62 (53, 71) years. Data is shown as median (25th, 75th interquartile range).

significant and shown in Figure 2. The SA-SDQ has a total of 12 items, out of which only one item [Q139: 'I have a problem with my nose blocking up when I am trying to sleep (allergies, infections)'] reached statistical significance (p=0.04). The RLS-SDQ has a total of 9 items, out of which one item (Q45: 'I feel that I have insomnia') reached statistical significance (p=0.05). The PSY-SDQ has a total of 9 items, out of which one item (Q101: 'Someone in my family has been hospitalized for a psychiatric illness or nervous breakdown') showed statistical significance (p=0.002). The NAR-SDQ has a total of 15 items, out of which one item (Q67: 'I get sudden muscular weakness when laughing, angry or in situations of strong emotions') showed statistical significance (p=0.03).

Discussion

It is increasingly recognized that OSA has significant attributable morbidity (and, possibly, mortality). Well recognized complications associated with OSA include systemic hypertension, pulmonary arterial hypertension, insulin resistance, metabolic syndrome and potentially atherosclerosis, mediated by sleep fragmentation, intermittent hypoxemia or oxidative stress mechanisms [14,15]. While much attention has been appropriately focused on the cardiovascular consequences of OSA, it seems also that OSA is associated with pulmonary conditions.

Until recent years, glucocorticosteroids were often used in treatment regimens for IPF population, despite the apparent lack of efficacy in this condition. Corticosteroids have well known negative effects on sleep quality, causing sleep-onset and sleep-maintenance insomnia, frequent nocturnal awakenings and alterations in sleep stage architecture, etc. [16,17]. Also, the well known corticosteroid-related fat deposition in the neck region may be a reason for the deterioration of underlying OSA during the course of IPF and the subsequent need for additional titration in order to assess the effective Continuous Positive Airway Pressure (CPAP).

Median SDQ* Score	IPF	IPF Controls	p
SA**	28.7	22.9	0.16
RLS#	27.1	24.7	0.56
PSY##	26.2	25.7	0.92
PSY## NAR@	26.5	24.2	0.56

*SDQ, Sleep disorders questionnaire
**SA, Sleep apnea
#RLS, Restless legs syndrome
##PSY, Psychiatric sleep disorder
@NAR, Narcolepsy

Table 2: Median SDQ Raw Scores in IPF patients vs. controls.

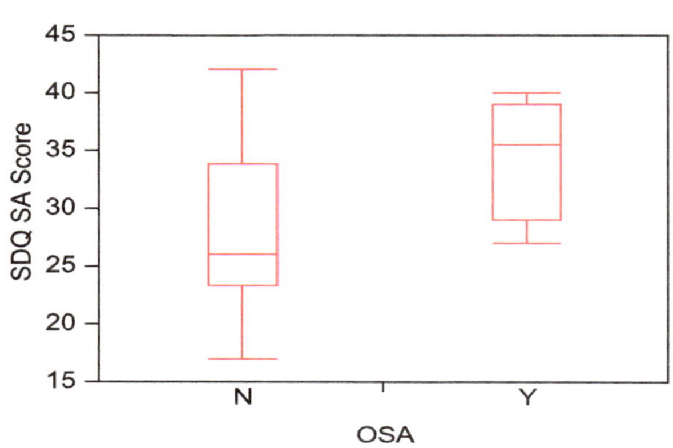

Figure 2: SDQ SA –score vs. OSA. (p=0.01). Sleep disorders questionnaire (SDQ), obstructive sleep apnea (OSA). N - OSA absent, Y - OSA present.

Depression and other mood disorders, seem to be commonly seen in IPF patients, especially in cases with a rapid disease progression, and might also have negative effects on sleep quality and architecture. Sleep fragmentation is common in IPF patients and is due to significant oxyhemoglobin desaturations during sleep, especially during Rapid Eye Movement (REM) sleep. Furthermore, increased arousals related to coughing, increased respiratory effort and reduced delta sleep (or slow wave sleep) was found [18]. These sleep disturbances had an effect on the subjective state/functionality, as measured by the Functional Outcomes of Sleep Questionnaire (FOSQ) and Pittsburgh *Sleep Quality Index* (PSQI) [18].

The present study examined the association between sleep apnea, restless legs syndrome, psychiatric sleep disorders and narcolepsy in patients with IPF. Overall, we did not find an increased incidence of sleep disorders in the IPF patients. Contrary to our study results, several recently published studies have found an increased association of Obstructive Sleep Apnea (OSA) in patients with IPF. The discrepancies can be explained by several factors, some of them being in fact current study weaknesses: [1] small sample size and lack of randomization; [2] lack of data related to prior use of glucocorticosteroids and weight history; [3] lack of standardization in evaluating sleep disorders (e.g., when is a polysomnogram ordered in patients with IPF?); [4] the IPF status of the individuals was self-reported. To the best of our knowledge, there are no articles in English literature examining the association between restless legs syndrome, psychiatric sleep disorders or narcolepsy and IPF.

In summary, using SDQ and a sample of patients with IPF and family member controls, we found that there was no increase in the incidence of sleep apnea, restless legs syndrome, psychiatric sleep disorders or narcolepsy in IPF. Concordant with prior studies, in our survey, patients with history of Obstructive Sleep Apnea (OSA) had higher SDQ-SA scores. Nevertheless, larger studies are needed to thoroughly evaluate the incidence of restless legs syndrome, psychiatric sleep disorders and narcolepsy in patients with IPF.

References

1. Young TM, Palta (1993) "The occurrence of sleep-disordered breathing among middle-aged adults." N Engl J Med 328: 1230-1235.
2. Young T, Peppard PE, Gottlieb DJ (2002) Epidemiology of obstructive sleep apnea: a population health perspective. Am J Respir Crit Care Med 165: 1217-1239.
3. Young T, Evans L, Finn L, Palta M (1997) Estimation of the clinically diagnosed proportion of sleep apnea syndrome in middle-aged men and women. Sleep 20: 705-706.
4. Raghu G, Weycker D, Edelsberg J, Bradford WZ, Oster G (2006) Incidence and prevalence of idiopathic pulmonary fibrosis. Am J Respir Crit Care Med 174: 810-816.
5. Rudd RM, Prescott RJ, Chalmers JC, Johnston ID; Fibrosing Alveolitis Subcommittee of the Research Committee of the British Thoracic Society (2007) British Thoracic Society Study on cryptogenic fibrosing alveolitis: Response to treatment and survival. Thorax 62: 62-66.
6. Raghu G, Collard HR, Egan JJ, Martinez FJ, Behr J, et al. (2011) An official ATS/ERS/JRS/ALAT statement: idiopathic pulmonary fibrosis: evidence-based guidelines for diagnosis and management. Am J Respir Crit Care Med 183: 788-824.
7. Mermigkis C, Stagaki E (2010) "How common is sleep-disordered breathing in patients with idiopathic pulmonary fibrosis?" Sleep Breath 14: 387-390.
8. Mermigkis C, Chapman J, Golish J, Mermigkis D, Budur K, et al. (2007) Sleep-

related breathing disorders in patients with idiopathic pulmonary fibrosis. Lung 185: 173-178.

9. Bradley TD, Brown IG, Grossman RF, Zamel N, Martinez D, et al. (1986) Pharyngeal size in snorers, nonsnorers, and patients with obstructive sleep apnea. N Engl J Med 315: 1327-1331.

10. Heinzer RC, Stanchina ML, Malhotra A, Fogel RB, Patel SR, et al. (2005) Lung volume and continuous positive airway pressure requirements in obstructive sleep apnea. Am J Respir Crit Care Med 172: 114-117.

11. Douglass AB, Bornstein R, Nino-Murcia G, Keenan S, Miles L, et al. (1994) The Sleep Disorders Questionnaire. I: Creation and multivariate structure of SDQ. Sleep 17: 160-167.

12. Laaban JP, Mounier L, Roque d'Orbcastel O, Veale D, Blacher J, et al. (2010) Cardiovascular risk factors in men and women with obstructive sleep apnoea syndrome. Respir Med 104: 1063-1068.

13. Peled N, Kassirer M, Shitrit D, Kogan Y, Shlomi D, et al. (2007) The association of OSA with insulin resistance, inflammation and metabolic syndrome. Respir Med 101: 1696-1701.

14. Chrousos GA, Kattah JC, Beck RW, Cleary PA (1993) Side effects of glucocorticoid treatment. Experience of the Optic Neuritis Treatment Trial. JAMA 269: 2110-2112.

15. Lozada F, Silverman S Jr, Migliorati C (1984) Adverse side effects associated with prednisone in the treatment of patients with oral inflammatory ulcerative diseases. J Am Dent Assoc 109: 269-270.

16. Bye PT, Issa F, Berthon-Jones M, Sullivan CE (1984) Studies of oxygenation during sleep in patients with interstitial lung disease. Am Rev Respir Dis 129: 27-32.

17. Perez-Padilla R, West P, Lertzman M, Kryger MH (1985) Breathing during sleep in patients with interstitial lung disease. Am Rev Respir Dis 132: 224-229.

18. Krishnan V, McCormack MC, Mathai SC, Agarwal S, Richardson B, et al. (2008) Sleep quality and health-related quality of life in idiopathic pulmonary fibrosis. Chest 134: 693-698.

Melatonin and REM Behavior Disorder

Chia-Mo Lin[1,2], Hsiao-Yean Chiu RNMS[3] and Christian Guilleminault[4]

[1,2]*Fu-Jen University Medical College and ShinKong Wu Ho-Su Hospital Sleep Center, Taipei, Taiwan*
[3]*Taipei Medical University, Taipei Taiwan*
[4]*Stanford University Sleep Medicine Division, Stanford, CA, USA*

Abstract

REM Sleep Behavior Disorder (RBD) is commonly associated with neurodegenerative diseases and leads to abnormal and often aggressive behavior during sleep, often causing injury to selfor the bed partner. Clonazepam and melatonin have been considered as treatments of RBD, but the underlying mechanism of action is unknown. Melatonin may restore the presence of physiological REM sleep muscle atonia. A clinical protocol was established to follow patients with RBD with clinical evaluation and polysomnography (PSG). A retrospective analysis was then performed on data from 28 RBD patients. From the obtained data, melatonin 6 mg has a positive effect on both clinical manifestation and PSG findings. Most subjects responded to melatonin 6 mg with a significant decrease or absence of abnormal behavior, and less than 20% of EMG bursts during total REM time during PSG, but one patient never responded to the drug even at up to 12 mg of melatonin and 3 mg of clonazepam. Depending on the patient, more disturbed sleep was noted with melatonin alone than with the combination of both melatonin and clonazepam, and a further decrease of "wake after sleep onset" was noted at polysomnography.

Keywords: Melatonin; REM behavior disorder; Treatment; Poor nocturnal sleep; Response to treatment

Introduction

Rapid Eye Movement (REM) Sleep Behavior Disorder (RBD) is a syndrome that was recognized many years ago by Japanese researchers in association with alcoholic delirium [1,2]. Jouvet and Delorme in Lyon, France lesioned the region of the peri-coeruleus in the upper brainstem in cats that was responsible for the initiation of the active inhibition of muscle tone during REM sleep, inducing a syndrome where cats were "acting out" their dreams with behavior similar to a cat trying to catch an invisible mouse or other oneiroid behaviors [3]. More recently, this descending pathway involving glycinergic and glutaminergic neurotransmitters has also been well mapped in rats by the Lyon school, as the rat anatomy of this descending pathway [4] is closer to the human anatomy than the one noted in cats. The syndrome called "REM without atonia" was also observed in olivo-ponto-cerebellar degeneration, a neuro-degenerative disorder, by Quera-Salva and Guilleminault in 1986 [5]. Then Schenck et al. noted the presence of REM without atonia in subjects who appeared to have no other neurological symptoms and the syndrome was called "RBD" [6]. Since then, RBD has been noted in Parkinson's patients and in patients with other neuro-degenerative disorders. Furthermore, the long-term follow-up of "idiopathic RBD cases" performed predominantly by Schenck et al. [6] has demonstrated the evolution of these idiopathic RBD patients toward the development of neuro-degenerative diseases, particularly Parkinson's, Multiple System Atrophy, or Dementia [7]. The histologic investigation of the brain of these patients revealed the presence of Lewy bodies and these different neuro-degenerative disorders with Lewy bodies at histology are classified today as "synucleinopathies" [8,9]. The aim of RBD treatment has been to eliminate the dangerous behavior associated with the abnormal persistence of muscle tone during REM sleep, leading to the acting out of dreams, and also to provide quiet and uninterrupted sleep.

Two drugs have been advocated as treatment: a benzodiazepine (clonazepam) and melatonin. Both drugs are given orally in the evening and have been reported to decrease or eliminate the violent behavior associated with RBD. However, the degree of response (complete vs. partial or incomplete), the dosages required, and the potential side effects remain unclear.

During 5 years (July 2007to July 2011) we used a clinical protocol to treat patients recognized with RBD. This clinical protocol covered the first 7 months following diagnosis of RBD and involved repeated polysomnography tests. Following the initial 7 months, patients may have been followed by neurologists or other specialists and/or may have been intermittently seen by the sleep medicine service (particularly when patients did not respond to treatment).

We retrospectively looked at the data obtained using our clinical protocol, and in specific cases we added follow-up information past the initial 7 months (these subjects were usually non-responders). The retrospective analysis of anonymous data was approved by the hospital IRB.

Clinical Protocol

Interview

There was a systematic interview of all patients seen in the sleep clinic on the presence of abnormal behavior during sleep. The interview was conducted not only with the patient but also with the bed partner or caregiver in elderly subjects. All symptoms associated with sleep disorders were explored and documented.

Most commonly, patients were referred for evaluation of snoring and the question of sleep-disordered breathing, but when symptoms of another sleep disorder were uncovered, further questions were asked to characterize the syndrome and its severity. If any reports of abnormal

***Corresponding author:** Chia-Mo Lin, MD, Shin Kong Wu Ho-Su Hospital Sleep Center, Sleep Center B2 No 95 Wen Chang Rd, Shilin District, Taipei, Taiwan
E-mail: aminus64@gmail.com

behaviors or vocalizations during sleep were elicited, further questions on dream enactment, degree of awareness, and bruises and trauma to self or bed partners were collected in a pre-established standardized grid covering the major sleep disorders.

Evaluation of co-morbidities and associated diseases was also systematically tabulated, including evaluation of any current medical treatment. Based on the results of the interview, the decision to perform a nocturnal polysomnographic (PSG) evaluation was made.

Polysomnography (PSG)

The following variables were systematically monitored: 4 EEG (including central, frontal, and occipital derivation), 2 electro-oculo gram, EMG leads including chin and legs, and 1 ECG lead. Respiration was monitored with nasal cannula pressure transducer, oral thermistor, chest and abdomen respiratory plethysmography bands, respiratory EMG leads, pulseoximetry, neck microphone, and position sensor. Patients were continuously video recorded during the nocturnal PSG.

Based on the results of the clinical interview and PSG, patients were labeled differently. If patients presented with Sleep-Disordered Breathing (SDB), they were first treated with nasal CPAP and the monitored nasal flow was derived from a Respironics PR1™ nasal CPAP machine replacing nasal cannula recording. Presence of abnormal EMG elevation during REM sleep was determined either at initial recording or during nasal CPAP recording.

Scoring of abnormal amount of EMG activity during REM sleep

At the time of initiation of the clinical protocol, monitoring of extra EMG leads involving legs and arms had been recommended to make a valid diagnosis, but the International Classification of Sleep Disorders2 (ICSD-2) [10] did not provide cut off values for the definition of "excessive amount of phasic or tonic EMG activity," nor did they indicate which muscle should be investigated in patients suspected of RBD. As a result, the same montage for PSG was used with the addition of flexor and extensor muscle monitoring at the wrist. The EMGs were recorded with surface electrodes placed about 2 cm apart and recorded with the low frequency filter set at 10 Hz and high frequency filter set at 100 Hz.

Scoring of the abnormal EMG activity was systematically undertaken. When low EMG activity allowed the identification of a clear onset of REM sleep, a REM sleep segment was scored. Rechtschaffen and Kales criteria [11] were used for further delineation of the onset and offset of REM and to identify NREM sleep, including the presence of K complexes and sleep spindles. When there was a large increase in the chin EMG, the REM sleep segment was defined based on the presence of a phasic event (i.e., rapid eye movement and abrupt burst of EMG activity in chin EMG) and on analysis of the EEG, using sleep spindles and K complexes to delineate the REM sleep segment. Once a sleep segment had been identified as REM, each 30-second period was sub-scored looking at all EMG bursts. Each muscle burst could last up to 5 seconds, independently of the involved muscle. If two muscles presented overlapping EMG bursts, the total time spent with high EMG activity extended from the beginning of the increase EMG activity of the first muscle to the end of the EMG activity of the second muscle. In these cases, the total segment of "high EMG activity" may have been longer than 5 seconds. The percentage of time spent with "high EMG" during REM sleep was calculated.

Follow-up procedures

Once the presence of abnormal behavior and EMG activity were confirmed, and any SDB had been controlled, patients were placed on the clinical protocol. The first two patients were initially treated differently but ultimately had similar treatment to the 26 other patients at 4-month follow-up (section below). During the first 4 weeks, bed partners were asked to keep a log of the number of nights with the presence of abnormal behavior and PSG with video recording was obtained at the end of this period. Follow-up was performed the following month and every other month thereafter up to the beginning of the 7th month. At each follow-up appointment, there was an interview with the patient and bed partner, collection of 4 weeks of sleep logs, and PSG with scoring of EMG in REM. Thus, three PSGs preceded by 4 weeks of sleep logs were obtained: at baseline, at the end of the 4th month, and at the end of the 6th month. With the exception of one patient who failed to respond to treatment, further follow-up after 7 months was performed by their neurologists with only intermittent referral back to the sleep clinic.

Melatonin prescription

Initial and follow-up treatment: In the 2 initial patients seen early in our treatment investigation, melatonin was started at a dosage of 3 mg given near bedtime. After 4 weeks of drug administration, bed partners reported no clear change in behavior a confirmed by sleep logs. A follow-up PSG indicated the continued presence of an abnormal amount of leg movements, muscle twitches, and EMG bursts. The impression was that melatonin at the dosage used gave no significant clinical response. These 2 patients were then placed on clonazepam 0.5 mg at bedtime and this was increased to 1 mg after 1 month. At the 2-month follow-up, bed partners reported much quieter sleep and the absence of abnormal behavior. As behavioral symptoms were again noted at 4 months after treatment onset, these 2 patients received melatonin at a dose of 6 mg in addition to the clonazepam, and are included in the 6 months of investigation (n=28). Thereafter, oral melatonin was always prescribed at a dose of 6 mg in all patients as the initial treatment dose (n=26). The drug was administered orally, about 30 minutes before usual bedtime.

After 4 months of treatment and the results of 4 weeks of sleep logs and one PSG, clonazepam 0.5 to 1 mg was added to the melatonin 6 mg prescription to all (n=28) subjects and the treatment was maintained until the end of the clinical protocol (i.e., at the beginning of the 7th month).

Past 7th month follow-up: After the end of the clinical protocol, as mentioned, one patient who had failed to respond to the medications continued with the same follow-up regimen consisting of 4 weeks of sleep logs and a PSG. Concomitantly, the dose of melatonin was increased at 9 months and at 12 months to 12 mg and the dose of clonazepam was increased to 3 mg.

Statistical Analysis

Statistical computations were performed using the SPSS 19.0. *P* values were one-sided with a significance level of 0.05. Data on demographic and disease characteristics were analyzed by descriptive statistics. For descriptive purposes, mean and standard deviation were used to address changes in dream-acting-out, percent of WASO, and percent of EMG during REM phase for three times: at Base Line (BL), at the end of the 4th month, and at the end of the 6th month. The Generalized Estimating Equation (GEE) was used to identify the changes in dream-acting-out, percent of WASO, and percent of

EMG after receiving melatonin treatment. The GEE, an extension of the generalized linear model, was developed by Zeger and Liang and is commonly used to analyze longitudinal data [12,13]. The unequal number of follow-up assessments among study subjects (26 and 2) was taken into consideration in the GEE analysis because the GEE model used the information obtained from each assessment as the analytical unit.

Results

Patients

The 28 patients presented in this retrospective report are listed in table 1. All patients were collected during the 5 years when the clinical protocol was applied. The suspicion of OSA was the cause of referral to the sleep clinic in 14 of the 16 patients diagnosed with OSA. Abnormal behavior during sleep was mentioned in only two of the referral letters for the patients. Patients were also referred for insomnia associated with neurological diseases, but all had family member reports of abnormal behavior during sleep. These were associated with dream enactment, patient unawareness, and some had injury with bruises and trauma to themselves and/or bed partners. The mean age of the group was 66.46 ± 9.1 years and the mean Body-Mass-Index (BMI) was 26.6 ± 2.3 kg/m^2. Twenty-eight percent were women.

Co-morbidities

Initial PSG showed that 16 patients (57%) presented with Obstructive Sleep Apnea (OSA) with a mean baseline Apnea-Hypopnea Index (AHI) of 29.5 ± 8 events/hour and a mean lowest oxygen saturation of 86 ± 3%. As severe OSAS may be associated with pseudo-RBD, all patients with OSAS were first treated with nasal Continuous Positive Airway Pressure (CPAP) with demonstration of complete resolution of this sleep-disordered breathing. With CPAP treatment, the minimum oxygen saturation was 93.3 ± 2.4%, but there was still a persistence of abnormal elevations of EMG tone during REM sleep and abnormal behavior related to dreaming. Ten patients had clinical signs of Parkinson's disease with 4 of them receiving dopamine agonists for their syndrome (pramipexole 2 to 4 mg/day) and 4 other patients exhibiting cognitive decline. Six of these patients were reported to have poor nocturnal sleep labeled as "insomnia". When performing investigations for RBD, the drugs prescribed for treatment of the associated neurological disorders were kept unchanged at the prescribed dosages. The dopamine agonist was at similar dosage from entry until the end of the 7th month.

Baseline

At entry, all bed partners reported the presence of vocalization and abnormal behavior during sleep. When awakened, these behaviors were associated with dream mentation, usually of a violent nature. The history of abnormal behavior during sleep had been present for a mean of 2.5 ± 3.2 years when patients were seen. All patients had experienced arm and leg movements during sleep, leading to mild trauma to bed partners in 23 out of 28 cases and bruises in all patients.

Sleep log investigation

Tables 1 and 2 show the results of the number of nights that abnormal behavior was observed during sleep during the 4 initial weeks of sleep logs. Abnormal behavior was often associated with some type of vocalization, but of variable intensity and duration, and there were some nights with movement but no vocalization. All patients with OSAS had nasal CPAP during sleep during this baseline data collection.

PSG investigation

The first PSG at the end of the 4 weeks of sleep logs showed an abnormal presence of chin and limb EMG tone during REM sleep with a variable presence of leg movements, small arm movements, and vocalization (Figures 1 and 2). Using the criteria outlined for the scoring of high EMG during REM sleep, all patients spent more than 20% of the total REM sleep time with elevated EMG, with the inclusion of the EMG bursts tabulated from all recorded muscles. However, only 14 subjects spent 50% or more of the total REM sleep time with elevated EMG. These 14 subjects included all patients with associated neurological disorders.

During this baseline nocturnal PSG, vocalization with or without abnormal behavior was observed in only 10 of the 28 patients.

Case #	Baseline No Drug	Melatonin 6mg at 4 months	Clonazepam 0.5-1mg & Melatonin 6mg at 7 months
1	5	0	0
2	12	-	0
3	14	0	0
4	17	2	1
5	4	0	0
6	7	0	0
7	9	0	0
8	5	0	0
9	6	0	0
10	8	0	0
11	13	3	1
12	10	0	0
13	4	0	0
14	11	0	0
15	12	-	0
16	8	0	0
17	7	0	0
18	6	0	0
19	14	2	1
20	5	0	0
21	3	0	0
22	8	0	0
23	17	14	2
24	11	2	0
25	7	0	0
26	4	0	0
27	9	1	0
28	10	1	0

Table 1: Number of Nights with Abnormal Behavior at home.

	Dream-acting -out		Nights of vocalizations	
	Mean	(SD)	Mean	(SD)
Baseline (n=28)	9.18	(5.13)	9.18	(5.13)
4th month				
Melatonin 6 mg (n=26)	1.08	(2.81)	0.61	(0.96)
6th month				
Melatonin 6 mg+Clonazepam 0.5-1 mg (n=28)	0.10	(0.05)	none	

Abbreviations: RBD= Rapid Eye Movement Sleep Behavior Disorder. SD= standard deviation.

Usage of General Estimation Equation shows that there were significant improvements in "dream-acting-out " from baseline to end of 4 month(B=0.39 p=0.0008) and to end of 6 months (B=9.18, p= 0.0001)

Table 2: Summary of distributions of frequencies of dream-acting-out, and nights of vocalizationsafter the treatment of melatonin (6 mg) or/and clonazepam (.5 to 1 mg) in RBD subjects.

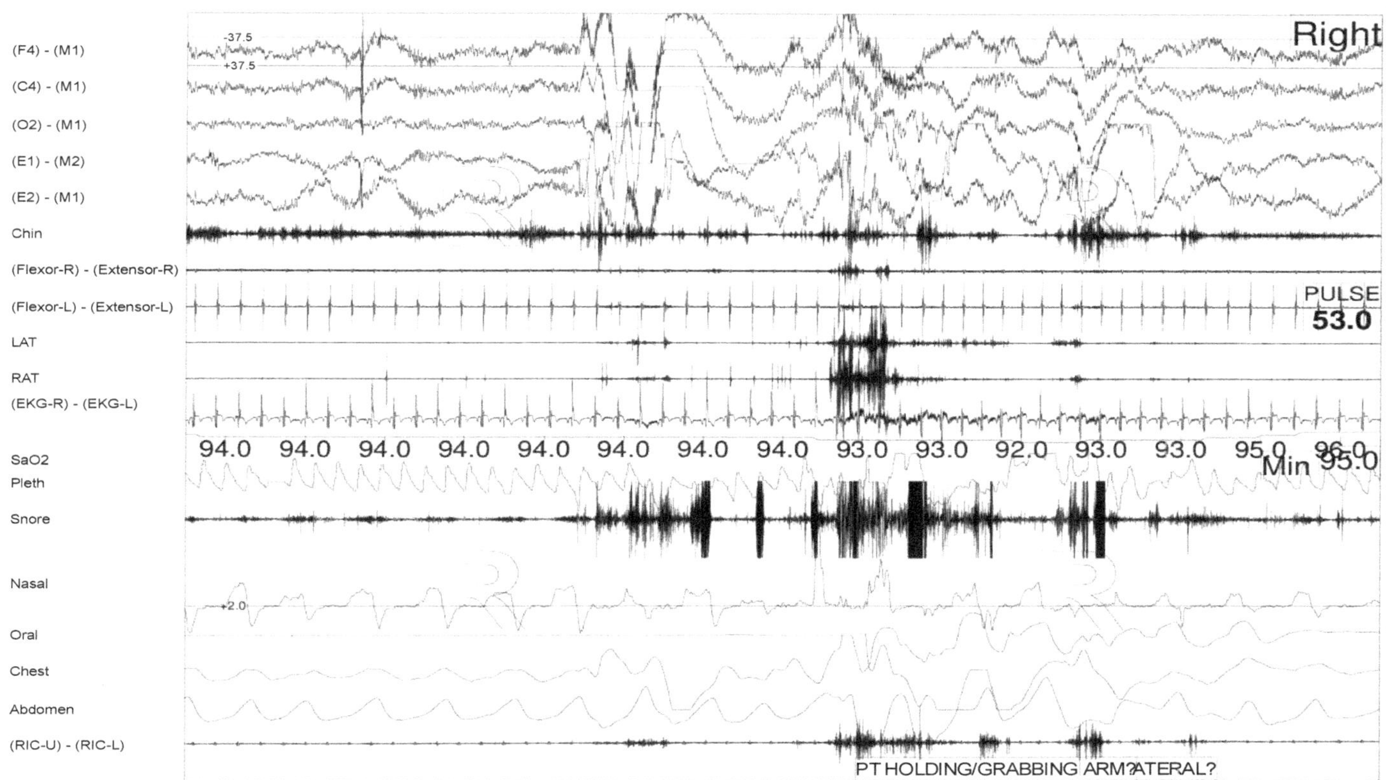

Figure 1: Polysomnogram (PSG) of a patient with REM-sleep Behavior Disorder. From top to bottom: three EEGs, right and left eye movements, 2 wrists EMG left and right leg EMG, ECG, pulse oximetry, finger plethysmography, microphone (snore), nasal pressure transducer, oral thermistor, chest and abdomen plethysmography bands, intercostal EMG. The 60 seconds recording obtained during REM sleep, as demonstrated by the rapid eye movements and the EEG, shows an abnormal amount of time with elevated EMG activity recorded by different EMG leads. The microphone indicates the presence of vocalization. Patient tried to grab something while dreaming (video- documentation).

Treatment and clinical response

All patients were treated with medication. The first 2 patients received melatonin 2 and 3 mg given near bedtime. After 8 weeks of drug administration, bed partners reported no change in the frequency of abnormal behavior and a follow-up PSG indicated the persistence of an abnormal amount of leg movements, muscle twitches, and EMG bursts. The percentages of total REM sleep time spent with elevated EMG were, respectively, 28 and 33%.With treatment, this improved to 26 and 25.4%. These patients were then treated with clonazepam 1 mg given at bedtime.

The next 26 patients received melatonin at a dose of 6 mg taken before bedtime. Table 2 shows the results obtained from the bed partner logs. Compared to baseline, there was a clear and significant improvement in all patients with treatment even though complete control of the abnormal behavior was not present in all cases. There was a significant decrease in the number of nights with reported clinical manifestations (Table 2). As can be seen in table 1, patients with a greater frequency of abnormal behavior at baseline were those, in general, who did not reach complete behavioral control during sleep with melatonin 6 mg.

Despite decreased abnormal behavior and vocalization, bed partners reported an impression that there were frequent short awakenings with the use of melatonin 6 mg. Therefore, "Wake After Sleep Onset" (WASO) was tabulated. Overall, there was a significant decrease in WASO compared to baseline. The percent of WASO during total sleep time decreased from 11.37 (SD=3.25) at baseline to 8.11 (2.48) (p=0.001Chi-square statistics) at the 4th month, but the standard deviation indicates that some subjects did not respond as well.

As clonazepam is considered to have hypnotic effects, clonazepam was also paired with melatonin in all patients. The addition of clonazepam further decreased the WASO compared to melatonin 6 mg taken in isolation, and at the end of the 6th month there was a significant reduction in the percent of time spent awake after sleep onset to 5.53 (SD=2.38) (Table 3 and Figure 3).

Evolution of the presence of high EMG during REM sleep

Repetitive PSG studies overtime indicated variable amounts of change in the percentage of elevated EMG tone during REM sleep (Table 4 and Figure 4). Compared to baseline, at the 4th month recording there were clear changes in the EMG pattern during REM sleep (Figures 5 and 6). However, as shown in figure 4, despite the fact that good control of abnormal behavior is reported by bed partners and demonstrated with sleep logs, there is actually a small, non-significant increase in the amount of time spent with high EMG at the 6-7th month recording compared to the previous recording. This is noted despite the administration of clonazepam and melatonin. There are no systematic follow-up PSG recordings after the end of the 6th month to demonstrate if this trend evolves. Only subjective reports were obtained at irregular intervals after the end of the systematic clinical protocol.

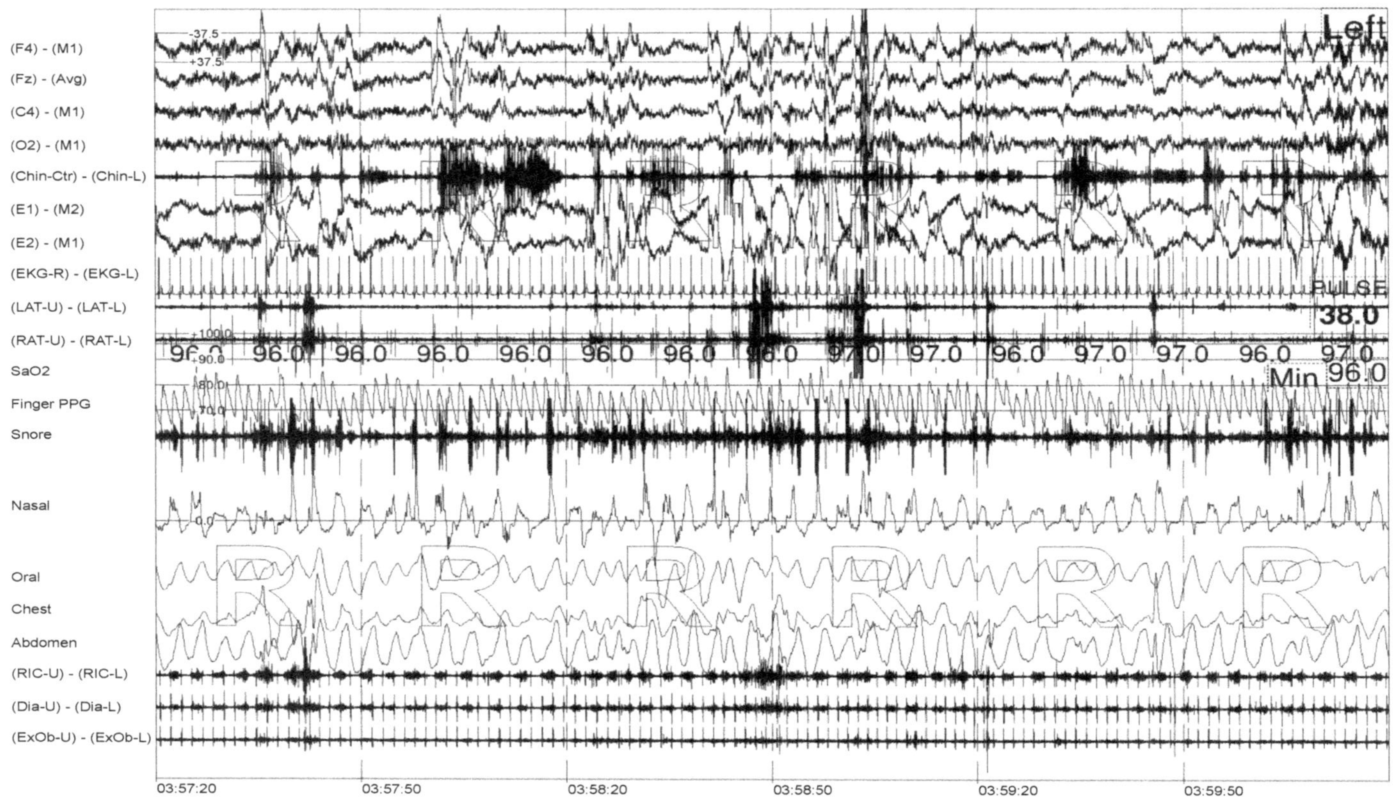

Figure 2: PSG of patient with obstructive sleep apnea treated with nasal CPAP and REM-sleep Behavior Disorder. Three minutes of polysomnographic recording during REM sleep with abnormal EMG activity.From top to bottom: Four EEGs, chin EMG, right and left eye movements, ECG, left and right leg EMG, pulse oximetry, finger plethysmography, microphone, nasal CPAP recording, chest and abdominal plethysmography bands, intercostal EMG, diaphragmatic EMG, and a upper limb EMG.Patient was treated with nasal CPAP receiving 15 cm H2O of nasal pressure but still presented with an abnormal amount of EMG activity and report of abnormal behavior during sleep.

	BL (n=28)		4th month (n=26)		6th month (n=28)	
	Mean	(SD)	Mean	(SD)	Mean	(SD)
WASO (%)	11.37	(3.25)	8.11	(2.48)	5.53	(2.38)

BL; baseline (no treatment but with nasal CPAP if with OSA), 4th month: melatonin 6 mg, 6th month melatonin 6 mg and clonazepam.5 to 1 mg
SD; standard deviation

Table 3: Percent of wake after sleep onset-WASO- during total sleep time at different time-points.

Failure

One subject diagnosed with "idiopathic RBD" and with no evidence of any other neurological disorder was never controlled by melatonin during the systematic clinical protocol. After an initial and short-lived decrease in the frequency of the events, the bed partner log indicates the recurrence of events despite subsequent dose increase. This subject was followed beyond the clinical protocol with additional month-long sleep logs and PSGs at the 9th and 12 months with increased medication doses, reaching 12 mg of melatonin and 3 mg of clonazepam near bedtime at the 12th month of evaluation. Despite these increased doses, the patient was never controlled. He slept on the floor in a sleeping bag and used arm and abdominal restraints to avoid injury from the persistent abnormal behavior.

Discussion

Our report is based on a clinical investigation and it is a retrospective study, with all the attendant limitations of this type of study. When we created our clinical protocol, there was no clear indication on the most appropriate treatment for RBD available, and both clonazepam and melatonin were used clinically as treatments. Long-term responses to treatment were not well described. Even today, when more information is available, systematic recordings are not necessarily repeated and many studies are based on sleep logs and bed partner reports. McCarter et al. [14] surveyed 45 patients seen at the Mayo clinic between 2008 and 2010 treated either with melatonin 6 mg or clonazepam 0.5 mg, and only 2 subjects received both treatments simultaneously. These authors found significant improvement in the RBD Visual Analogue Scale (VAS) with each treatment, but indicated that the patients receiving melatonin 6 mg had significantly reduced injuries and less frequent adverse effects. As this study is based on VAS, the issues of WASO and the impact on EMG augmentation in REM sleep cannot be addressed. Ferri et al. [15] also addressed the use of clonazepam in RBD, but these authors focused on the effects of the pharmaceutical agent on NREM sleep. They looked at the sleep recordings of drug-free idiopathic RBD patients and the changes observed following the administration of clonazepam on the REM sleep behavior disorder severity scale (RBDSS) [16] and on the NREM

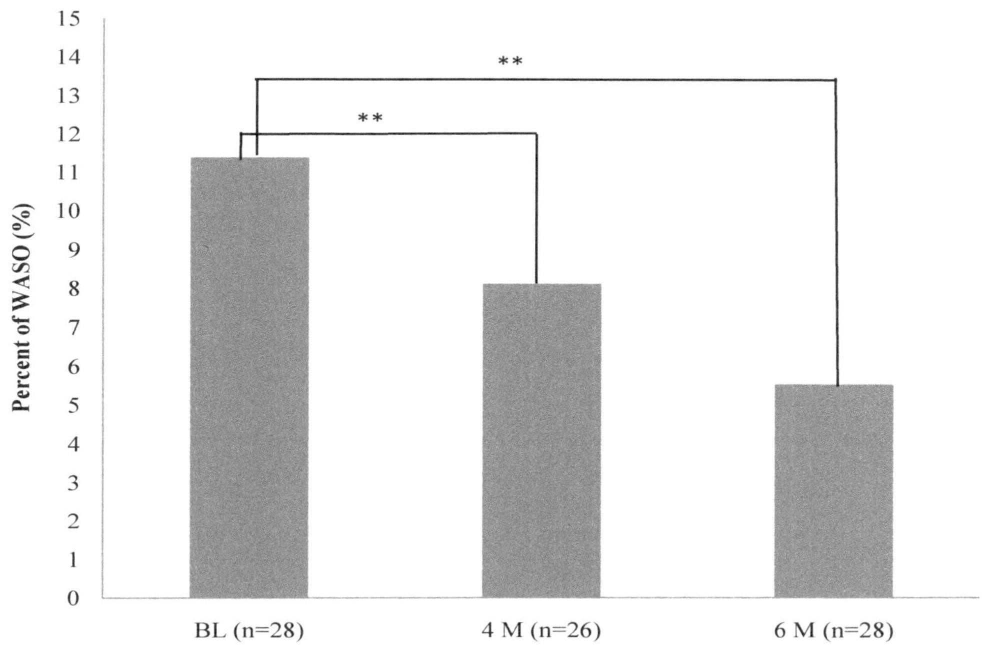

Legend: ** indicates p value <0.001. Abbreviations: WASO= wake after sleep onset. BL= baseline. 4M= 4th month. 6M= 6th month.

Figure 3: Comparison of percent of wake-after-sleep-onset-WASO- in RBD patients over time.

	BL (n=28)		4th month (n=26)		6th month (n=28)	
	Mean	(SD)	Mean	(SD)	Mean	(SD)
High EMG during REM (%)	46.98	(16.66)	1.37	(2.47)	2.55	(9.34)

At 4 months there were only 26 subjects taking melatonin 5 mg, but at end of 6th months the 28 subjects received both melatonin 6 mg and clonazepam (see text)

Table 4: Percentage of time spent with high EMG during total REM sleep time in different conditions (n=28).

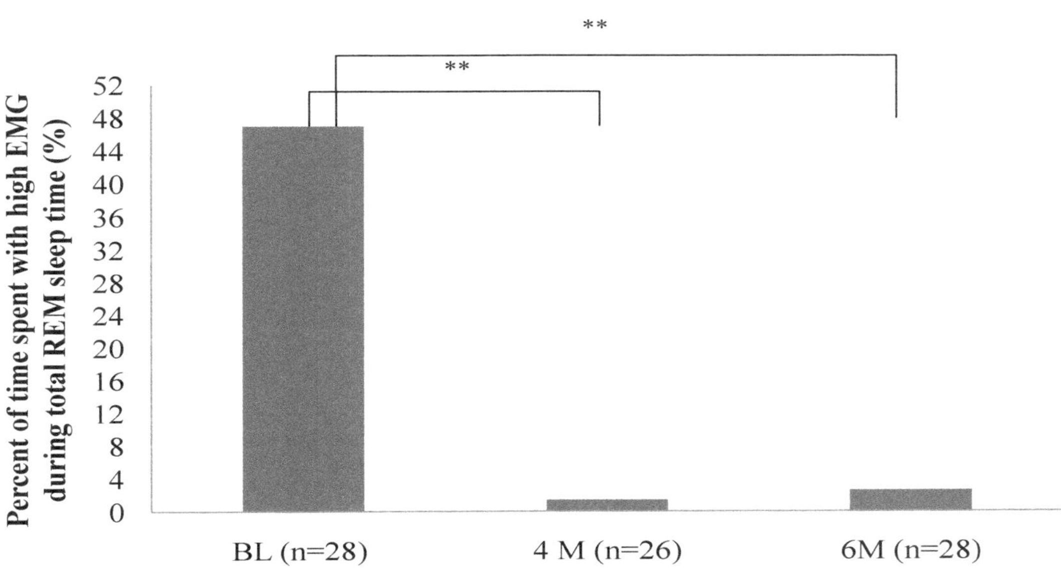

** indicates p value < 0.001. Abbreviations: EMG= electromyography. REM= rapid eye movement. BL=baseline. 4M= the 4th month. 6M= the 6th month. (GEE statistics were used)

Figure 4: Percentage of time spent with high EMG during total REM sleep time in different conditions. The calculation of "high EMG activity" took into consideration all monitored muscles and the percentage of time with high EMG activity spent during the total scored REM sleep period was calculated. The different REM sleep periods were then collapsed in a total REM sleep time, and a percentage of "high EMG activity" during total calculated REM sleep time was derived. There was a non-significant change between 4th and 6th months with increase in REM EMG at 6th month.

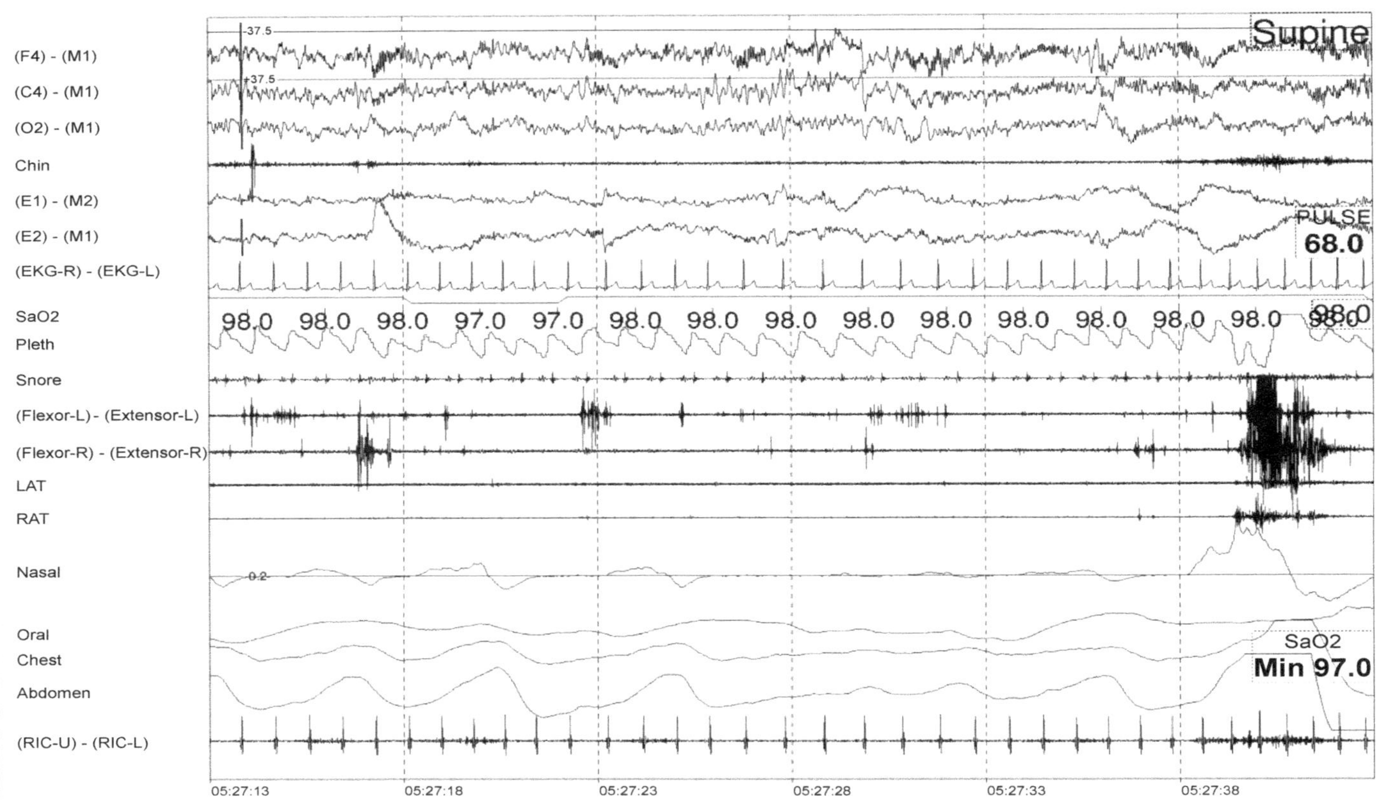

Figure 5: 30 seconds of PSG of RBD subject treated with melatonin 6 mg. From top to bottom: 3EEG, chin EMG, right and left eye movements, ECG oximetry, finger plethysmography, microphone (snore), left and right leg EMG, nasal pressure transducer, oral thermistor, chest and abdominal plethysmography belt There was a significant decrease in EMG activity compared to baseline with less than 20% of total REM time with EMG bursts, but the presented pattern could be noted intermittently. No abnormal behavior was reported by bed partner.

sleep recordings. These authors found that WASO was significantly decreased with clonazepam with an increase in stage 2 NREM sleep. The change in WASO is consistent with our finding that clonazepam decreased WASO further than melatonin alone. Our study included patients with neurological disorders, including those with Parkinson's disease, who usually have more disturbed sleep than what is usually noted in idiopathic RBD patients.

Scales have been validated since we established our clinical protocol and several could now be used. As recently reviewed by Lam et al. [17], the most attractive option to perform future follow-up studies on the treatment and evolution of RBD may be the RBD Questionnaire HongKong (RBDQ-HK) [18]. The most effective way to score the REM sleep EMG bursts has also been reviewed and improved in the recent past. Frauscher et al. [19] highlighted that until recently there was no consensus on how muscle activity during REM sleep should be scored. In 2012, the "Sleep Innsbruck-Barcelona Group" [19] proposed a way to monitor EMG activity during REM sleep and Frauscher et al. [20] also reviewed the different means of monitoring and scoring abnormal EMG activity (including computer-assisted methods). Our method of scoring was in line with what was suggested by Frauscher et al. in 2012 [19], but admittedly these methods were not exactly the same.

In our group of subjects, the diagnosis of REM behavior disorder was well established by patient history, 4 weeks of sleep logs, and repetitive PSG with video recordings. We found with our approach that at baseline there was a minimum of 20% of abnormal EMG activity during REM sleep. Moreover, melatonin at a dose of 6 mg always significantly decreased this percentage. This did not necessarily lead to a complete control of the abnormal behavior, however. In the future, one of the challenges related to follow-up of REM behavior disorder will be to establish the cut-off points based on PSGs that indicate the elimination of the risk of abnormal behavior during sleep.

Many of our patients had co-morbidities. The association of RBD with Parkinson's disease and with the presence of other neuro-degenerative diseases is well investigated. It is also known that OSA may be associated with RBD. The need to clearly control OSA before affirming the presence of RBD has been previously emphasized, and all our cases were first appropriately treated with nasal CPAP with demonstrated compliance. A fair number of subjects presented with both syndromes. The relationship between RBD and OSA has not been explored much. More than 50% of our patients had OSA and this was much more recognized than RBD in the letters of referral for sleep investigation. Except for the abnormal behavior during sleep, none of the OSA patients had any neurological symptoms and the RBD would commonly be called "idiopathic" in these subjects. They all demonstrated narrow naso-maxillary-mandibular complexes and secondary narrow upper airways, consistent with OSA. As mentioned, very little is known of the role of OSA in RBD. It is clear that both syndromes are seen in an aging population, and systematic questioning on dream-enactment behavior in OSA patients is justified. Such questioning is particularly important in patients investigated only for sleep-disordered breathing with the use of type III portable equipment

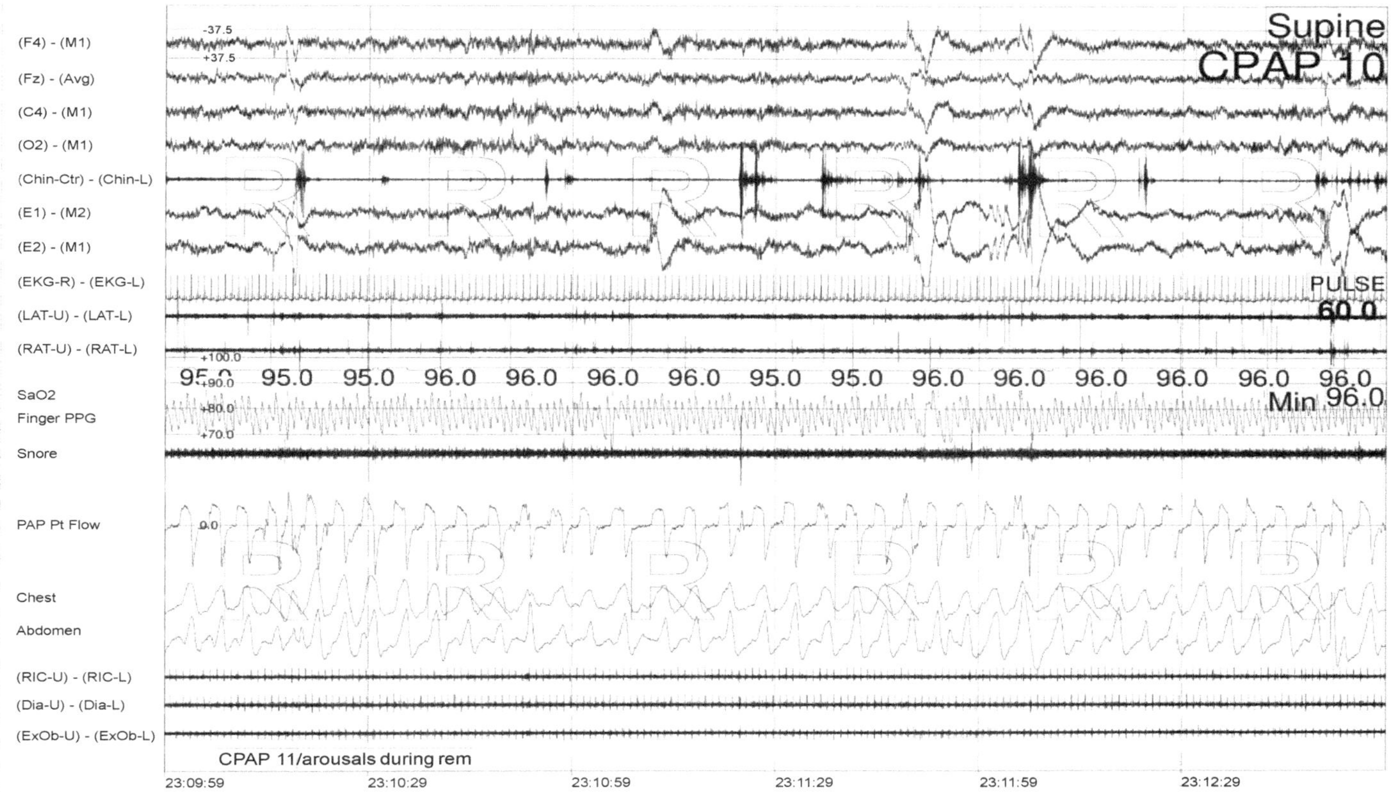

Figure 6: 3 minutes of PSG recording in a patient treated with CPAP and melatonin 6 mg. Patient has no abnormal behavior during sleep based on sleep log and clinical report. He presents with less than 20% of EMG activity during total REM time with intermittent bursts of EMG in association with REM. CPAP was set at 10 to 11 cm H2O of pressure. From top to bottom: Four EEGs, chin EMG, 2 eye movements, ECG, 2 leg EMGs, pulse oximetry, finger plethysmography, microphone (snore), CPAP flow recording (pressure at 10 cm H2O), thoracic and abdominal plethysmographic bands, intercostal EMG, diaphragmatic EMG, and upper limb EMG.

that will miss the presence of the associated patterns of elevated EMG during REM sleep.

Finally further investigation is needed to understand the underlying problems in patients that are non-responders to the usual treatments considered for RBD.

Acknowledgement

We thank Dr. Brandon R. Peters for his help in editing the manuscript.

References

1. Tachibana M, Tanaka K, Hishikawa Y, Kaneko Z (1975) A sleep study of acute psychotic states due to alcohol and meprobamate addiction. Adv Sleep Res2: 177–205.
2. Hishikawa Y, Sugita Y, Iijima S (1981) Mechanisms producing "stage-1 REM" and similar dissociation of REM sleep and their relation to delirium. AdvNeurolSci (Tokyo) 25: 1129–47.
3. Jouvet M, Delorme F (1965) Locus Coeruleusetsommeilparadoxal. CR SocBiol;159: 895–899.
4. Lupi D, Oster H, Thompson S, Foster RG (2008) The acute light-induction of sleep is mediated by OPN4-based photoreception. Nat Neurosci 11: 1068-1073.
5. Salva MA, Guilleminault C (1986) Olivopontocerebellar degeneration, abnormal sleep, and REM sleep without atonia. Neurology 36: 576-577.
6. Schenck CH, Bundlie SR, Ettinger MG, Mahowald MW. (1986) Chronic behavioral disorders of human REM sleep: a new category of parasomnia. Sleep 9: 293–308.
7. Schenck CH, Bundlie SR, Mahowald MW (1996) Delayed emergence of a parkinsonian disorder in 38% of 29 older men initially diagnosed with idiopathic rapid eye movement sleep behaviour disorder. Neurology 46: 388-393.
8. Olson EJ, Boeve BF, Silber MH (2000) Rapid eye movement sleep behaviour disorder: demographic, clinical and laboratory findings in 93 cases. Brain 123 : 331-339.
9. Boeve BF, Silber MH, Saper CB, Ferman TJ, Dickson DW, et al. (2007) Pathophysiology of REM sleep behaviour disorder and relevance to neurodegenerative disease. Brain 130: 2770-2788.
10. American Academy of Sleep Medicine (2005): International Classification of Sleep Disorders. (2ndedn). Worchester (IL)
11. Rechtschaffen A, Kales A (1968). A Manual of Standardized Terminology, Techniques and Scoring System for Sleep Stages of Human Subjects Los Angeles: BIS/BRI, UCLA.
12. Burton P, Gurrin L, Sly P (1998) Extending the simple linear regression model to account for correlated responses: an introduction to generalized estimating equations and multi-level mixed modelling. Stat Med 17: 1261-1291.
13. Zeger SL, Liang KY (1986) Longitudinal data analysis for discrete and continuous outcomes. Biometrics 42: 121-130.
14. McCarter SJ, Boswell CL, St Louis EK, Dueffert LG, Slocumb N, et al. (2013) Treatment outcomes in REM sleep behavior disorder. Sleep Med 14: 237-242.
15. Ferri R, Zucconi M, Marelli S, Plazzi G, Schenck CH, et al. (2013) Effects of long-term use of clonazepam on nonrapid eye movement sleep patterns in rapid eye movement sleep behavior disorder. Sleep Med 14: 399-406.
16. Sixel-Döring F, Schweitzer M, Mollenhauer B, Trenkwalder C (2011) Intraindividual variability of REM sleep behavior disorder in Parkinson's disease: a comparative assessment using a new REM sleep behavior disorder severity scale (RBDSS) for clinical routine. J Clin Sleep Med 7: 75-80.
17. Lam SP, Li SX, Zhang JZ, Wing YK (2013) Development of scales for the

assessment of REM behavior disorder. Sleep Med. Dx.doi.org/10.1016/j. sleep2012.09.008

18. Li SX, Wing YK, Lam SP, Zhang J, Yu MW, et al. (2010) Validation of a new REM sleep behavior disorder questionnaire (RBDQ-HK). Sleep Med 11: 43-48.
19. Frauscher B, Iranzo A, Gaig C, Gschliesser V, Guaita M, et al. (2012) Normative EMG values during REM sleep for the diagnosis of REM sleep behavior disorder. Sleep 35: 835-847.
20. Frauscher B, Ehrmann L, Högl B (2012) Defining muscle activities for assessment of REM sleep behavior disorder: From a qualitative to a quantitative diagnostic level. Sleep Med .

Effects of the CPAP Treatment on the NON-REM Sleep Microstructures in Patients with Severe Apnea-Hypoapnea Syndrome

Marcela Smurra[1], Susana Blanco[2*], Veronica Eguiguren[1] and Cecilia DiRisio[3]

[1]*Hospital Tornú, Argentina*
[2]*Faculty of Engineering, University of Belgrano-CONICET, Argentina*
[3]*Dosimetry Laboratory and Medical Technology, Faculty of Engineering, University of Belgrano, Argentina*

Abstract

Sleep quality is affected in patients with sleep apnea- hypopnea syndrome (SAHS) with nocturnal and diurnal consequences. Most of these patients who are treated with positive airway pressure (CPAP) return to normal sleep patterns. We could consider good sleepers those patients who present more sleep spindles in stage II, and slower wave sleep as a good sign of better sleep quality.

The objective in this research study was to compare the microstructure of stage II using the number of spindles and the increase of slow wave sleep before and after CPAP night titration.

We developed a wavelet filter using a spline cubic function from a wavelet mother, which was appropriate to be used over electroencephalographic signal. By means of this filter in a multi-resolution mode, the spindles were detected from the increase of the IV band power; the sampling rate of the device determined the filter characteristics. The staging of polysomnographic studies was made by an expert according AASM (American Academy of Sleep Medicine) and then processed by the filter to get the index of sleep spindles before-and-after CPAP during stage II as well as the relationship between fast and slow powers from the EEG signal. An increase in the power of the slow waves vs. fast activity was observed in all the cases as a feature of better sleep. The neuroprotective effect described in previous research works regarding the density of the sleep spindles seems to be detected in patients improving their sleep quality after the correction of the apnea-hypopnea syndrome using CPAP.

Keywords: Sleep spindles; Polisomnographic; Wavelets analysis; Slow wave sleep; CPAP

Introduction

The Sleep Apnea-Hypopnea Syndrome (SAHS) is a disorder characterized by recurrent episodes of either a partial or complete collapse of the upper airway during sleep. The resulting reduction of the airflow leads to alterations in gas exchange as well as recurrent arousals causing sleep fragmentation.

The prevalence rate is 3-7% and 2-5% in men and women respectively [1-3]. Clinically, somnolence is the most important symptom and it depends on the sleep fragmentation caused by microarousals related to respiratory effort and intermittent hypoxemia or both. With CPAP treatment, it is possible to achieve shorter times of reaction in vigilance tests as well higher levels in talking, visual and spatial memory tasks. It is also possible to improve depression and anxiety scores.

Spindles are structures of sleep EEG with a frequency range between 12 and 15 Hz, and with a duration of more than 0.5 seconds and a minimum width of 15 mV [4,5]. In previous studies comparing frequency patterns of spindles in patients with sleep apnea vs. control subjects, there was less frequency of sleep spindles within the former group, with no increase of spindles towards the end of the night [6].

Accordingly, the aim of the present work was to study the increase of spindles in phase II and slow wave sleep power vs fast wave sleep power frequency in patients with severe sleep apnea syndrome, quantifying them by indexes, before and after modifying the breathing pattern with CPAP treatment, considering these changes features of stable sleep.

Materials and Methods

We have performed the analysis of the sleep structure in the polysomnographic studies of 10 patients at baseline situation and post-calibration of CPAP to score sleep according to AASM standards [7].

Records were taken through the following standard:

1. Three channels of EEG: Two central (C3 and C4) and one occipital (O1) referenced to the left and right mastoids (A2 and A1) (systems 10-20) with sampling frequency of 349 Hz.
2. Two EOG channels with left and right eyelid electrodes.
3. Three EMG channels, two of them in sub-chin position and the other one in tibial location with a sampling frequency of 349 Hz.
4. EKG recorded from two electrode derivations in the second right and left intercostals space in paraesternal location with a sampling frequency of 349 Hz.
5. Oronasal flow sensors. One of them, of a thermistor type, and a nasal cannula with a pressure transducer to detect flow limitation through nasal pressure measurement.

***Corresponding author:** Susana Blanco, Faculty of Engineering, University of Belgrano-CONICET, Villanueva 1324, Buenos Aires, Argentina
E-mail: susana.blanco2006@gmail.com

6. A thoracic and abdominal piezoelectric band to record breathing effort.

7. A body position sensor.

8. Pulse oxymetry.

All records were carried out with 18-channel ATI Praxis equipment specially designed for polysomnography. (Polysomnograph equipment, Praxis 18-Line AMP18P-Lermed s.r.l Trade Mark).

Visual assessment of the alpha band power behavior with respect to the marked micro-awakenings was performed with the software associated with the AMP 18P. The remaining algorithms required to calculate the synchronization between ECG and EEG channels were developed with the help of MatLab 7.0.

Polysomnographic tracings in NREM stage were chosen and read sequentially in order to avoid the bias produced by the simultaneous observation of EEG and breathing events. At first, the EEG scoring was performed according to AAMS standards [7]; arousals are defined as an abrupt shift of EEG frequency including alpha, theta and/or frequencies greater than 16 Hz (but not spindles) that last at least 3 seconds, with at least 10 seconds of stable sleep preceding the change. Scoring of arousal during REM requires a concurrent increase in sub mental EMG lasting at least 1 second.

The respiratory events were classified as follows:

Apneas: There is a drop in the peak signal excursion by ≥ 90% of pre-event baseline using an oronasal thermal sensor (diagnostic study), PAP device flow (titration study) or an alternative apnea sensor (diagnostic study), during ≥ 10 seconds. Score an apnea as obstructive if it meets apnea criteria and is associated with continued or increased inspiratory effort throughout the entire period of absent airflow, as central if it meets apnea criteria and is associated with absent inspiratory effort throughout the entire period of absent airflow, and an apnea as mixed if it meets apnea criteria and is associated with absent inspiratory effort in the initial portion of the event, followed by resumption of inspiratory effort in the second portion of the event.

Hypopnea: The peak signal excursions drop by ≥ 30% of pre-event baseline using nasal pressure (diagnostic study), PAP device flow (titration study), or an alternative hypopnea sensor (diagnostic study) during ≥ 10 seconds. There is a ≥ 3% oxygen desaturation from pre-event baseline or the event is associated with an arousal.

Respiratory effort-related arousals, score a respiratory event as a respiratory effort-related arousal (RERA) if there is a sequence of breaths lasting ≥ 10 seconds characterized by increasing respiratory effort or by flattening of the inspiratory portion of the nasal pressure (diagnostic study) or PAP device flow (titration study) waveform leading to arousal from sleep when the sequence of breaths does not meet criteria for an apnea or hypopnea.

We have scored the severity of the disease according to the RDI (respiratory disturbance index) calculated as: numbers of respiratory events/Total sleep time x 60. More than 15 events/hour are considered an index of severity to determine the application of CPAP.

To obtain an optimal CPAP titration, we have taken into account the elimination of respiratory events or their reduction to reach a residual respiratory disturbance index not exceeding 5/h.

An adequate oxygenation and the lack of arousals partially ensure some improvement of sleep quality.

As a measure of this improvement in phase II sleep, we defined in this work the index IS=spindles number /time (minutes) and the index IW=SWP/FWP as the relationship between the power of slow and rapid waves with independence of the spindle frequency.

Mathematical Detection of Sleep Spindles and Cuantification of Swp Y Fwp

The wavelet transform gives us a powerful tool to analyze, from a time-frequency point of view, very diverse problems in applied sciences or pure mathematics [8-12].

A wavelet is a smooth and quickly vanishing oscillating function with good localization in both frequency and time.

A wavelet family $\psi_{a,b}(t)$ is a set of elemental functions generated by dilations and translations of a unique admissible mother wavelet $\psi(t)$:

$$\psi_{a,b}(t) = |a|^{-1/2}\psi(t-b/a)$$

Where $\mathbf{a, b} \in \mathbf{R}, \mathbf{a} \neq \mathbf{0}$ are the scale and translation parameters respectively and **t** is the time. As **a** increases, the wavelet becomes narrower. Thus we have a unique analytic pattern and its replicas at different scales and with variable localization in time.

Given a finite energy signal S(t), the different correlations $< \mathbf{S}, \psi_{a,b} >$ indicate how precisely the wavelet function locally fits this signal at every scale **a.** This correlation operation defines the transformation that synthesizes the numerical information obtained in this way. From a different viewpoint, the wavelets of a family play the role of elemental functions, representing the functions as a superposition of wavelets correlated with the function for different scales (different **a's**). This makes it possible to organize the information in some particular structure to distinguish, for example, trends or the shape associated with long scales of the local details from corresponding short scales.

For the special selection of the function ψ and a discrete net of parameters $a_j = 2^{-j}$ **and** $b_{j,k} = 2^{-j}k$, with $\mathbf{j, k} \in \mathbf{Z}$ and the scale 2^{-j} give us the shift parameter.

The subfamily

$$\Psi_{j,k}(t) = 2^{j/2}\Psi(2^j(t-k))j, k \in Z$$

constitutes an orthonormal basis of the Hilbert space L^2 (R). In this way, we can obtain discrete transformations, and it is possible to expand the signal in series of wavelets.

The discrete wavelet transform associated with ψ is simply seen as a restriction of the continuous wavelet. In this case, as it is well known, the information given by the discrete wavelet transform can be organized according to a hierarchical scheme of nested subspaces called multi resolution analysis in L^2 (R).

In the present analysis, we used a multirresolution scheme based on cubic orthogonal spline functions as a mother wavelet, with a discretized version of the integral wavelet transform given by Unser (Unser, 1996 [8]). We selected this wavelet due to the fact that it forms a base in L^2 (R) with a very convenient characteristic of symmetry and simplicity:

$$S(t) = \sum_K S_O(k)\phi(t-k)$$

where $\Phi(t)$ is the cubic cardinal spline.

For any resolution level N<0 we can write the decomposition of the signal as:

$$S(t) = \sum_K SN(k)\phi(2^N t-k) + \sum_{j=-N}^{-1}\sum_K C_j(k)\psi_{j,k}(t)$$

where $Cj(k)$ are the wavelet coefficients and the sequence $\{sN(k)\}$ represents the coarser signal data at resolution level N.

The second term is the wavelet expansion.

Since the family $\{\psi_{j,k}(t)\}$ is an orthonormal basis for L^2 (R), the concept of energy is linked with the usual notions derived from the Fourier theory. The sum $E_j = \sum_K |C_j(k)|^2$ gives us the energy of the details of S(t) at level j; and the total energy is given by $Etot = |S|^2 = \sum_{j<0} E_j$.

The polysomnographic system used for this research study let us obtain the raw data of each biological signal. Accordingly, we were able to develop the wavelet algorithm in the MATLAB programming environment.

We divided the EEG signals into 5 wavelet levels and we calculated a filter involving the characteristic frequencies of the sleep spindles (a burst with a spindle shape with frequencies between 11 and 15 Hz).

According to the characteristics of the multi-resolution scheme and sample rate of our equipment (349 Hz), spindles can be correlated to level 4 of a multi-resolution scheme.

Using the condition that the cubic spline functions constitute a base, each octave in which the signal is unfolded is linearly independent.

This enables us to calculate the energy of each octave independently by squaring the coefficients of the decomposition.

Using the power of the filtered signal in the band between 11 and 15 Hz as a way of viewing the spindles is both practical and graphic since the presence of a spindle is viewed as an increase of the resulting signal power.

In this manner it is simple to count spindles either manually or with peak-counting software. The software used for the wavelet analysis of the EEG signal was developed in Delphi language in order to connect it to the commercial software, with the authorization of the manufacturers and using windows to display and compare the signals.

As this multiresolution scheme let us calculate the energy of each octave independently, by squaring the coefficients of the wavelet decomposition, we define SPW summing the wavelet levels since 0.5 Hz to 8.0 Hz, and FWP summing the levels since 8.0 Hz to 30 Hz.

Results

The one-way ANOVA test was used to evaluate the differences between the indexes RDI, IS and IW in pre and post CPAP conditions. In the same way, by using the two-way ANOVA test, we evaluated the behavior of pre and post CPAP IS during the three different periods in which we divided every night of study. In all cases, we considered a 95% confidence level ($p<0.05$).

Table 1 shows the demographic characteristics of the patients and the respiratory disturbance index (RDI) pre and post CPAP results of the index. Statistical differences were observed when we compared the RDI (respiratory disturbance index) before and after CPAP.

Table 2 shows, for every patient, the indexes IS and IW before and after use of CPAP for the hole night.

There was an average percentage growth of the spindle rate per minute (IS) in all cases and an increase in the IW too. The use of CPAP leads to an increase in IW which is much higher than the increase of the index IS.

Statistical analysis (with $\alpha = 0.05$) showed significant differences between the indexes IS before and after CPAP.

The relationship between slow wave power vs. fast waves (IW) statistical analysis of the indices (with $\alpha=0.05$) showed significant differences pre and post CPAP.

To make a more detailed analysis, the nights were divided into thirds and spindles were counted in each. Table 3 shows the results for the IS index in each third of the night. Figure 1 show, plotted for the three thirds, pre and post CPAP IS indexes for each patient.

In the sample used, no significant differences were observed in the three night-time periods, either with or without CPAP, using the statistical variance F to a 95% confidence level. Significative differences were found for each third, pre and post CPAP.

Conclusion

The new proposed indexes, IS and IW, show a coherent behavior with the traditional RDI. These new indexes represent physiological information instead only statistical. We centralized our analysis in phase II.

Both indexes represent an indication of the physiological response to the CPAP use. Both are a representation of sleep quality but as it is well known, both have different neurological sources. It is interesting that both have a coherent response.

In our study, we detected a significant increase of the spindles/time index in patients with sleep breathing disorders, before and after the night of CPAP titration. There were no significant differences in the rate of spindles/time when we took into account three different times

P1	62	M	82	1,67	29,40	68	6,4
P2	70	F	51	1,55	21,23	24,3	4,67
P3	70	F	61	1,58	24,43	14,9	6
P4	66	F	118	1,58	47,27	36,5	5,2
P5	60	M	107	1,8	33,02	37,3	0,45
P6	75	M	128	1,76	41,32	56,6	24
P7	65	M	89	1,78	28,09	56	5,6
P8	47	F	85	1,69	29,76	25,8	2,5
P9	76	F	74	1,59	29,27	32,5	1,2
P10	69	M	82	1,63	30,86	20,6	2,7

Table 1: Patient data, BMI: body mass index, RDI: respiratory disturbance index pre and post CPAP.

1	1.2	1.5	3,5	13,1
2	1.2	1.9	1,8	25,2
3	0.87	1.6	2,5	15,7
4	1.18	1.30	2,7	20,6
5	1.61	1.74	2,1	15,4
6	1.18	2.14	3,5	5,2
7	2.	2.16	4,3	17,2
8	1.74	1.89	2,2	7,3
9	1.56	2.6	0,9	1,2
10	2.1	2.7	1	2,1

Table 2: ISPr :spindles number /time (minutes) pre CPAP, ISPospindles number / time (minutes) post CPAP. IWprand, IWporelationship between the power of slow and rapid waves pre and post CPAP.

P1	1,72	1,3
	1	1,27
	0,94	2,14
P2	1,53	1,9
	1,4	1,96
	1,78	1,82
P3	0,73	1,51
	1,06	1,76
	0,85	1,67
P4	1,2	1,03
	1,12	1,39
	1,18	1,37
P5	1,54	1,75
	1,57	1,57
	1,72	1,88
P6	1,2	2,21
	0,8	1,73
	1,41	2,16
P7	2	2,78
	1,8	2,3
	2,18	1,86
P8	1,55	1,7
	2,02	1,75
	1,81	2,5
P9	1,55	3,28
	1,53	2,27
	1,61	2
P10	2,13	2,35
	2,16	2,75
	2,27	2,75

Table 3: ISPo/r are the ISP index with and without CPAP during each third of the sleep time, for each patient.

at night. In the same sense, the increase of slow wave power vs. fast frequencies in EEG in studies with CPAP supports the hypothesis of the sleep protecting function in the transition of stage II to SWS.

The automatic spindle analysis has been technically solved with enough accuracy to detect these structures with antecedents in literature published since 1979, showing a good correlation between automatic and manual analysis and achieving 90% accuracy [13,14]. However, automatic scoring cannot take into consideration the differences in type and frequency of spindles [15]. In our study, we reached be very good results in identifying sleep structures using manual and automatic models to read polysomnographic tracings.

Old reports related sleep spindles as inhibitors of arousals and sleep preserver function; Hongo et al. [16] and Gaillard respectively [16,17] associated them with arousal inhibition. Accordingly, considering the K-complex as a possible transitory activation reaction, there is a description of an antagonistic effect with respect to the spindles, in other words, the higher the number of spindles, the fewer K-complexes. K-complexes represent an organismic state leading towards activation reaction [5]. Gora et al. [18] describe a "blunted" response to occlusion stimulus to elicit K-Complex in mild OSAS patients. We cannot detect a typical pattern in K-Complex distribution in relationship to Sleep Breathing Disorder before and after CPAP titration.

However, spindles participate in an activating effect through different ways generating thalamic activation processes for inhibiting access during NREM intrusive sounds, protecting the stability of sleep [19]. They also participate in sensory-motor processes and memory information [20].

The transition from low to high delta activity (starting in phase II with the progression from 3 to 4), which may indicate the deepness of sleep, supports the hypothesis of the relationship "sleep spindles-sleep stabilization", and sleep protecting function [15].

Patients with SAHS showed a lower level of neurocognitive information processing, initially related to sleep fragmentation and, secondly, to hypoxia episodes [19,20]. Hence, we hypothesized that other mechanisms, like the structural alterations of sleep that we observed in this study, can act as co-factors adding to transient arousal and hypoxia.

There are special situations to consider; in children, lower levels of sleep disruption were observed. NREM 2 sleep decreases but slow wave sleep is fairly preserved [21,22]. Sleep quality in obese patients is affected independently of the presence of sleep-related respiratory disorders with increased superficial sleep stages and decreased efficiency [23,24]. Even in patients with mild SAHS, a lower rate of sleep spindles, deep slow-wave sleep (SWS) and a greater index of arousal were observed in comparison with controls [25].

Although the efficacy of positive pressure for the elimination of respiratory events is fairly acknowledged, few details about its effect on sleep structure have been evaluated.

The slow spindle frequencies in apnea patients could indicate disturbed sleep and altered neural mechanisms in the structures regulating sleep spindle activity [26].

Loredo et al. [27] studied the effect of CPAP treatment on sleep quality in patients using the device for a short term and found no differences in those compared with sham CPAP [27].

More recently, an evaluation in the long term after an average 9-month CPAP use, the increase of deep slow wave sleep observed in the patients treated was similar to the proportion of SWS seen in the control group [28]. There was more SWS in prefrontal areas both before and after CPAP treatment, and SWS increased significantly more in prefrontal than central areas during treatment; even using a central location of electrodes, significant changes were obtained in SWS proportion [29].

The decrease of the tendency to present arousals in deep slow wave sleep would be the explanation for the increased neuromechanical stability of the upper airway at this stage of sleep [30-32] even though the compensatory ventilation response in either deep slow wave sleep or stage II does not appear to be different when assessed through the use of dial-down techniques from therapeutic levels of CPAP. The only finding that establishes a difference is that in phase II, the arousal threshold is lower than in the slow sleep pattern [33].

As far as we know, there are no bibliographic references about structural changes in sleep in relation to the effect of nasal positive pressure during the titration process in the same patient. The choice of indexes of spindles/minute, or the relationship SWS/fast frequencies seems to illustrate more clearly, according to our criteria, the change of EEG frequencies rather than their absolute variations as dynamic indicators of the changes generated by the treatment, showing significant modifications in the sleep microstructure as a sign of therapeutic success in the same patient.

However, it should certainly be emphasized that in our study, we can add sleep structural modifications to sleep and oximetric stability

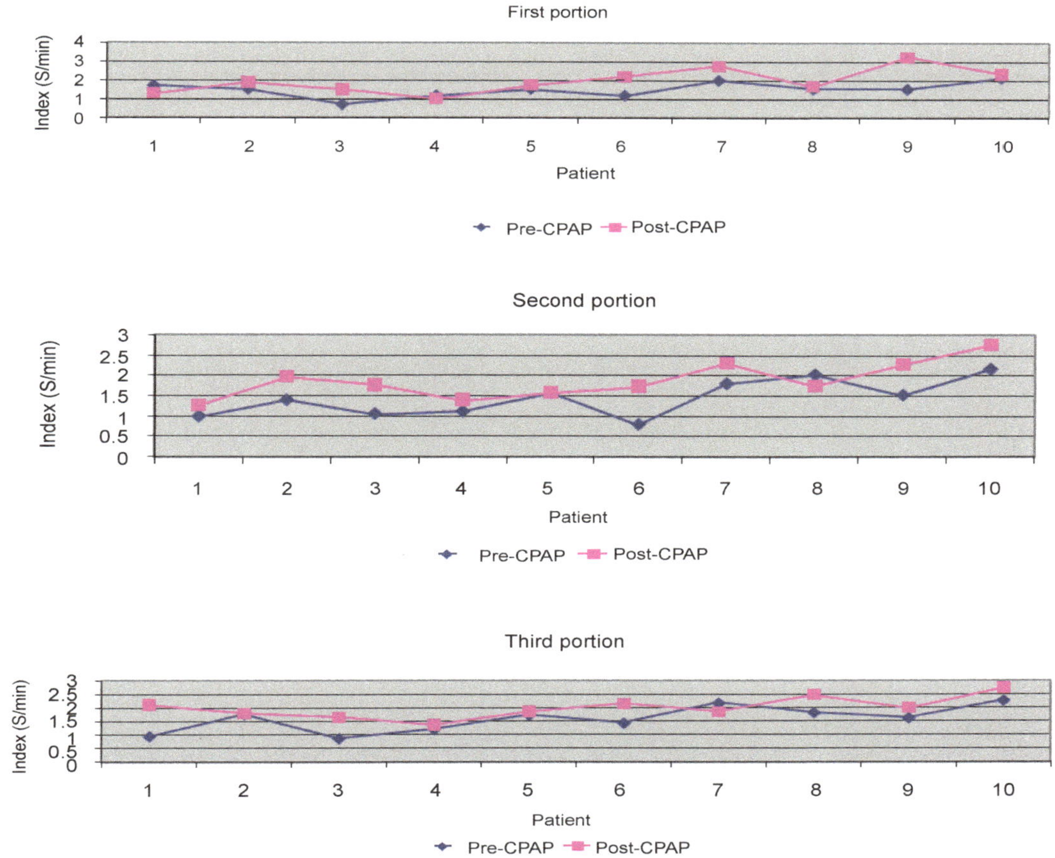

Figure 1: IS index for each patient and portion of sleep time.

to consider efficient CPAP titration, and with long term use of CPAP, the improvement in both the clinical and the neurocognitive courses can be achieved.

We think that a multirresolution scheme filter, using a mother wavelet cubic spline, is an appropriate tool to isolate sleep microstructures patterns. Furthermore, assessments should include the evaluation of the clinical impact of these changes in sleep structure, and the comparison of the acute effect of sleep deprivation in individuals without sleep breathing disorders.

References

1. Young T, Palta M, Dempsey J, Skatrud J, Weber S, et al. (1993) The occurrence of sleep-disordered breathing among middle-aged adults. N Engl J Med 328: 1230-1235.

2. Bixler EO, Vgontzas AN, Lin HM, Ten Have T, Rein J, et al. (2001) Prevalence of sleep-disordered breathing in women: effects of gender. Am J Respir Crit Care Med 163: 608-613.

3. Roure N, Mediano O, Durán-Cantolla J, García Río F, de la Peña M, et al. (2008) [Differences in clinical and polysomnographic variables between male and female patients with sleep apnea-hypopnea syndrome]. Arch Bronconeumol 44: 685-688.

4. Naitoh P, Antony-Baas V, Muzet A, Ehrhart J (1982) Dynamic relation of sleep spindles and K-complexes to spontaneous phasic arousal in sleeping human subjects. Sleep 5: 58-72.

5. Ehrhart J, Ehrhart M, Muzet A, Schieber JP, Naitoh P (1981) K-complexes and sleep spindles before transient activation during sleep. Sleep 4: 400-407.

6. Huupponen E, Himanen SL, Hasan J, Verri A (2003) Automatic analysis of electro-encephalogram sleep spindle frequency throughout the night. Med Biol Eng Comput 41: 727-732.

7. Berry RB, Brooks R, Gamaldo CE, Harding SM, Marcus CL, et al. (20120 American Academy of Sleep Medicine. The AASM Manual for the Scoring of Sleep and Associated Events: Rules, Terminology and Technical Specifications, Version 2.0. Darien, Illinois, American Academy of Sleep Medicine.

8. Unser M, Aldroubi A (1996) Review of Wavelets in Biomedical Applications. Proc of IEEE 84: 626-638.

9. Blanco S, D'Attellis CE, Isaacson SI, Rosso OA, Sirne RO (1996) Time-frequency analysis of electroencephalogram series. II. Gabor and wavelet transforms. Phys Rev E Stat Phys Plasmas Fluids Relat Interdiscip Topics 54: 6661-6672.

10. Blanco S, Kochen S, Rosso OA, Salgado P (1997) Applying time-frequency analysis to seizure EEG activity. IEEE Eng Med Biol Mag 16: 64-71.

11. Blanco S, Figliola A, Quiroga RQ, Rosso OA, Serrano E (1998) Time-Frequency analysis of electroencephalogram series (III): Information Transfer Function and Wavelets Packets. Physical Review E 57: 932-940.

12. Rosso OA, Blanco S, Yordanova J, Kolev V, Figliola A, et al. (2001) Wavelet entropy: a new tool for analysis of short duration brain electrical signals. J Neurosci Methods 105: 65-75.

13. Matsubayashi K, Ishiyama Y, Homma I, Ebe M (1981) Some characteristics of sleep spindles derived from automatic analysis. Sleep 4: 392-399.

14. Kumar A, Hofman W, Campbel K (1979) An Authomatic spindle analysis and detection system based on the evaluation of human ratings of the spindle quality. Walking and Sleeping 3: 325-33.

15. Kubicki S, Herrmann WM (1996) The future of computer-assisted investigation of the polysomnogram: sleep microstructure. J Clin Neurophysiol 13: 285-294.

16. Hongo T, Kubota K, Shimazu H (1963) EEG spindle and depression of gamma motor activity. J Neurophysiol 26: 568-580.

17. Gaillard JM, Aubert C (1975) Specificity of benzodiacepine action on human sleep confirmed, another contribution of authomatic analysis of polygraph recordings. Biol Spsychiatry 10: 185-197.

18. Gora J, Trinder J, Pierce R, Colrain IM (2002) Evidence of a sleep-specific blunted cortical response to inspiratory occlusions in mild obstructive sleep apnea syndrome. Am J Respir Crit Care Med 166: 1225-1234.

19. Schabus M, Dang-Vu TT, Albouy G, Balteau E, Boly M, et al. (2007) Hemodynamic cerebral correlates of sleep spindles during human non-rapid eye movement sleep. Proc Natl Acad Sci U S A 104: 13164-13169.

20. Verstraeten E (2007) Neurocognitive effects of obstructive sleep apnea syndrome. Curr Neurol Neurosci Rep 7: 161-166.

21. Cote KA, Epps TM, Campbell KB (2000) The role of the spindle in human information processing of high-intensity stimuli during sleep. J Sleep Res 9: 19-26.

22. Yang JSC, Nicholas CL, Nixon GM, Davey MJ, Anderson V, et al. (2010) Determining sleep quality in children with sleep disordered breathing: EEG spectral analysis compared with conventional polysomnography. Sleep 33: 1165-1172.

23. Vgontzas AN, Bixler EO, Tan TL, Kantner D, Martin LF, et al. (1998) Obesity without sleep apnea is associated with daytime sleepiness. Arch Intern Med 158: 1333-1337.

24. Resta O, Foschino Barbaro MP, Bonfitto P, Giliberti T, Depalo A, et al. (2003) Low sleep quality and daytime sleepiness in obese patients without obstructive sleep apnoea syndrome. J Intern Med 253: 536-543.

25. Ondze B, Espa F, Dauvilliers Y, Billiard M, Besset A (2003) Sleep architecture, slow wave activity and sleep spindles in mild sleep disordered breathing. Clin Neurophysiol 114: 867-874.

26. Himanen SL, Virkkala J, Huuponen E, Hasan J (2003) Spindle frequency remains slow in sleep apnea patients throughout the night. Sleep Med 4: 229-234.

27. Loredo JS, Ancoli-Israel S, Dimsdale JE (1999) Effect of continuous positive airway pressure vs placebo continuous positive airway pressure on sleep quality in obstructive sleep apnea. Chest 116: 1545-1549.

28. Heinzer R, Gaudreau H, Décary A, Sforza E, Petit D, et al. (2001) Slow-wave activity in sleep apnea patients before and after continuous positive airway pressure treatment: contribution to daytime sleepiness. Chest 119: 1807-1813.

29. Eskelinen V, Uibu T, Himanen SL (2007) nCPAP treatment of obstructive sleep apnea increases slow wave sleep in prefrontal EEG. Clin EEG Neurosci 38: 148-154.

30. Gleeson K, Zwillich CW, White DP (1990) The influence of increasing ventilatory effort on arousal from sleep. Am Rev Respir Dis 142: 295-300.

31. Berry RB, Bonnet MH, Light RW (1992) Effect of ethanol on the arousal response to airway occlusion during sleep in normal subjects. Am Rev Respir Dis 145: 445-452.

32. Berry RB, Asyali MA, McNellis MI, Khoo MC (1998) Within-night variation in respiratory effort preceding apnea termination and EEG delta power in sleep apnea. J Appl Physiol (1985) 85: 1434-1441.

33. Ratnavadivel R, Stadler D, Windler S, Bradley J, Paul D, et al. (2010) Upper airway function and arousability to ventilatory challenge in slow wave versus stage 2 sleep in obstructive sleep apnoea. Thorax 65: 107-112.

Excessive Daytime Sleepiness in Patients with Depressive Symptoms in a Nigerian Family Practice Setting

Shittu RO[1]*, Issa BA[2], Olanrewaju GT[2], Odeigah LO[1], Sule AG[1], Sanni MA[3] and Aderibigbe SA[4]

[1]*Department of Family Medicine, Kwara State Specialist Hospital, Nigeria*
[2]*Department of Behavioral Sciences, University of Ilorin Teaching Hospital, Nigeria*
[3]*Department of Hematology, Kwara State Specialist Hospital, Nigeria*
[4]*Department of Epidemiology and Community Health, University of Ilorin Teaching Hospital, Nigeria*

Abstract

Objectives: Clinically significant Excessive Daytime Sleepiness (EDS) is frequently encountered among patients with depressive symptoms, and a significant association was observed between depression, body mass index and EDS. Incidentally this sleep disorder is often overlooked. The aim of this study was to examine the association between excessive daytime sleepiness, depressive symptoms, body mass index and blood pressure in a Nigerian family practice setting.

Methods: This was a hospital based cross sectional study. Systematic sampling method was used in recruiting the patients. The PHQ-9 was administered to the respondents to screen for depressive symptoms. EDS was evaluated using the Epworth Sleepiness Scale (ESS). The international classification of BMI was used. Classification of hypertension was made according to (JNC 7).

Results: One hundred and seventy eight (44.5%) were found to have one form of depression or the other. There was female preponderance. Depression was prominent in the age group 51-60 years, more among the married than the single, as well as those with low socio economic status. There was strong statistical association between age, sex, marital status, level of education, occupation and monthly income (p-values 0.008, 0.000, 0.000, 0.003, 0.000 and 0.001 respectively). Forty five (25.3%) were hypertensive. Fifty nine (33.1%) scored 10 or more on the ESS which was clinically significant sleepiness. Forty seven (26.4%) were obese constituting (23.7%) of the poor sleepers. Ninety three (52.2%) were poor sleepers, sleeping less than the normal 7 hours.

Conclusion: In this study, significant EDS was found with patients with depressive disorders and higher body mass index. Therefore patients with a complaint of EDS should be thoroughly assessed for depression and obesity.

Keywords: Excessive daytime sleepiness; Depressive symptoms; Nigerian; Family practice setting

Introduction

The impact of sleep on psychomotor performance varies with the degree of sleepiness.

Mild sleepiness produces only minor disruptions of daily functions. Moderate sleepiness is associated with sleepy episodes occurring during activities. Severe sleepiness may impair function, causing a broad range of neuropsychological deficits like depression [1].

One major cause of sleepiness is insufficient sleep. Sleep deprivation and the resultant daytime sleepiness can result in depression, anger and confusion. Acute sleep deprivation also affects daytime alertness and mood [2].

Poor sleepers experience more problems with daytime functioning than good sleepers and highly depressed poor sleepers report greater impairment in function during the day. Examination of level of sleepiness among people with insomnia complaints and found that different levels of sleepiness were related to nocturnal sleep latencies.

Sleep debt secondary to sleep deprivation is one of the cardinal causes of EDS [3]. Other common causes include narcolepsy, idiopathic hypersomnia and obstructive sleep apnea and drugs that have sedative/ hypnotic properties [4]. Medical aetiology of EDS includes head trauma, cerebrovascular disease and brain tumors [5]. EDS and depressive symptoms may also be familial or hereditary.

The symptoms of EDS range from drowsiness and reduced performance to episodes of involuntary sleep in spite of efforts to remain awake [6]. Individuals who have EDS also have increased risk of motor vehicle crashes, industrial disasters and occupational errors [7-10]. EDS occurs among depressed individuals and is a predictor of and a risk factor for depression [11-14].

EDS is one of the main symptoms of depressive disorder [13]. Epidemiological studies have indicated a strong association between EDS and depression [11-13]. This sleep disturbance and others play a significant role as predictors of depression. They are indeed important when screening for depression onset. EDS frequently leads depressed patients to seek medical assistance, yet it is commonly under evaluated [15]. Therefore, the understanding and proper management of this sleep disturbance is required for proper clinical evaluation and eventual management of the patients.

There is paucity of data on EDS among depressed patients in Nigeria in particular and West Africa in general. The aim of this study

***Corresponding author:** Shittu RO, Department of Family Medicine, Kwara State Specialist Hospital, Sobi, Ilorin, Kwara State, Nigeria
E-mail: oorelopehospital@gmail.com

was therefore to evaluate EDS in outpatients with depressive symptoms and to study its relationship with Body Mass Index (BMI). This will also create the awareness that is required by physicians in the family practice setting show that number of people with EDS who are mismanaged will be reduced.

Methodology

This study was carried out at the Family Medicine Department of the Kwara State Specialist Hospital, Sobi, Ilorin, Nigeria, from 30th October to 30th November, 2013. The Patients Health Questionnaire (PHQ-9) [16] (Appendix A) which is a brief, 9 item, patients self-report depression assessment tool that was derived from the interview-based PRIME-MD [17] was used. It was specifically developed for use, in primary care general medical settings. Many depression screening and severity tools have been used in primary care, with good results. The PHQ-9, however, offers several advantages, because it is easily understood and it has very high face validity for patients and clinicians in primary care. Many other instruments use a 1-week time frame, but the PHQ-9 uses a 2 week time frame, which conforms to DSM-4 criteria. It is the only tool that was specifically developed for use as a patient self-administered depression diagnostic tool, rather than as a severity or screening tool. It is the only short self-report tool that can reasonably be used both for diagnosis of DSM-4 major depression as well as for tracking of severity of major depression over time [18]. Psychometric evaluation of the PHQ-9 revealed a sensitivity ranging from 62%-92% and a specificity between 74%-88% [16-18]. All subjects were screened for depression using PHQ-9. Scoring and level of depression was assessed viz: (1-4) Minimal depression, (5-9) Mild depression, (10-14) Moderate depression, (15-19) moderately severe depression, and (20-27) severe depression. Some direct depression care, such as care support, coordination, case management, and treatment was embarked on. Using the systematic random sampling, the PHQ-9 was administered to all the respondents, to screen for depression, until the estimated sample size of 178 was obtained. Respondents who scored one and more were assessed clinically for depression. The severity of the depression was further classified as minimal, mild, moderate and severe [15-17].

EDS was evaluated in the patients using the English Language version of the Epworth Sleepiness Scale (ESS) (Appendix B). This is a self-administered, eight-item, well-validated [18] and widely used subjective sleepiness scale. The patients were asked to score the likelihood of falling asleep in eight different situations. Scores on the ESS range from 0 to 24, with higher scores indicating greater likelihood of sleepiness. This questionnaire measures the propensity of patients to sleep or doze during active and passive situations commonly encountered during the wake period. The metrics of the ESS ranges from 0 to 24. ESS scores <10 were considered as indicative of less severe sleepiness and scores > 10 were deemed clinically significant sleepiness [19].

Height and weight were measured according to standardized procedures. Body Mass Index (BMI) was calculated as weight in Kg divided by height in m^2 (kg/m^2). The international classification of BMI was used. The principal cut-off points were as follows: moderate thinness (16.00-16.99), mild thinness (17.00-18.49), normal (18.50-24.99), pre-obese (25.00-29.99), obese class I (30.00-34.99), obese class II (35.00-39.99), obese class III (>40.00) [20].

An Accosson Mercury sphygmomanometer was used to measure the resting blood pressure of the subjects. Blood pressure was measured 3 times in the sitting position by trained and certified technicians using a standard mercury sphygmomanometer. The onsets of the first-phase (systolic) and fifth-phase (diastolic) Korotkoff sounds were recorded. The mean of the second and third measurements were used in the analyses. Classification of hypertension was made according to the seventh report of the Joint National Committee on Prevention, Detection, Evaluation and Treatment of high blood pressure (JNC 7). The following classification of blood pressure for adults aged ≥18 years was used.

Normal	Systolic: <120 mm Hg	Diastolic: <80 mm Hg
Pre-hypertension	Systolic: 120-139 mm Hg	Diastolic: 80-89 mm Hg
Stage 1 hypertension	140-159 mm Hg	Diastolic: 90-99 mm Hg
Stage 2 hypertension	≥ 160 mm Hg	Diastolic: ≥ 100 mm Hg

Completed questionnaire and measurements were entered into a computer data base. The data were analyzed using the epidemiological information (Epi-info) 2005 software package of Center for Disease Control and Prevention (CDC). The 2 by 2 contingency tables were used to carry out Chi-square test and to find out the level of significance and values less than 0.05 were regarded as statistically significant.

Results

Table 1 shows the association between socio-demographic variables and depression. Majority were females, depression was prominent in the age group 51-60 years, more among the married than the single as well as those with low socio economic status. There was strong statistical association between age, sex, marital status, level of education and occupation, (p-values 0.008, 0.000, 0.000, 0.003, and 0.000 respectively).

Table 2 displays the Epworth Sleeping Scale used to determine the level of Daytime Sleepiness and Depression. Fifty nine (33.1%) scored 10 and more which was considered clinically significant sleepiness.

Table 3 shows the association between Excessive Daytime Sleepiness and Duration of Sleep. Ninety three (52.2%) were poor sleepers with less than the normal 7 hours of sleep.

Table 4 displays the association between Excessive Daytime Sleepiness and Body Mass Index (BMI). Forty seven (26.4%) were obese. While 14 (23.7%) were poor sleepers.

Table 5 shows the association between Excessive Daytime Sleepiness and Blood Pressure. Forty five (25.3%) were hypertensive, out of which 16 (5.5%) were poor sleepers.

Discussion

Most of the patients were low-income middle-aged women. These results compare favorably with a previous work carried out in a major public hospital [21]. Women were reported to have depressive symptoms more frequently than men [22], as well as elderly and middle-aged adults in relation to youngsters [23]. This result differs considerably from the study of Eldevik where it was reported that men were affected to a greater extent than women [24].

The results showed that almost half of the patients with depressive symptoms in this study experienced clinically significant EDS. These findings are consistent with previous reports of a strong association between daytime sleepiness and depression [11,25].

Many of the patients (33.1%) had EDS defined as ESS score of ≥ 10. This was comparable to the work of Chellappa and colleagues [26] who reported 42.8% and to the (44.8%) reported by Mume et al. [27] but lower than 57.2% reported by Chellappa [26]. This result was higher

Variables	DEPRESSION				Total	P-value
	Minimal Depression	Mild Depression	Moderate Depression	Severe Depression		
Age						
21-30	15	6	2	1	**24**	**0.008**
31-40	13	8	0	2	**23**	
41-50	36	11	0	0	**47**	
51-60	31	20	0	0	**51**	
≥ 61	24	9	0	0	**33**	
Total	**119**	**54**	**2**	**3**	**178**	
Sex						
Male	33	3	0	3	**39**	0.000
Female	86	51	2	0	**139**	
Total	**119**	**54**	**2**	**3**	**178**	
Ethnicity						
Hausa	116	51	2	3	**172**	**0.567**
Yoruba	3	1	0	0	**4**	
Igbo	0	2	0	0	**2**	
Others	0	2	0	0	**2**	
Total	**119**	**54**	**2**	**3**	**178**	
Religion						
Christianity	21	6	0	0	**27**	**0.541**
Islam	98	48	2	3	**151**	
Total	**119**	**54**	**2**	**3**	**178**	
Marital Status						
Married	73	27	2	0	**102**	**0.000**
Single	7	2	0	3	**12**	
Divorced	5	1	0	0	**6**	
Separated	6	6	0	0	**12**	
Widow	28	18	0	0	**46**	
Total	**119**	**54**	**2**	**3**	**178**	
Level of Education						
Non-formal	71	37	0	0	**108**	**0.003**
Primary	16	6	0	0	**22**	
Secondary	16	7	0	2	**25**	
Tertiary	16	4	2	1	**23**	
Total	**119**	**54**	**2**	**3**	**178**	
Occupation						
Trader	38	18	0	0	**56**	**0.000**
Civil servant	19	4	2	2	**27**	
Self employed	45	28	0	0	**73**	
Unemployed	15	4	0	0	**19**	
Student	2	0	0	1	**3**	
Total	**119**	**54**	**2**	**3**	**178**	

Table 1: Association between Socio-Demographic Variables and Depression.

EDS	Level of Depression				Total	p-value
	Minimal Depression	Mild Depression	Moderate Depression	Severe Depression		
≤ 10	88	29	2	0	**119**	**0.003**
≥ 10	31	25	0	3	**59**	
Total	**119**	**54**	**2**	**3**	**178**	

Table 2: Association between Excessive Daytime Sleepiness and Depression.

than that obtained from analysis of the Geolong Osteoporosis Study, where 13% of the 844 women surveyed were found to have EDS, as measured by the Epworth Sleepiness Scale. Some other studies also found a significant association between EDS and depression [11]. Hayley et al. [28] reported that EDS patients had an increased likelihood of experiencing current and/or a lifetime history of depressive disorders compared to those without EDS. Overall, sleepiness may be attributed to depressive disorder [29].

There is thus ample evidence that EDS is a red flag of depression. EDS and depression have some genes in common and may be familial [5]. EDS has also been found to be strongly associated with suicidal ideation in depressed patients [30]. It is therefore clear that for complete clinical evaluation of depressive symptoms, evaluation of EDS is paramount. The clinician must therefore have a high index of suspicion of depressive disorder in patients who present with features of EDS. Incidentally, there are no facilities for objective and subjective evaluation of sleep complaints in Nigeria, making it difficult to make a cast iron diagnosis. It is therefore imperative for the authorities to

EDS	DURATION OF SLEEP				Total	p-value
	≥ 7	6.1-7hours	5-6hours	<5hours		
≤ 10	65	13	26	16	**119**	**0.023**
≥ 10	20	5	25	9	**59**	
Total	**85**	**17**	**51**	**25**	**178**	

Table 3: Association between Excessive Daytime Sleepiness and Duration of Sleep.

EDS	Body Mass Index		Total	p-value
	≤ 10	≥ 10		
Moderate thinness	0	3	**3**	**0.029**
Mild thinness	4	3	**7**	
Normal	46	21	**67**	
Pre-Obese	36	18	**54**	
Obese Class 1	23	4	**27**	
Obese Class 2	7	5	**12**	
Obese Class 3	3	5	**8**	
Total	**119**	**59**	**178**	

Table 4: Association between Excessive Daytime Sleepiness and Body Mass Index (Bml).

EDS	BLOOD PRESSURE				Total	p-value
	Normal	Pre-HTN	Stage 1	Stage 2		
≤ 10	66	24	14	15	**119**	**0.776**
≥ 10	28	15	8	8	**59**	
Total	**94**	**39**	**22**	**23**	**178**	

Table 5: Association between Excessive Daytime Sleepiness and Blood Pressure.

provide enough facilities and personnel in the field of sleep medicine to assist in this regard. Clinicians should be aware of the magnitude of the problem of EDS, especially among depressed patients, and should adopt holistic approach to assist them.

The current study demonstrated a significant association between EDS and Body Mass Index. Previous researches have established that EDS in non-pathological populations is not necessarily attributable to BMI and/or obesity [31]. Hayley et al. [28] reported that EDS and depression were independent of BMI. Thus, despite the established link between EDS and depression [32] and BMI and depression, future research assessing the prevalence of EDS while controlling for BMI to assess the mechanisms of this relationship will deepen and broaden our knowledge in this field. It has further been suggested that EDS may be related to the weight gain which is from the use of both antidepressant medication and neuroleptic medications, or a combination of these [33]. There is new evidence that a preceding maladaptive lifestyle and health factors often associated with the development of depression, such as obesity [34] contribute to maintain negative lifestyle and health outcomes which are recognized to share pathology with EDS, such as sleep disturbances.

Forty five (25.3%) were hypertensive, out of which 16 (5.5%) were poor sleepers. No significant association was found between EDS and blood pressure, contrary to Cui et al. [35] where the prevalence of self-reported EDS and mean values of systolic and diastolic blood pressure levels were significant.

Conclusion

In the present study, clinically significant EDS was frequently encountered among patients with depressive symptoms, and a significant association was observed between depression and EDS. Thus, careful investigation of daytime sleepiness in depressed patients is advised during clinical evaluation.

Incidentally, there are no facilities in Nigeria for proper evaluation of sleep complaints. Concerted effort should be made by appropriate authorities to establish facilities for dealing with sleep complaints. Besides, enough personnel in the field of sleep medicine in the country should be encouraged. It is expected that with adequate and proper facilities in place, the number of personnel in this field will gradually increase. In the meantime, clinicians should be aware of the magnitude of the problem of EDS, particularly, among depressed patients and be proactive in its management so as to reduce the burden of depressive disorder in the developing countries.

Declaration of Interest

No conflict of interest.

References

1. Rosenthal L, Roehrs TA, Rosen A, Roth T (1993) Level of sleepiness and total sleep time following various time in bed conditions. Sleep 16: 226-232.
2. Bonnet MH, Arand DL (1995) We are chronically sleep deprived. Sleep 18: 908-911.
3. Pagel JF (2009) Excessive daytime sleepiness. Am Fam Physician 79: 391-396.
4. Edd EM, Flores S (2009) Sleepiness or excessive daytime somnolence. Geriatr Nurs 30: 53-60.
5. Lessov-Schlaggar CN, Bliwise DL, Krasnow RE, Swan GE, Reed T (2008) Genetic association of daytime sleepiness and depressive symptoms in elderly men. Sleep 31: 1111-1117.
6. Bittencourt LR, Silva RS, Santos RF, Pires ML, Mello MT (2005) Excessive daytime sleepiness. Rev Bras Psiquiatr 27 Suppl 1: 16-21.
7. Ulfberg J, Carter N, Talbäck M, Edling C (1996) Excessive daytime sleepiness at work and subjective work performance in the general population and among heavy snorers and patients with obstructive sleep apnea. Chest 110: 659-663.
8. Lindberg E, Carter N, Gislason T, Janson C (2001) Role of snoring and daytime sleepiness in occupational accidents. Am J Respir Crit Care Med 164: 2031-2035.
9. Melamed S, Oksenberg A (2002) Excessive daytime sleepiness and risk of occupational injuries in non-shift daytime workers. Sleep 25: 315-322.

10. Garbarino S (2008) Sleep disorders and road accidents in truck drivers. G Ital Med Lav Ergon 30: 291-296.

11. Hublin C, Kaprio J, Partinen M, Heikkilä K, Koskenvuo M (1996) Daytime sleepiness in an adult, Finnish population. J Intern Med 239: 417-423.

12. Breslau N, Roth T, Rosenthal L, Andreski P (1996) Sleep disturbance and psychiatric disorders: a longitudinal epidemiological study of young adults. Biol Psychiatry 39: 411-418.

13. Silber MH (2001) Sleep disorders. Neurol Clin 19: 173-186.

14. Fava M (2004) Daytime sleepiness and insomnia as correlates of depression. J Clin Psychiatry 65 Suppl 16: 27-32.

15. Tylee A, Gastpar M, Lépine JP, Mendlewicz J (1999) DEPRES II (Depression Research in European Society II): a patient survey of the symptoms, disability and current management of depression in the community. DEPRES Steering Committee. Int Clin Psychopharmacol 14: 139-151.

16. Kroenke K, Spitzer RL, Williams JB (2003) The Patient Health Questionnaire-2: validity of a two-item depression screener. Med Care 41: 1284-1292.

17. Spitzer RL, Williams JB, Kroenke K, Linzer M, DeGruy FV 3rd, et al. (1997) Utility of a new procedure for diagnosing mental disorders in primary care. The PRIME-MD 1000 study. JAMA 272: 1749-1756.

18. Johns MW (1991) A new method for measuring daytime sleepiness: the Epworth sleepiness scale. Sleep 14: 540-545.

19. Kroenke K, Spitzer RL, Williams JB (2001) The PHQ-9: validity of a brief depression severity measure. J Gen Intern Med 16: 606-613.

20. Johns MW (1993) Daytime sleepiness, snoring, and obstructive sleep apnea. The Epworth Sleepiness Scale. Chest 103: 30-36.

21. Berry JM, Storandt M, Coyne A (1984) Age and sex differences in somatic complaints associated with depression. J Gerontol 39: 465-467.

22. Hara C, Lopes Rocha F, Lima-Costa MF (2004) Prevalence of excessive daytime sleepiness and associated factors in a Brazilian community: the Bambuí study. Sleep Med 5: 31-36.

23. Blazer DG (2000) Mood disorders: epidemiology. Comprehensive textbook of psychiatry, 7th ed, Philadelphia, Lippincott Williams & Wilkins, 1298-1308.

24. Eldevik MF, Flo E, Moen BE, Pallesen S, Bjorvatn B (2013) Insomnia, excessive sleepiness, excessive fatigue, anxiety, depression and shift work disorder in nurses having less than 11 hours in-between shifts. PLoS One 8: e70882.

25. Young TB (2004) Epidemiology of daytime sleepiness: definitions, symptomatology, and prevalence. J Clin Psychiatry 65 Suppl 16: 12-16.

26. Chellappa SL, Araújo JF (2006) Excessive daytime sleepiness in patients with depressive disorder. Rev Bras Psiquiatr 28: 126-129.

27. Mume CO (2010) Excessive daytime Sleepiness among depressed patients. Libyan J Med 5.

28. Hayley AC, Williams LJ, Berk M, Kennedy GA, Jacka FN, et al. (2013) The relationship between excessive daytime sleepiness and depressive and anxiety disorders in women. Aust N Z J Psychiatry. 47: 772-778.

29. Cano-Lozano MC, Espinosa-Fernández L, Miró E, Buela-Casas G (2003) A review of sleep disorders in depression. Rev Neurol 36: 366-375.

30. Johns M, Hocking B (1997) Daytime sleepiness and sleep habits of Australian workers. Sleep 20: 844-849.

31. Scott KM, McGee MA, Wells JE, Oakley Browne MA (2008) Obesity and mental disorders in the adult general population. J Psychosom Res 64: 97-105.

32. Guilleminault C, Brooks SN (2001) Excessive daytime sleepiness: a challenge for the practising neurologist. Brain 124: 1482-1491.

33. Stanton JM (1995) Weight gain associated with neuroleptic medication: a review. Schizophr Bull 21: 463-472.

34. Gallicchio L, Kalesan B (2009) Sleep duration and mortality: a systematic review and meta-analysis. J Sleep Res 18: 148-158.

35. Cui R, Tanigawa T, Sakurai S, Yamagishi K, Imano H, et al. (2008) Associations of sleep-disordered breathing with excessive daytime sleepiness and blood pressure in Japanese women. Hypertens Res 31: 501-506.

Subjective and Objective Measures of Sleep Quality in Advanced Cancer: A Possible Clinical Marker for Depression

Michael J Hasselberg[1]*, Anton P Porsteinsson[1], Lisa Boyle[1] and Kathy P Parker[2]

[1]Department of Psychiatry, University of Rochester School of Medicine and Dentistry, 601 Elmwood Ave., Rochester, NY 14642, USA
[2]University of Rochester School of Nursing, 255 Crittenden Blvd., Rochester, NY 14642, USA

Abstract

Purpose: It is estimated that between 30 and 75% of patients with cancer experience depression, poor nocturnal sleep, and daytime sleepiness. Research designed to specifically examine associations of depression with subjective and objective sleep measures is lacking. Thus the purpose of these analyses was to compare relationships among depression, subjective and polysomnographic measures of sleep.

Methods: Secondary data analysis design was used to assess sleep quality, and self-rated depression of patients with advanced cancer recruited from a university-based medical system. Responses to the Beck Depression Inventory-II (BDI-II), Pittsburgh Sleep Questionnaire Index (PSQI), and the Epworth Sleepiness Scale (ESS), and polysomnography data were analyzed using descriptive, correlation, and regression statistics.

Results: A total of 114 patients with advanced cancer completed the study. PSQI and ESS scores were positively correlated with BDI-II scores. Total nocturnal sleep time and a prolonged REM latency were also positively related to BDI-II scores. When controlling for selected demographic and clinical features, the relationships between polysomnographic variables and depression were no longer significant.

Conclusions: Depression was related to subjective sleep quality and daytime sleepiness suggesting that these problems occur together. In addition, higher levels of depression were associated with nocturnal sleep time and prolonged REM latency.

Keywords: Sleep quality; Pittsburgh Sleep Questionnaire Index; Epworth Sleepiness Scale; Depression, advanced cancer

Introduction

The relationship between sleep disturbances and depression is a well-recognized problem. It is estimated that 30% to 75% of patients with cancer will experience these symptoms during the course of the disease [1,2]. Sleep problems in particular have been associated with decreased quality of life and work productivity, fatigue, psychological distress, pain, impaired cognitive function, and disruptions in social interactions [3-8]. Poor sleep can also contribute to immunosuppression, which can have significant effects on the cancer process [9]. In advanced cancer populations problems with sleep have been linked to a person's desire for a hastened death, while depression has been found to be an independent predictor of early death [10,11].

Sleep disturbances in cancer patients are characterized by difficulty falling asleep, problems maintaining sleep, poor sleep efficiency, early awakening, and excessive daytime sleepiness [2,12,13]. It has been suggested that poor sleep in this population is associated with the biochemical changes occurring during neoplastic growth and the use of anticancer treatments [2,12,14]. Further research has shown that opioids used to treat cancer related pain can also affect a patients sleep quality and diurnal wakefulness [15,16]. Identified risk factors of sleep disturbances in individuals with cancer include: younger age, a general lack of energy, higher anxiety levels, and previous post-traumatic experience [17-19].

There is a distorted circadian rhythm in patients with advanced cancer, which was associated with complaints of poor sleep quality, fatigue, and insomnia [20]. Recent studies have shown that the more disrupted the daily sleep/wake circadian rhythm, the worse the depression [21,22]. Historically, sleep disturbances were viewed as a secondary condition that was caused by, or associated with, primary depression [23]. Current thinking suggests that these conditions have a bi-directional relation and can be considered comorbid disorders or symptom clusters [12,23-27].

The two-process model of sleep regulation has been widely used in both clinical practice and research of sleep in a variety of populations [28-30]. According to this model, there are two major processes that underlie sleep and waking, process S and process C. Process S, or the drive to sleep, is determined by prior sleep and waking and rises during wakefulness and declines during sleep. Slow wave sleep (EEG power - 0.75 to 4.5 Hz range) is a key indicator of process S. In depression, process S is deficient, which is reflected by a diminution of delta activity and slow wave sleep [31]. Sleep deprivation due to prolonged periods of wakefulness tends to enhance the deficiencies of process S associated with depression. Process C, or sleep propensity, determines the thresholds for sleep onset and termination, and is regulated by the master circadian oscillator, the suprachiasmatic nucleus (SCN). Depressed individuals experience a wide range of circadian rhythm disturbances, causing disruptions in process C, characterized by changes in sleep architecture, early morning waking and hypersomnia [32-34].

***Corresponding author:** Michael J. Hasselberg, Department of Psychiatry, University of Rochester, School of Medicine, 601 Elmwood Ave., Rochester, NY 14642, USA
E-mail: Michael_Hasselberg@urmc.rochester.edu

Although sleep disturbances and depression are prevalent, these conditions are often underrecognized, and undermanaged in patients with advanced cancer [35]. Sleep disturbances in particular, can be assessed both objectively and subjectively, but the objective and subjective measurements do not always correlate [12,36]. Patients with advanced cancer frequently complained of poor sleep despite having good sleep efficiency revealed through actigraphy [37]. Objective measures of sleep are not frequently used in cancer research, as investigators tend to rely more on subjective screening tools [38,39]. Diagnosing depression in cancer can be just as challenging due to the number of somatic symptoms frequently attributed to the cancer itself or anticancer treatments [40-43]. However, a factor analysis study of an oncology sample conducted by Passik and colleagues found that diurnal variation and insomnia did not cluster with somatic symptoms of depression, suggesting that sleep-related symptoms might be a unique clinical marker [44]. Thus, the purpose of this study was to compare and contrast relationships among depression, subjective measures of nocturnal sleep and daytime sleepiness, and polysomnographic measures of nocturnal and diurnal sleep.

Methods

A descriptive, correlational design was used to conduct a secondary data analysis of data obtained from a larger study examining sleep/wake patterns in patients with advanced cancer. The institutional review board approved the study. The purpose of the larger study was to describe the sleep/wake patterns of patients with advanced cancer using continuous ambulatory polysomnography (PSG) and to explore relationships with selected demographic and clinical variables [13]. All participants underwent continuous ambulatory PSG over a 42-hour period of time in their home setting and completed a sleep diary in which day and night were determined by participant reported "lights on" and "lights off" [13].

Sample

Patients were eligible for the study if they (a) had a diagnosis of advanced solid tumor malignancy (stages III and IV); (b) had no significant history of neurological disorders, alcohol/substance abuse, previous sleep apnea, or cerebral metastasis; and (c) had a Karnofsky Performance Score (KPS) equal to, or greater than 50. Patients were excluded from the study is they (a) had a recent hospital discharge; or (b) were unable to schedule in-home PSG until at least 5 days subsequent to the most recent chemotherapy and/or radiotherapy or 1 week after hospitalization.

The sample included 114 well-characterized patients with advanced solid tumor cancer (mean age 55.2 ± 9.0 years; 49% female) screened from medical oncology clinics within a large university health care system. Table 1 shows the demographic features of the sample. The majority of the sample was diagnosed with lung cancer (31.6%) followed by breast cancer (28.9%). The mean KPS was 76.3 (± 11.0). About 89% of the participants had been treated with chemotherapy, while only 39.5% of the sample received radiotherapy treatment. The clinical features of the sample can be found in Table 2.

Measures

Demographic and clinical data, medications, and laboratory information were obtained from medical record screening by the project manager, a registered nurse, in the original study. Depression was measured using the self-administered Beck Depression Inventory-II (BDI-II) prior to the first 24 hours of PSG. The BDI-II is the revised version of the Beck Depression Inventory, which has been updated to correspond with diagnostic criteria of depressive episodes from the Diagnostic and Statistical Manual of Mental Disorders IV-TR [45,46]. The BDI-II is comprised of 21 items, each consisting of four self-evaluative statements describing the intensity of depression symptom severity. The scores for each rating on the 21 items are then summed to yield a total value ranging from 0 to 63. According to the BDI-II manual, a total values score can be interpreted as minimal (0 to 13), mild (14 to 19), moderate (20 to 28), and severe (29 to 63) depression [46].

Objective measurement of nocturnal and daytime sleep was obtained using PSG recordings (Embla Systems, Broomfield, CO)

Variable	*n*	%
Age	114	100.0
Mean 55.2 ± 9.0 years		
Range (33 – 73 years)		
Gender		
Male	58	50.9
Female	56	49.1
Race		
White/Caucasian	45	39.5
African American	64	56.1
Other	5	4.4
Marital Status		
Married	50	43.9
Unmarried	64	56.1
Living Situation		
Lives alone	21	18.4
Lives with other	93	86.1
Employment Status		
Employed	17	14.9
Not employed	97	85.2
Disabled	59	51.8
Education		
High school of less	49	43.0
Above high school	65	57.0

Table 1: Demographic Features of the Sample.

Variable	*n*	%
Diagnosis		
Breast	33	28.9
Colon	18	15.8
Head & neck	12	10.5
Lung	36	31.6
Other	33	28.9
ECOG Scores		
0	21	18.4
1	71	62.3
2	22	19.3
Chemotherapy		
No	13	11.4
Yes	101	88.6
Radiotherapy		
No	69	60.5
Yes	45	39.5
Surgery		
No	113	99.1
Yes	1	0.9
Opioids		
No	30	26.3
Yes	84	73.7
Antidepressants		
No	78	68.4
Yes	36	31.6
Steroids		
No	109	95.6
Yes	5	4.4
Sedative/Hypnotics		
No	93	81.6
Yes	21	18.4

Note. ECOG = Eastern Cooperative Oncology Group

Table 2: Clinical Features of the Sample.

over a continuous 42 hours period of time with all recordings starting before 1800 hours on their first night and ending between 1200 hours and 1400 hours the day after the second night. Subjective measure of sleep quality was obtained using participant recorded sleep diaries and the Pittsburgh Sleep Quality Index (PSQI). The PSQI is a self-rated questionnaire, which assess sleep quality and disturbances over a one-month interval of time [47]. The questionnaire is comprised of nineteen individual items generating seven component scores (sleep quality, sleep latency, sleep duration, habitual sleep efficiency, sleep disturbances, use of sleeping medication, and daytime dysfunction), which are summed to yield one global score [47]. Subjective measure of daytime sleepiness was obtained using the Epworth Sleepiness Scale (ESS). The ESS is a self-administered questionnaire, which provides a measure of the subject's general level of daytime sleepiness [48]. Subjects are asked to rate their level of sleepiness on a scale of 0-3 in eight different proposed situations to be summed together to provide a total score over the whole range of daytime sleepiness [48]. Both the PSQI and ESS were self-administered prior to the first 24 hours of PSG. The details of the design and methods of the larger study have been published elsewhere [13].

Data Analysis

Descriptive statistics were used to summarize the data. There were no significant differences between nocturnal PSG variables for the first and second nights, so the data were pooled together. Nocturnal PSG measures calculated included: Total Sleep Time (TST); sleep efficiency; percentage of TST spent in stages 1,2,3, and 4, and Rapid Eye Movement Sleep (REM); latency to the first 60 seconds of continuous sleep; and the latency to the first epoch of REM sleep. Daytime PSG sleep measures calculated included: TST; percentage of time spent in sleep stages; and an index of awakenings lasting at least 60 seconds. Nonparametric analysis was used because most variables did not meet the assumptions of parametric procedures. The spearman rho (r_s) and partial (r_p) correlation procedures were used to detect significant relationships between BDI-II scores, and sample characteristics, subjective measures of nocturnal sleep and daytime sleepiness, and PSG measures of nocturnal and diurnal sleep. Although parametric assumptions were not met, according to the central limit theorem the sample size in this study permitted the use of hierarchical linear regression analyses to further explore the relationship between depression (BDI-II scores) and significantly correlated predictor variables. SPSS (SPSS Inc, Chicago, IL) was the statistical package used. The level of significance was set at $\alpha = 0.05$.

Results

Depression measures

The mean total score for the BDI-II (n = 114) was 13.0 ± 8.0 (SD). 60.5% of the participants scored in the minimal range (0-13), 22.8% scored in the mild range (14-19), 12.3% scored in the moderate range (20-28), and 4.4% scored in the severe range (29-63).

The relationship between various demographic, clinical characteristics and depression was examined using correlation statistics. The variable of age was found to have a significant correlation ($r_s = -0.23$; $p < 0.02$) with total BDI-II scores suggesting that younger age was associated with higher levels of depression. The analysis of the association between categorical variables and depression found that female patients reported significantly more depression ($r_s = 0.20$, $p < 0.05$) than male patients. When controlling for age and gender, patients taking opioid ($r_p = 0.21$, $p < 0.04$) and antidepressants ($r_p = 0.31$, $p < 0.01$) experienced statistically significantly more depression compared to those patients not taking these medications.

Nocturnal and daytime sleep/waking measures

The mean total score for the PSQI (n = 114) was 7.0 ± 3.3 (SD). The nocturnal PSG sleep measures appear in Table 3. The sample averaged approximately 6.4 hours of sleep per night. The majority of nocturnal sleep occurred in non-rapid eye movement (NREM) stage 2 (73.8%) followed by NREM stage 1 (10.9%). An absence of NREM stages 3 and 4 was noted in most participants. Nocturnal sleep latency was within normal limits (<30 minutes) but the REM latency was prolonged at 129.0 minutes ± 97.4 minutes, which is suggestive of nocturnal sleep fragmentation.

The mean total score for the ESS (n = 114) was 7.7 ± 4.3 (SD). The daytime PSG sleep measures appear in Table 4. During the daytime, participants slept on average 89.3 minutes ± 94.2 minutes. The majority of daytime sleep occurred in NREM stage 2 (59.9%) followed by NREM stage 3 (20.1%), while a minority of sleep occurred in REM (4.2%). An absence of NREM stages 3 and 4 was noted in all participants.

Nocturnal and daytime sleep/waking measures and depression

Table 5 shows the relationships between sleep measures with BDI-II. Increasing depression was positively correlated to worse subjective sleep quality ($r_s = 0.51$; $p < 0.01$) but not worse sleep efficiency as would be normally expected. Level of depression severity also was not an indicator of nocturnal sleep onset latency. Once participants fell asleep, those with higher levels of depression took longer time to reach first onset of REM sleep ($r_s = 0.23$; $p < 0.02$) but this relationship was no longer significant when controlling for antidepressant and opioid medication use. During the nocturnal sleep period, participants with higher levels of depression tended to have longer periods of total sleep time ($r_s = 0.19$; $p < 0.05$). Neither, the amount of time spent in different stages of nocturnal sleep nor the number of arousals occurring throughout the night were not found to be associated with level of

Variable	Mean (SD)	Normal*
	382.3(96.5)	340–466
Total Sleep Time (min)	29.7(41.7)	< 30
Sleep Latency (min) to first 60 seconds of sleep		
Sleep Efficiency (%) referred to sleep period	77.2(12.8)	86–100
NREM (%)		
Stage 1		
Stage 2	10.9(5.9)	3–12
Stage 3	73.8(8.4)	51–72
Stage 4	0.3(1.0)	0-17
REM (%)	0.0	0-17
REM Latency (min)	15.0(7.8)	17-25
Arousal Index (events/hour)	129.0(97.4)	65-104
	63.9(18.0)	Not available

Note. min = minutes; sec = seconds; REM = rapid eye movement; NREM = non-REM; * According to Williams et al., 1974

Table 3: Nocturnal Sleep Parameters (Two nights pooled).

Variable	Mean (SD)
Total Sleep Time (min)	89.3(94.2)
NREM (%)	
Stage 1	20.1(18.8)
Stage 2	59.9(30.4)
Stage 3	0.0
Stage 4	0.0
REM (%)	4.2(7.7)

Note. min = minutes; REM = rapid eye movement; NREM = non-REM

Table 4: Daytime Sleep Parameters.

Dependent: BDI-II	Spearman's	P-value
Total ESS score	0.23	0.02
Global PSQI score	0.51	0.00
Nocturnal Total Sleep Time (min)	0.19	0.05
Nocturnal REM Latency (min)	0.23	0.01

Note. BDI-II = Beck Depression Inventory-II; ESS = Epworth Sleepiness Scale; PSQI = Pittsburgh Sleep Questionnaire Index; min = minutes; REM = rapid eye movement

Table 5: Significant Correlations Between Sleep Variables with BDI-II.

depression severity. During the day, those participants with higher levels of depression reported higher levels of general daytime sleepiness ($r_s = 0.23$; $p < 0.03$). However, this relationship could not be confirmed through PSG as none of the daytime objective sleep measures were significantly correlated with the BDI-II.

In order to further examine the relationship between depression and sleep/wake measures, total BDI-II scores was hierarchically regressed with variables entered in three blocks. Significantly correlated demographic and clinical characteristics including age, gender, and use of antidepressant and opioid medications, were entered in the first block and accounted for 20.8% of the variance ($p < 0.01$). The subjective sleep measures, total PSQI and ESS scores, were entered in the second block and accounted for an additional 12.1% of the variance ($R^2 = 0.329$, $p < 0.01$). The objective sleep measures of nocturnal REM latency and average nocturnal total sleep time were entered in the third block and only accounted for 0.9% of the variance and was not significantly different from the second block. Overall the regression model accounted for 33.8% of the variance in depression but found that the selected polysomnographic sleep variables were not significant predictors of depression.

Discussion

The American Psychiatric Association has developed the fifth edition of Diagnostic and Statistical Manual of Mental Disorders (DSM-V), with assistance of DSM-V sleep-wake nosology. The primary purpose of the DSM-V sleep-wake nosology is to improve the recognition of sleep disorders that are associated with other health conditions by incorporating quantitative physiologic measures (polysomnographic and neurobiologic) into the diagnostic classification system, and dimensional measures of severity [49]. This is the first study to our knowledge to employ both subjective and continuous PSG quantitative measures to examine the relationship between sleep/waking and depression in a sample of patients with cancer.

Similar to previous reports, the sleep/wake pattern in our sample was characterized by poor sleep maintenance, reduced quality of sleep, and difficulty with the ability to initiate and maintain sleep states [1,2,4-6,8,12,14-16,21,27,37,38]. Overall 39.5% of our sample reported mild to severe symptoms of depression, contrary to other studies that found a higher prevalence of depression symptoms [11,17].

Sleep disturbances are a common complaint for most depressed patients and belong to the core symptoms of depressive disorders [31]. Our study found that subjective complaints of poor sleep quality and excessive daytime sleepiness were significantly related to the severity of depression. Although this finding was congruent with previous results the measure of sleep disturbance cannot be encapsulated by subjective assessments alone [11,16,17,32,37]. Previous research examining both subjective and objective sleep measures using actigraphy in depressed patients with cancer have produced mixed results [12,36,37]. Similar to results reported by Gibbins and colleagues [37], our study found that depression was positively correlated to poor subjective sleep quality but was not correlated to the objective measure of sleep efficiency. However, our study did find that increased levels of depression were associated with longer periods of total nocturnal sleep time and a prolonged REM latency after sleep.

Although this study did not attempt to infer causal effects of sleep/wake variables on depression, the descriptive results obtained can be applied to the conceptual context of the two-process model of sleep regulation [28-30]. Process S refers to the homeostatic process of sleep regulation, which is a dependent function of prior sleep and waking duration. Process S was derived from studies examining slow wave sleep activity and reflects that the need for sleep builds throughout the day and dissipates during the night. Most participants in our study were unable to attain slow wave sleep activity. This result was expected, as patients with depression tend to have a diminution of slow wave sleep [31]. Though, it was surprising that the absence of time spent in slow wave sleep was not significantly correlated with the severity of depression. This observation might be explained by the potential confounding factors in the sample including medication use, age, and pain levels. Participant perception of excessive daytime sleepiness was significantly related to higher levels of depression. It is unclear whether daytime sleepiness is predictor of depression or whether it is the reverse. The lack of slow wave sleep can prevent the dissipation of sleep need and increase daytime sleep tendency. The relationship between the lack of slow wave sleep and severity of depression might have been mediated by daytime sleepiness.

Process C refers to the circadian process of sleep regulation, which determines the thresholds for sleep onset and termination, and is regulated by the SCN. REM sleep is markedly influenced by process C, as the incidence of REM sleep has been used as a phase indicator of circadian oscillation [28-30]. In normal sleep, there is a decreasing trend of REM sleep propensity during the daytime hours while during the night it is the reverse [30]. In our study, there was a small percentage of REM sleep that occurred during the day, which typically does not occur in healthy individuals. We also found that prolonged REM latency after sleep onset was correlated with higher levels of depression. This result is incongruent with previous psychobiological research that has shown that a shorter REM latency period is typically associated with depression [31]. This difference was probably related to the use of antidepressants, especially selective serotonin reuptake inhibitor medications, by many of the participants in our sample. It has also been generally assumed that total sleep time is determined to a large extent by circadian factors [29,30]. Although the mean total sleep time in this sample was noted to be within a normal range, it should be noted that participants with longer periods of nocturnal total sleep time had significantly higher levels of depression. This result was also probably related to the use of antidepressant and opioid medications in our sample.

The findings of this study suggest that the interaction between Process S and Process C is altered in advanced cancer patients with depression. The almost total absence of slow wave sleep and prolonged REM latency may have contributed to the poor sleep quality, and daytime sleepiness in the sample. This increase in daytime sleepiness and poor sleep quality suggest that the homeostatic need for sleep was not dissipated at night, and/or the circadian ability to decrease sleep propensity during the day and increase sleep propensity during the night was attenuated.

The question of which comes first, depression or sleep disturbance remains unknown. Healthcare professionals need to be aware of the presence of symptom clusters when evaluating sleep and depression in patients with cancer [50]. Symptom clusters suggest that sleep disturbances might be part of multiple interrelated symptoms including depression, which have a synergistic adverse effect on quality of life [7,12,50]. A major limitation of this study was that the secondary data analysis design bounded our analyses to the variables collected by the original investigators. This restricted our ability to examine other variables usually found in cancer symptom clusters, which may have contributed to depression severity and/or sleep disturbances. The concept of depression was also restricted to a cross-sectional measure of the BDI-II, prohibiting the ability to draw inferences concerning subtypes or longitudinal course of depression in the sample. Our regression analysis suggests that younger age and poor subjective sleep quality were significant predictors of depression but we were unable to determine causal, mediating, or moderating relationships. Due to our relatively small sample size (n = 114) the use of path analysis or structural equation modeling techniques to further examine these relationships would not be appropriate. Future research using larger sample sizes is needed to estimate possible causal relations between the variables found in cancer symptom clusters. Research is also needed to determine if subjective sleep appraisals are predicted by certain psychological factors in patients with advanced cancer [51].

Conculsions

To our knowledge, the results of this exploratory study provide the first comprehensive description of the relationship between sleep/wake state and depression of patients with advanced cancer using both subjective and polysomnographic measures. The results suggest that subjective sleep quality and daytime sleepiness, increased total nocturnal sleep time, and prolonged REM latency have a profound impact on depression severity, highlighting the need for careful screening of both subjective and objective measures of sleep. The clinical significance of these results should be interpreted with caution due to confounding sample characteristics and further work is needed to identify the underlying mechanisms of sleep regulatory processes associated with depression in advanced cancer.

Acknowledgement

Funding: Supported in part by grant from the National Institute of Nursing Research, RO1 NR 008125 award to Kathy P. Parker.

References

1. Clark J, Cunningham M, McMillan S, Vena C, Parker K (2004) Sleep-wake disturbances in people with cancer part II: evaluating the evidence for clinical decision making. Oncol Nurs Forum 31: 747-771.

2. Lee K, Cho M, Miaskowski C, Dodd M (2004) Impaired sleep and rhythms in persons with cancer. Sleep Med Rev 8: 199-212.

3. Anderson KO, Getto CJ, Mendoza TR, Palmer SN, Wang XS, et al. (2003) Fatigue and sleep disturbance in patients with cancer, patients with clinical depression, and community-dwelling adults. J Pain Symptom Manage 25: 307-318.

4. Chen ML, Yu CT, Yang CH (2008) Sleep disturbances and quality of life in lung cancer patients undergoing chemotherapy. Lung Cancer 62: 391-400.

5. Dirksen SR, Epstein DR, Hoyt MA (2009) Insomnia, depression, and distress among outpatients with prostate cancer. Appl Nurs Res 22: 154-158.

6. Shuman AG, Duffy SA, Ronis DL, Garetz SL, McLean SA, et al. (2010) Predictors of poor sleep quality among head and neck cancer patients. Laryngoscope 120: 1166-1172.

7. Stepanski EJ, Walker MS, Schwartzberg LS, Blakely LJ, Ong JC, et al. (2009) The relation of trouble sleeping, depressed mood, pain, and fatigue in patients with cancer. J Clin Sleep Med 5: 132-136.

8. Vargas S, Wohlgemuth WK, Antoni MH, Lechner SC, Holley HA, et al. (2010) Sleep dysfunction and psychosocial adaptation among women undergoing treatment for non-metastatic breast cancer. Psychooncology 19: 669-673.

9. O'Donnell JF (2004) Insomnia in cancer patients. Clinical Cornerstone 6: S6-S14.

10. Lloyd-Williams M, Shiels C, Taylor F, Dennis M (2009) Depression--an independent predictor of early death in patients with advanced cancer. J Affect Disord 113: 127-132.

11. Mystakidou K, Parpa E, Tsilika E, Pathiaki M, Galanos A, et al. (2007) Depression, hopelessness, and sleep in cancer patients' desire for death. Int J Psychiatry Med 37: 201-211.

12. Berger AM, Parker KP, Young-McCaughan S, Mallory GA, Barsevick AM, et al. (2005) Sleep wake disturbances in people with cancer and their caregivers: state of the science. Oncol Nurs Forum 32: E98-126.

13. Parker KP, Bliwise DL, Ribeiro M, Jain SR, Vena CI, et al. (2008) Sleep/Wake patterns of individuals with advanced cancer measured by ambulatory polysomnography. J Clin Oncol 26: 2464-2472.

14. Roscoe JA, Kaufman ME, Matteson-Rusby SE, Palesh OG, Ryan JL, et al. (2007) Cancer-related fatigue and sleep disorders. Oncologist 12 Suppl 1: 35-42.

15. Mercadante S, Girelli D, Casuccio A (2004) Sleep disorders in advanced cancer patients: prevalence and factors associated. Support Care Cancer 12: 355-359.

16. Mystakidou K, Parpa E, Tsilika E, Pathiaki M, Patiraki E, et al. (2007) Sleep quality in advanced cancer patients. J Psychosom Res 62: 527-533.

17. Mystakidou K, Parpa E, Tsilika E, Gennatas C, Galanos A, et al. (2009) How is sleep quality affected by the psychological and symptom distress of advanced cancer patients? Palliat Med 23: 46-53.

18. Price MA, Zachariae R, Butow PN, deFazio A, Chauhan D, et al. (2009) Prevalence and predictors of insomnia in women with invasive ovarian cancer: anxiety a major factor. Eur J Cancer 45: 3262-3270.

19. Rogers LQ, Courneya KS, Robbins KT, Rao K, Malone J, et al. (2008) Factors associated with fatigue, sleep, and cognitive function among patients with head and neck cancer. Head Neck 30: 1310-1317.

20. Levin RD, Daehler MA, Grutsch JF, Quiton J, Lis CG, et al. (2005) Circadian function in patients with advanced non-small-cell lung cancer. Br J Cancer 93: 1202-1208.

21. Du-Quiton J, Wood PA, Burch JB, Grutsch, JF, Gupta D, et al. (2010). Actigraphic assessment of daily sleep-activity pattern abnormalities reflects self-assessed depression and anxiety in outpatients with advanced non-small cell lung cancer. Psycho-Oncology 19: 180-190.

22. Palesh OG, Collie K, Batiuchok D, Tilston J, Koopman C, et al. (2007) A longitudinal study of depression, pain, and stress as predictors of sleep disturbance among women with metastatic breast cancer. Biol Psychol 75: 37-44.

23. Weinberger T, Forrester A, Markov D, Chism K, Kunkel EJ (2010) Women at a dangerous intersection: diagnosis and treatment of depression and related disorders in patients with breast cancer. Psychiatr Clin North Am 33: 409-422.

24. Donovan KA, Jacobsen PB (2007) Fatigue, depression, and insomnia: evidence for a symptom cluster in cancer. Semin Oncol Nurs 23: 127-135.

25. Hoyt MA, Thomas KS, Epstein DR, Dirksen SR (2009) Coping style and sleep quality in men with cancer. Ann Behav Med 37: 88-93.

26. McMillan SC, Tofthagen C, Morgan MA (2008) Relationships among pain, sleep disturbances, and depressive symptoms in outpatients from a comprehensive cancer center. Oncol Nurs Forum 35: 603-611.

27. Sateia MJ, Lang BJ (2008) Sleep and cancer: recent developments. Curr Oncol Rep 10: 309-318.

28. Borbély AA (1982) A two process model of sleep regulation. Hum Neurobiol 1: 195-204.

29. Borbély AA, Achermann P (1999) Sleep homeostasis and models of sleep regulation. J Biol Rhythms 14: 557-568.

30. Daan S, Beersma DG, Borbély AA (1984) Timing of human sleep: recovery process gated by a circadian pacemaker. Am J Physiol 246: R161-183.

31. Riemann D, Berger M, Voderholzer U (2001) Sleep and depression--results from psychobiological studies: an overview. Biol Psychol 57: 67-103.

32. Boyce P, Barriball E (2010) Circadian rhythms and depression. Aust Fam Physician 39: 307-310.

33. Gorwood P (2010) Restoring circadian rhythms: a new way to successfully manage depression. J Psychopharmacol 24: 15-19.

34. Gouin JP, Connors J, Kiecolt-Glaser JK, Glaser R, Malarkey WB, et al. (2010) Altered expression of circadian rhythm genes among individuals with a history of depression. J Affect Disord 126: 161-166.

35. Palesh OG, Roscoe JA, Mustian KM, Roth T, Savard J, et al. (2010) Prevalence, demographics, and psychological associations of sleep disruption in patients with cancer: University of Rochester cancer center-community clinical oncology program. J Clin Oncol 28: 292-298.

36. Young-McCaughan S, Mays MZ, Arzola SM, Yoder LH, Dramig SA, et al. (2003) Research and commentary: Change in exercise tolerence, activity and sleep patterns, and quality of life in patients with cancer participating in a structured exercise program. Oncology Nursing Forum 30: 441-454.

37. Gibbins J, McCoubrie R, Kendrick AH, Senior-Smith G, Davies AN, et al. (2009) Sleep-wake disturbances in patients with advanced cancer and their family carers. J Pain Symptom Manage 38: 860-870.

38. Ancoli-Israel S, Moore PJ, Jones V (2001) The relationship between fatigue and sleep in cancer patients: a review. Eur J Cancer Care (Engl) 10: 245-255.

39. Passik SD, Whitcomb LA, Kirsh KL, Theobald DE (2003) An unsuccessful attempt to develop a single-item screen for insomnia in cancer patients. J Pain Symptom Manage 25: 284-287.

40. Akechi T, Nakano T, Akizuki N, Okamura M, Sakuma K, et al. (2003) Somatic symptoms for diagnosing major depression in cancer patients. Psychosomatics 44: 244-248.

41. Cathcart F (2006) Psychological distress in patients with advanced cancer. Clin Med 6: 148-150.

42. McDaniel JS, Musselman DL, Porter MR, Reed DA, Nemeroff CB (1995) Depression in patients with cancer. Diagnosis, biology, and treatment. Arch Gen Psychiatry 52: 89-99.

43. Rao A, Cohen HJ (2004) Symptom management in the elderly cancer patient: fatigue, pain, and depression. J Natl Cancer Inst Monogr : 150-157.

44. Passik SD, Lundberg JC, Rosenfeld B, Kirsh KL, Donaghy K, et al. (2000) Factor analysis of the Zung Self-Rating Depression Scale in a large ambulatory oncology sample. Psychosomatics 41: 121-127.

45. American Psychiatric Association (1994) Diagnostic and statistical manual of mental disorders (4th ed.). Washington, DC.

46. Beck AT, Steer RA, Brown GK (1996) Manual for the Beck Depression Inventory-II. San Antonio, TX: Psychological Corporation.

47. Buysse DJ, Reynolds CF 3rd, Monk TH, Berman SR, Kupfer DJ (1989) The Pittsburgh Sleep Quality Index: a new instrument for psychiatric practice and research. Psychiatry Res 28: 193-213.

48. Johns MW (1991) A new method for measuring daytime sleepiness: the Epworth sleepiness scale. Sleep 14: 540-545.

49. Reynolds III CF, Redline S (2010) The DSM-V sleep-wake disorders nosology: An update and an invitation to the sleep community. J Clin Sleep Med 6: 9-10.

50. Dodd MJ, Miaskowski C, Paul SM (2001) Symptom clusters and their effect on the functional status of patients with cancer. Oncol Nurs Forum 28: 465-470.

51. Williams RL, Karacan I, Hursch CJ (1974). EEG of human sleep: Clinical applications. New York, NY: John Wiley & Sons.

Interventions to Improve CPAP Adherence and Outcomes: Role of Theory and Behavioral Change Techniques

Carl Stepnowsky[1,2]*, Tania Zamora[1], Christine Edwards[1], Lin Liu[1,3], and Zia Agha[1,2]

[1]*Health Services Research & Development Unit, Veterans Affairs San Diego Healthcare System, San Diego, CA, USA*
[2]*Department of Medicine, University of California, San Diego, USA*
[3]*Department of Family and Preventive Medicine, University of California, San Diego, USA*

Abstract

Study Background: Low patient adherence to nasal Continuous Positive Airway Pressure (CPAP) limits treatment effectiveness. A wide variety of CPAP adherence intervention studies have been performed to date, with many showing some improvement in CPAP adherence. Better understanding of the theoretical foundations, specific behavioral change techniques, and modes of intervention delivery can help provide guidance for future interventional efforts and reflects efforts underway in the general treatment adherence literature.

Methods: The CPAP adherence literature was reviewed to identify those studies that included a specific intervention designed to increase CPAP use. Twenty-nine studies were included in this review. Published coding schemes were used.

Results: The average effect size of the CPAP adherence interventions in adults who are new users of CPAP was 0.52 (SD=0.42, range: 0-1.52). This moderate effect size did not appear to be related to the number of behavioral change techniques, use of theory, or to mode of delivery.

Conclusion: Future research efforts should build on previous interventional studies, with the ultimate goal of identifying those techniques that can help improve CPAP adherence and patient outcomes.

Keywords: Behavioral change; Continuous positive airway pressure; Sleep apnea; Treatment adherence

Introduction

Obstructive Sleep Apnea (OSA) is a disorder characterized by repeated breathing cessations during sleep, which can result in potentially serious consequences affecting cardiovascular, physiological, neurocognitive, emotional, and psychosocial functioning [1]. Nasal Continuous Positive Airway Pressure (CPAP) [2] is the treatment of choice for this condition [3], with meta-analytic studies reporting that CPAP improves both objectively and subjectively measured daytime sleepiness [4] and health-related quality of life [5]. CPAP has also been shown to normalize sleep architecture [6] and reduce blood pressure [7]. Many, if not most, patients have difficulty adhering to CPAP therapy despite its documented efficacy. It is estimated that over 50% of those started on CPAP will not be using it one year later [3]. Of those patients continuing to use it one year later, most are not using CPAP for the entire night, as prescribed. Published adherence rates from studies in the United States range from 3.3 to 5.3 hours per night [8-11]. One study showed that only 6% of patients used the machine for > 7 hours per night on at least 70% of the nights [8]. It seems reasonable to claim that CPAP adherence can be significantly improved.

Treatment adherence is a critically important area of research for helping to maximize the potential health and financial benefits of this highly efficacious therapy. The health outcomes of OSA patients depend largely on their adherence to appropriate treatment recommendations. In chronic disease literature, patient nonadherence is a pervasive problem that can lead to the continued onset and progression of chronic illnesses and to more difficult clinical management. The same can be said of CPAP treatment nonadherence. Those OSA patients who stop using CPAP and do not start another treatment remain at risk for the consequences of untreated OSA. Studies that examine the relationship between amount of CPAP use and response to treatment have generally found that the less CPAP use is associated with fewer benefits [12-14], and conversely, more CPAP use results in an increase in benefits. One of the most important financial costs of CPAP nonadherence is the indirect cost of lost productivity and decreased quality of life for patients who are under- or untreated and continue to live with the effects of a chronic sleep disorder. In addition, while we are not aware of any studies that have specifically examined the monetary cost to the healthcare system of CPAP nonadherence, it seems reasonable to assert that a percentage of the diagnostic and treatment initialization costs, as well as any direct costs to the patient, may be considered costs of nonadherence.

There have been a number of previous reviews that summarize the findings of CPAP adherence intervention studies [15-19]. However, the specific Behavioral Change Techniques (BCT) employed in these interventional studies have not been standardized, nor have they been well studied for efficacy. There is a movement in the behavioral change literature to better define these techniques so that they might be standardized [20,21], thereby allowing for the replication of the intervention and for identification of effective interventions. This can be accomplished by examining the following factors: the theoretical basis of the CPAP adherence interventions, the behavior change techniques utilized in those interventions, and the modes of intervention delivery [20,21].

***Corresponding author:** Carl Stepnowsky, VA San Diego Healthcare System, 3350 La Jolla Village Drive (111N-1), San Diego, CA 92161, USA
E-mail: cstepnowsky@ucsd.edu

The goals of this paper, therefore, are to (1) to provide background information in these three areas (theoretical basis, BCT, and mode of intervention delivery) and (2) to present the results of a literature review of published CPAP adherence interventions in each of these three areas.

Theoretical basis

Theory-based behavioral change interventions are thought to be more effective than those that do not use, or are not based on, theory. It should be noted that while "model" and "theory" are often used interchangeably in the literature, a brief comment about their distinction might be useful. Theories help to explain or understand events by illustrating or describing the relationships between variables. Models, on the other hand, tend to pull from one or more theories, and even other models, to help explain a particular problem or issue [22]. This will help to explain why the Health Belief Model, for example, looks very different now than when it was first conceptualized, and also why for example, various authors interpret and use Social Cognitive Theory differently in their models.

Using theory to guide research is important for a number of reasons: (1) theories help to describe (and explain) how behaviors change and symptoms improve through the use of behavioral change programs; (2) theories guide program development and facilitate testing of the intervention; and (3) they help to firmly link an intervention to a theoretical foundation. Finally, grounding adherence interventions in theory are important to help the literature build a foundation and grow over time. Because of the importance of theoretical foundations, one recent study examined the extent to which theory has been used (i.e., operationalized, informed, applied, and tested) in the empirical health behavior research literature [23]. The study included 193 studies across different health behaviors and found that 35.7% mentioned theory. Of these studies, most (68.1%) used theory to "inform" the research project. Theory was used to a significantly lesser extent for the following purposes: applying theory (18%), building theory (9.4%), and testing theory (3.6%).

However, while most researchers would agree that use of theory leads to more effective Interventions, it should be noted that there is some debate about the importance of theory [24,25]. For example, Jeffery has argued that the behavioral change literature of the last 25 years has been dominated by cognitive decision making and cognitive variables, yet (a) it has come up short in terms of consistently predicting behavioral outcomes very well, (b) there is little evidence that cognitive schema help to cause behavioral change, and (c) cognitive processes are hard to directly change. However, more recent evidence based on meta-analysis suggests that medium-to-large change in intention (i.e., cognition) leads to a small-to-medium change in health behaviors [26]. This ongoing debate is mentioned here because it is important that our field be well aware of current theories' potential limitations, with an eye toward newer developments that may have a greater impact on behavioral change.

There are many ways one might categorize the interventions employed in an attempt to improve CPAP adherence. Because one goal of this review is to understand the theoretical foundation and associated techniques or strategies of the existing CPAP adherence interventions, we classified interventions as primarily concerned with providing educational, clinical, or behavioral change support. Educational support includes providing information for informational or knowledge purposes, but does not include education related to skills or psycho-educational purposes (i.e., behavioral change). Similarly, clinical support will refer to medical support and decision making offered by medical providers, and typically includes mask changes, pressure changes, or other kinds of medical support. It often includes increased access to medical professionals. Behavioral change will refer to those interventions that specifically attempt to change the way a patient thinks or acts using some defined behavioral change theory or model, with the express purpose of increasing the amount of CPAP use.

Behavioral change theory and models: There are a wide variety of behavioral change theories and models available to use, each with advantages and disadvantages (for a good review, see [22]). Models that have already been described within the CPAP literature include Social-Cognitive Theory, Transtheoretical Model, Health Belief Model, Triandis Theory of Behavioral Change, and the Health Action Process Model (see Appendix). A recent review of the most commonly used health behavior change models used in the general medical literature found the following order of use: Transtheoretical Model (27.5%), Social-Cognitive Theory (27.5%), and Health Belief Model (20%) [23].

One problem in the general treatment adherence literature, as related to the use of theory and models, is the lack of empirical studies. In a recent large meta-analysis, DiMatteo found that nearly 87% of the general adherence literature consisted of reviews, description of conceptual frameworks and models, and suggestions for improving patient adherence [27]. In other words, empirical studies make up only 13% of the general adherence literature. DiMatteo's review is important because it reviewed and analyzed over 16,000 English language citations and in all likelihood represents the largest review of its kind [27].

Modes of delivery: Interventions are delivered to the patients in three ways: individual or group format; use of supplemental educational tools; and use of remote technologies. Because of various ways an intervention may be delivered, a taxonomy for organizing modes of delivery is required. Webb et al. [28] have proposed a taxonomy focused on the physical manner in which participants receive the intervention (i.e., individual or group) and the nature of the person delivering the intervention (i.e., medical professional or trained facilitator). Another coding scheme, or organizing taxonomy, has focused on the delivery of interventions using health information technologies. It includes the use of supplemental modes of delivery (e.g., use of email; telephone; text messaging; cd-rom; videoconferencing/ teleconferencing; and video education) and the use of automated functions (e.g., automated tailored feedback; automated follow-up messages; as-needed remote access to an advisor to request advice; scheduled remote contact with an advisor; and peer-to-peer access) [28].

Specific Behavioral Change Techniques

Specific BCTs represent the "active" components of the interventions and refer to the strategies employed within the interventions that promote behavioral change. There have been attempts in the past to classify BCTs. On a broad basis, the developers of the Transtheoretical Model generated a list of the "processes of change" that enabled categorization of the ways in which shifts in behavior occur. These change processes are the covert and overt activities and experiences that individuals engage in when they attempt to modify their behaviors. The ten processes of change are consciousness raising, counter conditioning, dramatic relief, environmental reevaluation, helping relationships, reinforcement management, self-liberation, self-reevaluation, social liberation, and stimulus control. However, each process is a broad category encompassing multiple techniques, methods, and interventions that are traditionally associated with disparate theoretical orientations.

There have been various attempts to identify specific BCTs within particular domains, for example: physical activity [29,30], weight management [31], and HIV-related condom use [32]. Additionally, there has been a call for more comprehensive categorization of specific BCTs across various illness domains [26]. One of the most comprehensive efforts to date has been that by Abraham and Michie [20], who empirically developed a theory-linked taxonomy of BCTs. The result was a list of BCTs with standardized, operational definitions that provides a useful starting point for identifying the BCTs used in CPAP adherence interventions. This taxonomy will be used to guide our review; its methods are described in the next section.

Summary

While most behavior change research describes a specific intervention approach that may or may not be based on theory, there appears to have been little examination of the specific behavior change elements or techniques that comprise those interventions. Clearly, the majority of CPAP adherence interventional research is based on intervention with multiple components. A better understanding of what components are included in an intervention, and ultimately, the critical components that lead to behavioral change, is what may be needed to develop interventions that are more effective. There is good reason for taking these steps; when an intervention is described as being comprised of, for example, "classes," "workshops," or "counseling sessions," such general descriptions can mask procedurally distinct change components and may fail to adequately describe techniques such that they are not reproducible. In addition to promoting identification of specific intervention techniques, improved (or even standardized) descriptions of intervention content would facilitate the fidelity of intervention operationalization in replication studies and applications. To the extent that the effective change techniques that help to increase CPAP adherence can be identified, the opportunity to advance our field through the dissemination of efficacious interventions and techniques is increased. The second goal of this paper is to present the results of a literature review of published CPAP adherence interventions in each of these three areas (theoretical basis, BCT, and mode of intervention delivery) per the recommendations of Michie and colleagues [20,21].

Methods

Literature review

The CPAP adherence literature was reviewed to identify those studies that included a specific intervention designed to increase CPAP use. Studies were included in this review if they were considered to be an evaluation of an intervention to improve CPAP adherence (even if a case series or single group design), in order to be comprehensive. PubMed was searched using the terms "continuous positive airway pressure," "compliance," and their variants. Each abstract was reviewed and articles that met the criteria of testing or evaluating an intervention whose goal was to increase CPAP adherence or use were retrieved. This search was supplemented by examining each of the article's reference lists and any relevant review articles.

Study selection

Relevant CPAP adherence interventions are defined as those interventions that are designed with an educational, clinical support, or behavioral change approach with the expressed purpose of helping the OSA patient initially start CPAP therapy and/or maintain use over time. Studies that were focused on one aspect of CPAP adherence (e.g., feelings of claustrophobia or difficulty breathing with CPAP) were included, given the intended broad scope of this review. Pediatric studies were also included. We did not include studies that (1) only examined a technological intervention (e.g., the effect of humidification, the effect of pressure modification, or evaluation of a new mask type) but had no behavioral component; (2) were focused on providing descriptions of CPAP adherence rates (but that did not include description of an intervention or an evaluation of that intervention); (3) focused solely on examining predictors of CPAP adherence, but without an explicit intervention. In all, 29 studies met inclusion and exclusion criteria (see Table 1).

Use of theory

The use of theory was coded using item 1 of the theory coding scheme developed by Michie and Prestwich [21]: whether or not "methods/theories that specify relations among variables in order to explain or predict behavior are mentioned."

Behavioral change techniques

All the specific BCTs that were coded included CPAP intervention studies, including those that did not follow a specific behavioral model or theory. A 26-item list of behavioral change techniques was utilized per Abraham and Michie [20]. Their recommendation for implementing the coding scheme is to not code for behavioral change techniques if they overlap with the comparison intervention, the rationale being that any effect of the behavioral change technique would not be unique.

Mode of delivery

This review first classifies whether an intervention was delivered on an individual or group basis, as the mode of delivery may have an impact on outcomes. Secondarily, studies were classified according to whether they were primarily delivered "in person" or "remotely." In person refers to face-to-face contact (whether in the clinic or in the home). Remote refers to the use of some form of electronic means of communication at a distance, examples of which include the following: email, telephone, text messaging, or videoconferencing/teleconferencing. In addition to classifying mode of delivery into delivery format (individual or group) and delivery method (in person or remote), supplemental forms of education were coded as well, for example, web-based interactive modules or use of video education.

Data analysis

Descriptive and count data were used to describe the number of studies that cited a theoretical basis, the number of BCTs used per study, and the number of modes of delivery used throughout this literature. The d-index, used as a measure of effect size for the CPAP intervention studies, was defined as the difference between the means of the two groups being compared divided by the mean standard deviation (for CPAP adherence, in hours per night). An effect size was calculated for studies examining one group pre-intervention and post intervention. Mean effect sizes for the studies that employed a Randomized Controlled Trial design (RCT) were reported separately. An alpha level of 0.05 was used. Cohen recommended one classification of categorizing effect sizes: d=0.2 (small), d =0.5 (medium) and d =0.8 (large) [33].

Results

Use of theory

Theories and models were used relatively infrequently in the reviewed CPAP adherence intervention studies (Table 2). Out of the 29 studies, 11 unique (37%) studies mentioned a theory or a model (from Table 1: studies 6, 7, 12, 16, 18, 20, 21, 23, 24, 27, and 29). Richards et

	Study	Design	Effect Size (d)	Intervention and control group descriptions	Approach [a]	Theoretical Model [b]	Format [c] (*method*)
1	Fletcher and Luckett [57]	Cross-over	0.03	Basic: Video education, CPAP titration. Telephone Support: CPAP trouble-shooting via telephone.	Clinical Support	Not specified	Individual (*remote*)
2	Chervin et al. [58]	RCT	Lit: 1.11 Tele: 0.47	Basic: CPAP instruction & set-up. Literature support: Educational pamphlet and CPAP use guidelines written by PI's. Telephone support: Weekly follow-up phone calls.	Clinical Support	Not specified	Individual (*remote*)
3	Likar et al. [59]	Self-selected cohort	0.40	Basic: Nurse instruction of CPAP and OSA, 6-month follow-up, invited to contact with concerns. Group support: Basic, plus optional 2-h support meetings.	Clinical Support	Not specified	Group
4	Hoy et al. [60]	RCT	0.63	Basic support: OSA education by nurse & video; CPAP acclimatization; 24-hour help line; 1-mo f/u. Intensive support: Basic + home education with partner involvement; CPAP titration at home; multiple check-up home visits by nurses.	Clinical Support & Additional Educational Support	Not specified	Individual (*in person*)
5	Hui et al. [61]	RCT	0.00	Basic support: CPAP education via nurse & OSA brochure; telephone support. Intensive support: Basic + video education; multiple physician & nurse f/u visits and phone calls.	Clinical Support	Not specified	Individual (*in person*)
6	Aloia et al. [34]	RCT	1.14	Usual care: Overnight titration, physician follow-up. Cognitive-Behavioral Intervention: Usual + 2 one-to-one sessions by a clinical psychologist.	Behavioral Change	Cognitive-Behavioral Theory	Individual (*in person*)
7	Koontz et al. [62]	Retro-spective	N/A [e]	Consultation and Recommendation (CR) Session vs. CR + Behavioral Therapy (BT) vs. CR with BT referral, but BT not utilized	Behavioral Change	Behavioral Therapy	Individual (*in person*)
8	DeMolles et al. [63]	RCT	0.55	Usual care: Usual medical care alone. TLC-CPAP: Telephone-linked communications for CPAP was an interactive, touch-pad response system.	Clinical Support	Not specified	Individual (*remote*)
9	Palmer et al. [64]	Pre- vs. post- design	CAR: 0.16 NHV: 0.37	Consultant Annual Review (CAR): by consultant clinic appointment. Nurse Home Visit (NHV): by specialist nurse	Clinical Support	Not specified	Individual (*in person*)
10	Smith et al. [65]	One group pre/post	N/A [e]	Standard sleep apnea education program: Booklet provision and nurse-led group education.	Educational Support	Not specified	Group
11	Wiese et al. [66]	RCT	N/A [e]	Usual Care: MD provided information with Respiratory Therapist support. Educational Video: 15 min, author scripted video.	Educational Support	Not specified	Individual (*in person*)
12	Golay et al. [67]	One-group pre/post	0.33	Therapeutic Educational Program: CPAP hands on workshop; educational courses and spousal roundtables.	Educational, Clinical, & Behavioral Support	Health Belief Model	Group
13	Lewis et al. [68]	RCT	0.24	Standard follow-up: Phone number provided for needed support. Extra early support: Consisted of a video (20-min), telephonic support 2-5 days post-start, MD visit 1-2 weeks.	Clinical support	Not specified	Individual (*in person*)
14	Smith et al. [69]	RCT	1.0	Control group: telehealth intervention on importance of vitamins. Telehealth group: telehealth intervention using video teleconferencing between nurse and patient focusing on CPAP use.	Clinical Support	Not specified	Individual (*remote*)
15	Taylor et al. [70]	RCT	0.03	Traditional Care vs. Telemedicine Support: Health Buddy computer that allowed for informational support and problem trouble-shooting.	Clinical Support	Not specified	Individual (*remote*)
16	Aloia et al. [11]	RCT	SE: 0.36 MET: 0.23	Standard Care: Provision of print materials and MD visits at diagnosis and 8-10 weeks post. Simple Education (SE): completely didactic intervention and focused on OSA and CPAP Motivational Enhancement Therapy (MET): based on principles of motivational interviewing.	Behavioral Change	Motivational Enhancement	Individual (*in person*)
17	Ballard et al. [71]	One group	0.05	Two-phase intervention: Phase I focused on standard interventions including mask optimization, humidification, topical nasal therapy, and OSA education; Phase II was for persistently noncompliant patients and included randomization to CPAP or BiPAP.	Clinical Support	Not specified	Individual (*in person*)
18	Means et al. [72]	One group	1.52	Graded exposure therapy. This study was based on a previously published protocol and represents the report of a clinical case series	Behavioral Change	Graded Exposure Therapy	Individual (*in person*)
19	Meurice et al. [73]	RCT	0.0	Standard education vs. Reinforced education: included standard education plus written support. This study added the component of who was delivering education (prescriber and homecare network)	Educational Support	Not specified	Individual (*in person*)
20	Richards et al. [74]	RCT	1.09	Usual Care vs. Cognitive Behavioral group approach: Primarily group education (didactics via slide presentation, video and booklet) with CBT components (correction of distorted beliefs, promotion of positive treatment outlook).	Educational with Behavioral Change component	Cognitive-Behavioral Theory; Social-Cognitive Theory	Group

21	Slifer et al. [75]	Case series	6.0 [e]	Behavioral Therapy: comprised of counterconditioning, shaping, and education.	Behavioral Change	Behavioral Therapy	Individual (*in person*)
22	Stepnowsky et al. [76]	RCT	0.65	Control group: Usual care of 1-week phone call and 1-month clinic visit. Telemonitoring group: Based on the premise of therapist having daily access to CPAP adherence and efficacy data, and acting on that data proactively.	Clinical Support	Not specified	Individual (*remote*)
23	Stepnowsky et al. [77]	Single group	N/A [e]	Self-Management: comprised of OSA & CPAP education, self-monitoring, decision-making, and problem-solving	Educational & Behavioral Change	Cognitive-Behavioral Therapy	Group
24	Smith et al. [78]	RCT	0.84	Control group: placebo focused on daily vitamins. Music and habit-forming intervention: Didactics on OSA and CPAP benefits; problem-solving guide; nightly use reminder placards; and 20 min music audiotape for sleep onset with CPAP.	Educational and Behavioral Change	Triandis Theory of Behavior	Individual (*in person*)
25	Damjanovic et al. [79]	RCT	0.49	Standard support vs. Intensive support consisted of optimizing mask fit, using moisturizers as needed, and identification of early low compliance.	Clinical Support	Not specified	Individual (*in person*)
26	Fuchs et al. [81]	Two-group design	1.08	Patient Information Program (PIP): 2 hour standardized educational lecture + summary booklet. Control group: PIP nonattendance. Nonrandomized, uncontrolled study.	Educational Support	Not specified	Group
27	Roecklin et al. [81]	RCT	0.17	Standard Information: 3 AASM pamphlets Personalized Feedback: inclusive of OSA severity and OSA risks.	Educational Support	Motivational Approach	Individual (*in person*)
28	Sparrow et al. [83]	RCT	N/A [e]	Attention placebo control: Usual medical care alone. TLC-CPAP: Telephone-linked communications for CPAP was an interactive, touch-pad response system.	Clinical Support	Not specified	Individual (*remote*)
29	Trupp et al. [83]	RCT	0.53 [e]	Educational Message Framing: positive vs. negative framing	Educational Support	Prospect Theory	Individual (*in person*)

Note. RCT = randomized controlled trial. [a] Approach allowed for the classification of the experimental intervention as primarily being Educational, Clinical Support or Behavioral Change. [b] For those studies labeled with a theoretical model as "not specified," one could presume that more education and/or more support was the guiding principle behind these studies. [c] Format was classified as the intervention being delivered individually or in group format. Individual format was further divided into "in person" or "remote," with "remote" referring to the use of some sort of electronic communication (e.g., telephone; telephone-linked communications; telemedicine device; telemonitoring). [d] Pediatric study. [e] *Notes on Effect Size.* (1) Koontz et al. (2003) was a retrospective chart review and did not use a well-defined control group against which to make comparisons; however, if one considered the intervention group from within-subject perspective, effect sizes would be large (with BT increasing adherence from 0.77 hrs/nt to 5.51 hrs/nt, and CR+BT increasing adherence from 1.72 hrs/nt to 7.47 hrs/nt) (note: SD was not reported for this data); (2) Smith et al. (2004) did not report adherence data; (3) Wiese et al. (2004) did not report sufficient data for ES calculation (video education did result in greater attendance at one-month follow-up visit (72.9% vs. 48.9%; p=0.02); (4) Meurice *et al.* 2007 found no differences among type of education and deliverer of the education (prescriber and homecare team); (5) Slifer *et al.* 2007 was a case series of 4 children; it should be noted that Figure 2 of the paper presents adherence data for each child and shows large improvements in PAP use over 26 to 60 nights; (6) Stepnowsky *et al.* (2007) presents pilot data on a single group of new OSA patients, with mean adherence = 5.5 ± 2.5 hrs/nt; (7) Sparrow *et al.* (2010) does not report mean or standard deviation so the effect size was unable to be calculated (authors did not respond to inquiries); (8) Trupp *et al.* (2011) did not report the mean and SD for the adherence data, so effect size was calculated based on the p-value.

Table 1: Review of Psychoeducational Interventions Designed to Increase CPAP Adherence

al. (study 20) mentioned both Cognitive-Behavioral Theory and Social-Cognitive Theory and was therefore counted twice. Aloia and colleagues [34] (study 6) mentioned that their study is based on Cognitive-Behavioral Theory; however, given a later study by the same group, it would appear the 2001 study may have been a pilot of the Motivational Enhancement Training intervention [11]. Two pediatric studies cited using Behavioral Therapy (studies 7 and 21). In terms of the amount of text describing the interventional methods, the two pediatric studies were the most comprehensive.

Behavioral change techniques

Out of the possible 26 different behavioral change techniques, the two most common techniques were "provide general information" and "provide instruction." This is not unexpected, given that OSA patients require significant amounts of information and education regarding OSA and CPAP, as well as detailed initial and ongoing instruction on CPAP use. The third most commonly used technique was "provide information on consequences," fourth was "provide general encouragement," and fifth was "prompt barrier identification." Table 3 provides a rank ordering of the frequency with which specific behavioral change techniques were employed.

The next most common behavioral change techniques were "provide feedback on performance" (6th); "prompt practice" (7thT, where "T" refers to "tie"); and "model or demonstrate the behavior" (7thT). It was surprising that the provision of feedback was not used more often because of the common availability of CPAP data downloads and the important information they provide regarding CPAP adherence and efficacy. It is unlikely that the year of study plays a role, as only four of the 29 intervention studies were published before 2000. It was also surprising that demonstration and prompt practice (i.e., using CPAP in presence of provider in initial visit) were not more commonly used techniques because of the benefit of being sure the patient can tolerate the air pressure prior to home use. Three or fewer studies utilized techniques 7, 10-12, 14, 15, 18-20, and 25. And no studies utilized techniques 3, 4, 16, 21-24, or 26.

In terms of BCT use by study, the mean number of BCTs used across the 29 studies was 4.3 ± 2.0 (mean ± SD) per intervention, the minimum number of BCTs used per intervention was one, and the maximum was nine. Figure 1 shows the distribution of studies by number of BCTs. The most common number of BCTs per study was 4. Clearly, BCTs used per study ranged from one BCT per study, representing simple, one-component interventions, up through multicomponent studies. When the same data were examined only for those studies that employed a two-group (typically randomized controlled trial) design, the mean number of BCTs was nearly the same as for the entire group: 4.3 ± 2.0 (mean ± SD) (range: 1-9) per intervention. The d-index measure of effect size is

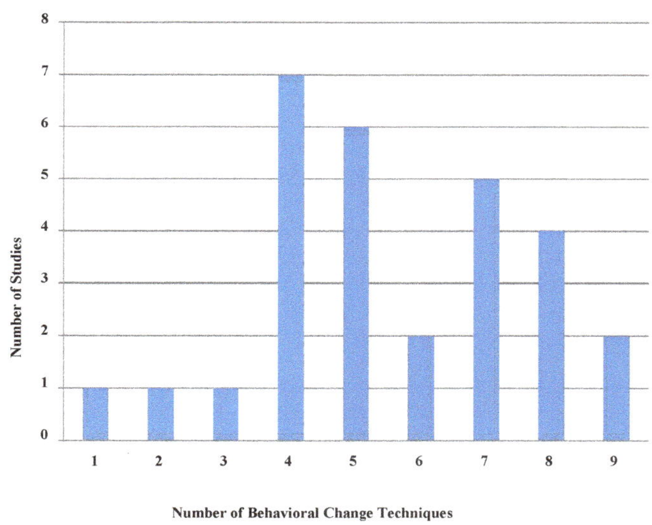

Figure 1: Number of Behavioral Changes Techniques Used Per Study (n=29).

reported in Table 1 for each study. The mean dindex across all studies in the review was 0.72 ± 1.13 (range: 0 - 6). When the outlier effect size for the one case-series pediatric study was excluded, the mean d-index was 0.52 ± 0.42 (range: 0- 1.52). This d-index then represents the mean d-index of CPAP adherence interventions for adults with OSA who were new users of CPAP. When only the studies that employed a two group (typically randomized, controlled trial, or RCT) were included, the mean d-index was 0.56 ± 0.39 (range: 0 - 1.14). In terms of Cohen's effect size, a medium effect size is considered to be 0.50, which helps provide some context for the CPAP adherence intervention effect sizes found in this review [33].

Across all studies, the correlation between the d-index and the number of BCTs was positive such that the higher the number of BCTs, the higher the effect size, though it did not reach statistical significance (r=0.365; p=0.061; n=27). In only those RCT studies, the correlation between the d-index and number of BCTs was not statistically significant (r = 0.304;p=0.205; n=19).

The studies were then classified according to primary CPAP adherence intervention type (clinical support, educational support, or behavioral change). Across all studies in the review, the d-index was statistically different across intervention type (F(2,24)=4.445; p=.023). These results held when the one case series pediatric study (with a d-index of 6.0) was excluded (F(2,23)=4.349; p=0.025) such that behavioral interventional studies had the highest effect size (0.96 ± 0.48), followed by educational interventions (0.43 ± 0.42) and clinical support interventions (0.41 ± 0.33). However, these results changed when only RCT studies were examined, with the d-index not significantly different across type of CPAP adherence intervention (F(2,16)=1.281; p=.305; behavioral change interventions: 0.83 ± 0.42; clinical interventions: 0.52 ± 0.37; and educational interventions: 0.43 ± 0.42).

The number of BCTs by CPAP adherence intervention type was also examined. For all studies, the difference approached statistical significance (F(2,29)=3.009; p=.065), with the most BCTs found in behavioral interventional studies (5.4 ± 1.7 BCTs), followed by clinical support (4.4 ± 2.1 BCTs) and educational support: 3.0 ± 1.3 BCTs). When examining only RCTs, there was not a statistically different number of BCTs by intervention type (F(2,18)=2.479; p=.112), with nearly the same distribution of BCTs by intervention type: behavioral interventional studies (5.5 ± 0.60 BCTs), followed by clinical support (4.3 ± 2.0 BCTs) and educational support: 3.2 ±1.3 BCTs).

The relationship between format type (group vs. individual) and the d-index and number of BCTs was examined next. Across all studies, format type was not related to the d-index (t=-0.455; p=0.653) but was associated with the number of BCTs (t=-2.046; p=0.050). These results held when examining only RCT studies, with format type not related to the d-index (t=-0.800;p=0.435), but was related to the number of BCTs (t=-2.154; p=0.044) such that group format had 5.75 ± 1.0 BCTs while the individual format had 3.8 ± 1.7 BCTs.

Lastly the relationship between use of theory and the d-index and number of BCTs was examined. Across all studies, use of theory was not related to the d-index (t=-1.546; p=0.135) or to the number of BCTs (t=-1.752; p=0.090). These results held when examining only RCT studies, with use of theory not related to the d-index (t=-0.533; p=0.601) or to the number of BCTs (t=-.432; p=0.671).

Mode of delivery

Table 1 shows the intervention delivery format (group or individual) and delivery method (in person or remote). Six out of the 29 CPAP interventions utilized a group-based format (smallest group = 3 patients; largest group = 12 patients). In most cases, spouses were encouraged to participate in the group-based format. Of the 6 group interventions, one used a supplemental video to provide education, and none appeared to use supplemental forms of electronic communication. Twenty-three out of the 29 interventions utilized individual-based interactions. Of the 23 interventions, 7 utilized remote interactions as the primary contact method. It is important to note that none of the studies were conducted entirely via remote, as all started with in-person interactions at the outset. In addition, all 7 interventions provided mechanisms to schedule in-person meetings should they be needed. Of the 7 studies that used remote interactions, three studies used telephone (with one study using telemonitoring to obtain CPAP adherence and efficacy data, and then calling patients via telephone); two used telephone-linked communications (i.e., interactive voice response, or IVR); one used a telemedicine device called Health Buddy; and one used videoconferencing. The only form of supplemental education used, video education, was used in 9 out of the 29 interventions. Few studies (2 out of 9) described the video education intervention in detail. For those studies that reported video length, it ranged from 14 to 20 minutes. One study indicated that ResMed was the video manufacturer, and in another case, it appeared that the video was scripted and taped by the study authors.

Discussion

Low patient adherence to nasal Continuous Positive Airway Pressure (CPAP) treatment limits treatment effectiveness. A number of CPAP adherence interventional approaches have been studied to date, including clinical support, educational support, and behavioral change interventions. The average effect size of the studies on new adult OSA patients who were newly prescribed CPAP was 0.52 (SD=0.42, range: 0-1.52), suggesting that CPAP adherence interventions have a moderate effect on increasing the amount of nightly use with CPAP. The number of Behavioral Change Techniques (BCTs) used in each intervention did not appear to be associated with the effect size. However, those studies designated as being primarily focused on behavioral change did have higher effect sizes than either clinical or educational support intervention studies when all studies were included; when only RCTs

Theory	Number of Studies	Study Numbers[a]
Cognitive Behavioral Therapy/Theory	3	6, 20, 23
Behavioral Therapy	2	7, 21
Motivational Interviewing Theory	2	16, 27
Social Cognitive Theory	1	20
Health Belief Model	1	12
Triandis Theory of Behavior	1	24
Graded Exposure Therapy	1	18
Prospect Theory	1	29
Total	12	

Note. [a] Study numbers are from Table 1.
Running head: INTERVENTIONS TO IMPROVE CPAP ADHERENCE 32

Table 2: Theoretical Basis of CPAP Adherence Intervention Studies

Rank #	Behavioral Change Technique[a]	Count[b]
1	Provide general information (1)	24
2	Provide instruction (8)	18
3	Provide information on consequences (2)	15
4	Provide general encouragement (6)	11
5	Prompt barrier identification (5)	10
6	Provide feedback on performance (13)	9
7T[c]	Model or demonstrate the behavior (9)	7
7T	Prompt practice (17)	7
8T	Set graded tasks (7)	3
8T	Prompt self-monitoring of behavior (12)	3
9T	Prompt specific goal setting (10)	2
9T	Prompt review of behavioral goals (11)	2
9T	Provide contingent rewards (14)	2
9T	Use follow-up prompts (18)	2
9T	Provide opportunities for social comparison (19)	2
9T	Motivational interviewing (25)	2
10T	Teach to use prompts/cues (15)	1
10T	Plan social support/social change (20)	1
--	Provide information about others' approval (3)	0
--	Prompt intention formation (4)	0
--	Agree on behavioral contract (16)	0
--	Prompt identification as a role model (21)	0
--	Prompt self-talk (22)	0
--	Relapse prevention (23)	0
--	Stress Management (24)	0
--	Time Management (26)	0

Note. [a] Name of specific Behavioral Change Technique along with its identification number in parentheses from the original Abraham & Michie (2008) BCT coding scheme. The text in the Results section identifies some of the BCTs in this table by their number. [b] Count refers to the number of CPAP adherence studies that used that specific BCT. [c] "T" indicates that two or more techniques were tied in terms of the count,

Table 3: Behavioral Change Techniques Used In CPAP Adherence Studies: Count and Rank Order

were examined, this relationship did not hold. Finally, whether an intervention was delivered in group or individual format, or whether it stated it was based on a theoretical foundation, did not appear related to the effect size. Group formats were associated with a greater number of BCTs than individual format.

Better understanding of the theoretical foundation and BCTs used in this literature may help provide direction for future efforts. The findings of this review suggest that a relatively small percentage of CPAP adherence studies (~25%) are based on, or use, theory. However, relative to the general medical literature on the use of theory in adherence interventions (~35%), this percentage is only ~10% less. It would appear that most studies, both in the CPAP adherence literature (~75%) and in the general medical literature (~65%), either do not use, or do not report using, a theoretical basis.

Given the needs of new OSA patients prescribed CPAP therapy, it was not surprising that the most commonly used BCTs are concerned with providing general information, instruction, and information on consequences. Given that OSA is a chronic illness that occurs while one is asleep, providing basic information and education regarding OSA and its consequences is clearly a necessary step. And given that CPAP is a complex treatment regimen, it is reasonable that most interventions include providing CPAP-related instruction, both initially and on an ongoing basis.

Clinical experience and the research literature suggest that barriers are common reasons why OSA patients limit, or do not use, CPAP. The fifth most commonly used BCT concerns barrier identification, and it was used in only 10 out of the 29 reviewed studies. Barrier identification allows for improved troubleshooting and problem-solving.

Providing feedback on performance was identified in only 9 out of the 29 reviewed studies, which was surprising given the CPAP adherence and efficacy data recorded by the CPAP units, and the ease with which this information can be obtained by providers and shared with OSA patients. Our own research has found this to be a central part of what we do in terms of providing patients with objective feedback on how well CPAP may be working for them, and it engenders patient-centered, collaborative care.

While it is clear that not every BCT can be incorporated into a CPAP adherence intervention, 30% of the possible BCTs that comprised this specific coding scheme were not utilized in any CPAP adherence intervention. One reasonable possibility for this is that the published literature provides limited descriptions of the interventions themselves. This review was based only on what was described in the articles and did not seek to obtain intervention manuals or ask for further information from study authors (as some of the studies are more than 10 years old). It may very well have been that more BCTs would have been identified had these steps been taken. Indeed, the interventional methods sections of the reviewed CPAP adherence papers ranged in length from one to thirteen paragraphs. Clearly, more description allowed for the possibility of reporting greater numbers of BCTs. Another possibility is that our field is not utilizing one or more BCTs that might be effective for CPAP adherence. Future research would do well to consider those BCTs that are untested for CPAP adherence. Readers should be cautioned that the current review included a wide range of studies, including across age ranges (pediatric and adult), across study design types (i.e., those designed for all new users and those designed for more specific subsets of users), and utilizing multiple formats.

This raises the issue of future directions for our field. Clearly, as was established in other health domains, improved reporting of the specific BCTs is needed. While there is clear guidance on reporting clinical trials, both generally as per the CONSORT statement [35,36] and specifically on reporting behavioral trials [37], the recommended level of description or clarity requested for the "content or elements" for a behavioral change intervention remains problematic. The CONSORT statement states that evaluators should report the "precise details of interventions " [36], but the problem remains that there is no standardized or commonly agreed upon vocabulary with which to describe the techniques used in behavioral change trials. This results in a whole host of consequences, including not being able to identify the "active" component of an intervention or not being able to reproduce the intervention. Using the relatively new taxonomy of BCTs, as developed by Abraham and Michie [20], provides a good first step toward being able to use common and standardized descriptions within our field. Given that CPAP adherence is a unique complex behavioral treatment regimen, it may very well be that each BCT will need some modification (or qualifications) to be most applicable and useful to our field.

Future reporting of CPAP adherence intervention trials would do well to follow the guidelines for behavioral scientists in reporting behavioral trials for interventions [37]: (1) the content or elements of the intervention (e.g., oral communication, written material, videos, others), (2) the characteristics of those delivering the intervention (e.g., level of education or amount of training required), (3) the characteristics of the recipients, (4) the setting (e.g.,worksite, community, medical center), (5) the mode of delivery (e.g., face-to-face, individual, group), (6) the intensity (e.g., contact time), (7) the duration (e.g., number of sessions over a given period), and (8) adherence to delivery protocols. It should be noted that there was a recent effort to disseminate behavioral treatments for sleep disorders, including several CPAP adherence interventions, in a recently published book [38].

Lastly, it should be noted that globally there are ever increasing cost pressures in healthcare, whether the costs are borne by individuals, governments, or third-party payers. In the United States, the Centers for Medicare and Medicaid Services have issued a CMS Local Coverage Determination adherence criterion for continued reimbursement of CPAP after 90 days of use. This example of reimbursement linked to use level suggests there is an urgent need to identify those interventions, and specifically BCTs, that foster the greatest level of use in OSA patients relatively early in the treatment initialization process, whether within the 3-month period defined by CMS in the US, or the various standards in other countries. Furthermore, it may be that policy-related efforts are also needed to help influence health service delivery factors, as follows: (1) examining how OSA care is currently organized and how it might be improved to better facilitate good chronic illness care and (2) examining how reimbursement is currently structured. For example, there may be a good rationale for cost-shifting away from expensive diagnostic testing for routine OSA screening and moving those savings to CPAP treatment initialization and follow-up efforts, which is significantly underfunded currently in the US. This critical point is made because the reality of implementing efficacious CPAP interventions is largely dependent on adequate reimbursement. Finally, it may be that utilizing a stepped care approach that best matches various kinds of BCTs to those who need them, and when they need them, is a viable future direction [39].

Appendix

Social cognitive theory: Social Cognitive Theory (SCT) posits multiple influences on behavior, with an emphasis on personal (e.g., cognitive) and environmental (e.g., social) factors [40]. Variables derived from this model include self-efficacy, outcome expectations, social support, and knowledge. Self-efficacy refers to the beliefs in one's abilities to engage in a particular behavior [41]. Outcome expectations refer to beliefs that engaging in a particular behavior will result in certain outcomes [41]. Because these judgments occur in and are influenced by social situations, social support is a key variable of the model. Social support refers to the availability and usefulness of the tangible support of family, friends, and medical staff. Though knowledge alone rarely translates into health-related behavior change, SCT [42] holds that accurate information provides the basis for such change. SCT has provided the basis for both specific and general chronic disease self-management programs. Self-management refers to the day-to-day tasks an individual must undertake to control or reduce the impact of disease on health status.

Cognitive behavioral therapy: Cognitive-Behavioral Therapies (CBT) do not necessarily represent a specific theoretical foundation, but a general therapeutic approach that aims to solve problems concerning problematic cognitions, behaviors, and emotions through a goal-oriented, systematic procedure. By definition, CBTs draw from an assortment of therapeutic approaches, including cognitive, behavioral, and educational. Within each of these approaches, various theoretical foundations may or may not be made explicit. Indeed, defining the scope of what constitutes CBT is a difficulty that has persisted throughout its history [43]. While it is convenient to label an interventional approach as being "CBT," for our field to advance, specification of the following is necessary: underlying theoretical model, the proposed relationships between measured constructs or predictors and the outcome, and BCTs. CBT has been shown to be effective for a variety of problems, including treatment adherence.

Transtheoretical model: The Transtheoretical Model (TM) is a multidimensional approach to behavior change that integrates behavior change processes and principles from across leading theories [44]. The core construct, around which the other dimensions are organized, is the stages of change, which represents ordered categories along a continuum of motivational readiness to change a specific behavior. Five categories comprise the stage of change construct and include pre-contemplation, contemplation, preparation, action, and maintenance. Pre-contemplation is the stage at which there is little or no intention to change behavior in the near future. Many individuals in this stage are unaware of their options. In the contemplation stage, individuals seriously consider changing their behavior, but have not yet made a commitment to take action. The preparation stage combines both intention and behavioral aspects. The individual in the preparation stage has clear intentions to change behavior and has made some behavioral attempts. In the action stage, individuals modify their behavior, experiences, or environment in order to make the change. The individual in the action stage has made overt behavioral changes that have required considerable time and energy, and has typically done so for a defined period of time, often 1 month or more. Maintenance is the stage in which the individual has engaged in behavior change for a defined period of time, typically 6 months or more.

The model asserts that patients engage in a decisional "balance sheet" of comparative potential gains and losses, termed the decisional balance. The decisional balance is a summary index of the pros and cons of engaging in the behavior. This balance varies depending in which stage the individual may be classified, and is said to get at the "why" of behavior change. For example, it has been shown that the number of cons significantly outweigh the number of pros for an individual in the pre-contemplation stage of change, while the number of pros outweigh the number of cons for an individual in the maintenance stage of change [45].

Health belief model: The Health Belief Model (HBM) was initially developed to help predict the engagement in a single health behavior [46], for example, obtaining a vaccination or wearing a bicycle helmet [47]. However, given the need for behavior change models to help understand more complex behavior, the HBM borrowed other concepts developed in other areas and included them in its model. HBM also allows for the inclusion of demographic, psychological, and social influences on adherence [48]. HBM has been applied to the prediction of compliance outside of the sleep research literature [48-

50], and within the sleep research literature, has been applied to CPAP adherence prediction [19,51]. Future research will determine how well it can be applied to the development and testing of CPAP adherence interventions.

Health action process approach: The Health Action Process Approach (HAPA) suggests that the adoption, initiation, and maintenance of health behaviors are conceived as a process that consists of at least a motivation phase and a volition phase [52]. The latter is further subdivided into a planning phase, action phase, and maintenance phase. It is claimed that perceived self-efficacy plays a crucial role at all stages, along with other cognitions [41]. For example, risk perceptions serve predominantly to set the stage for a contemplation process early in the motivation phase but do not extend beyond. Similarly, outcome expectancies are chiefly important in the motivation phase when individuals balance the pros and cons of certain consequences of behaviors, but they lose their predictive power after a personal decision has been made. However, if one does not believe in one's capability to perform a desired action, one will fail to adopt, initiate, and maintain it. Therefore, the HAPA model is closely related to both Social Cognitive Theory and the Health Belief Model. While SCT is comprised of outcome expectations and perceived selfefficacy, perception of risk in not one of its core concepts. From Bandura's perspective, perception of risk would probably be best conceptualized as a physical outcome expectation. It may be that perception of risk can play a role in mediating some kinds of health behavior change, and it may, after it is appropriately modeled and empirically tested, prove to be a useful construct for its potential role in understanding CPAP adherence. The HAPA Model is included because one set of assessment tools for CPAP adherence research appears to be in large part based on this model: self-efficacy measure for sleep apnea [53].

Triandis theory of behavioral change: Social psychologist Harry Triandis attempted to develop an integrated model of "interpersonal" behavior [54] over thirty years ago. He recognized the important role played by both social and emotional factors in forming intentions, as well as the importance of past behavior on future behavior. On the basis of these observations, he proposed a theory in which intentions are immediate antecedents of behavior, which is consistent with many other models. However, he proposed two main distinctions from other models: (1) that habits also mediate behavior (in an attempt to incorporate the role of past behavior) and (2) that both of these influences (intentions and habits) are moderated by facilitating conditions (i.e., objective environmental factors that enable persons to engage in the behavior). CPAP adherence researchers have used this theory to provide a foundation for the importance of habit formation and environmental modification to facilitate health-related behaviors. Researchers using Triandis Theory have found empirical support that following routines that guide treatment use and sensitizing patients to benefits and nontreatment risks result in improved adherence [55,56].

Acknowledgement

This research was supported in part by Department of Veterans Affairs, Veterans Health Administration, Office of Research and Development, and the Research Service of the San Diego Veterans Affairs Healthcare System (VA HSRD IIR 02-275 and 07-163, and AHRQ R18017246).

References

1. Bassiri, A.G. and C. Guilleminault, Clinical features and evaluation of obstructive sleep apnea-hypopnea syndrome, in Principle and Practice of Sleep Medicine, M. Kryger, T. Roth, and W.C. Dement, Editors. 2000, W.B. Saunders & Co.: Philadelphia, PA. p. 869- 78.
2. Sullivan CE, Issa FG, Berthon-Jones M, Eves L (1981) Reversal of obstructive sleep apnoea by continuous positive airway pressure applied through the nares. Lancet 1: 862-865.
3. Loube DI, Gay PC, Strohl KP, Pack AI, White DP, et al. (1999) Indications for positive airway pressure treatment of adult obstructive sleep apnea patients: a consensus statement. Chest 115: 863-866.
4. Patel SR, White DP, Malhotra A, Stanchina ML, Ayas NT (2003) Continuous positive airway pressure therapy for treating sleepiness in a diverse population with obstructive sleep apnea: results of a meta-analysis. Arch Intern Med 163: 565-571.
5. Wright J, Johns R, Watt I, Melville A, Sheldon T (1997) Health effects of obstructive sleep apnoea and the effectiveness of continuous positive airways pressure: a systematic review of the research evidence. BMJ 314: 851-860.
6. McArdle N, Kingshott R, Engleman HM, Mackay TW, Douglas NJ (2001) Partners of patients with sleep apnoea/hypopnoea syndrome: effect of CPAP treatment on sleep quality and quality of life. Thorax 56: 513-518.
7. Pepperell JC, Ramdassingh-Dow S, Crosthwaite N, Mullins R, Jenkinson C, et al. (2002) Ambulatory blood pressure after therapeutic and subtherapeutic nasal continuous positive airway pressure for obstructive sleep apnoea: a randomised parallel trial. Lancet 359: 204-210.
8. Kribbs NB, Pack AI, Kline LR, Smith PL, Schwartz AR, et al. (1993) Objective measurement of patterns of nasal CPAP use by patients with obstructive sleep apnea. Am Rev Respir Dis 147: 887-895.
9. Reeves-Hoche MK, Meck R, Zwillich CW (1994) Nasal CPAP: an objective evaluation of patient compliance. Am J Respir Crit Care Med 149: 149-154.
10. Stepnowsky CJ Jr, Marler MR, Ancoli-Israel S (2002) Determinants of nasal CPAP compliance. Sleep Med 3: 239-247.
11. Aloia MS, Smith K, Arnedt JT, Millman RP, Stanchina M, et al. (2007) Brief behavioral therapies reduce early positive airway pressure discontinuation rates in sleep apnea syndrome: preliminary findings. Behav Sleep Med 5: 89-104.
12. Stepnowsky CJ Jr, Moore PJ (2003) Nasal CPAP treatment for obstructive sleep apnea: developing a new perspective on dosing strategies and compliance. J Psychosom Res 54: 599-605.
13. Stepnowsky CJ, Dimsdale JE (2002) Dose-response relationship between CPAP compliance and measures of sleep apnea severity. Sleep Med 3: 329-334.
14. Weaver TE, Maislin G, Dinges DF, Bloxham T, George CF, et al. (2007) Relationship between hours of CPAP use and achieving normal levels of sleepiness and daily functioning. Sleep 30: 711-719.
15. Engleman HM, Wild MR (2003) Improving CPAP use by patients with the sleep apnoea/hypopnoea syndrome (SAHS). Sleep Med Rev 7: 81-99.
16. Weaver TE, Grunstein RR (2008) Adherence to continuous positive airway pressure therapy: the challenge to effective treatment. Proc Am Thorac Soc 5: 173-178.
17. Weaver TE (2006) Adherence to positive airway pressure therapy. Curr Opin Pulm Med 12: 409-413.
18. Smith I, Nadig V, Lasserson TJ (2009) Educational, supportive and behavioural interventions to improve usage of continuous positive airway pressure machines for adults with obstructive sleep apnoea. Cochrane Database Syst Rev : CD007736.
19. Olsen S, Smith S, Oei T, Douglas J (2008) Health belief model predicts adherence to CPAP before experience with CPAP. Eur Respir J 32: 710-717.
20. Abraham C, Michie S (2008) A taxonomy of behavior change techniques used in interventions. Health Psychol 27: 379-387.
21. Michie S, Prestwich A (2010) Are interventions theory-based? Development of a theory coding scheme. Health Psychol 29: 1-8.
22. Glanz, K., B. Rimer, and F. Lewis, Health Behavior and Health Education: Theory, Research and Practice. 3rd ed. 2002, San Francisco, CA: John Wiley & Sons, Inc.
23. Painter JE, Borba CP, Hynes M, Mays D, Glanz K (2008) The use of theory in health behavior research from 2000 to 2005: a systematic review. Ann Behav Med 35: 358-362.

24. Oxman AD, Fretheim A, Flottorp S (2005) The OFF theory of research utilization. J Clin Epidemiol 58: 113-116.

25. Jeffery RW (2004) How can Health Behavior Theory be made more useful for intervention research? Int J Behav Nutr Phys Act 1: 10.

26. Webb TL, Sheeran P (2006) Does changing behavioral intentions engender behavior change? A meta-analysis of the experimental evidence. Psychol Bull 132: 249-268.

27. DiMatteo MR (2004) Variations in patients' adherence to medical recommendations: a quantitative review of 50 years of research. Med Care 42: 200-209.

28. Webb TL, Joseph J, Yardley L, Michie S (2010) Using the internet to promote health behavior change: a systematic review and meta-analysis of the impact of theoretical basis, use of behavior change techniques, and mode of delivery on efficacy. J Med Internet Res 12: e4.

29. Hillsdon M, Foster C, Thorogood M (2005) Interventions for promoting physical activity. Cochrane Database Syst Rev : CD003180.

30. Conn VS, Valentine JC, Cooper HM (2002) Interventions to increase physical activity among aging adults: a meta-analysis. Ann Behav Med 24: 190-200.

31. Hardeman W, Griffin S, Johnston M, Kinmonth AL, Wareham NJ (2000) Interventions to prevent weight gain: a systematic review of psychological models and behaviour change methods. Int J Obes Relat Metab Disord 24: 131-143.

32. Albarracín D, Gillette JC, Earl AN, Glasman LR, Durantini MR, et al. (2005) A test of major assumptions about behavior change: a comprehensive look at the effects of passive and active HIV-prevention interventions since the beginning of the epidemic. Psychol Bull 131: 856-897.

33. Cohen, J., *Statistical power analysis for the behavioral sciences*. 2nd ed. 1988, Hillsdale,NJ: Lawrence Erlbaum Associates.

34. Aloia MS, Di Dio L, Ilniczky N, Perlis ML, Greenblatt DW, et al. (2001) Improving compliance with nasal CPAP and vigilance in older adults with OAHS. Sleep Breath 5: 13-21.

35. Schulz KF, Altman DG, Moher D; CONSORT Group (2010) CONSORT 2010 statement: updated guidelines for reporting parallel group randomized trials. Ann Intern Med 152: 726-732.

36. Moher D, Schulz KF, Altman DG; CONSORT GROUP (Consolidated Standards of Reporting Trials) (2001) The CONSORT statement: revised recommendations for improving the quality of reports of parallel-group randomized trials. Ann Intern Med 134: 657-662.

37. Davidson KW, Goldstein M, Kaplan RM, Kaufmann PG, Knatterud GL, et al. (2003) Evidence-based behavioral medicine: what is it and how do we achieve it? Ann Behav Med 26: 161-171.

38. Perlis, M., M. Aloia, and B. Kuhn, Behavioral Treatments for Sleep Disorders: A Comprehensive Primer of Behavioral Sleep Medicine Interventions. 2010, San Diego, CA: Academic Press.

39. Von Korff M, Moore JE, Lorig K, Cherkin DC, Saunders K, et al. (1998) A randomized trial of a lay person-led self-management group intervention for back pain patients in primary care. Spine (Phila Pa 1976) 23: 2608-2615.

40. Bandura, A., Social foundations of thought and action. A social cogntive theory. 1986, Englewood Cliffs, NJ: Prentice Hall.

41. Bandura, A., Self-Efficacy: The Exercise of Control. 1997, New York, NY: W.H. Freeman and Company.

42. Bandura, A., Social cognitive theory and exercise of control over HIV infection. Preventing AIDS: theories and methods of behavioral interventions, ed. R.J. DiClemente and J.L. Peterson. 1994, New York, NY: Plenum Press. 25-59.

43. Dobson, K.S. and D.J.A. Dozois, Historical and Philosophical Bases of the Cognitive- Behavioral Therapies, in Handbook of Cognitive Behavioral Therapies, K.S. Dobson, Editor. 2001, Guilford Press: New York, NY. p. 3-39.

44. Prochaska JO, DiClemente CC (1983) Stages and processes of self-change of smoking: toward an integrative model of change. J Consult Clin Psychol 51: 390-395.

45. Prochaska JO, Velicer WF, Rossi JS, Goldstein MG, Marcus BH, et al. (1994) Stages of change and decisional balance for 12 problem behaviors. Health Psychol 13: 39-46.

46. Becker, M., The health belief model and sick role behavior. Health Education Monographs, 1974. 2: p. 409-419.

47. Quine L, Rutter DR, Arnold L (2001) Persuading school-age cyclists to use safety helmets: Effectiveness of an intervention based on the Theory of Planned Behaviour. Br J Health Psychol 6: 327-345.

48. Connor, M. and P. Norman, Predicting health behavior: Research and practice with social cognition models. 1996, Buckingham: Open University Press.

49. Clark, N. and M. Becker, Theoretical models and strategies for improving adherence and disease management. 2nd ed. The handbook of health behavior change, ed. S. Shumaker, et al. 1998, New York: Springer Publishing Company.

50. Juniper KC, Oman RF, Hamm RM, Kerby DS (2004) The relationships among constructs in the health belief model and the transtheoretical model among African-American college women for physical activity. Am J Health Promot 18: 354-357.

51. Sage, C., A. Southcott, and S. Brown, The Health Belief Model and compliance with CPAP treatment for obstructive sleep apnoea. Behavior Change, 2001. 18(3): p. 177-185.

52. Schwarzer, R. and R. Fuchs, Self-Efficacy and Health Behaviours, in Predicting Health Behaviour: Research and Practice with Social Cognition Models, M. Conner and P. Norman, Editors. 1996, Open University Press: Philadelphia, PA. p. 163-196.

53. Weaver TE, Maislin G, Dinges DF, Younger J, Cantor C, et al. (2003) Self-efficacy in sleep apnea: instrument development and patient perceptions of obstructive sleep apnea risk, treatment benefit, and volition to use continuous positive airway pressure. Sleep 26: 727-732.

54. Triandis, H., Interpersonal behavior. 1977, Monterrey, CA: Brooks/Cole.

55. Murray, K. and G. Haubl, Explaining cognitive lock-in: the role of skill- based habits. J Consum Res, 2007. 24.

56. Lauver D (1992) A theory of care-seeking behavior. Image J Nurs Sch 24: 281-287.

57. Fletcher EC, Luckett RA (1991) The effect of positive reinforcement on hourly compliance in nasal continuous positive airway pressure users with obstructive sleep apnea. Am Rev Respir Dis 143: 936-941.

58. Chervin RD, Theut S, Bassetti C, Aldrich MS (1997) Compliance with nasal CPAP can be improved by simple interventions. Sleep 20: 284-289.

59. Likar LL, Panciera TM, Erickson AD, Rounds S (1997) Group education sessions and compliance with nasal CPAP therapy. Chest 111: 1273-1277.

60. Hoy CJ, Vennelle M, Kingshott RN, Engleman HM, Douglas NJ (1999) Can intensive support improve continuous positive airway pressure use in patients with the sleep apnea/hypopnea syndrome? Am J Respir Crit Care Med 159: 1096-1100.

61. Hui DS, Chan JK, Choy DK, Ko FW, Li TS, et al. (2000) Effects of augmented continuous positive airway pressure education and support on compliance and outcome in a Chinese population. Chest 117: 1410-1416.

62. Koontz KL, Slifer KJ, Cataldo MD, Marcus CL (2003) Improving pediatric compliance with positive airway pressure therapy: the impact of behavioral intervention. Sleep 26: 1010-1015.

63. DeMolles DA, Sparrow D, Gottlieb DJ, Friedman R (2004) A pilot trial of a telecommunications system in sleep apnea management. Med Care 42: 764-769.

64. Palmer S, Selvaraj S, Dunn C, Osman LM, Cairns J, et al. (2004) Annual review of patients with sleep apnea/hypopnea syndrome--a pragmatic randomised trial of nurse home visit versus consultant clinic review. Sleep Med 5: 61-65.

65. Smith SS, Lang CP, Sullivan KA, Warren J (2004) A preliminary investigation of the effectiveness of a sleep apnea education program. J Psychosom Res 56: 245-249.

66. Jean Wiese H, Boethel C, Phillips B, Wilson JF, Peters J, et al. (2005) CPAP compliance: video education may help! Sleep Med 6: 171-174.

67. Golay A, Girard A, Grandin S, Métrailler JC, Victorion M, et al. (2006) A new educational program for patients suffering from sleep apnea syndrome. Patient Educ Couns 60: 220-227.

68. Lewis KE, Bartle IE, Watkins AJ, Seale L, Ebden P (2006) Simple interventions

improve re-attendance when treating the sleep apnoea syndrome. Sleep Med 7: 241-247.

69. Smith CE, Dauz ER, Clements F, Puno FN, Cook D, et al. (2006) Telehealth services to improve nonadherence: A placebo-controlled study. Telemed J E Health 12: 289-296.

70. Taylor Y, Eliasson A, Andrada T, Kristo D, Howard R (2006) The role of telemedicine in CPAP compliance for patients with obstructive sleep apnea syndrome. Sleep Breath 10: 132-138.

71. Ballard RD, Gay PC, Strollo PJ (2007) Interventions to improve compliance in sleep apnea patients previously non-compliant with continuous positive airway pressure. J Clin Sleep Med 3: 706-712.

72. Means MK, Edinger JD (2007) Graded exposure therapy for addressing claustrophobic reactions to continuous positive airway pressure: a case series report. Behav Sleep Med 5: 105-116.

73. Meurice JC, Ingrand P, Portier F, Arnulf I, Rakotonanahari D, et al. (2007) A multicentre trial of education strategies at CPAP induction in the treatment of severe sleep apnoea-hypopnoea syndrome. Sleep Med 8: 37-42.

74. Richards D, Bartlett DJ, Wong K, Malouff J, Grunstein RR (2007) Increased adherence to CPAP with a group cognitive behavioral treatment intervention: a randomized trial. Sleep 30: 635-640.

75. Slifer KJ, Kruglak D, Benore E, Bellipanni K, Falk L, et al. (2007) Behavioral training for increasing preschool children's adherence with positive airway pressure: a preliminary study. Behav Sleep Med 5: 147-175.

76. Stepnowsky CJ, Palau JJ, Marler MR, Gifford AL (2007) Pilot randomized trial of the effect of wireless telemonitoring on compliance and treatment efficacy in obstructive sleep apnea. J Med Internet Res 9: e14.

77. Stepnowsky CJ, Palau JJ, Gifford AL, Ancoli-Israel S (2007) A self-management approach to improving continuous positive airway pressure adherence and outcomes. Behav Sleep Med 5: 131-146.

78. Smith CE, Dauz E, Clements F, Werkowitch M, Whitman R (2009) Patient education combined in a music and habit-forming intervention for adherence to continuous positive airway (CPAP) prescribed for sleep apnea. Patient Educ Couns 74: 184-190.

79. Damjanovic D, Fluck A, Bremer H, Müller-Quernheim J, Idzko M, et al. (2009) Compliance in sleep apnoea therapy: influence of home care support and pressure mode. Eur Respir J 33: 804-811.

80. Fuchs, F.S., A. Pittarelli, E.G. Hahn, and J.H. Ficker, Adherence to continuous positive airway pressure therapy for obstructive sleep apnea: impact of patient education after a longer treatment period. Respiration, 2010. 80(1): p. 32-7.

81. Roecklein KA, Schumacher JA, Gabriele JM, Fagan C, Baran AS, et al. (2010) Personalized feedback to improve CPAP adherence in obstructive sleep apnea. Behav Sleep Med 8: 105-112.

82. Sparrow D, Aloia M, Demolles DA, Gottlieb DJ (2010) A telemedicine intervention to improve adherence to continuous positive airway pressure: a randomised controlled trial. Thorax 65: 1061-1066.

83. Trupp RJ, Corwin EJ, Ahijevych KL, Nygren T (2011) The impact of educational message framing on adherence to continuous positive airway pressure therapy. Behav Sleep Med 9: 38-52.

Morbidity and Predicted Mortality in Older Adults with Central Sleep Apnea

Saban-Hakki Onen [1,2]*, Virgine Dauphinot[3], Nalaka S Gooneratne[4,5], Ghislaine Watchueng[1], Jian-Sheng Lin[2] and Fannie Onen[6,7]

[1]Hospices Civils de Lyon, Hôpital Antoine Charial, Centre Gériatrique de Médecine du Sommeil, F-69340 Francheville, France
[2]Inserm U1028, Université Lyon1, F-69373 Lyon Cedex 08, France
[3]Hospices Civils de Lyon, CMRR Biostatistiques, Hôpital des Charpennes, F-69100 Villeurbanne, France
[4]Center for Sleep and Circadian Neurobiology and Division of Sleep Medicine, School of Medicine, University of Pennsylvania, Philadelphia, PA, USA
[5]Division of Geriatric Medicine, School of Medicine, University of Pennsylvania, Philadelphia, PA, USA
[6]CHU Bichat Claude Bernard, APHP, Service de Gériatrie, F-75018 Paris, France
[7]INSERM U669, Université Paris Descartes, 75014 Paris, France

Abstract

Objectives: To assess cardiovascular morbidity and prognostic mortality risk in older patients with CSA in comparison to those with OSA and without any SDB (apnea-hypopnea index <15/hour).

Background: Sleep-Disordered Breathing (SDB), including both Central Sleep Apnea (CSA) and Obstructive Sleep Apnea (OSA), is a prevalent condition in older adults. In contrast to OSA, the information concerning the morbidity and mortality associated with CSA is scarce and inconsistent.

Methods: We analyzed a prospectively collected database of consecutive patients aged 70 and over referred for suspicion of SDB. All patients underwent an overnight polysomnography and a clinical assessment. Cardiovascular morbidities and prognostic index for 4-year mortality (PIM) were abstracted from patient records.

Results: The data derived from 207 patients (79.7 ± 5.7 years) was divided into three groups according to the apnea classification (20 CSA, 121 OSA, and 66 no-SDB). Stroke (7/20, p= 0.02) and hypertension (19/20, p=0.003) were more frequent in CSA patients than OSA and no-SDB patients. The mean PIM score of patients with CSA (10.7 ± 3.3) was higher than those with OSA (7.8 ± 3.1) and no-SDB (8.4 ± 2.9), even after adjustment for potential confounders including gender and SpO_2 (p <0.001).

Conclusion: CSA is associated with stroke and hypertension and an increased prognostic mortality risk compared to OSA and no-SDB in older patients. The knowledge of morbidities and mortality risk associated with CSA may help in planning preventive and therapeutic strategies to improve patients' global health status and quality of life.

Keywords: Central sleep apnea; Obstructive sleeps apnea; Sleep-disordered breathing; Mortality; Older adult

Brief Summary

Current knowledge/study rationale

Sleep-Disordered Breathing (SDB) in general and Central Sleep Apnea (CSA) in particular are known to increase with advancing age. The information concerning the morbidity and mortality associated with CSA in older populations is scarce and inconsistent. It is not known if CSA-related mortality is greater than Obstructive Sleep Apnea (OSA) related mortality in the elderly.

Study impact

Our study using a prognostic mortality risk index demonstrates that CSA diagnosed by full polysomnography is a major and independent risk factor for mortality in older adults. Untreated CSA compared with OSA is also significantly associated with stroke and hypertension.

Introduction

The prevalence of Sleep-Disordered Breathing (SDB), defined as an Apnea-Hypopnea index (AHI) of 15 or greater, is 23% in the community-dwelling older over the age of 70 [1]. Central Sleep Apnea (CSA), a form of SDB, can affect more than one third of these elderly patients with SDB [1]. The prevalence, severity and costs of CSA will likely escalate as the older adult population increases in number and lives longer.

CSA is characterized on the polysomnogram by recurrent cessation of respiration during sleep with no associated ventilatory effort. In contrast obstructive sleep apnea (OSA) is defined as repetitive episodes of upper airway obstruction with ongoing respiratory efforts [2]. In OSA patients the repetitive upper airway collapse occurs during sleep because negative pressure generated during inspiration is not effectively counteracted by splinting by pharyngeal dilators, especially when narrowing occurs as a result of excessive soft tissue (e.g. obesity, loss of soft tissue elasticity related to age) or vulnerable craniofacial anatomy (e.g. edentulous older adults). In both cases, the Continuous Positive Airway Pressure (CPAP) is the most widely used treatment even in older adults. Furthermore, bilevel positive airway pressure (BiPAP) in a spontaneous-timed mode and Adaptive Servo-Ventilation (ASV) which generates positive airway pressure with variable pressure in response to a patient's expiration are increasingly recommended in order to ameliorate central respiratory events related to chronic heart failure.

***Corresponding author:** Dr Saban-Hakki ONEN, Hôpital Antoine Charial 40, avenue de la Table Pierre 69340, FRANCHEVILLE - FRANCE
E-mail: saban-hakki.onen@chu-lyon.fr

There is a limited body of information concerning the morbidity and mortality associated with CSA in older populations. In previous cohort studies concerning older patients, chronic heart failure is mentioned as the most common comorbid condition, yet the specific mortality rate associated with untreated CSA or untreated OSA is not well understood [3,4]. Since there is a high prevalence of CSA in the elderly, we can expect that CSA may increase the risk of both cardiovascular morbidity (not only chronic heart failure) and mortality risk in that age group.

We hypothesized that in older patients, CSA is associated with increased cardiovascular morbidity and mortality risk when compared to OSA and no-SDB, independent of potential confounders. To address this hypothesis, we conducted a cross-sectional study in 207 consecutive older adult patients seen in our geriatric sleep disorders center that underwent an in-hospital polysomnography and clinical assessment.

Materials and Methods

Study design and patient population

This is a cross-sectional, observational study using a Lyon University Hospital, Geriatric Sleep Center (Lyon, France) clinic population. Following approval from the Local Ethics Committee, a review of the medical records was performed.

Consecutive patients referred to our sleep center and who met our inclusion criteria (see below) during a three year period were enrolled. Patients were all referred by geriatricians or family physicians because of suspected SDB (either OSA or CSA) with symptoms of snoring, witnessed apneas, excessive daytime sleepiness, or obesity.

Inclusion criteria were: (1) Caucasian men or women (the study sample was limited to Caucasian patients as the prevalence of non-Caucasian patients in our clinic was too low to allow for meaningful subgroup analyses by race/ethnicity), (2) age 70 years and over, (3) hospital based complete polysomnography, (4) extensive geriatric assessment including an evaluation of medical history and comorbid conditions, and (5) stable clinical situation with no medication adjustment for at least 2 weeks prior to the polysomnography.

The exclusion criteria were: (1) acute heart failure, (2) acute respiratory failure, (3) previously diagnosed SDB, (4) currently on CPAP treatment or nocturnal oxygen supplementation.

Polysomnography

Each polysomnography included at least the following recordings: three channel electroencephalography, chin electromyography, bilateral electro-oculography, chest and abdomen respiratory effort, nasal and oral airflow via a thermocouple, snoring, pulse oximetry, ECG and body position. Sleep staging and arousals were scored using standard methods [5].

Apneas were defined as the complete cessation of airflow for at least 10 seconds.

Hypopnoeas were defined as an airflow amplitude reduction of >50% from baseline lasting at least 10 seconds, accompanied by the presence of arousal or oxygen desaturation of at least 4% [6].

Apneas were classified as obstructive if they were associated with continued chest or abdominal movement, or central if there was a cessation of chest and abdominal movement. In addition, mixed apneas were identified if both central and obstructive components were present. The AHI was defined as the total number of apnea and/or hypopnea episodes divided by the number of hours of sleep.

The diagnosis of both CSA and OSA required an AHI of 15 or more events per hour [2]. Patients with AHI<15 were classified as no-SDB. Patients were considered to have CSA or OSA if more than 50 percent of the events determined were central or obstructive events, respectively [7].

Assessment of mortality risk

The potential mortality risk was assessed using the Prognostic Index for 4-year Mortality validated in older adults [8]. An intake form was used to collect information in patient files. The index is composed of 12 independent predictors of mortality: 2 demographic variables (age: 60-64 years, 1 point; 65-69 years, 2 points; 70-74 years, 3 points; 75-79 years, 4 points; 80-84 years, 5 points; ≥ 85 years, 7 points and male sex, 2 points), 6 comorbid conditions (diabetes, 1 point; cancer, 2 points; lung disease, 2 points; heart failure, 2 points; current tobacco use, 2 points; and BMI <25, 1 point), and difficulty with 4 functional variables (bathing, 2 points; walking several blocks, 2 points; managing money, 2 points, and pushing large objects, 1 point). The prognostic index total scores range from 0 (lowest risk) to 26 (highest risk). This prognostic index, incorporating age, sex, self-reported comorbid conditions, and functional measures, accurately stratified community-dwelling older adults into groups at varying risk of mortality: 0 to 5 points predicted a less than 4% risk, 6 to 9 points predicted a 15% risk, 10 to 13 points predicted a 42% risk, and 14 or more points predicted a 64% risk [8].

Abstraction of clinical data

Data on the demographic characteristics, body mass index (BMI, kg/m^2), medical history and cardiovascular comorbidities were extracted from standard medical records at the time of polysomnography. Major sedative drug (e.g. opioid pain relief drugs, sodium oxybate) consumption was checked. In addition, each patient's 4-year prognostic mortality index was calculated based on information available at the time of polysomnography.

Medical history chart abstraction was performed using the following standardized algorithm. Hypertension was defined as a documented diagnosis, treatment of such, or whether the recorded resting blood pressure was ≥ 140/90 mmHg three times in the previous month. Stroke and Transient Ischemic Attack (TIA) were defined as a documented history of stroke or TIA. Ischemic heart disease was defined as a documented history of angina pectoris and/or myocardial infarction and/or coronary angioplasty and/or coronary artery bypass surgery. Atrial Fibrillation (AF) was defined as a documented history of permanent, paroxysmal or persistent AF (at least 2 episodes in the previous 3 months). The diagnosis of chronic heart failure was based on a history of dyspnea and symptomatic exercise intolerance with signs of pulmonary congestion or peripheral edema or documentation of left ventricular enlargement or dysfunction by chest x-ray film, echocardiography, or radionuclide ventriculography. Diabetes mellitus diagnosis was based on a history of diabetes, current treatment (oral therapy and/or insulin) or a fasting glucose value ≥ 7 mmol/l.

Statistical analysis

Descriptive characteristics and polysomnography measures were compared between patients with CSA, OSA and those without sleep apnea (no-SDB). Means were compared using analyze of variance (ANOVA); the difference in the proportions was tested using the Chi-squared test. The 4-year mortality risk index was compared according to the sleep apnea status using univariate and multivariate ANOVA.

Multiple pairwise comparisons were performed using Scheffe's test, to compare each group with every other one to determine which group differed significantly. Potential confounding covariates were tested in the model: gender, BMI, AHI, SpO_2<90%, hypertension and stroke. Means with their 95% confident intervals (CI), p value of the ANOVA F test and p value of the Sheffe's tests are presented. A p value <0.05 was considered as significant. Statistical analyses were performed with SPSS version 15.0 for Windows (SPSS Software, Chicago, USA).

Results

The study population included 207 patients, grouped by diagnostic status as follows: 20 patients with CSA, 121 patients with OSA, and 66 patients with no-SDB.

Characteristics of the study sample are presented in Table 1. The mean age was 79.7 ± 5.7 years, and there was no significant difference between groups. Patients with CSA had significantly higher proportions of men (90%), stroke or TIA (35%), and hypertension (95%) compared to patients with no SDB (38%, 9% and 56% respectively). BMI was higher among patients with OSA compared to those with no-SDB. No significant differences were observed for age, ischemic heart disease, AF, diabetes mellitus and CHF. In all groups, no patient was identified using chronically or during sleep study opioid pain relief drugs and sodium oxybate which both may contribute to the depression of respiratory drive (Table 1).

Between CSA and OSA patients, no significant differences were noted concerning total AHI, mixed apnea index, hypopnea index, mean SpO_2, lowest SpO_2, and sleep time with SpO_2<90% (Table 2).

Table 3 presents 4-year mortality index univariate and stepwise multivariate analysis. The mean 4-year mortality index was significantly higher among patients with CSA compared to patients with OSA or no SDB (12.0 ± 3.5; 8.1 ± 3.1; 7.1 ± 2.9 respectively; p<0.001). The results remained significant after controlling for gender and SpO_2<90% (p<0.001); no other variables were significant covariates in the multivariate model. There was a trend toward a higher mean of 4-year mortality index among patients with CSA compared to patients with OSA, but the difference did not reach statistical significance.

Discussion

This study highlights two main findings in an older population referred for investigation of SDB. First, patients with CSA had significantly higher proportions of stroke and hypertension compared to patients with no-SDB. Second, there was an association between the CSA and increased prognostic mortality index values. This association remained significant after adjustment for clinical parameters known to affect survival prognosis.

Variables	No-SDB (n=66)	OSA (n=121)	CSA (n=20)	*p* Value
Age, year	79.1 ± 6.0	79.9 ± 4.7	80.7 ± 5.4	0.42
Male gender	25 (38%)	69 (57%)	18 (90%)¶	<0.001
BMI, kg/m²	27.0 ± 5.5	30.8 ± 6.3†	28.5 ± 4.7	<0.001
Stroke or TIA	6 (9%)	23 (19%)	7 (35%)§	0.02
Ischemic Hearth D.	12 (18%)	26 (21%)	6 (30%)	0.52
Atrial fibrillation	7 (11%)	20 (17%)	6 (30%)	0.11
Diabetes mellitus	8 (12%)	29 (24%)	5 (25%)	0.13
CHF	6 (9%)	16 (13%)	6 (30%)	0.06
Hypertension	37 (56%)	87 (72%)	19 (95%)*	0.003

Values are expressed as means ± SD or No. (%) unless otherwise stated. No-SDB, subjects without sleep disordered breathing. CSA, subjects with central sleep apnea. OSA, subjects with obstructive sleep apnea. BMI, body mass index. TIA transient ischemic attack, CHF chronic heart failure.
¶p < 0.001 (No-SDB subjects vs. patients with CSA)
†p < 0.001 (No-SDB subjects vs. patients with OSA)
§p = 0.02 (No-SDB subjects vs. patients with CSA)
*p = 0.003 (No-SDB subjects vs. patients with CSA)

Table 1: Clinical characteristics and cardiovascular comorbidities.

Variables	No-SDB (n=66)	OSA (n=121)	CSA (n=20)	*p* Value
Total AHI, No./h	7.6 ± 4.1	42.9 ± 19.6†	47.1 ± 16.6†	<0.001
CSA index, No./h	0.8 ± 1.5	3.3 ± 4.7	25.4 ± 13.6‡	<0.001
OSA index, No./h	2.6 ± 2.5	26.2 ± 17.4§	7.0 ± 5.8	<0.001
MSA index, No./h	0.1 ± 0.4	3.5 ± 6.9†	6.1 ± 6.1†	<0.001
H index, No./h	4.1 ± 3.3	9.9 ± 8.7†	8.5 ± 5.4	<0.001
Mean SpO_2, %	93.4 ± 2.3	92.3 ± 3.2¶	92.5 ± 2.1	0.03
Lowest SpO_2, %	81.9 ± 8.5	72.6 ± 11.5*	75.2 ± 7.8**	<0.001
Time with SpO_2<90%, %	9.1 ± 18.1	17.5 ± 21.3	20.4 ± 17.1***	0.01

Values are expressed as means SD unless otherwise stated.
AHI, apnea hypopnea index. CSA, central sleep apnea. OSA, obstructive sleep apnea. MSA, mixed sleep apnea. H, hypopnea. See Table 1 for abbreviation not used in the text.
†p < 0.001 (patients with OSA or CSA vs subjects with no-SDB)
‡p < 0.001 (patients with CSA vs patients with OSA or no-SDB)
§p < 0.001 (patients with OSA vs patients with CSA or no-SDB)
¶p = 0.03 (patients with OSA vs subjects with no-SDB)
*p < 0.001 (patients with OSA vs subjects with no-SDB)
**p = 0.04 (patients with CSA vs subjects with no-SDB)
***p = 0.02 (patients with CSA vs subjects with no-SDB)

Table 2: Polysomnography Measures.

Mortality Index	No-SDB (n=66)	OSA (n=121)	CSA (n=20)	*p* Value	*p* value No-SDB vs CSA	*p* value No-SDB vs OSA	*p* value CSA vs OSA
Univariate*	7.1 ± 2.9	8.1 ± 3.1	12.0 ± 3.5	<0.001	<0.001	0.1	<0.001
Multivariate†	7.9 ± 2.8	7.9 ± 3.1	10.8 ± 3.3	<0.001	<0.001	0.1	<0.001

*Univariate model for mortality index; R^2=9 %. †Stepwise multivariate model adjusted for gender (p<0.001), and SpO_2 <90% (p<0.001). The other variables (BMI, AHI, hypertension and stroke) were tested in the model and were not significant. The mean age was not significantly different between groups (Table 1), so age was not included in different models. The multivariate analysis contributed significantly to the explanation of the model; R^2=35%.

Table 3: Four-year mortality index univariate and stepwise multivariate analysis in patients with central sleep apnea (CSA), obstructive sleep apnea (OSA) and free of sleep apnea syndrome (no-SDB).

Cardiovascular morbidity

From a pathophysiological point of view, both ventilatory instability and depression of the brainstem respiratory centers may cause central sleep apnea. The ventilatory system is at particular risk of instability when the resting $PaCO_2$ approaches the $PaCO_2$ apneic threshold. In other words, reduction of $PaCO_2$ just a few mm Hg below the $PaCO_2$ set point can result in central apneas. Some other additional factors, such as metabolic alkalosis, low functional residual capacity, upper airway instability, and hypoxia, may further contribute to respiratory instability and CSA [9]. Post-hypocapnia hyperventilation is believed to be the main underlying pathophysiological mechanism for CSA associated with congestive heart failure. CSA associated with long-acting opioid drug use for at least two months [10] or brainstem lesions such as stroke are due to depression of the brainstem respiratory centers or disturbances of peripheral chemoreceptors or both.

We did not observe chronic opioid drug use in our population; however CSA was significantly associated with stroke. According to Bassetti et al. [11] SDB is common particularly in elderly stroke male patients with diabetes, but the authors did not discuss if there was a specific association between CSA and stroke. In a cohort study, among 132 patients who recently had stroke, Sahlin et al. [12] found that 23

OSA patients were at a greater risk of early death, while the 28 with CSA did not have an increased mortality risk. The risk of death was independent of age, sex, BMI, hypertension, diabetes mellitus and AF. In this cohort, the prevalence of CSA was greater than the prevalence of OSA.

CSA was associated with hypertension in our study as well. This may be due to increased sympathetic activity from recurrent apneas and hypoxia, similar to what is seen in obstructive sleep apnea. Of note, other research has shown a limited association between SDB and hypertension in older adults [13].

Depending on the population studied, OSA and/or CSA occur in 24% to 82% of heart failure patients [14]. In our study, the association between CHF, OSA and CSA did not reach statistical significance, although it showed a trend towards significance (p=0.06). This finding may be explained by the clinically stable nature of the study patient population, possible unrecognized heart failure or the old age of our sample with possible survival bias. Although CSA is probably a consequence of heart failure, once established it may play an important role in heart failure progression, morbidity, and mortality [15]. As yet, however, causality has not been proven [16].

Our findings were also consistent with previously published work which shows an association between SDB and conditions such as diabetes [17] and atrial fibrillation [18,19].

Mortality

The present study demonstrates that in older adults, CSA is associated with an increased risk of mortality based on a prognostic mortality index scale. This mortality index risk is independent of common confounding factors, such as gender and SpO_2. Our results confirm and extend findings from previous studies performed in younger populations, or samples that may be biased because of CPAP treatment. Of note, the prognostic mortality index is greater in CSA patients compared to OSA or no-SDB patients. According to Lee et al. [8], mortality index scores around 8, similar to those observed in no-SDB and OSA patients are associated with a 15% 4-year mortality risk, and scores around 11 as observed in CSA patients are associated with a 42% mortality risk.

In studies focused on younger adults, CSA has been associated with increased mortality [20,21]. Later research noted that older patients with CSA plus congestive heart failure have a mortality rate greater than those with just congestive heart failure, or CSA or OSA alone [4]. However, investigators of this cohort were not able to determine precisely if any of the patients received oxygen supplementation or CPAP treatment during the 17-year follow up period. Using CPAP to treat OSA in patients with chronic heart failure may also alleviate the heart disease and possibly lengthen survival.

In contrast, other cohort studies, after controlling for common confounding factors in younger patients with CSA and congestive heart failure [22] or CSA and stroke [12] did not observe higher mortality rates in comparison to those with no-SDB. However, in latter cohorts followed for up to 10 years, some CSA patients continued with CPAP therapy at home for up to five years.

Strengths and limitations

The strengths of our study include the availability of hospital-based full polysomnography data, which is the "gold standard" for SDB diagnosis. Previous cohort studies using cardiorespiratory polygraphy to distinguish between OSA and CSA may lead to some inaccuracy and may underestimate the sleep apnea severity due to their inability to distinguish wake from sleep [23].

Our patients were old "old adults" with a mean age of about 80 years. These patients are, on average, about 11 to 14 years older than those in previous studies [3,4]. Some limitations have to be mentioned as well. Patients with unstable clinical conditions were not included. In other words, our sleep center did not recruit patients with acute heart failure or acute ischemic heart disease and, therefore, cannot exclude CSA associated with these comorbid conditions and related mortality. According to Johanson et al. [24], OSA, in persons >75 years does not appear to be associated with cardiovascular disease (CVD) disease or mortality, whereas CSA might be a pathological marker of CVD and impaired systolic function associated with higher mortality. In this cohort of 331 community-dwelling elderly underwent a one-night cardiorespiratory polygraphy (without EEG) and followed-up 7 years, authors did not mention if OSA and CSA patients were treated with CPAP, BiPAP or ASV. The cross-sectional nature of our study precludes inferences about causality between CSA and comorbid conditions. Although our overall sample was large, categorization of CSA, OSA and no-SDB resulted in small groups of CSA, OSA and no-SDB that limited statistical power to determine potential group-related differences in comorbid conditions. Mortality itself was not directly assessed, and was determined instead as a prognostic mortality risk. However, this prediction calculation of the mortality risk [8] has been used in over a dozen research publications, including older adults with diabetes mellitus [25] and functional disability [26]. One benefit of this prognostic mortality risk approach is that it minimizes the potential effect of subsequent SDB treatment on overall survival. In contrast most prior cohort studies have not been able to adequately measure SDB treatment during the period of study follow-up. Clearly, CPAP, BiPAP and ASV treatments can have an impact on study outcomes and may lead to an underestimate of both OSA and CSA effects on mortality.

Conclusions

Previous studies assessing mortality in patients with CSA have been controversial and have had important limitations, including the use of cardiopulmonary polygraphy (instead of complete polysomnography) and unmeasured CSA treatment with CPAP or oxygen therapy during the study follow-up period. In our study, CSA compared to OSA and no-SDB was associated with stroke and hypertension. Furthermore, we noted an increased prognostic mortality risk independent of potential confounders. With regard to increased mortality risk the relative number of co-morbid conditions was also higher in CSA patients, than in patients with OSA or no-SDB. Thus, CSA may be both risk factor and consequence of cardiovascular co-morbidities and vulnerability. Future research is necessary to determine if treatment of CSA in the elderly can lead to reduced morbidity and mortality from these conditions.

Acknowledgments

We thank Chantal Langrand, sleep technician, for her careful management of our older patients.

This study was supported by a research grant (HRA-0012011) from the International Association of Sleep Research in Gerontology. The funding source had no role in the design or conduct of the study, data management or analysis, or manuscript preparation or review.

References

1. Johansson P, Alehagen U, Svanborg E, Dahlström U, Broström A (2009) Sleep disordered breathing in an elderly community-living population: Relationship to

cardiac function, insomnia symptoms and daytime sleepiness. Sleep Med 10: 1005-1011.

2. AASM (American Academy of Sleep Medicine), International Classification of Sleep Disorders, second ed.: Diagnostic and Coding Manual. American Academy of Sleep Medicine, Darien, IL 2005.
3. Bliwise DL, Bliwise NG, Partinen M, Pursley AM, Dement WC (1988) Sleep apnea and mortality in an aged cohort. Am J Public Health 78: 544-547.
4. Ancoli-Israel S, DuHamel ER, Stepnowsky C, Engler R, Cohen-Zion M, et al. (2003) The relationship between congestive heart failure, sleep apnea, and mortality in older men. Chest 124: 1400-1405.
5. Iber C, Ancoli-Israel S, Chesson A, Quan SF (2007) The AASM manual for the scoring of sleep and associated events: rules, terminology, and technical specification, first ed. American Academy of Sleep Medicine, Westchester, IL.
6. (1999) Sleep-related breathing disorders in adults: recommendations for syndrome definition and measurement techniques in clinical research. The Report of an American Academy of Sleep Medicine Task Force. Sleep 22: 667-689.
7. Bradley TD, Logan AG, Kimoff RJ, Sériès F, Morrison D, et al. (2005) Continuous positive airway pressure for central sleep apnea and heart failure. N Engl J Med 353: 2025-2033.
8. Lee SJ, Lindquist K, Segal MR, Covinsky KE (2006) Development and validation of a prognostic index for 4-year mortality in older adults. JAMA 295: 801-808.
9. Bradley TD (2002) Crossing the threshold: implications for central sleep apnea. Am J Respir Crit Care Med 165: 1203-1204.
10. Alattar MA, Scharf SM (2009) Opioid-associated central sleep apnea: a case series. Sleep Breath 13: 201-206.
11. Bassetti CL, Milanova M, Gugger M (2006) Sleep-disordered breathing and acute ischemic stroke: diagnosis, risk factors, treatment, evolution, and long-term clinical outcome. Stroke 37: 967-972.
12. Sahlin C, Sandberg O, Gustafson Y, Bucht G, Carlberg B, et al. (2008) Obstructive sleep apnea is a risk factor for death in patients with stroke: a 10-year follow-up. Arch Intern Med 168: 297-301.
13. Fletcher EC (2003) Sympathetic over activity in the etiology of hypertension of obstructive sleep apnea. Sleep 26: 15-19.
14. Javaheri S, Parker TJ, Liming JD, Corbett WS, Nishiyama H, et al. (1998) Sleep apnea in 81 ambulatory male patients with stable heart failure. Types and their prevalences, consequences, and presentations. Circulation 97: 2154-2159.
15. Garcia-Touchard A, Somers VK, Olson LJ, Caples SM (2008) Central sleep apnea: implications for congestive heart failure. Chest 133: 1495-1504.
16. Roebuck T, Solin P, Kaye DM, Bergin P, Bailey M, et al. (2004) Increased long-term mortality in heart failure due to sleep apnoea is not yet proven. Eur Respir J 23: 735-740.
17. Basoglu OK, Sarac F, Sarac S, Uluer H, Yilmaz C (2011) Metabolic syndrome, insulin resistance, fibrinogen, homocysteine, leptin, and C-reactive protein in obese patients with obstructive sleep apnea syndrome. Ann Thorac Med 6: 120-125.
18. Leung RS, Huber MA, Rogge T, Maimon N, Chiu KL, et al. (2005) Association between atrial fibrillation and central sleep apnea. Sleep 28: 1543-1546.
19. Mehra R, Stone KL, Varosy PD, Hoffman AR, Marcus GM, et al. (2009) Nocturnal Arrhythmias across a spectrum of obstructive and central sleep-disordered breathing in older men: outcomes of sleep disorders in older men (MrOS sleep) study. Arch Intern Med 169: 1147-1155.
20. Findley LJ, Zwillich CW, Ancoli-Israel S, Kripke D, Tisi G, et al. (1985) Cheyne-Stokes breathing during sleep in patients with left ventricular heart failure. South Med J 78: 11-15.
21. Hanly PJ, Zuberi-Khokhar NS (1996) Increased mortality associated with Cheyne-Stokes respiration in patients with congestive heart failure. Am J Respir Crit Care Med 153: 272-276.
22. Luo Q, Zhang HL, Tao XC, Zhao ZH, Yang YJ, et al. (2010) Impact of untreated sleep apnea on prognosis of patients with congestive heart failure. Int J Cardiol 144: 420-422.
23. Chesson AL Jr, Berry RB, Pack A; American Academy of Sleep Medicine; American Thoracic Society; American College of Chest Physicians (2003) Practice parameters for the use of portable monitoring devices in the investigation of suspected obstructive sleep apnea in adults. Sleep 26: 907-913.
24. Johansson P, Alehagen U, Svanborg E, Dahlström U, Broström A (2012) Clinical characteristics and mortality risk in relation to obstructive and central sleep apnoea in community-dwelling elderly individuals: a 7-year follow-up. Age Ageing 41: 468-474.
25. Brown SE, Meltzer DO, Chin MH, Huang ES (2008) Perceptions of quality-of-life effects of treatments for diabetes mellitus in vulnerable and nonvulnerable older patients. J Am Geriatr Soc 56: 1183-1190.
26. Gitlin LN, Hauck WW, Dennis MP, Winter L, Hodgson N, et al. (2009) Long-term effect on mortality of a home intervention that reduces functional difficulties in older adults: results from a randomized trial. J Am Geriatr Soc 57: 476-481.

Tai Chi Improves Sleep Quality in Healthy Adults and Patients with Chronic Conditions

Gowri Raman[1], Yuan Zhang[2], Vincent J Minichiello[3], Carolyn D'Ambrosio[4] and Chenchen Wang[5]*

[1]Center for Clinical Evidence Synthesis, Institute for Clinical Research and Health Policy Studies, Tufts Medical Center, Tufts University School of Medicine, Boston, MA, USA
[2]School of Nursing, University of Massachusetts, Lowell, MA, USA
[3]Department of Family Medicine, University of Wisconsin, Madison, WI, USA
[4]Pulmonary, Critical Care and Sleep Medicine Division, Tufts Medical Center, Tufts University School of Medicine, Boston, MA, USA
[5]Center for Integrative Medicine, Division of Rheumatology, Tufts Medical Center, Tufts University School of Medicine, Boston, MA, USA

Abstract

Background: Physical activity and exercise appear to improve sleep quality. However, the quantitative effects of Tai Chi on sleep quality in the adult population have rarely been examined. We conducted a systematic review and meta-analysis evaluating the effects of Tai Chi on sleep quality in healthy adults and disease populations.

Methods: Medline, Cochrane Central databases, and review of references were searched through July 31, 2013. English-language studies of all designs evaluating Tai Chi's effect on sleep outcomes in adults were examined. Data were extracted and verified by 2 reviewers. Extracted information included study setting and design, population characteristics, type and duration of interventions, outcomes, risk of bias and main results. Random effect models meta-analysis was used to assess the magnitude of treatment effect when at least 3 trials reported on the same sleep outcomes.

Results: Eleven studies (9 randomized and 2 non-randomized trials) totaling 994 subjects published between 2004 and 2012 were identified. All studies except one reported Pittsburg Sleep Quality Index. Nine randomized trials reported that 1.5 to 3 hour each week for a duration of 6 to 24 weeks of Tai Chi significantly improved sleep quality (Effect Size, 0.89; 95% Confidence Interval [CI], 0.28 to 1.50), in community-dwelling healthy participants and in patients with chronic conditions. Improvement in health outcomes including physical performance, pain reduction, and psychological well-being occurred in the Tai Chi group compared with various controls.

Limitations: Studies were heterogeneous and some trials were lacking in methodological rigor.

Conclusions: Tai Chi significantly improved sleep quality in both healthy adults and patients with chronic health conditions, which suggests that Tai Chi may be considered as an alternative behavioral therapy in the treatment of insomnia. High-quality, well-controlled randomized trials are needed to better inform clinical decisions.

Keywords: Tai Chi; Sleep quality; Quality of Life

Introduction

Adequate sleep is critical for optimum human functioning. Insomnia is a common sleep disorder affecting 30% of adults in the United States, with 10% having insomnia severe enough to cause daytime consequences [1]. Considerable evidence suggests that short-term sleep deprivation can negatively impact an individual's alertness, mood, attention, and ability to concentrate, whereas long-term sleep deprivation is associated with chronic fatigue, obesity and diabetes, cardiovascular diseases and increased mortality [2-7]. Recent large-scale cohort studies have established a relationship between sleep deprivation and mortality [7,8]. Poor or deprived sleep can result in increased workplace injuries and accidents, reduced work efficiency, poor employee physical and mental health, and an increased economic loss to the society [9-11]. Each year, insomnia associated with lost productivity in the workplace is estimated to cost 63.2 billion U.S. dollars [1].

Treatment approaches to improve sleep quality include both non-pharmacological strategies, such as modifying the sleep environment and improving sleep hygiene, as well as pharmacological strategies. Recent studies have started to explore the effects of mind-body therapies, such as Tai Chi, in addition to conventional treatment approaches to improve sleep quality in various populations.

Tai Chi originated in China as a martial art, focusing on the mind and body as an interconnected system, on breathing, and on keeping a calm state of mind with a goal toward deep states of relaxation. Recent evidence demonstrates the benefits of Tai Chi in treating chronic pain, psychological health, osteoarthritis, rheumatoid arthritis, Parkinson's disease, cardiovascular health, and overall health related quality of life [12-20]. Tai Chi is becoming increasingly popular in many countries as a form of exercise to promote fitness and well-being. Insomnia may stem from somatized tension or anxiety, and therefore, Tai Chi practice may be a logical therapeutic approach for people seeking to improve their sleep quality. Nevertheless, convincing quantitative evidence to estimate treatment effects has been lacking. No meta-analysis addressing any sleep outcomes with Tai Chi has ever been published. To better inform patients and physicians, we systematically reviewed

***Corresponding author:** Chenchen Wang, Division of Rheumatology, Tufts Medical Center, Box 406, Tufts University School of Medicine Boston, MA 02111, USA
E-mail: cwang2@tuftsmedicalcenter.org

the quantitative relationship between Tai Chi and sleep quality by critically appraising and synthesizing the evidence from published English studies of healthy and chronically ill populations.

Methods

Data sources and study selection

Medline and Cochrane Registry for Clinical Trials were searched until July 31, 2013 using the search terms for Tai Chi ("Tai Chi", "Taijiquan", "T'ai Chi Ch'uan") and search terms for insomnia ("sleep", "insomnia", "Pittsburg Sleep Quality Index-PSQI"). Studies of all designs including Randomized Controlled Trials (RCTs), clinical trials, and observational studies were deemed eligible. Bibliographies of reviews were perused to identify additional articles.

English language studies conducted in adults (≥ 18 years) with or without health problems were selected. Studies that examined any style of Tai Chi as an intervention compared to a control group were eligible. Sleep-related outcomes of interest included global measure and individual components of PSQI. The PSQI was originally designed for use in clinical populations as a simple and valid assessment of both sleep quality and sleep disturbance [21]. The seven components assessed with the PSQI questionnaire include: subjective sleep quality, sleep latency, sleep duration, habitual sleep efficiency, sleep disturbances, use of sleeping medication, and daytime dysfunction. A global PSQI score greater than five has a diagnostic sensitivity of 89.6% and specificity of 86.5% in distinguishing good and poor sleepers [21]. Other outcomes of interest in this review include quality-of-life, cognitive performance, functional mobility, and pain.

Data extraction and study quality assessment

We screened abstracts and further examined full-text articles according to pre-specified eligibility criteria. Extracted data included information on study and participant characteristics, intervention and comparator characteristics (intensity, frequency, duration, and style of Tai Chi practice), follow-up, PSQI outcomes, and other sleep-related outcomes. Data about pain and quality-of-life were also extracted. One reviewer extracted data into structured forms that were reviewed by a second reviewer for completeness and accuracy. Risk of bias was graded using Cochrane Risk of Bias tool [22]. Individual items evaluating risk of bias included: random sequence generation, allocation concealment, blinding of participants and personnel, blinding of outcome assessment, incomplete outcome data, and selective outcome reporting.

Data synthesis and statistical analysis

Quantitative meta-analysis was conducted when at least 3 trials provided comparative data on outcomes of interest. Data were synthesized at the end of the last follow-up. When calculating the standardized Effect Size (ES) for each study, a correlation of 0.50 was used between baseline and final values to account for repeated measurement within each study. The Hedges g value, the bias-corrected standardized mean difference, and the corresponding standard error were computed for each study. In view of significant heterogeneity, random-effect models were used for pooling. The overall mean ES was computed using a random-effects model that assumes the existence of no single true population effect and allows for random between -study variance in addition to sampling variability. The magnitude of the ES (clinical effects) indicates: (0-0.19) = negligible effect, (0.20-0.49) = small effect, (0.50-0.79) = moderate effect, (0.80+) = large effect. Included trials used the difference between the treatment and control group means.

Heterogeneity was estimated with the I^2 statistic and $I^2 > 75\%$ indicates significant heterogeneity.

Statistical heterogeneity was also assessed using the X^2 test. Statistical analyses were conducted using Stata version SE/11.2 (Stata Corp., College Station, TX).

Results

We reviewed 36 English language abstracts and retrieved 13 full-text articles for detailed evaluation (Figure 1). Two of 13 studies were eliminated for not reporting relevant sleep outcome data. Ultimately, 11 studies that included a total of 994 participants were identified for data abstraction and critical appraisal. We did not search for any unpublished and non-English literature.

Table 1 describes the study design and number of studies and participants for sleep outcomes. Of the 11 studies, there were 9 RCTs, 2 non randomized comparative studies published between 2004 and 2012. They were conducted in 5 countries (USA, Spain, Japan, Vietnam, and Iran). Seven studies were conducted in the US. There were 632 healthy individuals (5 studies) and 362 patients with chronic conditions (6 studies) which included fibromyalgia (3 studies), heart failure (1 study), and cerebrovascular disorder (1 study). Mean age ranged from 21 to 77 years, and 58% of participants were female. Various controls were compared among the 9 RCTs, with 4 RCTs having multiple types of controls. Both non randomized comparative studies from the same US investigators used special recreation as controls among college students. Most studies employed subjective sleep measures, including the PSQI Scale and Epworth Sleepiness Scale (ESS). Only one RCT reported collecting objective sleep measure of Electrocardiogram (ECG)-derived estimation of cardiopulmonary coupling.

Table 2 qualitatively assesses methodology quality for 9 RCTs.

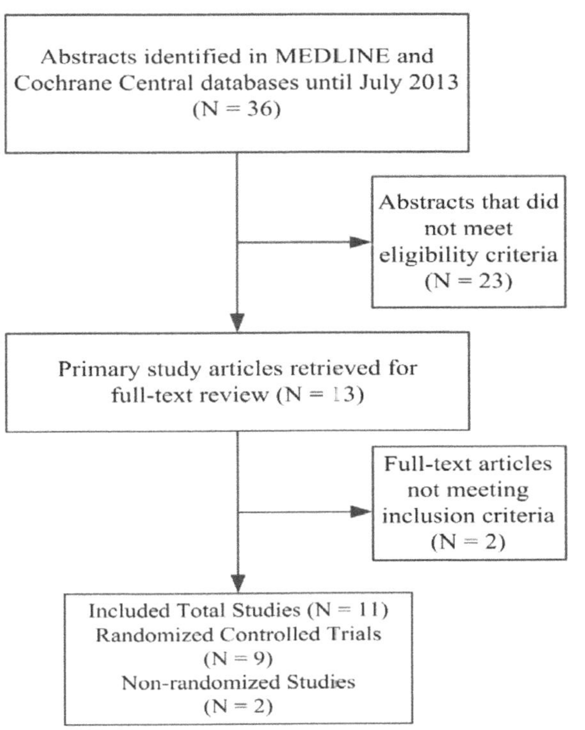

Figure 1: Study Flow Diagram.

Source Country RCTs	Population Subjects (N) Women (%)	Mean Age (yr)	Intervention Duration (Follow-up)	Tai Chi Frequency (Style) Intervention	Control Intervention	Outcomes related to Sleep	Additional Outcomes	Main Conclusion (Effect of Tai Chi vs. Control)
Jones, 2012 USA	Fibromyalgia 101 93%	54	12 wk (12 wk)	1.5 hr, 2x/wk (Modified 8-form Yang style)	Education 1.5 hr, 2x/wk	PSQI	FIQ; BPI; Arthritis Self-efficacy questionnaire; balance; functional mobility	Improved sleep quality, FIQ, pain, arthritis self-efficacy, and functional mobility.
Wang, 2010 USA	Fibromyalgia 66 87%	50	12 wk (24 wk)	1 hr, 2x/wk (10-form Classic Yang style)	Education and stretch exercises 1hr, 2x/wk	PSQI	FIQ; Patient /Physician global assessment score; 6-min walk; BMI; SF-36; CES-D; CPSS; VAS	Improved sleep quality, FIQ, depression, pain and quality of life.
Calandre, 2009 Spain	Fibromyalgia 81 90%	50	6 wk (18 wk)	1 hr, 3x/wk (Pool-based)	Stretching of main body muscles in warm water	PSQI	FIQ; BDI; STAI; SF-12	No significant differences between groups, but improved post-intervention scores for sleep and FIQ in Tai Chi group.
Wang, 2010 Japan	Elderly with cerebrovascular disorder 34 65%	77	12 wk (12 wk)	50 min, 1x/wk (Classical Yang style)	Non-resistance training and resistance training	PSQI	GHQ; P300 amplitude and latency (obtained by auditory stimulus system)	Improved sleep quality, general health, anxiety/ insomnia, and severe depression.
Yeh, 2008 USA	Patients with heart failure 18 50%	59	12 wk (12 wk)	1 hr, 2x/wk (5-core Master ChengManCh'ing's Yang style) plus instructional video	Pharmacological therapy, dietary and exercise counseling	Sleep (sleep spectrogram on ECG)	MLHFQ; 6-min walk-test; symptom-limited exercise test; BNP; peak VO2; catecholamine measurements	Improved sleep state, 6-min walk distance, and quality of life
Nguyen, 2012 Vietnam	Older adults 96 50%	69	24 wk (24 wk)	1 hr, 2x/wk (24-form style)	Routine daily activity	PSQI	FES; TMT	Improved sleep quality, cognitive performance, and balance.
Irwin, 2008 USA	Older adults 112 63%	70	16 wk (25 wk)	40 min, 3x/wk (westernized and Standardized version of Tai Chi)	Health education (2 hr/wk)	PSQI	BDI (qualitative)	Improved sleep quality, especially in older adults.
Li, 2004 USA	Older adults with moderate sleep complaints 118 81%	75	12 wk (24 wk)	1 hr, 3x/wk (Simplified Yang style, 8-form Easy Tai Chi)	Low-impact exercise (1 hr, 3x/wk)	PSQI; ESS	Physical performance; SF-12	Improved sleep quality, physical performance and health.
Hosseini, 2011 Iran	Older adult residents in nursing home 62 52%	69	12 wk (12 wk)	Gradually increased from 5min/session to 25 min/session, 3x/wk (10-stage Tai Chi)	No exercise	PSQI	None	Improved sleep quality.
NRS Caldwell, 2011 USA	College students 208 37%	21	15 wk (15 wk)	50 min, 2x/wk (Chen-style)	Special recreation (2.5 hr, 1x/wk or 1.25 hr, 2x/wk)	PSQI	Five Facet Mindfulness Questionnaire; Four Dimensional Mood Scale; Perceived Stresss Scale; Self-Regulatory Self-Efficacy Scale	Improved sleep quality, mindfulness, and mood, reduced perceived stress.
Caldwell, 2009 USA	College students 98 51%	21	15 wk (15 wk)	50 min, 2x/wk (Chen-style)	Special recreation or Pilates 50 min, 2x/wk	PSQI	Self-regulatory efficacy; Four Dimensional Mood Scale; Strength and Balance	A trend towards improvement in sleep quality, self-efficacy, and mood.

BDI = Beck Depression Inventory, BNP = B-type Natriuretic Peptide, BPI = Brief Pain Inventory, CES-D = Center for Epidemiologic Studies Depression, CPSS = Chronic Pain Self-Efficacy Scale, ESS = Epworth Sleepiness Scale; FIQ = Fibromyalgia Improvement Questionnaire, FES = Falls Efficacy Scale, GHQ = General Health Questionnaire, MLHFQ = Minnesota Living with Heart Failure Questionnaire, NRS = Non-randomized Studies, PSQI = Pittsburg Sleep Quality Index, RCT = Randomized Controlled Trial, TMT = Trail Making Test, SF = Short Form, VAS = Visual Analog Scale, wk = week

Table 1: Characteristics of Randomized Controlled Trials and Observational Studies Examining Tai Chi and Sleep Outcomes.

Overall 4 of 9 RCTs were graded good, 1 moderate, and 4 poor quality. Specifically, 6 RCTs reported on randomization sequence generation; 3 described an appropriate allocation concealment method, 5 reported on blinding for outcome assessors. All nine RCTs described withdrawals and dropouts. Dropout rates were moderate with 4 RCTs reporting dropouts 15 to 22%, and that the remaining 5 RCTs reported attrition <15%. One non randomized comparative study reported high dropouts of 23%, while the other did not report data on attrition.

None of the studies reported any other physical activities and exercise other than Tai Chi during study intervention period.

Meta-analysis results

We included 8 of 9 RCTs that provided data on sleep quantitative measures that used the global score of PSQI in the meta-analysis. Figure 2 displays the overall effects of Tai Chi on PSQI. Below, we describe results for studies that provided data for meta-analysis and those excluded from meta-analysis.

Eight of 9 RCTs with 660 participants assessed the effects of Tai Chi on sleep quality in both healthy adults and disease populations using the PSQI questionnaire. We found statistically significant improvements in PSQI with Tai Chi intervention compared with various controls

Source	Random sequence generation	Allocation concealment	Blinding of participants and personnel	Blinding of outcome assessment	Incomplete outcome data	Selective outcome reporting	Overall Risk of bias
Jones, 2012	+	?	+	+	+	+	+
Wang, 2010 (US)	+	+	+	+	+	+	+
Calandre, 2009	+	?	-	-	+	+	?
Wang, 2010 (Japan)	-	?	-	+	-	+	-
Yeh, 2008	-	-	-	-	-	+	-
Nguyen, 2012	-	?	?	?	-	+	-
Irwin, 2008	+	+	+	+	+	+	+
Li, 2004	+	+	+	+	+	+	+
Hosseini, 2011	-	-	-	-	-	+	-

+ = low risk of bias; — = high risk of bias; ? = unclear risk of bias

Table 2: Risk of Bias in Randomized Controlled Trials.

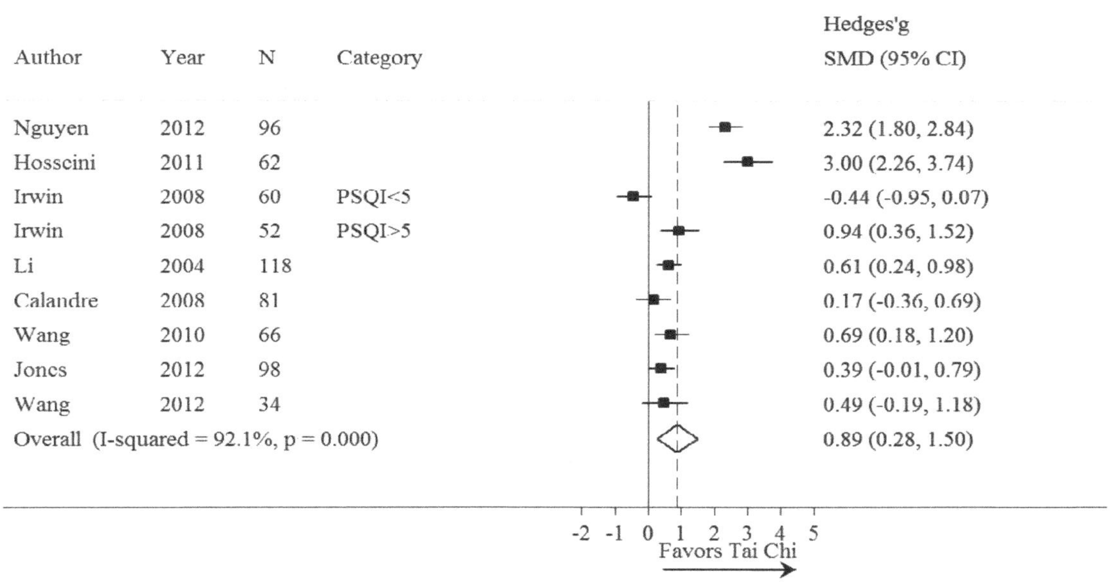

Figure 2: Effect of Tai Chi on Pittsburg Sleep Quality Index in Randomized Controlled Trials.

(Effect size, 0.89; 95 % CI, 0.28 to 1.50) (Figure 2), with an I^2 of 92%. Additional outcome measures examined in RCTs included pain, stress, depression, anxiety and quality of life as well as physical function performance. Tai Chi was performed between 6 and 24 weeks (40 to 90 minutes each session, 1 to 3 times per week).

One RCT with 18 participants did not report data on PSQI and therefore, was not included in the meta-analysis [26]. Using objective measures of sleep spectrogram on ECG, this remaining RCT conducted among participants with chronic heart failure showed significantly enhanced sleep stability, walk distance and quality-of-life after a 12 week Yang style Tai Chi intervention that involved a practice frequency of one hour, twice a week [26].

Two non-randomized comparative studies were not included in the meta-analysis due to lack of sufficient quantitative data, and the participants in these studies were healthy college students. These studies reported that a single 50 minutes, twice a week, Chen-style Tai Chi intervention significantly improved sleep quality in healthy college students [31,32].

Other outcomes

RCTs varied considerably in the types of questionnaires used for evaluation of other outcomes including, pain, quality of life, and depression. Four RCTs reported sleep outcomes in detail, of which 3 RCTs reported improvement in sleep outcomes including sleep latency, sleep duration, and use of sleep medications [24,28,29]; 1 RCT found no significant difference [25]. Additional improvements with Tai Chi intervention were observed for the outcome of pain [12,23,24] and functional mobility in 5 RCTs [12,23,26,27,29].

Results were mixed for the outcomes of cognitive ability, depression, and quality-of-life. Significant improvements in cognitive ability with Tai Chi occurred in healthy older adults [27]; however, no significant difference was observed between Tai Chi and control groups in patients with a cerebrovascular disorder [25]. Two RCTs found significant improvement in depression scores [12,25], however 2 other RCTs found no significant difference between Tai Chi and control groups in depression scores [24,28]. Five RCTs evaluated four different quality-of-life measures [12,24-26,29]. Notably, while the overall or physical functioning component of quality-of-life scores improved with Tai Chi intervention versus controls in all 5 RCT s, mental functioning scores showed no difference between groups in 2 RCTs [24,29]. Tai Chi intervention in two non randomized studies showed improvements in outcomes of mood and perceived stress among healthy college students, but had no effect on stre ngth and balance.

Discussion

Tai Chi, a form of low impact mind-body exercise, has spread worldwide over the past three decades. This meta-analysis strengthens a growing body of evidence and updates our previous investigations of the effects of Tai Chi on health outcomes in terms of improved sleep quality.

Specifically, 8 of the 9 RCTs from our quantitative meta-analysis and qualitative evidence synthesis reported that a Tai Chi practice "dose" of 1.5 to 3 hours each week significantly improves overall improvement of sleep quality and enhances functional ability in healthy older adults and patients with chronic conditions. While the subjects with illness may get more benefit than the healthy subjects, we were unable to distinguish significant effects between subjects with and without underlying diseases because only two RCTs reported data on healthy subjects.

Our review is consistent with several other reviews of mind-body therapies for sleep. For example, Sarris and Byrne [33] explored the effects of complementary medicine on the treatment of insomnia. Their review [33] supported evidence that mind-body therapies (Tai Chi and yoga) and manual therapies (acupuncture and acupressure) improve sleep quality. Another review by Irwin, Cole, and Nicassio [34] showed similar robust improvements in sleep quality, sleep latency, and the ability to remain asleep with the use of cognitive-behavioral treatment, relaxation, and behavioral-only treatment in older adults. Indeed, Tai Chi may act in a similar way to cognitive behavioral therapy for insomnia, in that it allows the patient to have a better mind-body connection.

With other forms of exercise, the mind-body connection or control is not always incorporated. For example, compared to a meta-analysis of the effect of exercise training (SMD=0.47, 95% CI 0.08 to 0.86) on improving sleep quality in middle-aged and older adults with sleep problems [35], our study shows that Tai Chi intervention has a better effect (SMD=0.89, 95% CI 0.28 to 1.50). Thus, it appears that Tai Chi has more advantages than regular exercise because of its mind-body attributes.

Although the exact biological mechanisms remain unknown, Tai Chi, a multi-component therapy integrating physical, psychosocial, emotional, spiritual, and behavioral elements, may act through intermediate pathways (e.g., neuroendocrine, immune function, neurochemical, and analgesic) to improve health outcomes [36,37]. It has been hypothesized that mind-body therapies improve sleep outcomes by restoring the homeostatic balance of sympathetic/parasympathetic function by reducing sympathetic activity and stimulating the parasympathetic nervous system. In addition, by focusing on movement or body positioning through controlled breathing and quieting the mind, Tai Chi might stimulate the release of endogenous neurohormones or other health recovery mechanisms [38], and promote deep states of relaxation, thereby proving to be an effective strategy in the treatment of insomnia.

From our review and meta-analysis, we understand that Tai Chi has been useful in treating insomnia and improving sleep quality in both adults and the elderly population, in both healthy people and people with chronic medical problems, as well as in people from different countries. Insomnia causes many negative health and economic outcomes [1-11] and it is prevalent as both a solitary condition and as co-morbidity in a variety of other diseases.

Therefore, it is important to explore an inexpensive and effective way, such as Tai Chi, to treat insomnia and to improve sleep quantity and quality in various populations.

There are several limitations to the available literature base examining the effect of Tai Chi on sleep quality. First, only English language published studies are included in this review. Studies published in other languages should be considered in the future for another systematic review and meta-analysis. Second, the parameters of the study population and intervention are widely variable. There are only 11 studies in this review and these studies vary markedly with regard to recruited populations, control groups, and outcome assessment. They also only examine a short duration of Tai Chi practice (6 to 24 weeks), and as a result the long-term effect of Tai Chi intervention needs to be explored in the future. The eligible studies also include small sample sizes and some of the studies lack a sufficient follow-up period. Third, there are methodology limitations in the reviewed studies, including, lack of allocation concealment and lack of blinding. Fourth, very little information is available on whether mind-body therapies promote objective measures of healthy sleep. For example, none of the studies presented information on objective evaluation of polysomnography in participants.

Even though most of the studies have scientific rigor to support the positive effect of Tai Chi on improving sleep quality, we found that there was a mild to moderate dropout rate from each study. Therefore, we suggest that prior to considering Tai Chi as a treatment option, clinicians discuss with their patients that Tai Chi practice requires discipline and perseverance to achieve the desired outcomes. This is exemplified by the duration and frequency of practice in all eleven studies, which usually require practicing Tai Chi for approximately an hour, two or three times a week and continuing this practice for 12 to 24 weeks. As is the essence of many behavioral therapies, Tai Chi may have profound salutogenic effects on improving sleep quality, and these effects come only with consistent practice.

In conclusion, evidence accrued from 11 clinical trials indicates that Tai Chi appears to be an effective behavioral therapy to treat insomnia and improve sleep quality among healthy subjects and patients with chronic conditions. Future high-quality, well-controlled, longer duration RCTs are needed to better inform clinical decisions about using Tai Chi to treat insomnia and improve sleep quality.

Funding Support

The National Center for Complementary and Alternative Medicine of the National Institutes of Health for Dr. Wang.

Reference

1. Kessler RC, Berglund PA, Coulouvrat C, Hajak G, Roth T, et al. (2011) Insomnia and the performance of US workers: results from the America insomnia survey. Sleep 34: 1161-1171.

2. Wehrens SM, Hampton SM, Kerkhofs M, Skene DJ (2012) Mood, alertness, and performance in response to sleep deprivation and recovery sleep in experienced shiftworkers versus non-shiftworkers. Chronobiol Int 29: 537-548.

3. Fletcher CE (2001) Hospital RNs' job satisfactions and dissatisfactions. J Nurs Adm 31: 324-331.

4. Buscemi D, Kumar A, Nugent R, Nugent K (2007) Short sleep times predict obesity in internal medicine clinic patients. J Clin Sleep Med 3: 681-688.

5. Yaggi HK, Araujo AB, McKinlay JB (2006) Sleep duration as a risk factor for the development of type 2 diabetes. Diabetes Care 29: 657-661.

6. Mullington JM, Haack M, Toth M, Serrador JM, Meier-Ewert HK (2009) Cardiovascular, inflammatory, and metabolic consequences of sleep deprivation. Prog Cardiovasc Dis 51: 294-302.

7. Kripke DF, Garfinkel L, Wingard DL, Klauber MR, Marler MR (2002) Mortality associated with sleep duration and insomnia. Arch Gen Psychiatry 59: 131-136.

8. Patel SR, Ayas NT, Malhotra MR, White DP, Schernhammer ES, et al. (2004) A prospective study of sleep duration and mortality risk in women. Sleep 27: 440-444.

9. Berger AM, Hobbs BB (2006) Impact of shift work on the health and safety of nurses and patients. Clin J Oncol Nurs 10: 465-471.

10. Léger D, Massuel MA, Metlaine A; SISYPHE Study Group (2006) Professional correlates of insomnia. Sleep 29: 171-178.

11. Roth T, Jaeger S, Jin R, Kalsekar A, Stang PE, et al. (2006) Sleep problems, comorbid mental disorders, and role functioning in the national comorbidity survey replication. Biol Psychiatry 60: 1364-1371.

12. Wang C, Schmid CH, Rones R, Kalish R, Yinh J, et al. (2010) A randomized trial of tai chi for fibromyalgia. N Engl J Med 363: 743-754.

13. Wang C, Bannuru R, Ramel J, Kupelnick B, Scott T, et al. (2010) Tai Chi on psychological well-being: systematic review and meta-analysis. BMC Complement Altern Med 10: 23.

14. Wang C, Schmid CH, Hibberd PL, Kalish R, Roubenoff R, et al. (2008) Tai Chi for treating knee osteoarthritis: designing a long-term follow up randomized controlled trial. BMC Musculoskelet Disord 9: 108.

15. Wang C, Schmid CH, Hibberd PL, Kalish R, Roubenoff R, et al. (2009) Tai Chi is effective in treating knee osteoarthritis: a randomized controlled trial. Arthritis Rheum 61: 1545-1553.

16. Yeh GY, Wang C, Wayne PM, Phillips R (2009) Tai chi exercise for patients with cardiovascular conditions and risk factors: a systematic review. J Cardiopulm Rehabil Prev 29: 152-160.

17. Wang C (2008) Tai Chi improves pain and functional status in adults with rheumatoid arthritis: results of a pilot single-blinded randomized controlled trial. Med Sport Sci 52: 218-229.

18. Li F, Harmer P, Fitzgerald K, Eckstrom E, Stock R, et al (2012) Tai Chi and postural stability in patients with Parkinson's disease. N Engl J Med 366: 511-519.

19. Yeh GY, McCarthy EP, Wayne PM, Stevenson LW, Wood MJ, et al. (2011) Tai chi exercise in patients with chronic heart failure: a randomized clinical trial. Arch Intern Med 171: 750-757.

20. Blake H, Hawley H (2012) Effects of Tai Chi exercise on physical and psychological health of older people. Curr Aging Sci 5: 19-27.

21. Buysse DJ, Reynolds CF 3rd, Monk TH, Berman SR, Kupfer DJ (1989) The Pittsburgh Sleep Quality Index: a new instrument for psychiatric practice and research. Psychiatry Res 28: 193-213.

22. Higgins JP, Altman DG, Gøtzsche PC, Jüni P, Moher D, et al. (2011) The Cochrane Collaboration's tool for assessing risk of bias in randomised trials. BMJ 343: d5928.

23. Jones KD, Sherman CA, Mist SD, Carson JW, Bennett RM, et al. (2012) A randomized controlled trial of 8-form Tai ch improves symptoms and functional mobility in fibromyalgia patients. Clin Rheumatol 31: 1205-1214.

24. Calandre EP, Rodriguez-Claro ML, Rico-Villademoros F, Vilchez JS, Hidalgo J, et al. (2009) Effects of pool-based exercise in fibromyalgia symptomatology and sleep quality: a prospective randomised comparison between stretching and Ai Chi. Clin Exp Rheumatol 27: S21-28.

25. Wang W, Sawada M, Noriyama Y, Arita K, Ota T, et al. (2010) Tai Chi exercise versus rehabilitation for the elderly with cerebral vascular disorder: a single-blinded randomized controlled trial. Psychogeriatrics 10: 160-166.

26. Yeh GY, Mietus JE, Peng CK, Phillips RS, Davis RB, et al. (2008) Enhancement of sleep stability with Tai Chi exercise in chronic heart failure: preliminary findings using an ECG-based spectrogram method. Sleep Med 9: 527-536.

27. Nguyen MH, Kruse A (2012) A randomized controlled trial of Tai chi for balance, sleep quality and cognitive performance in elderly Vietnamese. Clin Interv Aging 7: 185-190.

28. Irwin MR, Olmstead R, Motivala SJ (2008) Improving sleep quality in older adults with moderate sleep complaints: A randomized controlled trial of Tai Chi Chih. Sleep 31: 1001-1008.

29. Li F, Fisher KJ, Harmer P, Irbe D, Tearse RG, et al. (2004) Tai chi and self-rated quality of sleep and daytime sleepiness in older adults: a randomized controlled trial. J Am Geriatr Soc 52: 892-900.

30. Hosseini H, Esfirizi MF, Marandi SM, Rezaei A (2011) The effect of Ti Chi exercise on the sleep quality of the elderly residents in Isfahan, Sadeghieh elderly home. Iran J Nurs Midwifery Res 16: 55-60.

31. Caldwell K, Emery L, Harrison M, Greeson J (2011) Changes in mindfulness, well-being, and sleep quality in college students through taijiquan courses: a cohort control study. J Altern Complement Med 17: 931-938.

32. Caldwell K, Harrison M, Adams M, Triplett NT (2009) Effect of Pilates and taiji quan training on self-efficacy, sleep quality, mood, and physical performance of college students. J Bodyw Mov Ther 13: 155-163.

33. Sarris J, Byrne GJ (2011) A systematic review of insomnia and complementary medicine. Sleep Med Rev 15: 99-106.

34. Irwin MR, Cole JC, Nicassio PM (2006) Comparative meta-analysis of behavioral interventions for insomnia and their efficacy in middle-aged adults and in older adults 55+ years of age. Health Psychol 25: 3-14.

35. Yang PY, Ho KH, Chen HC, Chien MY (2012) Exercise training improves sleep quality in middle-aged and older adults with sleep problems: a systematic review. J Physiother 58: 157-163.

36. Davidson RJ, Kabat-Zinn J, Schumacher J, Rosenkranz M, Muller D, et al. (2003) Alterations in brain and immune function produced by mindfulness meditation. Psychosom Med 65: 564-570.

37. Irwin MR, Olmstead R, Oxman MN (2007) Augmenting immune responses to varicella zoster virus in older adults: a randomized, controlled trial of Tai Chi. J Am Geriatr Soc 55: 511-517.

38. Jahnke R, Larkey L, Rogers C, Etnier J, Lin F (2010) A comprehensive review of health benefits of qigong and tai chi. Am J Health Promot 24: e1-1e25.

Comparative Action of Sedative Hypnotics on Neurophysiology of Sleep

Ashish Kumar U[1] and Princy Louis Palatty[2*]

[1]3rd Year MBBS Student, Father Muller Medical College, Kankanady, Mangalore, Karnataka, India
[2]Department of Pharmacology, Father Muller Medical College, Kankanady, Mangalore, Karnataka, India

Abstract

In spite of tremendous advances in medical science, sleep has not been understood completely. The causes for many of parasomnias are still not evident. Even then these parasomnias are treated with different drugs, one of the major groups among them being sedative hypnotics. The use of sedative hypnotics are always associated with adverse effect, and there is many a times loss of the normal sleep architecture. This causes problems both during drug intake and with the withdrawal of drugs. Hence the need for today is the use of sedative hypnotics with minimum alteration in sleep architecture. The changes in the sleep architecture with the administration of sedative hypnotics can be recorded with the changes in the normal sleep EEG pattern. In this review effort has been made in elaborating the various sleep EEG pattern changes, resulting with the use of different groups of sedative hypnotic drugs with a brief note on their respective mechanism of action and pharmacological properties.

Keywords: Sedative hypnotics; Neurophysiology of sleep; EEG pattern; Benzodiazepines

Introduction

Sleep is regarded physiologically as absence of alertness and wakefulness. The biological clock/ circadian rhythm or the central pace maker which is located at the supra chiasmatic nuclei in the hypothalamus regulates diurnal variation of physiological functions of the body. The wand that regulates this variation is melatonin (the hormone from pineal gland).

Sleep is defined as a reversible period of oblivion with minimum alertness and is essential to mankind (also animals). Alternatively sleep has also been defined as a state of consciousness that is different from alert wakefulness by a loss of critical reactivity to event stimuli in the environment. Scientists now agree that sleep is not passive or inactivity rather it involves the active reorganisation of the brain. Despite a great amount of research is done on sleep there remain grey areas in this field.

Method

This review explores the actions of various sedatives hypnotics on the neurophysiology of sleep. A PubMed literature search was conducted exploring the mechanism of action of various sedative hypnotics presently available and the correlation with the neurophysiology of sleep. The present review compiled all data to bring fourth relevant aspects for the improved understanding of sleep physiology. Most of the articles reviewed were repetitive and only the significant gleaned and presented in this review. A unique paper of old [1967] titled "neurophysiology of the states of sleep" by Michel Jouvet was a stimulating introspection of the knowledge of sleep then, but prophetic in its conjecture. The study type was explorative description.

Areas of Interest

Neuro physiology of sleep

The normal sleep pattern consists of six to eight cycles of sleep that transcends from light sleep to deep sleep. Sleep is characterised into two types, Non Rapid Eye Movement (NREM) sleep and rapid eye movement sleep (REM) sleep.

NREM sleep; there is sequential transition of sleep from stage one to four in NREM sleep. One NREM sleep last approximately 20 minutes. It is characterised by dominant parasympathetic activity with reduced metabolic rate, heart rate, cardiac output, peripheral vascular resistance etc. NREM sleep is of a peaceful nature, and EEG shows basically alpha rhythm with sleep spindles. Muscle tone diminishes progressively. There is no movement of eye ball in NREM sleep. In stage four NREM sleep there is more preponderance of ischemic cerebro vascular stroke. Growth hormone secretion occurs in stage three and four of NERM sleep [1]. The American academy of sleep medicine alternatively classifies NREM sleep into three stages-N1, N2, N3. N3 includes stage 3 and stage 4 of the conventional classification also called the slow wave sleep.

REM sleeps; REM sleep last approximately 30 minutes but progressively increases in the latter sleep cycles. In an uninterrupted normal sleep the person awakens from REM sleep in the morning. REM sleep is characterised by sympathetic activity. In REM sleep all the voluntary muscles except extra ocular muscles are found flaccid. As 75% of the dreams occur during REM sleep, it is usually associated with corresponding rise in heart rate, muscle, respiratory rate etc. The EEG in the REM sleep resembles that in awake person i.e. beta rhythm. The brain shows increased oxygen consumption. Obstructive sleep apnoea there is extreme hypotonia of the muscles of the moderate respiratory passages. Hypertensive hypoxic cardio vascular events occur during REM sleep due to the secretions of catecholamines. REM sleep does not affect growth hormone secretion. REM sleep constitutes 25% of the total sleeping time.

A normal man spend one third of his life in sleep. Adequate sleep is necessity of healthy life. Insomnia indicates lack of sleep which may

***Corresponding author:** Princy Louis Palatty, Professor, Department of Pharmacology, Father Muller Medical College, Kankanady, Mangalore, Karnataka, India E-mail: drprincylouispalatty@gmail.com

be due to variability in initiation or maintenance of sleep. Parasomnias are a group of sleep disorders that are associated with sleep such as sleepwalking, bruxism, night terrors, sleep paralysis, enuresis etc.

Lack of sleep leads to poor concentration, motor in coordination, attention deficit, irritability, restlessness, raised blood pressure and heart rate etc.

Electrophysiology of sleep

Sleep is classified into stages based on the electroencephalogram (EEG) readings, electro ocular gram reading (EOG) and electromyogram (EMG) readings-i.e. into NREM sleep and REM sleep.

The EEG wave patterns has been divided into 4 types

1. α wave; high amplitude, 8- 14 cycles per second
2. β wave; low amplitude, 15-35 cycles per second
3. Θ wave; low amplitude, 4-7 cycles per second
4. δ wave; high amplitude, 0-5 -3 cycles per second

In stage 1 of NREM sleep alpha waves are predominant being interspersed with Θ waves. Stage two shows Θ waves with interspersed spindles. While the stage 3 of NREM sleep shows Θ,δ waves, stage 4 shows predominance of δ activity.

The electrical activity of the sleeping brain has a recurrent evolution preceding from two opposite modes- the slow wave sleep and the activated sleep also called the paradoxical sleep.

The EEG aspect of Slow Wave Sleep (SWS) consist of 11 to 16 cycles/ sec of high amplitude spindles that are often synchronous with the cortex and present at the level of the frontal and reticular formation and associative areas. The spindles are usually followed by 1 to 4 cycles/ sec high voltage slow waves, also recorded at the sub cortical level.

On the other hand the EEG recording of a paradoxical sleep shows tonic activity characterised by a neo cortical diencephalic and mesencephalic low voltage fast activity (20-30 cycles/ sec), being similar to the cortical desynchronization that usually follows arousal or attention states. However, the EEG recording during a paradoxical sleep is differentiated from that due to arousal or attention states by the presence of some electrical local cortical and subcortical activity [2-4]. The continuous presence of theta rhythm during paradoxical sleep is characteristic [5-12].

Site of Action of Sedative Hypnotics

Sedative produces calming and drowsiness. It decreases activity and moderates excitement. Hypnotics are a drug that induce sleep and maintains sleep just like natural sleep. Sedative hypnotics are a group of drugs that are widely used in clinical care. Sedation on the other hand, is the very common adverse effect of most drugs especially those that have generalised CNS depressant action. Examples, antihistaminic, anti psychotics, alcohol.

Sedative hypnotics are used widely in clinical care as in, the treatment of insomnia, sedatives, anxiolytics, muscle relaxants etc.

The need of the day is the use sedative hypnotics that do not or causes least alteration in the normal sleep architecture. There is an increasing emphasis on quality of sleep along with the quantity of sleep which was the main emphasis before (Table 1).

Sedative hypnotic drugs cause grades of CNS depression i.e. drowsiness (sedation), sleep (hypnotic), unconsciousness, coma, fatal respiratory depression, death. The index of CNS depressant activity is noted from cognitive deficit and attention to environmental stimuli.

Benzodiazepines	Alprazolaam,brotizolam,chlordiazepoxide, clobazam clonazepam,clorazepate, diazepam, estazolam, flumazenil, lorazepam, oxazepam, triazolam
Z compounds (benzodiazepine receptor agonist)	Zolpidem, zopiclone, zaleplon, eszopiclone
Barbiturates	Phenobarbitone, mephobarbitone
Newer agents	Melatonin agonists, orexin antagonists
Miscellaneous	paraldehyde, chloral hydrate, meprobromate

Table 1: Classification of sedative hypnotics.

GABAa Receptor

There are three types of GABA receptors- GABAa and GABAb and GABAc. The most important among the three is the GABAa receptor which is a ligand gated chloride channel. The GABAa receptor has three subunits-alpha, beta and gamma. GABAa receptor could be either pentameric or tetrameric protein in which the subunits assemble around a central pore. The GABAa receptor has separate binding sites for GABA, benzodiazepine, and barbiturates. There are six subgroups of alpha subunit and three each of beta and gamma, indicating the presence of large group of GABAa receptor types.

Benzodioazepines

Chlordiazepoxide and diazepam were the first benzodiazepines to be introduced in 1960, replacing the order barbiturate group of sedative hypnotics.

The basic structure of benzodiazepines consists of benzene ring fused to seven member diazepine ring. All effects of benzodiazepines are based on their action on the specific receptors present in the CNS, which includes effects like sedation, hypnosis, anterograde amnesia, decreased anxiety, muscle relaxation and anticonvulsant activity. Most of the benzodiazepines are absorbed completely on oral administration and are highly protein bound in the plasma. Even with excessive doses of BZD usages surgical anaesthesia cannot be achieved, unless other drugs are added. The benzodiazepines receptors agonists have least potecyl of respiratory depression and are the preferred sedative hypnotics today. Benzodiazepines are use full in the treatment of insomnia, by decreasing the time needed to enter stage 1 of NREM sleep, decrease awakefullness. Benzodiazepines are safer as compared to barbiturates due to lesser depression of respiration, heart and blood pressure and also due to the presence of a effective antidote flemazenil, in cases of toxicity. On long term use of benzodiazepines, there is usually development of tolerance. Cross tolerance is also known to occur with alcohol.

Mechanism of action

Benzodiazepines act by interacting with the inhibitory neurotransmitter receptor activated directly by GABA. There are predominately two types of GABA receptors-GABAa and GABAb. Benzodiazepines act by binding to the ionotropic GABA a receptors and have not action on the GABA b receptors. The binding site of benzodiazepines are distinct from that of GABA binding. Benzodiazepines do not act on the GABA a receptor directly but they potentiate the action of GABA on GABA a receptors. Benzodiazepines increase the chloride current in response to GABA activation by increasing the frequency of chloride channel opening.

Action of benzodiazepines on electro physiology of sleep

Benzodiazepines decreases the time spent in stage 1 NREM sleep, while the time spent in stage 3 and stage 4 of NREM sleep is decreased considerably. However the time taken from the onset of spindle sleep to REM sleep is increased because of increase in the time spent in the stage 2 of NREM sleep, that being the major fraction of NREM stage of sleep. Benzodiazepines increase NREM sleep [13]. While REM sleep period is decreased by most of the benzodiazepines, although the number of cycles of REM sleep is increased. With chronic use of benzodiazepine the affect on various stages of sleep declines, and if such a chronic use is discontinued there can be rebound of the pattern of drug induced changes of sleep parameter. The withdrawal symptoms may also include agitations, depression, abdominal pain, Insomnia, seizures. Dependence to benzodiazepines can be prevented and controlled through dose tapering, medication switching and/ or medication augmentation.

Benzodiazepines cause anterograde amnesia, and hence can cause illusion of anaesthesia in pre anaesthetic doses.

The changes in the neurophysiology of sleep with the administration of drugs belonging to the benzodiazepine group remains minimal with only mild changes relating to the potency of the individual drugs. Known as the 'benzodiazepine signature', there is usually a 10-15 Hz increase and lower-frequency (<10 Hz) suppression relative to the preceding drug-free night [14]. In a study aimed at observing the effects of haloxazolam, flunitrazepam, and triazolam, on the EEG pattern of subjects, showed that the three drugs induced EEG changes of similar pattern. It was observed that higher frequency (including the sigma and beta bands) activity increased and lower frequency activity reduced with the administration of drugs [15]. Triazolam (0.25 mg) induces changes in the EEG spectra which are typical for benzodiazepine receptor agonists characterised by EEG power density in non-REM sleep reduced in the frequency range of 1.25-10.0 Hz and enhanced in the range of sleep spindles (12.25-13.0 Hz) [16].

Z Compounds

These compounds though not structurally related to benzodiazepines act by binding to and activating the benzodiazepine receptor site in the GABA a receptors. Drugs in this class include zolpicone, zolpidem, zaleplon etc. Z drugs are now replacing benzodiazepines. They are specific sedative hypnotics and hence lack anticonvulsant, ant anxiety, muscle relaxant properties. They cause minimum hangover when compared to the benzodiazepines.

Action of Benzodiazepine Receptor Agonist on Electro Physiology of Sleep

Unlike benzodiazepines these drugs have little effect on the stages of sleep. Zolpidem and zaleplon suppress REM sleep to a lesser extent as compared to the benzodiazepines, and hence are considered superior [13]. Zolpidem and zaleplon don't show rebound insomnia on abrupt discontinuation [17]. On administration of zolpidem in mince the change in EEG pattern is found to be distinct from that see due to benzodiazepines, and this affect is due to the action of zolpidem on alpha 1 GABAa receptor [18]. The EEG profile of heath volunteers administered with zolpidem was characterised by a decrease of alpha activity and an increase in delta and beta activity. The effect on beta activity was marked within the first hour and then disappeared [19]. The drug also reduced REM sleep but did not significantly affect other sleep stages and subjective sleep parameter [20].

Barbiturates

One among the pioneers groups of sedative hypnotics, Barbiturates have been replaced now by the much safer benzodiazepines. Barbiturates consists of 2,4,6- trioxohexahydropyrimidine and alkyl or aryl groups at the position 5, which confers the molecule the central sedative hypnotic property. On oral administration the absorption is almost complete and is distributed widely. Before excretion by the kidney almost all barbiturates undergo complete metabolism or conjugation in the liver. Barbiturate cause respiratory depression which is lethal at high doses, compared to the benzodiazepines which have minimal effect on respiration, heart rate and blood pressure.

Mechanism of action

Barbiturates act by binding to the barbiturate receptor in the GABA a receptor, distinct from that of GABA and benzodiazepine receptors and enhancing the inhibitory neurotransmission. In contrast to benzodiazepines, barbiturates cause increased duration of chloride channel opening. They also have a direct stimulatory effect on GABA receptors by acting as a GABA agonist and causing inhibitory action directly.

Action of barbiturates on electro physiology of sleep

Barbiturates also alter the sleep stages in manner almost similar to the benzodiazepines. Rapid eye movement (REM) sleep during barbital treatment was reduced to half the time as compared to that seen in drug free subjects [21].

A quantitative analysis of beta-rhythms can differentiate the effects of barbiturates and benzodiazepine drugs on the EEG [22].

Newer and Miscellaneous Group of Sedative Hypnotics

Chloral hydrate, paraldehyde, triclophos etc are included in the miscellaneous group of sedative hypnotics which are only of historical importance today. Chloral hydrate banned today in many countries for it addiction potency is capable of inducing sleep and modifying the sleep EEG, improving organization of sleep spindles and generalized paroxysms [23]. However there is a lack of sufficient data to describe the EEG changes in sleep due to paraldehyde and others.

Melatonin agonists the newer sedative hypnotic is structurally similar to melatonin- the hormone secreted from the pineal gland, the biological clock. The secretions from the pineal gland play an important role in synchronizing the sleep- wake cycle with the circadian rhythm. The melatonin agonists have hence played an important role in the treatment of jet lag. Melatonin agonists have little effect on sleep latency and duration of sleep. The effect on the electrophysiology of sleep is also minimal. Although melatonin agonists are unlikely to have the adverse effect of conventional sedative hypnotic, its long term safety is not clear.

Receptor antagonists of the neurotransmitter orexin are another group of newer sedative hypnotics, called orexin antagonists. Orexin regulates arousal, appetite, wakefulness [24]. This newer group of drugs has been found useful in the treatment of sleep pathology such as insomnia [25,26]. In a study which involved intracerebro ventricular orexin A administration, differently affected fronto-occipital EEG waves in the different frequent bands. The power of the Delta and alpha waves decreased while that of theta and beta waves increased.

Potential Drug Targets

The sedative hypnotic effect of the present day drugs are not optimal and beset with adverse reaction and change in sleep architecture. The quest for new drugs and probable target is on. The elusive endogenous benzodiazepine could be a potential target.

Conclusion

Sedative hypnotic are one among the most commonly used drugs in clinical practice such as for the treatment of insomnia, as anti convalescents etc. They are associated with a large number of side effect and hence there is a need for understanding their action on various systems thoroughly, one of them being the changes the induce in electrical activity of the brain during sleep.

The neuro physiology of sleep leaves a lot of lacunae that impedes the understanding of sleep. The drug group availed are not optimal in the treatment of sleep disorders. The lookout for potential targets and molecules still continues. Optimizing the presently available sedative hypnotics concurrent with functional imaging and somnographic techniques would be the order of the day.

References

1. Takahashi Y, Kipnis DM, Daughaday WH (1968) Growth hormone secretion during sleep. J Clin Invest 47: 2079-2090.
2. BUENDIA N, GOODE M, SIERRA G, SEGUNDO JP (1963) Responsiveness and discrimination during sleep. Experientia 19: 208-209.
3. Okuma T, Fujimori M (1963) Electrographic and Evoked Potential Studies During Sleep in the Cat (The Study On Sleep, I). Seishin Shinkeigaku Zasshi 17: 25-50.
4. Tokizane, T (1965) Hypothalamic control of cortical activity and some observations during different states of sleep. In Aspects anatomo-fonctionnels de la physiologie du sommeil, a Symposium, edited by M. Jouvet. Paris Centre Natl Rech Sci 15l -184.
5. Cadilhac J, Passouant-Fontaine T, Passouant P (1961) Modification de l'activite de l'hippocampe suivant les divers stades du sommeil spontane chez le chat. Rev Neurol 105: 171-176.
6. Grastyan E, Karmos G (1961) A study of a possible "dreaming" mechanism in the cat. Acta Physiol Acad Sci Hung 20: 41-50.
7. Jouvet M. Recherches sur les structures nerveuses et les mecansimes responsables des differentes phases du sommeil physiologique. Arch Ital Biol 100: 125-206.
8. Lena C, Parmeggiani PL (1964) Hippocampal Theta Rhythm and Activated Sleep. Helv Physiol Pharmacol Acta 22: 120-135.
9. Lena C, Parmeggiani PL (1964) [Hippocampus and activated sleep]. Boll Soc Ital Biol Sper 40: 130-133.
10. Parmeggiani PL, Zanocco G (1963) A Study on the Bioelectrical Rhythms of Cortical and Subcortical Structures During Activated Sleep. Arch Ital Biol 101: 385-412.
11. Passouant P, Cadilhac J (1962) Les rythmes theta hippocampiques au cours du sommeil. In Physiologie de l'hippocampe, edited by P. Passouant Paris Centre Natl, Rech Sci: 331-345.
12. Feinberg I, Maloney T, Campbell IG (2000) Effects of hypnotics on the sleep EEG of healthy young adults: new data and psychopharmacologic implications. J Psychiatr Res 34: 423-438.
13. Feige B, Voderholzer U, Riemann D, Hohagen F, Berger M (1999) Independent sleep EEG slow-wave and spindle band dynamics associated with 4 weeks of continuous application of short-half-life hypnotics in healthy subjects. Clin Neurophysiol 110: 1965-1974.
14. Tan X, Uchida S, Matsuura M, Nishihara K, Kojima T (2003) Long-, intermediate- and short-acting benzodiazepine effects on human sleep EEG spectra. Psychiatry Clin Neurosci 57: 97-104.
15. Aeschbach D, Cajochen C, Tobler I, Dijk DJ, Borbély AA (1994) Sleep in a sitting position: effect of triazolam on sleep stages and EEG power spectra. Psychopharmacology (Berl) 114: 209-214.
16. Voderholzer U, Riemann D, Hornyak M, Backhaus J, Feige B, et al. (2001) A double-blind, randomized and placebo-controlled study on the polysomnographic withdrawal effects of zopiclone, zolpidem and triazolam in healthy subjects. Eur Arch Psychiatry Clin Neurosci 251: 117-123.
17. Tobler I, Kopp C, Deboer T, Rudolph U (2001) Diazepam-induced changes in sleep: role of the alpha 1 GABA(A) receptor subtype. Proc Natl Acad Sci U S A 98: 6464-6469.
18. Patat A, Trocherie S, Thebault JJ, Rosenzweig P, Dubruc C, et al. (1994) EEG profile of intravenous zolpidem in healthy volunteers. Psychopharmacology (Berl) 114: 138-146.
19. Brunner DP, Dijk DJ, Münch M, Borbély AA (1991) Effect of zolpidem on sleep and sleep EEG spectra in healthy young men. Psychopharmacology (Berl) 104: 1-5.
20. Hinman DJ, Okamoto M (1984) Sleep patterns in cats during chronic low-dose barbiturate treatment and withdrawal. Sleep 7: 69-76.
21. Feshchenko VA, Veselis RA, Reinsel RA (1997) Comparison of the EEG effects of midazolam, thiopental, and propofol: the role of underlying oscillatory systems. Neuropsychobiology 35: 211-220.
22. Castro CB, Chisté MA, Vizioli JF, Córdova NM, Ohlweiler L, et al. (1994) [Comparison between the EEG of natural sleep and the induced by chloral hydrate in relation to paroxysmal changes and baseline rythm]. Arq Neuropsiquiatr 52: 326-329.
23. Sakurai T, Amemiya A, Ishii M, Matsuzaki I, Chemelli RM, et al. (1998) Orexins and orexin receptors: a family of hypothalamic neuropeptides and G protein;coupled receptors that regulate feeding behavior. Cell 92: 573-585.
24. Roecker AJ, Coleman PJ (2008) Orexin receptor antagonists: medicinal chemistry and therapeutic potential. Curr Top Med Chem 8: 977-987.
25. Cao M, Guilleminault C (2011) Hypocretin and its emerging role as a target for treatment of sleep disorders. Curr Neurol Neurosci Rep 11: 227-234.
26. Toth A, Balatoni B, Hajnik T, Detari L (2012) EEG effect of orexin A in freely moving rats. Acta Physiol Hung 99: 332-343.

Chronic Insomnia, Pharmacotherapy and the Cognitive Behavioral Approaches

Mohammad Torabi Nami*

Department of Neuroscience, School of Advanced Medical Science and Technology, Shiraz University of Medical Sciences, Shiraz, Iran

Abstract

Insomnia is a common complaint of patients presenting to primary care physician and sleep medicine experts. Approximately 10-20% of the general population worldwide has reported symptoms of chronic insomnia of which 25% have primary insomnia. Insomnia is more prevalent among females and the elderly subjects (over 65 years). Pharmacotherapy for insomnia is mainly focused on hypnotics such as benzodiazepine receptor agonists (BzRAs), antihistamine drugs, tricyclic antidepressants like doxepin, and a melatonin receptor agonist (ramelteon). However, these very often used medications are shown to have potential untoward effects outweighing their benefits in many instances. Once the underlying disorder affecting sleep is appropriately addressed, cognitive behavioral therapy, singly or combined with drug therapy, is demonstrated to be amongst the most efficacious treatment strategies in some cases with refractory insomnia.

Keywords: Insomnia; Cognitive and behavioral therapy; Pharmacotherapy; Sleep hygiene; Recommendations

Insomnia; Not Only a Prevalent But also a Consequential Sleep Disorder

The different aspects of the complex physiological process of sleep are yet to be understood and despite all so far efforts, sleep remains one of the great mysteries of science [1-3]. Insomnia which is resulted from problems with sleep initiation and maintenance is considered as one of the most prevalent health issue and a widely encountered challenge in clinical practice [4-6]. Due to many potential causes for insomnia, unfamiliarity with non-pharmacological treatments, and existing concerns about the challenges faced with pharmacological approaches, many health care professionals seem reluctant to efficiently address insomnia in their practice [4,6]. Physicians should expand their awareness on the advances in treating insomnia due to its potential effects on function and general health [6].

We may even quantify to what extent insomnia has negatively affected one's quality of life. Some recently validated and currently available sleep-health indices such as the Glasgow Sleep Impact Index (GSII) make measuring the impact of insomnia on sleep-related quality of life impairment possible [7]. Meanwhile, further attempts should be done to develop further psychometric and clinical evaluation tools available to assess the neurocognitive and health-related burden of chronic insomnia [8,9].

Although the pathophysiological aspects of insomnia are described in the literature [6], many contributing mechanisms for this disorder have remained unraveled. The question of "nature or nurture" has also existed for insomnia. Both sleep-wake related mechanisms and stress-response-related gene-environment interactions are shown to play a role in our brain plasticity [10]. There are some recent theories on the epigenetic mechanisms involved in insomnia and gene-environment interactions which regulate this disorder [11].

Based on the International Classification of Sleep Disorders (ICSD), 2nd edition, insomnia is characterized as "difficulty initiating and/or maintaining sleep, early awakening or non-restorative sleep despite adequate opportunity" [12]. This needs be accompanied by at least one of the following complaints during the day: fatigue and daytime sleepiness, lapses in attention, concentration or impaired memory function, poor performance in social, occupational or academic perspectives, irritability or dysregulation in mood, motivation, energy or initiative. Moreover, insomniacs are notably prone to errors or accidents at work or while driving [6,9]. Reports indicate that insomniacs suffer from tension headaches or GI distress due to sleep loss and worries about sleep [5,6,9,10,12].

The ICSD differentiates insomnia either as primary or secondary [12]. Primary insomnia includes idiopathic insomnia, psycho-physiological insomnia and paradoxical insomnia. Secondary insomnia includes insomnia secondary to psychosocial stressors, psychiatric disorders, medical disorders, various sleep disorders, drug and substance abuse and prescription medications. Misuse of some medications which are thought to help sleep may profoundly lead to poor sleep and unfavorable neuro-cognitive consequences [12-15].

Over the past few years the term comorbid insomnia is preferentially used instead of secondary insomnia. Comorbid insomnia implies that insomnia in subjects with other health conditions is as significant as the underlying disorder and hence requires independent assessment and treatment [13].

Distressed emotion, lack of energy and profound fatigue, sleepiness and impaired functioning during the daytime, are shown to be some cardinal consequences of insomnia. Furthermore, impairment is social and occupational performance adversely affects the quality of life. As reports indicate, insomniacs tend to be at increased risk for mental health problems, substance abuse and cardiovascular morbidity [6].

***Corresponding author:** Mohammad Torabi Nami, MD, PhD, Department of Neuroscience, School of Advanced Medical Science and Technology, Shiraz University of Medical Sciences, Shiraz, Iran E-mail: torabinami@sums.ac.ir

When physicians tend to approach this condition, taking a thorough clinical history is often the least thing needed to identify the contributing factors [5]. Where hypnotic medications are perceived efficacious, they must be carefully monitored for adverse effects [4,16,17]. In parallel, behavioral therapeutic approaches should be used whenever indicated and possible [18,19]. The focus of this review is putting together the current options and strategies for the treatment of insomnia and discussing the concurrent approaches (i.e. pharmacotherapy in presence of cognitive-behavioral approaches) which may provide a better outcome in some cases with insomnia.

Pharmacological Approaches in Treating Insomnia, Merits and Demerits

Recent critical reviews and meta-analyses have elaborated on the advantages and disadvantages of pharmacotherapy in insomnia [4,5]. Although efficacious in many instances, sleep aid medications must be carefully monitored for their potential adverse effects. Some approved hypnotics including benzodiazepine receptor agonists (BzRAs), antihistamine drugs, tricyclic antidepressants like doxepin, and a melatonin receptor agonist (ramelteon) are being widely used for insomnia management, whereas some other still approved medications for insomnia such as barbiturates and chloral hydrate are far from recommendation due to their potential toxicity [4]. Meanwhile; anxiolytic benzodiazepines [20], sedating antidepressants [20], atypical anti-psychotics [21], and anticonvulsants [4,20] are being increasingly used in insomnia although not approved for this indication. Given these medications' safety issues relative to their modest efficacy in many instances, there remain persistent concerns for the routine use of hypnotic medications in insomnia. When the primary clinical diagnosis is insomnia, the short-course prescription of hypnotics may become warranted while their long-term use possibly results in lack of efficacy and physical or psychological dependence [5,17,20]. Considering the untoward effects of hypnotics, elderly patients with insomnia and those with underlying medical problem with complex pill regimens should preferably receive behavioral therapies for insomnia rather than add-on hypnotic medications [17]. The popular over-the-counter melatonin is shown to more exert regulatory effects on disrupted chronobiology rather than possessing hypnotic properties [4]. Meanwhile, the advent of a new class of evolving drugs for primary insomnia known as dual orexin receptor antagonists (DORA) are underway and their primary efficacy and safety results are intriguing [22].

Cognitive and Behavioral Approaches in Insomnia

Sleep logs

Sleep logs, when completed properly, are useful not only in the assessment of insomnia but also in its management and monitoring progress.

Sleep logs provide information on sleep patterns of patients in their own environments. They also assist to assess the impact of therapeutic interventions, help to monitor progress over a period of time and help patients to realize that insomnia may not be as frequent or as severe as they had thought (e.g. paradoxical insomnia) [17].

Sleep hygiene

Sleep hygiene refers to a set of instructions that help patients fall and stay asleep. Sleep hygiene measures, on their own are not effective in the treatment of insomnia [16]. However, they provide a framework for other therapeutic interventions. Some of sleep hygiene measures that can be recommended to patients include maintaining a regular waking time and removing from the bedroom anything that could impair sleep. Patients are usually advised to strictly avoid alcohol, caffeine, nicotine and heavy exercise several hours before bed time. Patients should neither take large meals before going to sleep nor go to bed hungry or thirsty, and finally they should avoid naps during the day [23].

Stimulus control

The goal of stimulus control is to assist patients re-associate bed with sleep. Some of the recommended behaviors include not going to bed until ready to sleep, using bed only for sleep (sex is an exception). Patients should avoid reading, watching TV or eating in bed and are recommended to set an alarm to get up at the same time every morning [23,24].

Biofeedback

There is compelling interest in using biofeedback as a technique to train individuals in order to improve their health by means of developing better awareness or voluntary control over the physiological processes which are affected by anxiety or stress. In this technique, the level of anxiety or stress is measured by fixing electrodes or sensors on the scalp, forehead, around the trunk and on the fingertips that record biological signals. The biofeedback setup and the type of sensors used depend of what specific technique is applied.

With regard to the treatment of insomnia, two types of biofeedback including electromyography (EMG) biofeedback and sensory-motor rhythm (SMR) biofeedback are commonly applied. EMG biofeedback is found to be effective in anxious individuals who have sleep-onset insomnia, and SMR biofeedback is found to be effective in non-anxious individuals who have sleep maintenance insomnia. The therapist acts as a coach by facilitating patient relaxation, which further reduces stress and anxiety [8,16,25]. Relaxation is a key component in biofeedback [25].

Sleep restriction

Sleep restriction is based on the premise that time spent in bed awake makes insomnia worse. When appropriately applied, sleep restriction is shown to improve sleep efficiency by almost 85% and to consolidate sleep. Subjects are trained to stay in bed only when they are asleep. They are then allowed to increase "time in bed" by 15-20 minutes each night, only if their sleep efficiency exceeds 90%. Consequently, the time they spend in bed should be 15-20 minutes each night in case their sleep efficiency is below 90% [24].

Cognitive and Behavioral Therapy for Insomnia (CBTi)

Other than sleep hygiene consideration in changing life style and behaviors enacted before going to bed, CBTi is an effective non-pharmacological approach to treat insomnia [16,17,19]. The main behavioral and cognitive ingredients of CBTi are as follow:

1. Stimulus control: the rationale is to establish associative links between bed and sleep, overcoming the existing conditioned inability to sleep. e.g. The 15 minutes rule for getting out of bed.
2. Sleep timings: patients are encouraged to maintain a sleep schedule compatible with their sleep regulating systems also during weekends avoiding compensative attempts to sleep.
3. Reduction of the time spent in bed, i.e. sleep restriction.
4. Relaxation: simple techniques like progressive muscular

relaxation and meditation are promoted within the CBTi program.

5. Cognitive restructuring and control: experience-based revision of worries about insufficient sleep; simple strategies to avoid the presence of intrusive thoughts in bed before sleeping.

6. Paradoxical intentions: the effort to stay awake can be used to contrast the effort to sleep, typically reported by insomniacs.

The therapeutic process in CBTi encompasses restoration of dysregulation in processes C and S plus behavioral and cognitive changes. The goal of cognitive therapy for insomnia is to identify and correct dysfunctional beliefs and attitudes relating to sleep. Patients can be taught facts and techniques such as: 1-sleep needs differ and not everyone needs eight hours of sleep a night, 2- learn not to worry or get frustrated if you are not sleeping, 3- learn to do thinking and worrying during the day instead of at night– in bed at night, use thought stopping and thought switching to reduce worries, 4- lying in bed resting peacefully is nearly as restorative as sleep, and it is much more restorative than lying there thinking and worrying and 5- for patients who have not been helped by other methods, paradoxical injunction can be used (to reduce the anticipated anxiety associated with trying hard to sleep, patients are requested to stay awake as long as possible) [17-19,25,26].

The combination of cognitive and behavioral therapies for insomnia (CBTi) with pharmacotherapy has not only been shown to be more effective, but also the effects last longer compared to pharmacological treatment alone [18]. In some instances, the concurrent therapy using both pharmacological and behavioral approaches is the only way to help symptoms [18]. The full-fledged treatment package which comprises both pharmacotherapy and behavioral interventions may then be de-escalated to cognitive behavioral therapy alone in long run [4,5,16,20,25]. The above therapeutic measures have also demonstrated to positively influence polysomnographic variables [27]. The improved variables following appropriate treatment of insomnia include increased total sleep time (lights out to lights on time spent asleep) and sleep efficiency (total sleep time divided by the time in bed in minutes expressed in percentage) and decreased sleep onset latency (time in minutes to the first epoch of sleep from lights out) and wake time after sleep onset (time in minutes awake after the first epoch of sleep) [27,28].

Comment

Primary care physicians seem to need to optimize their knowledge and practice with regard to pharmacological and non-pharmacological approaches in treating insomnia. CBTi has been found to offer valuable therapeutic benefits when applied for the right patients and in the right setting. Apart from the need to run basic etiopathophysiological studies to further explore the underlying causes of insomnia and other neuroscience researches to further elucidate the nature of this disorder some more actions are needed to provide primary care physicians with management updates on prevalent disorders such as insomnia. Incorporating practical lessons for the management of insomnia, hypersomnia and other common sleep disorders into the continuous medical education courses designed for health care professionals (CME), is expected to result in a more evidence-based practice when they encounter sleep-related complaints raised by their patients.

References

1. Rosenbluth G, Landrigan CP (2012) Sleep science, schedules, and safety in hospitals: challenges and solutions for pediatric providers. Pediatr Clin North Am 59: 1317-1328.

2. Dresler M, Spoormaker VI, Beitinger P, Czisch M, Kimura M, et al. (2013) Neuroscience-driven discovery and development of sleep therapeutics. Pharmacol Ther.

3. Ferri R, Bruni O (2013) Psychophysiology and cognitive neuroscience of sleep and sleep disorders. Int J Psychophysiol 89: 149-150.

4. Buysse DJ (2013) Insomnia. JAMA 309: 706-716.

5. Merrigan JM, Buysse DJ, Bird JC, Livingston EH (2013) JAMA patient page. Insomnia. JAMA 309: 733.

6. Roth T (2007) Insomnia: definition, prevalence, etiology, and consequences. J Clin Sleep Med 3: S7-10.

7. Kyle SD, Crawford MR, Morgan K, Spiegelhalder K, Clark AA, et al. (2013) The Glasgow Sleep Impact Index (GSII): a novel patient-centred measure for assessing sleep-related quality of life impairment in Insomnia Disorder. Sleep Med 14: 493-501.

8. Buysse DJ, Germain A, Moul DE, Franzen PL, Brar LK, et al. (2011) Efficacy of brief behavioral treatment for chronic insomnia in older adults. Arch Intern Med 171: 887-895.

9. Sarsour K, Kalsekar A, Swindle R, Foley K, Walsh JK (2011) The association between insomnia severity and healthcare and productivity costs in a health plan sample. Sleep 34: 443-450.

10. Summers MO, Crisostomo MI, Stepanski EJ (2006) Recent developments in the classification, evaluation, and treatment of insomnia. Chest 130: 276-286.

11. Palagini L, Biber K, Riemann D (2013) The genetics of insomnia - Evidence for epigenetic mechanisms? Sleep Med Rev.

12. American Academy of Sleep Medicine (2005) International classification of sleep disorders, (2ndedn). Diagnostic and coding manual. American Academy of Sleep Medicine, Westchester.

13. Culpepper L (2006) Secondary insomnia in the primary care setting: review of diagnosis, treatment, and management. Curr Med Res Opin 22: 1257-1268.

14. Carney CE, Edinger JD (2006) Identifying critical beliefs about sleep in primary insomnia. Sleep 29: 444-453.

15. Nami M, Madadi G (2009) Medication Induced Poor Sleep And Neurocognitive Consequences In Allergic Rhinitis: A Brief Review. The Internet Journal of Family Practice 9: 2.

16. Bootzin RR, Perlis ML (1992) Nonpharmacologic treatments of insomnia. J Clin Psychiatry 53 Suppl: 37-41.

17. Lande RG, Gragnani C (2010) Nonpharmacologic approaches to the management of insomnia. J Am Osteopath Assoc 110: 695-701.

18. Morin CM, Vallières A, Guay B, Ivers H, Savard J, et al. (2009) Cognitive behavioral therapy, singly and combined with medication, for persistent insomnia: a randomized controlled trial. JAMA 301: 2005-2015.

19. Irwin MR, Cole JC, Nicassio PM (2006) Comparative meta-analysis of behavioral interventions for insomnia and their efficacy in middle-aged adults and in older adults 55+ years of age. Health Psychol 25: 3-14.

20. Buscemi N, Vandermeer B, Friesen C, Bialy L, Tubman M, et al. (2007) The efficacy and safety of drug treatments for chronic insomnia in adults: a meta-analysis of RCTs. J Gen Intern Med 22: 1335-1350.

21. Khazaie H, Rezaie L, Darvishi F, Najafi F, Avis K (2013) Treatment of paradoxical insomnia with atypical antipsychotic drugs. A comparison of olanzapine and risperidone. Neurosciences (Riyadh) 18: 64-69.

22. Winrow CJ, Renger JJ (2013) Discovery and development of orexin receptor antagonists as therapeutics for insomnia. Br J Pharmacol.

23. Torabi Nami M (2011) "Sleep Hygiene" The Gateway for Efficient Sleep: A Brief Review. WMC BRAIN 9: 002245.

24. Vincent N, Lewycky S, Finnegan H (2008) Barriers to engagement in sleep restriction and stimulus control in chronic insomnia. J Consult Clin Psychol 76: 820-828.

25. Mitchell MD, Gehrman P, Perlis M, Umscheid CA (2012) Comparative effectiveness of cognitive behavioral therapy for insomnia: a systematic review. BMC Fam Pract 13: 40.

26. Morawetz D (2003) Insomnia and depression: which comes first?. Sleep Research Online 5: 77-81.

27. Ferri R, Gschliesser V, Frauscher B, Poewe W, Hogl B (2013) On â€œpolysomnography reveals unexpectedly high rates of organic sleep disorders in patients with prediagnosed primary insomniaâ€ (Sleep Breath 2011 doi 10.1007/s11325-011-0608-8). Sleep Breath 17: 1-2.

28. Van Der Kloet D, Giesbrecht T, Franck E, Van Gastel A, De Volder I, et al. (2013) Dissociative symptoms and sleep parameters--an all-night polysomnography study in patients with insomnia. Compr Psychiatry 54: 658-664.

Sleep Abnormalities in Guillain Barre Syndrome: A Clinical and Polysomnographic Study

Karkare K, Sinha S*, Taly AB and Rao S

Departments of Neurology and Biostatistics, National Institute of Mental Health and NeuroSciences (NIMHANS), Bangalore

Abstract

Purpose: We analyzed the polysomnographic (PSG) profile and various factors contributing to sleep disturbances in patients with GB Syndrome.

Methodology: This prospective hospital based study included 30 adults with GB syndrome (mean: 34.30 ± 1.40 years; M:F=24:6). All patients underwent evaluation with phenotypic details, nerve conduction studies, sleep questionnaires and over-night polysomnography (PSG). Three (10%) patients had baseline sleep disturbances with a Pittsburgh Sleep Quality Index (PSQI) of >5 and all the 3 patients continued to have poor sleep during hospitalization. Sixteen (53.3%) patients had poor sleep during their hospital stay as assessed by Richards score. Sleep disturbances as per St Mary's sleep score depicted similar observations over 10 nights. Overnight PSG was carried out within 1st to 12 day of hospitalization (mean: 6.83 ± 3.07; median: 6.5).

Results: During overnight PSG several patients did not have all the stages of sleep: stage 1-2 patients, stage 3-6 patients, stage 4-13 patients and REM stage -7 patients. Other notable PSG observations were: increased stage 1 and stage 2 sleep, reduced stage 4 and REM sleep, decreased sleep efficiency of <85% -28; increased sleep onset latency of >30 min -4; duration of sleep of <6 hours -20; and increased arousal (arousals >5/hour) -6. Majority of arousals were due to respiratory events and oxygen desaturation. Three patients had abnormal periodic leg movement (PLM) arousal index (>5/hours). Sub-analysis revealed that depressed patients had lesser duration of sleep (p=0.049). There no REM related behavioral disorder noted.

Conclusions: To conclude, sleep disturbances and altered sleep architecture in GB syndrome during hospitalization are common and may be multifactorial.

Keywords: Guillain barre syndrome; Polysomnography; Sleep disturbances

Introduction

Sleep is an important predictor of quality of life and has been the subject of current research in many systemic and neurological disorders. Similar to the disorders of Central Nervous System (CNS), sleep disturbances have also been studied in a few disorders of Peripheral Nervous System (PNS) like diabetic neuropathy, myotonic dystrophy, and myasthenia gravis. Sleep disturbances in these disorders are ascribed to sensory phenomenon, respiratory events and mental burden of the disease e.g. pain and depression in diabetic neuropathy [1], restless leg syndrome in alcohol induced neuropathy [2] and multifocal motor neuropathies [3], respiratory muscle weakness and sleep disordered breathing in neuromuscular disorders like amyotrophic lateral sclerosis [4], and myasthenia gravis [5]. In myotonic dystrophy, excessive day time sleepiness is postulated to be due to defect in central dysregulation of sleep rather than sleep apnea [6].

Patients with Guillain Barre syndrome (GBS) experience sensory disturbances including pain, motor disability, require prolonged hospital stay and exhibit anxiety regarding uncertain nature of the disease and may be expected to have sleep disturbances. Cochen et al. in their study involving patients of GBS, admitted in ICU setup, had shown REM behavioral disorders, REM onset sleep, REM with atonia and abnormal eye movements in NREM sleep [7]. From this center, Karkare et al. had noted both quantitative and qualitative sleep disturbances in a cohort of 60 patients with GB syndrome [8]. The sleep disturbances were possibly due to anxiety, pain, paresthesia, and severity of immobility and it improved after the 1st week of inpatient care.

We analyzed the polysomnographic (PSG) profile in patients with GB syndrome and studied various factors contributing to sleep disturbances.

Patients and Methods

This prospective hospital based study involved 30 patients with GB syndrome (mean: 34.3 ± 1.4 years; median: 31; M:F=24:6) evaluated at the Department of Neurology of a tertiary care university hospital (NIMHANS, Bangalore, India). The diagnosis was based on the National Institute of Neurological and Communicative Disorders and Stroke (NINCDS) criteria for GB syndrome [9]. Ethical approval was obtained from the Institutional ethics committee. Informed consent was obtained from the patient and/or care giver. Patients with respiratory distress, who didn't consent, or who were evaluated within 48 hours of admission were excluded. Respiratory distress in patients with GB syndrome was detected with standard bedside clinical methods like single breath count, respiratory rate, laboured breathing, use of accessory muscle, paradoxical breathing, and sometimes low

***Corresponding author:** Dr Sanjib Sinha, Additional Prof of Neurology NIMHANS, Bangalore: 560 029, Karnataka, India E-mail: sanjib_sinha2004@yahoo.co.in

oxygen saturation and impaired blood gas reports. Information was noted on a predesigned digital data sheet. The study was divided into following parts:

Clinical evaluation and laboratory tests

Information regarding the demographic characters, duration and severity of illness, presence of paresthesia, pain, weakness and their duration, and antecedent event was obtained. Details of blood pressure, single breath count, chest expansion and routine neurological examination were recorded. Pain and paresthesia were measured using Wong and Baker Face scale [10]. Patients were explained about the scale and were required to give a score separately for pain and paresthesia. Verbal rating scale was also used with 0 as having no pain and 10 reflecting most severe pain [11]. Severity of GBS was assessed using Hughes severity score [12], Modified Rankin score [13]. Anxiety and depression were measured using hospital anxiety and depression scale (HADS) [14]. Investigations included: hemogram, serum biochemistry including creatine phosphokinase (CPK), potassium, RA, ANA, HBsAg and HIV; Urine for porbhobilinogen and Bence Jones protein; and CSF analysis. All patients underwent routine motor and sensory nerve conduction studies on right side (median, ulnar, common peroneal and sural nerves) using standard procedures.

Assessment of sleep

It was done using the following scales: Pittsburgh Sleep Quality Index (PSQI) at admission [15]; and daily with Richard Campbell Sleep score [16]; and St Mary's Hospital Sleep Questionnaire [17]. Data from 30 patients was collected on 10 consecutive days with the sleep questionnaires following admission in the hospital. The first questionnaire was administered within 48 hours of admission.

i) **Pittsburgh Sleep Quality Index** (PSQI) is a self-rated questionnaire which assesses sleep quality and disturbances over a 1-month time interval. Nineteen individual items generate 7 "component" scores: subjective sleep quality, sleep latency, sleep duration, habitual sleep efficiency, sleep disturbances, use of sleeping medication, and daytime dysfunction. Each component score ranges from 0 (no difficulty) to 3 (severe difficulty). The component scores are summed to produce a global score (range of 0–21);

ii) **Richard Campbell Sleep score** consists of pictorial representation of 5 questions wherein patient marks or indicate mark on a line of 100 mm length with two ends of the line define extremes of answers of a particular question. Total Score is calculated by averaging the score on each line and is divided as good sleep (0-33 mm); moderate sleep (33-66 mm) and poor sleep (> 66 mm). In the current study, the original Richards score was modified for better understanding by the patient population i.e. score 0 was attributed to good sleep and score 100 to poor sleep, unlike the original scale, where scores are reverse; and

iii) **St Mary's Hospital Sleep Questionnaire** consists of 14 questions regarding sleep onset, onset latency, number of awakenings, duration of sleep in day and night, depth of sleep, satisfaction after sleep, and causes of disturbed sleep if any. The score ranges from 6 to 39 with the higher score indicating better sleep.

Polysomnographic evaluation

All subjects underwent PSG at the sleep laboratory in the department of Neurology according to the American Association of Sleep Medicine guidelines [18]. The PSG was reported following the AASM 2007 guidelines by a joint sitting of the investigators (KK, SS).

Statistical analysis

Data was analyzed using descriptive statistics such as Mean, SD, Minimum, Maximum values for continuous variables and frequency and percentage for categorical variables. Comparison between clinical variable groups and continuous sleep variables was done using independent sample'*t*' test. Association between categorical variables was analyzed by means of Chi Square test or Fisher's exact test. A $p<0.05$ was considered statistically significant.

Results

Seventeen patients with GB syndrome presented in the 1st week, 8 in 2nd week and 6 in 3rd week of illness. Six patients were in the progressive phase at presentation. Antecedent events observed in 21/30 patients were: fever-70%, diarrhea-30%, and respiratory symptoms-12.5%. The distribution of limb weakness was: distal upper limb - 27, distal lower limb - 28, proximal upper limb - 25, and proximal lower limb - 28. Sensory symptoms included paresthesia in upper limb – 30, paresthesia in lower limb - 28, and pain - 30. Bulbar symptoms present in 23/60 patients were dysphagia - 5, poor cough - 6, dysphonia - 4. Neurological deficits consisted of facial paresis - 13, impaired joint position sense - 7, impaired vibration sense- 6, impaired pain - 4, and papilledema – 1. The severity of disease as per Hughes score and Modified Rankin's score is shown in table 1. Based on the HADS scale, anxiety and depression were present in 12 and 11 patients respectively. Serum CPK values ranged from 51 to 1688 IU/L (median: 265). The CSF cell count varied from 0 to 7 cells/cu.mm (mean: 0.85 ± 1.6) and protein ranged from 22 to 424 mg/dl (mean: 144.3 ± 108.3).

All patients were subjected to large volume plasma exchange on alternate day and 25 patients were given symptomatic therapy for pain viz. non-steroidal anti-inflammatory drugs (NSAIDs) -15 and antineuralgic agents – 22 (carbamazepine – 20; pregabalin - 2, duloxetine - 2, amitriptyline - 1 and tramadol - 1). Five patients did not receive symptomatic treatment.

Sleep disturbances

Pittsburgh Sleep Quality Index (PSQI): All patients were assessed by PSQI to ascertain their baseline sleep pattern i.e. before the onset of illness. Three (10%) patients had baseline sleep disturbances with a PSQI of >5 (Range 0-11, mean 1.62 ± 2.3). All the three patients

	Day 1 N (%)	Day 10 N (%)
	Hughes grade	
4	19 (63.3)	15 (50)
3	6 (20)	7 (23.3)
2	3 (10)	4 (10)
1	2 (6.6)	2 (6.6)
	Modified Rankin's score	
5	11 (36.6)	10 (33.3)
4	10 (33.3)	9 (30)
3	7 (23.3)	7 (23.3)
2	1 (3.3)	2 (6.6)
1	1 (3.3)	2 (6.6)
0	0	0

Table 1: Severity of illness on first (day 1) & last day (day10) of the study.

continued to have poor sleep during the acute phase of illness i.e. 10 days of hospitalization.

Richards Campbell score: Sixteen (53.3%) patients had poor sleep during their hospital stay as assessed by Richards score. The mean of the Richards score for all 60 patients on 10 nights was also calculated. It was observed that the sleep score was highest (poor sleep) on day 3 of evaluation and improved towards the last 3 days of evaluation i.e. 8th through 10th day. When the data was analyzed with respect to nights, abnormal Richard scores of >33 was recorded on 138 nights (46%) and a highly abnormal score of >66 was observed on 69 nights (23%) (Table 2).

St. Mary's score: Assessment of sleep disturbances was also performed by St. Mary's hospital sleep in any patients. Patients were also categorized on the basis of components of St. Mary's score viz. sleep onset latency, number of arousals and duration of sleep (Table 2). When these individual components were plotted with respect to day of illness, it was noted that the disturbances were maximum in the first week of illness.

Overnight polysomnography

The day of polysomnographic assessment ranged from 1st to 12th day of hospitalization and initial assessment (mean: 6.83 ± 3.07; median: 6.5).

Sleep macrostructure: The details of total time in bed, total sleep time, sleep efficiency, sleep onset, latency to various stages are provided in table 3. Sleep efficiency among patients was low with sleep efficiency of <85% being present in 28/30 patients. Twenty patients had sleep duration of less than 6 hours. Sleep onset latency >30 minutes was present in 4/26 patients. It is noteworthy that several patients did not have all the stages of sleep: stage 1-2 patients, stage 3-6 patients, stage 4-13 patients and REM stage -7 patients. A significant observation was reduction of percentage (<5%) of REM sleep in 5 patients. There was no 'REM related behavior' noted.

Arousals: During the overnight PSG, 8 patients had frequent arousals. Maximum arousals were due to respiratory events and oxygen desaturation. (Table 4) The number of arousals among these patients was: ≤ 10:12; 11 to 20:10, 21 to 30:6 and >30:2. Six patients had abnormal arousal index i.e. >5 arousals/hour.

Periodic and isolated leg movements in sleep: Though seven patients had frequent periodic leg movements (PLMS), only three had abnormal PLMS index (5/hour) (Table 4).

Saturation parameters, heart rate and respiratory events in sleep and wake stages: The details are provided in tables 4 and 5. The abnormal apnea index i.e. apnea >5/hour was present in 3 out of 30 patients. Twenty one out of 30 patients had oxygen desaturation. Maximum frequency of desaturation events was in one patient (no.11) noted up to 116 times with a mean duration of desaturation being 49 seconds and desaturation index of 54.2 in him.

Correlation of factors responsible for sleep disturbances

The total sleep time was calculated in younger (<40 years: <6 hours-13; >6 hours: 10) and older (>40 years: <6 hours-7; >6 hours: 0) and it was noted that none of the older patients slept >6 hours (p=0.03). The sleep latency (<30 mins or >30 mins) and total sleep time were not affected by factors like anxiety, severity of illness (Hughes scale: 1-3 vs. 4-5; Rankin scale: 1-3 vs. 4-5), visual analogue scale for paresthesia (Vapar ≤ 5 or >5); Visual analogue scale for pain (Vap ≤ 5 or >5); and Verbal rating scale for pain (Verp ≤ 5 or >5). However presence of

Sleep Question Score	Day of hospitalization	1	2	3	4	5	6	7	8	9	10
Richards Campbell score	Mean ± SD	42.8 ± 36.8	43.8 ± 28.7	47.4 ± 31.5	48.08 ± 32.8	44.02 ± 29.5	43.2 ± 30.01	38.6 ± 27.3	35.1 ± 27.9	35.71 ± 27.68	35.04 ± 29.5
	>33	14	13	17	16	15	15	**15**	12	10	11
St Mary's sleep score	Mean ± SD	23.9 ± 9.1	22.6 ± 9.04	21.4 ± 9.06	23.03 ± 9.2	21.3 ± 9.4	22.1 ± 9.3	23.7 ± 8.6	25.57 ± 8.7	26.64 ± 8.7	25.7 ± 8.9
	Sleep onset latency>30 min	9	10	12	9	10	10	7	7	4	9
	Frequent arousals (>2)	12	12	14	13	14	15	12	9	8	7
	Duration of sleep <6 hrs	14	17	18	18	18	18	17	15	15	12

Table 2: Richards Campbell & St Mary's sleep score on consecutive 10 nights.

Sleep parameters	Minimum	Maximum	Mean	SD
Time In Bed (TIB) (min)	266.70	541.30	466.86	59.91
Total Sleep Time (min)	48	495.50	297.49	106.81
Sleep Efficiency (%)	18	96.50	61.88	18.65
Sleep Onset (min)	0	116	22.94	26.18
Latency to stage 1 (min) [n=28]	1.5	394.7	110.2	112.2
Latency to stage 2 (min) [n=30]	0	271.00	36.6	54.5
Latency to stage 3 (min) [n=24]	12	325.3	72.8	62.3
Latency to stage 4 (min) [n=17]	0	165.00	73.2	48.4
Latency to stage REM (min) [n=23]	0	273.00	136.5	76.3
% in stage 1 [n=28]	2	38	11.78	8.38
% in stage 2 [n=30]	39.2	100	71.52	14.31
% in stage 3 [n=24]	0.30	22.90	8.52	5.11
% in stage 4 [n=17]	1.10	23.20	7.01	6.75
% in stage REM [23]	1.40	18.30	8.57	5.21

Table 3: Polysomnographic variables showing sleep macrostructure in patient population.

Arousal events	Minimum	Maximum	Mean±SD
Arousal number	3	104	18 ± 18.41
Arousal index	0.5	18.2	4.36 ± 4.29
Arousal due to desaturation	0	52	2.10 ± 9.46
Arousal due to apnea	0	57	3.47 ± 10.63
Arousal due to snoring	0	4	0.13 ± 0.73
Arousal due to desaturation- index	0	24.30	0.93 ± 4.42
No. of PLMs	0	49	6.4 ± 11.84
PLMs index	0	7.30	1.23 ± 1.97
No. of Isolated leg movements	0	14	3.20 ± 4.13
Isolated leg movements index	0	2.90	0.64 ± 0.75
No. of Isolated leg movements with arousal	0	2	0.20 ± 0.48
Arousal due to PLMs	0	4	0.7 ± 1.15
Arousal due to PLM - index	0	0.9	0.16 ± 0.25
Arousal due to apnea - index	0	26.60	1.25 ± 4.84
Arousal due to snore index	0	0.9	0.03 ± 0.16
Apnea index total	0.0	44.40	3.47 ± 9.43
Hypopnea index total	0.0	15.40	2.01 ± 3.63
Apnea- hypopnea index total	0.0	59.80	5.5 ± 12.62
Arousal due to obstructive apnea	0.0	2.80	0.32 ± 0.65
Arousal due to mixed apnea	0.0	15.40	0.52 ± 2.81
Arousal due to central apnea	0.0	8.40	0.40 ± 1.61
Arousal due to hypopnea - index	0.0	2.30	0.15 ± 0.43

Table 4: Arousals in sleep and the events responsible for arousals.

Saturation parameters and Heart rate	Minimum	Maximum	Mean ± SD
Awake minimum saturation	87	96	92.70 ± 7.48
Awake maximum saturation	96	103	98.86 ± 1.43
Awake average saturation	91.30	98.30	95.60 ± 1.76
Sleep minimum saturation	61	95	96.93 ± 7.81
Sleep maximum saturation	95	104	98.36 ± 1.56
Sleep average saturation	90.20	98.20	94.91 ± 2.13
Awake minimum heart rate	42	104	67.60 ± 15.14
Awake maximum heart rate	84	182	117.50 ± 18.94
Sleep minimum heart rate	40	103	66.43 ± 13.92
Sleep maximum heart rate	94	151	105.67 ± 24.39
Sleep average heart rate	48.30	111.60	80.08 ± 14.65

Table 5: Saturation parameters and heart rate in sleep and wake stages.

depression did not influence sleep latency it certainly reduced sleep total time (p=0.049).

Discussion

Sleep disturbances have been recorded in patients with diabetic neuropathy, multifocal motor neuropathy [3] and are attributed to pain, paraesthesia, restless leg syndrome and depression [1,19]. GB syndrome is the most severe form of polyneuropathy with variable sensory symptoms and motor disability and the need for hospitalization with uncertainty of the course of the disease. Thus sleep disturbances are expected in GB syndrome. This study evaluated polysomnographic (PSG) profile of 30 patients with GBS shortly after hospitalization, irrespective of the day of illness.

Phenotype

All patients had quadriparesis with distal (90-93%) more than proximal weakness (77-91%). Sensory symptoms viz. paresthesia (90%) and pain (95%) were rather frequent, probably due to prospective and daily evaluation of sensory symptoms for ten consecutive days. Other phenotypic features were similar to earlier reports [20-22].

Questionnaire based sleep disturbances

A total of 16 patients had poor sleep during their hospital stay as assessed by Richards scale. Three of these patients had baseline poor quality of sleep (PSQI>5) thus 13 patients with baseline good sleep developed sleep disturbances during the acute phase of illness. Richard's scale consists of visual analogue scale. It is easy to administer and enables objective comparison between patient populations. According to Richards score, 16 patients had a poor sleep. Of the 297 nights studied (data of 3 nights were not available due to early discharge from hospital) poor sleep was reported on 138 nights (46%). Sleep disturbances in hospitalized patients could be due to various factors like paresthesia, pain, immobility, anxiety/depression, plasmapheresis, untimely injections, shift from one ward to other, hospital schedule like checking of vitals, diagnostic procedures, type of facility like general or special ward with privacy matters, disturbances from other patient e.g. shouting and snoring, death of the other patient(s) and others. Patients were asked these questions every day and also given option to cite any other reason that believe could have caused sleep disturbances.

In this study, St Mary's Hospital sleep Questionnaire was used to evaluate nature of sleep disturbances. An abnormal sleep onset latency of >30 min was noted on day 3. The common reasons reported by patients were pain, paresthesia, and immobility causing difficulty to turn around in bed or need for going to toilet. The environmental disturbances like hospital schedule, presence of other patients, new place, and transfer were less frequently reported in the current study. This is in contrast to other studies where sleep in hospitalized patients was significantly affected due to environmental disturbances [23]. Most of the studies about sleep disturbances in hospitalized patients have evaluated patients in acute care settings like post cardiac surgery patients or in intensive care units. Interestingly, patients with less sensory symptoms and minimal motor disability complained more about the environmental disturbances. The effect of pain on sleep latency has been studied in various studies [24]. Frequent awakening i.e. arousals of >2 in night time was considered abnormal. The maximum number of patients experienced frequent awakenings on day six of the study. On an average, 12 patients had sleep fragmentation. Most of the patients attributed sleep fragmentation to pain (7/10 nights), paresthesia (7/10 nights), anxiety/depression (5/10 nights), frequent desire to pass urine, cough, and environmental disturbances.

Polysomnography

The results of PSG revealed reduced sleep efficiency in patient population. Sleep efficiency of >85% is considered normal. Only 2 patients had good sleep. Frequent arousals, long latency to sleep after arousal or prolong sleep onset were responsible for reduced sleep efficiency. All the patients had >2 arousals during the sleep.

In this study, sleep architecture of patients was deranged with increase in Stage 1 and 2, reduced REM and stage 4 percentages. Seven patients had absent REM. All these changes may happen in persons suffering from depression or chronic pain disorders [24].
On assessing sleep parameters among depressed and non-depressed individuals, total sleep time was decreased in depressed individuals. However, other parameters like sleep fragmentation and duration of sleep were equally distributed in depressed and non depressed group. This differential effect of depression requires further studies. Similarly, there was no difference in sleep parameters in groups with presence of anxiety, disability, higher pain and paresthesia scores. This suggests that GBS per se may give rise to certain sleep abnormalities independent of the co-morbid factors. The current study has revealed abnormal sleep

onset latency in 4 out of 30 patients. These patients were in age of 16 to 25 years. This supports the observations in the meta-analysis that PSG recorded sleep onset latency is unchanged irrespective of the age [25]. The distribution of these factors in sleep related abnormalities are equal implying unknown mechanism in GBS may be responsible for sleep disturbances that require exploration.

Cochen et al. evaluated 139 patients of GB syndrome with or without mental status abnormalities admitted to ICU [7]. The abnormalities were: with sleep onset REM (83%), abnormal eye movements during non-REM sleep (57%), high percentages of REM sleep without atonia (92 ± 22%), REM sleep behavior disorders and autonomic dysfunction (100%), and reminiscent of a status dissociatus. The patients in this cohort were not admitted to ICU and did not have REM associated behavioral issues or any other mental status abnormalities during sleep.

Pathophysiology of sleep disturbances in GB syndrome

The exact mechanism of sleep disturbances in GB syndrome is unknown and speculative. There could be variable combination of peripheral and central mechanisms. These patients experience sensory disturbances including pain, have recent onset motor disability, require prolonged hospital stay and exhibit anxiety regarding uncertain course of the disease and may be expected to have sleep disturbances.

The CSF hypocretin-1 (a hypothalamic neuropeptide deficient in narcolepsy) levels, measured in 20 patients, were lower in patients of GBS with hallucinations (555 ± 132 pg/ml) than in those without (664 ± 71 pg/ml, p=0.03). The authors proposed involvement of lateral hypothalamus in GB syndrome that governs the sleep architecture. This may be due to its location where the blood brain barrier is exposed to antibodies circulating in blood. Thus GB syndrome may also have putative antibodies against central targets [26]. There are studies reporting CNS involvement in GB Syndrome [27]. It has been postulated that dreamlike and other hallucinatory experiences may occur when there is a disruption in the "corollary discharge" system that allows us to discriminate between self-generated and externally generated neural activity [28]. The sensory and motor denervation that occurs in GB syndrome might allow the same confusion between internally and externally generated thoughts and sensations that occur in sleep, resulting in thoughts having a dreamlike or hallucinatory quality [29]. The possible explanations for CNS involvement in GBS include watershed infarction, demyelination, reversible posterior leukoencephalopathy, and adverse effects of immunoglobulin, status dissociaticus [27,30]. These aspects were not studied here.

This comprehensive study is first of its kind where qualitative and quantitative evaluation of sleep disturbances was done in GB syndrome in a prospective manner. Sleep disturbances and altered architecture in GBS may be multifactorial and may include many unidentified factors which require further studies. Inclusion of control group will strengthen the result. Treatment of underlying causes like pain, anxiety; early institution of specific treatment for GB syndrome like plasma exchange or IVIg and reassurance might be some of the steps in alleviating the sleep disturbances. Systematic enquiry, evaluation and treatment of sleep disturbances may reduce morbidity and improve quality of life.

References

1. Zelman DC, Brandenburg NA, Gore M (2006) Sleep impairment in patients with painful diabetic peripheral neuropathy. Clin J Pain 22: 681-685.
2. Pourfar M, Feigin A (2009) The numb and the restless: peripheral neuropathy and RLS. Neurology 72: 950-951.
3. Lo Coco D, Cannizzaro E, Lopez G (2009) Restless legs syndrome in a patient with multifocal motor neuropathy. Neurol Sci 30: 401-403.
4. Arnulf I, Similowski T, Salachas F, Garma L, Mehiri S, et al. (2000) Sleep disorders and diaphragmatic function in patients with amyotrophic lateral sclerosis. Am J Respir Crit Care Med 161: 849-856.
5. Amino A, Shiozawa Z, Nagasaka T, Shindo K, Ohashi K, et al. (1998) Sleep apnoea in well-controlled myasthenia gravis and the effect of thymectomy. J Neurol 245: 77-80.
6. Gulfidan C, Tayyibe S, Mustafa Y, Zuhal A, Esra A, et al. (2007) Myotonic Dystrophy and Sleep Apnea. Indian J Chest Dis 49: 173-175.
7. Cochen V, Arnulf I, Demeret S, Neulat ML, Gourlet V, et al. (2005) Vivid dreams, hallucinations, psychosis and REM sleep in Guillain-Barré syndrome. Brain 128: 2535-2545.
8. Karkare K, Sinha S, Taly AB, Rao S (2013) Prevalence and profile of sleep disturbances in Guillain-Barre Syndrome: a prospective questionnaire-based study during 10 days of hospitalization. Acta Neurol Scand 127: 116-123.
9. Asbury AK, Cornblath DR (1990) Assessment of current diagnostic criteria for Guillain-Barré syndrome. Ann Neurol: S21-24.
10. Wong DL, Baker CM (1988) Pain in children: comparison of assessment scales. Pediatr Nurs 14: 9-17.
11. Garra G, Singer AJ, Taira BR, Chohan J, Cardoz H, et al. (2010) Validation of the Wong-Baker FACES Pain Rating Scale in pediatric emergency department patients. Acad Emerg Med 17: 50-54.
12. Winer JB, Hughes RA, Osmond C (1988) A prospective study of acute idiopathic neuropathy. I. Clinical features and their prognostic value. J Neurol Neurosurg Psychiatry 51: 605-612.
13. (1988) United Kingdom transient ischaemic attack (UK-TIA) aspirin trial: interim results. UK-TIA Study Group. Br Med J (Clin Res Ed) 296: 316-320.
14. Herrmann C (1997) International experiences with the Hospital Anxiety and Depression Scale--a review of validation data and clinical results. J Psychosom Res 42: 17-41.
15. Buysse DJ, Reynolds CF 3rd, Monk TH, Berman SR, Kupfer DJ (1989) The Pittsburgh Sleep Quality Index: a new instrument for psychiatric practice and research. Psychiatry Res 28: 193-213.
16. Richards KC, O'Sullivan PS, Phillips RL (2000) Measurement of sleep in critically ill patients. J Nurs Meas 8: 131-144.
17. Ellis BW, Johns MW, Lancaster R, Raptopoulos P, Angelopoulos N, et al. (1981) The St. Mary's Hospital sleep questionnaire: a study of reliability. Sleep 4: 93-97.
18. Iber C, Ancoli-Israel S, Chesson A, Quan SF (2007) The AASM manual for the scoring of sleep and associated events: rules, terminology, and technical specification. (1stedn), American Academy of Sleep Medicine. Westchester, IL.
19. Benbow SJ, Wallymahmed ME, MacFarlane IA (1998) Diabetic peripheral neuropathy and quality of life. QJM 91: 733-737.
20. Taly AB, Veerendrakumar M, Das KB, Gupta SK, Suresh TG, et al. (1997) Sensory dysfunction in GB syndrome: a clinical and electrophysiological study of 100 patients. Electromyogr Clin Neurophysiol 37: 49-54.
21. Pentland B, Donald SM (1994) Pain in the Guillain-Barré syndrome: a clinical review. Pain 59: 159-164.
22. Karkare K, Taly AB, Sinha S, Rao S (2011) Temporal profile of pain and other sensory manifestations in Guillain-Barre' syndrome during ten days of hospitalization. Neurol India 59: 712-716.
23. Young JS, Bourgeois JA, Hilty DM, Hardin KA (2008) Sleep in hospitalized medical patients, part 1: factors affecting sleep. J Hosp Med 3: 473-482.
24. Call-Schmidt TA, Richardson SJ (2003) Prevalence of sleep disturbance and its relationship to pain in adults with chronic pain. Pain Manag Nurs 4: 124-133.
25. Floyd JA, Medler SM, Ager JW, Janisse JJ (2000) Age-related changes in initiation and maintenance of sleep: a meta-analysis. Res Nurs Health 23: 106-117.
26. Kanbayashi T, Ishiguro H, Aizawa R, Saito Y, Ogawa Y, et al. (2002) Hypocretin-1 (orexin-A) concentrations in cerebrospinal fluid are low in patients with Guillain-Barré syndrome. Psychiatry Clin Neurosci 56: 273-274.

27. Maier H, Schmidbauer M, Pfausler B, Schmutzhard E, Budka H (1997) Central nervous system pathology in patients with the Guillain-Barré syndrome. Brain 120: 451-464.

28. Feinberg I (1978) Efference copy and corollary discharge: implications for thinking and its disorders. Schizophr Bull 4: 636-640.

29. Rosenlicht N, Lee K (2000) Hallucinations in Guillain-Barré syndrome. Am J Psychiatry 157: 2056-2057.

30. Peralta A, Bentes C, Santos R (2006) Clinical and polysomnographic status dissociatus in Guillain-Barre syndrome. Clin Neurophysiol 117: 106-107.

Sleep Duration, Insomnia Symptoms, and Emotion Regulation among Black Women

Christie Racine[1], Kaushal Kalra[2], Mirnova Ceide[3], Natasha J. Williams[1], Ferdinand Zizi[1], Mauro V Mendlowicz[4,5] and Girardin Jean-Louis[1*]

[1]Center for Healthful Behavior Change, Department of Population Health, NYU Langone Medical Centre, NY, USA
[2]Department of Family Practice, SUNY Downstate Medical Centre, NY, USA
[3]Albert Einstein College of Medicine of Yeshiva University, Department of Psychiatry and Behavioural Sciences, NY, USA
[4]Department of Psychiatry and Mental Health, Universidade Federal Fluminense, NY, USA
[5]Institute of Psychiatry, Universidade Federal do Rio de Janeiro, NY, USA

Abstract

Introduction: This study explored the associations between sleep duration and emotion regulation among urban black women (mean age = 59 ± 7 yrs).

Method: Eligible women (n = 523) provided sociodemographic data during face-to-face interviews. We used the Comprehensive Assessment and Referral Examination Physical to measure health status; women also estimated their habitual sleep duration. We utilized a modified version of Weinberger's conceptual model of repression, the Index of Self-Regulation (ISE) to measure emotion regulation. ISE scores were derived by amalgamating the defensive subscale from the Social Desirability Scale and the anxiety subscale from the State-Trait Anxiety Inventory.

Results: The median habitual sleep duration was 7 hours; 20% of the women were short sleepers (<6 hours) and 6% were long sleepers (>8 hours). Short sleepers, rather than long sleepers, had a greater likelihood of reporting insomnia symptoms than those sleeping 6-8 hours [63.4% vs. 28.1%; X^2 = 41.87, p<0.001]. In the first logistic regression model, the odds of being a short sleeper for low regulators were 3 times greater than for high regulators [OR = 3.22 95% CI: 2.05-5.06; p<0.0001]. In multivariate-adjusted analysis, OR was reduced to 2.06, but remained significant. In the second logistic model, the likelihood of being a long sleeper among low regulators were 37% greater than for high regulators, but results were not significant [OR = 1.37, 95% CI: 0.62-3.01; NS].

Discussion: Short and long sleep duration are associated with reduced ability for emotion regulation. Women sleeping 6-8 hrs might be more adept at regulating emotions in their daily lives. Insomnia symptoms might mediate associations between emotion regulations and sleep durations.

Keywords: Sleep duration; Emotion regulation; Anxiety; Women; Race/ethnicity

Introduction

Several published reports have suggested that black race/ethnicity is independently associated with extreme sleep durations [1-3]. Short sleep, defined as sleeping less than 6 hours, which is decried as a public health hazard, is more prevalent among blacks [3,4]. Long sleep, sleeping greater than 8 hours, which is often associated with psychological illnesses, is likewise more prevalent among blacks [3-5]. While epidemiologic findings favour worse physical and psychological health outcomes individuals sleeping abnormally less or more than the population mode (7 hours), [5-9] little has been done to examine what specific illnesses might be associated with short or long sleep among blacks, an understudied population regarding adverse effects of inadequate sleep durations.

There is ample literature evidencing associations between extreme sleep durations and medical co-morbidities. Epidemiologic and clinical data has indicated that short or long sleepers are at high risk for obesity,[10] diabetes, [10,11] hypertension, [10] and cardiovascular disease [10,11]. There is a dearth of published studies addressing relationships of short/long sleep durations to psychological health. This is important since psychological illnesses negatively affect the sleep process [12-15]. Generally, depression, loneliness, and stress are related to sleep [16-18] Among women, in particular, increased depression and anxiety are associated with increased sleep complaints [19] To our knowledge, there are no published studies that have specifically addressed relationships of short/long sleep durations to psychological health among blacks. In a previous study, we noted that black women exhibiting a low level of emotion regulation [20,21] were more likely to report symptoms of insomnia [22]. Unfortunately, data on sleep duration were not available permitting the determination of whether blacks experiencing short or long sleep might have reduced ability to regulate their emotion.

The present study tested the hypothesis that emotion regulation would predict inadequate sleep (sleeping less than 6 hours or longer than 8 hours) among black women. Emotion regulation refers to individuals' ability to distance themselves psychologically from events discretely appraised as negative or situations that threaten their self-concept. The present study utilized a modified version of Weinberger's conceptual model of repression to capture individuals' level of emotion regulation [21]. We also explored whether the presence of insomnia symptoms would mediate associations between emotion regulation and sleep duration.

***Corresponding author:** Girardin Jean-Louis, Center for Healthful Behavior Change, Department of Population Health New York University School of Medicine, 227 East 30th Street, 6th Floor, Room 641, New York, NY 10016
E-mail: Girardin.Jean-Louis@nyumc.org

Methods

Data for the present analyses came from a community-based study assessing physical and psychological health among older adults in Brooklyn, NY. The study sample comprises 523 black women (mean age = 59 ± 7 yrs). The present analyses focused on associations of short sleep (< 6 hrs) and long sleep (> 8 hrs) with emotion regulation.

Procedures

Trained, quality-controlled interviewers administered several scales/questionnaires during face-to-face interviews conducted in the volunteer's home or a location of their choosing (usually a church or a senior center). Interviews lasted approximately 1.5 hours, and women completing the study received $25 for participating. The Internal Review Board at Long Island University approved the study.

Measures for the present analysis included sociodemographic and medical factors: age, education, income, and BMI. Physical health was measured with the Comprehensive Assessment and Referral Evaluation (CARE). Repressive coping was assessed with the Index of Self-Regulation of Emotion (ISE). According to Hoyle and Bradfield, self regulation, the means by which people manage their attention, thoughts, motivation, feelings, and behavior, is a unique and important predictor of consequential personal, social, and economic outcomes [23].

The CARE has been widely used to assess physical health of older individuals in minority communities. It has shown good construct validity [24] as well as concurrent and predictive validity; [25] sub-scales included in our analyses were: somatic complaint, sleep disorder, leg problems, heart disease, respiratory disease, arthritis, vision problems, and hypertension (Cronbach α = 0.86; 0.85; 0.86; 0.83; 0.72; 0.91; 0.85; and 0.92, respectively). Additionally, women were asked to estimate habitual sleep duration (using full hour units i.e., 5 hours, 6 hours, 7 hours, etc.); no information on specific sleep disorders was elicited during the interview.

The Index of Self-Regulation constitutes a modified version of Weinberger's conceptual model of repression [21]. According to Mendolia's research, the model stipulates that the interaction of individual differences in emotional responsiveness and situational threats to self-concept contributes to one's tendency to regulate emotional responsiveness. This model of repressive behavior posits that repressive copers are hypersensitive to both negative and positive emotional events, but they distance themselves from these events only when the situation threatens their self-concept [26-28]. Repressive coping refers to a person's belief that he or she is capable of conforming to rigid standards of self-control [20].

Mendolia's model represents an extension of conventional categorical measures of repression, which might not yield an accurate representation of observed variations in repressive coping [26]. This revised model accounts for the motivation and conditions in which repressors use a perceptual defense in response to negative and positive emotional events. In our analysis, ISE scores were derived following Mendolia's conceptualization, which amalgamates the defensive scale of the Social Desirability Scale (α = 0.73) [20] and the anxiety subscale of the State-Trait Anxiety Inventory (α = 0.75) [29]. Scores ranged from 0 to 52, with higher scores representing greater defensiveness/ repressive coping. According to this classification scheme, individuals have a repressive coping style when they are highly defensive (e.g., high score on the social desirability) scale, but also low in trait anxiety (e.g., low score on the manifest anxiety scale). Details on the derivation of ISE scores as used in our analysis have been reported elsewhere.[30]

The stress index scale used initially by the National Survey of Black Americans was administered to our participants [31]. Respondents rated on a 4-point scale the degree to which a set of items provoked stress in the past month or two. These stress-induced life events were health, money, job, and problems with family or marriage, problems with people outside the family, children, crime, police, love life, and racial conflict. Scores ranged from 0 to 29, and higher scores denoted greater stress levels (α = 0.81).

Statistical Analysis

To describe the sample, we used frequency and measures of central tendency. In preliminary analyses, Pearson and Spearman correlations were used to explore relationships between variables of interest. Chi's square test was employed to assess differences in categorical variables. For descriptive purposes, the sleep measure classified participants into three groups: those reporting short sleep (<6 hrs) or long sleep (>8 hrs) referenced to those reporting sleeping 6 to 8 hours. These cut-off points were chosen based on previous research showing health risks associated with short and long sleep durations [32-35]. The Index of Self-Regulation of emotion was dummy-coded as high regulator vs. low regulator using a median split.

To test the hypothesis that emotion regulation was associated with short sleep [<6 hrs] and long sleep [>8 hrs], we utilized logistic regression modeling. For both models: A) short sleep and B) long sleep, first we performed univariate logistic regression analyses to determine associations of emotion regulation with short or long sleep. Next, we performed multivariate logistic analyses to ascertain likely effects of several covariates including age, education, income, BMI, and a history of hypertension, respiratory disease, arthritis, heart disease, and vision problems. We also assessed the contribution of insomnia symptoms (i.e., difficulty initiating sleep, difficulty maintaining sleep and/or early morning awakening) in the logistic models. Before constructing the models, we assessed bivariate associations between hypothesized predictors and the dependent variable; only factors showing a p value < 0.05 were entered in the final model [36]. All analyses were performed using SPSS 18.0.

Results

Of the sample, 80% had at least a high school diploma. The median income of those women was $10,000, and the median BMI was 29 kg/m^2. Thirty-eight percent of the women reported heart disease; 66%, arthritis; 23%, respiratory disease; 60% hypertension; and 50%, vision problems. Thirty-six percent reported insomnia symptoms: difficulty initiating sleep, difficulty maintaining sleep, or early morning awakening. The median habitual sleep time was 7 hours; 20% of the women were short sleepers (<6 hrs) and 6% were long sleepers (>8 hrs). In Table 1, we compare the total number of women reporting differing sleep durations based on their classification as a low or high regulator.

Using Chi square tests, we found that women sleeping less than 6 hours habitually had a greater likelihood of reporting insomnia symptoms than those sleeping 6-8 hours [63.4% vs. 28.1%; $X^2 = 41.87$, $p < 0.001$]. We observed no significant difference in the likelihood of experiencing insomnia symptoms between women sleeping longer than 8 hours and those sleeping 6-8 hours [32.1% vs. 32.0%; $X^2 = 2.87$, NS].

We constructed two logistic regression models. Results of the

Self-Reported Sleep Duration Based on Level of Emotion Regulation (n = 523)		
Sleep	Emotion Regulation	
	Low Regulator (38%)	Hi Regulator (62%)
≤ 5 hours	60 (59.4)	41 (40.6)
6 hours	32 (38.6)	62 (61.4)
7 hours	42 (30.2)	97 (69.8)
8 hours	46 (29.9)	108 (70.1)
≥ 9 hours	11 (39.3)	17 (60.7)

Table 1: Comparison of low regulators and high regulators based on reported sleep duration; values represent number and percent of cases for each sleep category.

first logistic regression model showed that the odds of being a short sleeper for low regulators were 3 times greater than for high regulators [OR = 3.22 95% CI: 2.05-5.06; p <0.0001]. As shown in Table 2, in multivariate-adjusted analysis OR was reduced to 2.06, but remained significant; differences in age, education, income, BMI, stress level, and a history of hypertension, heart disease, respiratory disease, arthritis, and vision problems were adjusted. Results of the second logistic model showed that the likelihood of being a long sleeper among low regulators was 37% greater than for high regulators; however, results were not significant [OR = 1.37, 95% CI: 0.62-3.01; NS]. Results for each factor entered in the multivariate logistic models are shown in Table 2.

As expected, when the insomnia factor was added to the short sleep model, the odd associated with being a short sleeper for low regulators was significantly reduced [OR = 1.44, 95% CI: 0.82-2.52, NS]. We did not explore the addition of the insomnia factor to the long sleep model, as results of the initial model were not significant.

Discussion

Linking sleep with emotion regulation is not a novel concept. Many studies have shown that those two factors are intimately related, likely in a bidirectional fashion [37,38]. Although emotion regulation may vary across the lifespan, [39,40] relationships with sleep persist [37]. In the biological sciences recent data, on the interaction between sleep and emotion regulation has provided evidence supporting the view of a sleep-dependent emotional brain processing [41,42]. With emerging interest in the associations of emotions with sleep, a question has arisen as to the possible effects of reduced sleep time on the ability to regulate emotions, since sleep duration has declined over the years [5-9]. The present study demonstrates that women sleeping less or more than the population healthy sleep range (6-8 hours) might experience difficulty regulating their emotions.

The main finding of our analysis is that women classified as low regulators were at increased odds of being short or long sleepers, relative to women exhibiting a high level of regulating their emotions. Specifically, our first regression model showed that the odds of being a short sleeper for low regulators were 3 times greater than for high regulators. Likewise, our second logistic model showed that there was a 37% greater likelihood for low regulators to report sleeping longer than the average sleep time. Of note, when we adjusted for differences in sociodemographic and medical factors, the model explaining associations of emotion regulation with short sleep remained significant, although the adjusted odds ratio was reduced (OR = 2.06). That the model for long sleep was not significant, even before the inclusion of confounders, may be attributed to lack of statistical power to detect significance associations. Only 6% of the women reported long sleep durations, whereas 20% indicated short sleep durations.

As reduced sleep time is often associated with the presence of insomnia, we performed a separate analysis adjusting for potential effects of insomnia symptoms on relationships between emotion regulation and short sleep duration. In the present study, 36% of the women reported insomnia symptoms (i.e., difficulty initiating sleep, difficulty maintaining sleep, or early morning awakening). As expected, when the insomnia factor was added to the short sleep model, the likelihood of being a short sleeper for low regulators was 44% greater than for high regulators. These findings suggest that much of the effect of emotion regulation on short sleep seems to be mediated by the presence of insomnia symptoms. This is consistent with our previous analysis of community-based physical and psychological health data obtained from 1,274 women [22]. That analysis showed significant associations between emotion regulation and insomnia symptoms for both black [r_s = -0.43, p<0.0001] and white women [r_s = -0.18, p <0.0001]. Hence, although short sleep is independently associated with emotion regulation, one cannot discount the importance of insomnia symptoms in analysis examining effects of emotion regulation on short sleep durations.

Interestingly, we observed no significant difference in the likelihood of experiencing insomnia symptoms comparing women sleeping longer than 8 hours and those sleeping 6-8 hours. There is evidence suggesting that some individuals classified as long sleepers may experience insomnia symptoms, resulting from various medical [43,44] and psychological conditions [45,46]. It is of interest to examine effects of emotion regulation on long sleep duration in larger samples, providing data allowing adequate statistical control.

Our focus on individuals of black race/ethnicity was guided by data evidencing that short and long sleep durations are more prevalent among blacks, [3] and that blacks reporting sleep problems have significantly poorer physical health than other ethnic groups [47]. Future studies should investigate whether associations between emotion regulation and sleep durations would be similar for women from other racial/ethnic groups. In our previous study, we found that women of black race/ethnicity exhibited greater ability to regulate their emotions, relative to white women [22]. This differential racial/ethnic effect, in part, explained why black women reported fewer insomnia complaints than their white counterparts.

Our study has notable limitations. First, since we used an observational design, we could not establish the mechanism by which emotion regulation is associated with short or long sleep duration.

Associations of Emotion Regulation, Sociodemographic, Medical Factors with Sleep Duration				
	Model A: Short Sleep		Model B: Long Sleep	
Variables	OR	95% C.I.	OR	95% C.I.
Low Emotion Regulation	2.06**	1.22-3.48	1.87	.74-4.75
Age	1.04	.99-1.08	.92	.86-.99
Education	1.11	.82-1.49	1.38	.76-2.52
Income	1.00	.99-1.02	1.00	1.00-1.02
Stress	1.01	.97-1.05	1.10*	1.01-1.19
BMI	1.00	.96-1.04	.96	.89-1.04
Heart Disease	.57	.32-1.02	.67	.25-1.96
Hypertension	1.41	.82-2.43	.83	.32-2.17
Respiratory Disorders	.61	.35-1.06	1.11	.35-3.58
Arthritis	.88	.49-1.58	1.37	.49-3.77
Vision Problems	.53	.29-.99	2.63	.92-7.48

Table 2: Regression coefficients of the sleep duration measure on emotion regulation (High Regulator vs. Low Regulator), sociodemographic factors, and medical factors. The sleep measure included individuals who reported short sleep durations (<6 hrs) or long sleep (>8 hrs) vs. those sleeping 6-8 hours habitually; ** p<0.001.* p<0.05.

Second, we did not use a population-based representative sample of US adults. Thus, our results are not generalizable to other racial/ethnic groups. Notwithstanding these limitations, our study has several strengths. Many studies in the past have not specifically examined associations between emotion regulation and sleep durations, particularly among black women, an understudied population. Another strength of our study is that it examines association of emotion regulation with both short sleep and long sleep; previous studies have not examined long sleep as a correlate of emotion dysregulation. Future studies should explore those associations among Hispanic and Asian populations as well.

Acknowledgement

This research was supported by funding from the NIH (R01HL95799, R25HL105444, and R01MD004113).

References

1. Hale L, Do DP (2007) Racial differences in self-reports of sleep duration in a population-based study. Sleep 30: 1096-1103.
2. Stamatakis KA, Kaplan GA, Roberts RE (2007) Short sleep duration across income, education, and race/ethnic groups: population prevalence and growing disparities during 34 years of follow-up. Ann Epidemiol 17: 948-955.
3. Nunes J, Jean-Louis G, Zizi F, Casimir GJ, von Gizycki H, et al. (2008) Sleep duration among black and white Americans: results of the National Health Interview Survey. J Natl Med Assoc 100: 317-322.
4. Schoenborn CA (1986) Health habits of U.S. adults, 1985: the "Alameda 7" revisited. Public Health Rep 101: 571-580.
5. Qureshi AI, Giles WH, Croft JB, Bliwise DL (1997) Habitual sleep patterns and risk for stroke and coronary heart disease: a 10-year follow-up from NHANES I. Neurology 48: 904-911.
6. Kripke DF, Simons RN, Garfinkel L, Hammond EC (1979) Short and long sleep and sleeping pills. Is increased mortality associated? Arch Gen Psychiatry 36: 103-116.
7. Wingard DL, Berkman LF (1983) Mortality risk associated with sleeping patterns among adults. Sleep 6: 102-107.
8. Kripke DF, Assmus JD (1999) A duration ≥ 8 hours for sleep is not safer! Sleep Research Online 2: 144.
9. Patel SR, Ayas NT, Malhotra MR, White DP, Schernhammer ES, et al. (2004) A prospective study of sleep duration and mortality risk in women. Sleep 27: 440-444.
10. Buxton OM, Marcelli E (2010) Short and long sleep are positively associated with obesity, diabetes, hypertension, and cardiovascular disease among adults in the United States. Soc Sci Med 71: 1027-1036.
11. Krueger PM, Friedman EM (2009) Sleep duration in the United States: a cross-sectional population-based study. Am J Epidemiol 169: 1052-1063.
12. Kales JD, Kales A, Bixler EO, Soldatos CR, Cadieux RJ, et al. (1984) Biopsychobehavioral correlates of insomnia, V: Clinical characteristics and behavioral correlates. Am J Psychiatry 141: 1371-1376.
13. Patel SR, Malhotra A, Gottlieb DJ, White DP, Hu FB (2006) Correlates of long sleep duration. Sleep 29: 881-889.
14. Grandner MA, Drummond SP (2007) Who are the long sleepers? Towards an understanding of the mortality relationship. Sleep Med Rev 11: 341-360.
15. Strine TW, Chapman DP, Ahluwalia IB (2005) Menstrual-related problems and psychological distress among women in the United States. J Womens Health (Larchmt) 14: 316-323.
16. Riemann D, Berger M, Voderholzer U (2001) Sleep and depression--results from psychobiological studies: an overview. Biol Psychol 57: 67-103.
17. Cacioppo JT, Hawkley LC, Berntson GG, Ernst JM, Gibbs AC, et al. (2002) Do lonely days invade the nights? Potential social modulation of sleep efficiency. Psychol Sci 13: 384-387.
18. Akerstedt T, Kecklund G, Axelsson J (2007) Impaired sleep after bedtime stress and worries. Biol Psychol 76: 170-173.
19. Voderholzer U, Al-Shajlawi A, Weske G, Feige B, Riemann D (2003) Are there gender differences in objective and subjective sleep measures? A study of insomniacs and healthy controls. Depress Anxiety 17: 162-172.
20. Crowne, Marlowe (1960) A new scale of social desirability independent of psychopathology. J Consult Psychol 24: 349-354.
21. Weinberger DA, Schwartz GE, Davidson RJ (1979) Low-anxious, high-anxious, and repressive coping styles: psychometric patterns and behavioral and physiological responses to stress. J Abnorm Psychol 88: 369-380.
22. Jean-Louis G, Magai C, Consedine NS, Pierre-Louis J, Zizi F, et al. (2007) Insomnia symptoms and repressive coping in a sample of older Black and White women. BMC Womens Health 7: 1.
23. Hoyle R, Bradfield E (2010) Measurement and Modeling of Self-Regulation: Is standardization a reasonable goal? National Research Council Workshop on Advancing Social Science Theory: The Importance of Common Metrics. Washington, DC: National Institute on Drug Abuse and Department of Psychology and Neuroscience - Duke University. 1-39, 2010.
24. Teresi JA, Golden RR, Gurland BJ, Wilder DE, Bennett RG (1984) Construct validity of indicator-scales developed from the Comprehensive Assessment and Referral Evaluation interview schedule. J Gerontol 39: 147-157.
25. Teresi JA, Golden RR, Gurland BJ (1984) Concurrent and predictive validity of indicator scales developed for the Comprehensive Assessment and Referral Evaluation interview schedule. J Gerontol 39: 158-165.
26. Mendolia M (2002) An index of self-regulation of emotion and the study of repression in social contexts that threaten or do not threaten self-concept. Emotion 2: 215-232.
27. Mendolia M, Moore J, Tesser A (1996) Dispositional and situational determinants of repression. J Pers Soc Psychol 70: 856-867.
28. Mendolia M (1999) Repressors' Appraisals of Emotional Stimuli in Threatening and Nonthreatening Positive Emotional Contexts. Journal of Research in Personality 33: 1-26.
29. Bieling PJ, Antony MM, Swinson RP (1998) The State-Trait Anxiety Inventory, Trait version: structure and content re-examined. Behav Res Ther 36: 777-788.
30. Consedine NS, Magai C, Neugut AI (2004) The contribution of emotional characteristics to breast cancer screening among women from six ethnic groups. Prev Med 38: 64-77.
31. Jackson JS, Brown TN, Williams DR, Torres M, Sellers SL, et al. (1996) Racism and the physical and mental health status of African Americans: a thirteen year national panel study. Ethn Dis 6: 132-147.
32. Singh M, Drake CL, Roehrs T, Hudgel DW, Roth T (2005) The association between obesity and short sleep duration: a population-based study. J Clin Sleep Med 1: 357-363.
33. López-García E, Faubel R, León-Muñoz L, Zuluaga MC, Banegas JR, et al. (2008) Sleep duration, general and abdominal obesity, and weight change among the older adult population of Spain. Am J Clin Nutr 87: 310-316.
34. Patel SR, Hu FB (2008) Short sleep duration and weight gain: a systematic review. Obesity (Silver Spring) 16: 643-653.
35. Marshall NS, Glozier N, Grunstein RR (2008) Is sleep duration related to obesity? A critical review of the epidemiological evidence. Sleep Med Rev 12: 289-298.
36. Hosmer DW, Taber S, Lemeshow S (1991) The importance of assessing the fit of logistic regression models: a case study. Am J Public Health 81: 1630-1635.
37. Dahl RE (1999) The Consequences of Insufficient Sleep for Adolescents: Links Between Sleep and Emotional Regulation. Phi Delta Kappan 80: 354-359.
38. Baglioni C, Spiegelhalder K, Lombardo C, Riemann D (2010) Sleep and emotions: a focus on insomnia. Sleep Med Rev 14: 227-238.
39. Magai C, Consedine NS, Krivoshekova YS, Kudadjie-Gyamfi E, McPherson R (2006) Emotion experience and expression across the adult life span: insights from a multimodal assessment study. Psychol Aging 21: 303-317.
40. Kliegel M, Jäger T, Phillips LH (2007) Emotional development across adulthood: differential age-related emotional reactivity and emotion regulation in a negative mood induction procedure. Int J Aging Hum Dev 64: 217-244.
41. Walker MP (2009) The role of sleep in cognition and emotion. Ann N Y Acad Sci 1156: 168-197.
42. Walker MP, van der Helm E (2009) Overnight therapy? The role of sleep in emotional brain processing. Psychol Bull 135: 731-748.

43. Magee CA, Iverson DC, Caputi P (2009) Factors associated with short and long sleep. Prev Med 49: 461-467.

44. Gallicchio L, Kalesan B (2009) Sleep duration and mortality: a systematic review and meta-analysis. J Sleep Res 18: 148-158.

45. van Mill JG, Hoogendijk WJ, Vogelzangs N, van Dyck R, Penninx BW (2010) Insomnia and sleep duration in a large cohort of patients with major depressive disorder and anxiety disorders. J Clin Psychiatry 71: 239-246.

46. Vincent N, Cox B, Clara I (2009) Are personality dimensions associated with sleep length in a large nationally representative sample? Compr Psychiatry 50: 158-163.

47. Baldwin CM, Ervin AM, Mays MZ, Robbins J, Shafazand S, et al. (2010) Sleep disturbances, quality of life, and ethnicity: the Sleep Heart Health Study. J Clin Sleep Med 6: 176-183.

Dream Content Alalysis at the Initiation of CPAP for Obstructive Sleep Apnea

Sinziana Lovin[1]*, Carmen Rusu[2], Mihai Mutica[3], Anamaria Necula[4] and Costinela Georgescu[5]

[1]*University Lower Danube, Faculty of Medicine, Galati, Romania*
[2]*Psychotherapy practice, Galati Romania*
[3]*Hospital of Pychiatry, Galati, Romania*
[4]*Hospital of Pneumology, Timisoara, Romania*
[5]*University Lower Danube, Faculty of Medicine, Galati, Romania*

Abstract

Obstructive Sleep Apnea Hypopnea Syndrome (OSAHS) is a condition characterized by repeated episodes of airway obstruction during sleep, causing intermittent asphyxia and sleep fragmentation. The goal of this study was to assess dream content analysis before and during the first night of treatment for OSAHS using Continuous Positive Pressure (CPAP). We included 38 patients diagnosed using complete overnight polysomnography (PSG), who received CPAP therapy during a second night under PSG. Dream content (word count, thematic units, and emotional content) and the percent of REM sleep were analyzed after both nights. There was an increase in the percent of REM under CPAP (from 16,7% to 26,8%). There was an increase in the number of thematic units (1,36 without CPAP versus 1,82 under CPAP) and in the word count (30,52 without CPAP versus 45,22 under CPAP) and a change in the dream content (unpleasant content in 50% without CPAP versus 37,5% under CPAP). Under CPAP, more patients recalled their dreams than without CPAP (94,2% versus 57,9%). In conclusion, at the initiation of CPAP for OSAHS, there is a rebound of REM sleep associated with a quantitative increase in dream recall and a change in dream content.

Keywords: Obstructive Sleep Apnea Hypopnea Syndrome (OSAHS); Polysomnography; Continuous Positive Airway Pressure (CPAP)

Introduction

Obstructive Sleep Apnea Hypopnea Syndrome (OSAHS) is caused by repeated episodes of upper airway obstruction during sleep, associated with intermittent oxygen desaturation and sleep disruption. The main features of OSAHS are nocturnal breathing pauses and daytime somnolence caused by sleep fragmentation [1].

OSAHS is defined by the presence of 5 or more apneas (pauses exceeding 10 seconds) or hypopneas (significant flow reduction) per hour of sleep in symptomatic (somnolent) patients. The severity of OSAHS is expressed in terms of AHI (apnea hypopnea index per hour of sleep). OSAHS is mild for an AHI between 5 and 15 per hour, moderate for an AHI between 15 and 30 and severe for an AHI exceeding 30/h.

The gold standard for the diagnosis of OSAHS is polysomnography, a complex investigation including measurement of: electric brain activity during sleep, respiratory flow, pulse oxymetry and other parameters. The standard treatment for OSAHS is nocturnal ventilation with Continuous Positive Airway Pressure (CPAP), a mechanical aid which maintains airway patency and prevents intermittent asphyxia and sleep fragmentation [2].

Dreams are associated with the REM stage of the human sleep, characterized by rapid eye movements, intense unconscious brain activity, and muscle atonia. The only muscular activity in REM is represented by the oculomotor, cardiac and diaphragmatic movements. Since the ventilation is assured by the diaphragm alone in REM stage, patients with ventilatory impairments (such as emphysema, kyphoscoliosis, obesity etc) are at risk for desaturations especially during this stage. The oxygen desaturations produce micro-arousals responsible for sleep fragmentation and for a selective REM sleep deprivation. Patients with sleep disturbed breathing are REM deprived and present a rebound of the REM stage at the initiation of the therapy for their sleep disturbed breathing [3].

The literature addressing dream content in patients with OSAHS shows controversial data. Much of the literature shows that OSAHS patients report mostly dreams with negative emotional content. In some studies, patients with OSAHS report their dreams to be predominantly negatively toned prior to continuous positive airways pressure (CPAP) therapy and more negatively toned on non-CPAP nights compared to CPAP treatment nights [4,5]. Other studies report an inverse correlation between the severity of OSAHS and the negative content of the dreams and a higher amount of dream recall under CPAP therapy than without treatment [6,7]. The study published by Carrasco in 2006 [5] concludes dream recall is decreasing with CPAP, which is in contradiction to the other results in the literature.

Objective

To study dream content in patients with severe OSAHS at the initiation of nocturnal Continuous Positive Airway Pressure (CPAP) treatment for OSAHS in relation to the Rapid Eye Movement (REM) sleep stage.

Methods

Multichannel video-polysomnography was used to diagnose

***Corresponding author:** Sinziana Lovin, Faculty of Medicine, University Lower Danube, Galati, Romania, E-mail: sinziana_lovin@yahoo.com

OSAHS and to supervise the initiation of CPAP. We have included 38 consecutive patients with severe OSAHS and an indication for CPAP, who presented spontaneous awakenings in REM sleep during both nights (the diagnostic night and the first night under CPAP), and who relalled dreams during at least one of the nights. The second night under PSG (and the first night with CPAP) was not directly recorded after the first (diagnostic) night; the period between the two nights was 1 to 3 weeks. Exclusion criteria were: inability to speak, severe mental disorders, previous treatment for OSAHS (such as surgery or mandibular advancement splint), and patient refusal. The dream recall was elicited verbally by the medical staff who supervised the polysomnographic recordings. The dream recall was done immediately after the spontaneous awakening from REM sleep. Video recordings were used to analyze dream content (word count, number of thematic units, emotional content). A change in the thematic unit was considered when the main setting of the dream, the main character or the course of action changed. The emotional content was considered either positive, negative or neutral according to the theme expressed by the patient (the interpretation was made by an experienced clinical pshychologist) or according to the spontaneous interpretation offered by the patient. The percent of REM and the severity of OSAHS expressed by the number of respiratory events per hour of sleep (apnea-hypopnea index - AHI) were assessed using the polysomnography software.

The statistical analysis was performed using SPSS -18 and Excel for Windows Vista. Informed consent was obtained from all the patients included in the study. The review board of the Faculty of Medicine Galati approved the project before inception.

Results

In our group, there were 21 men and 17 women. The mean age was 57 years and the mean AHI was 52,05/h.

There were more thematic units in the dreams described under CPAP than during the night without CPAP (1,82 thematic units under CPAP versus 1,36 thematic units without CPAP; t Student's p<0.01), the patients used more words to describe their dreams under CAP (45,22 words under CPAP versus 30,52 words after the night without CPAP; t Student's p<0.05) and the percent of REM sleep was higher under CPAP than during the diagnostic night (26,81% REM sleep under CPAP versus 16,71% REM sleep without CPAP; t Student's p<0.01). Table 1 shows the characteristics of the whole group and the mean parameters before and under CPAP.

More patients recalled their dreams under CPAP than without CPAP: of the 38 patients, 32 recalled their dream content under CPAP (84.2%) versus 22 during the night without CPAP (57.9%). The dream content was less unpleasant under CPAP: 12 patients (37.5% of the recallers) reported unpleasant dream content under CPAP versus 11 patients (50% of the recallers) without CPAP. The dream content was neutral in 8 patients (25% of the recallers) under CPAP versur 8 patients (36% of the recallers) without CPAP. The dream content was pleasant in 12 patients (37.5% of the recallers) under CPAP versus 3 patients (14% of the recallers) without CPAP Figure 1.

Wher we compared men to women, the only parameter which has shown a significant diference was age (mean age in women was 61,64 years versus 53,85 years in men; t Student's p<0.05). The rest of

Parametert	Mean ± SD	
	Without CPAP	Under CPAP
Age	57.34 ± 10.34	
AHI	52.05 ± 14.43	
Men	21	
Women	18	
Word count	30.52 ± 18.37	45.22 ± 16.07
Thematic units	1.36 ± 0.56	1.82 ± 0.85
% REM	16.71 ± 4.68	26.81 ± 6.13

Table 1: The characteristics of group and the mean parameters before and under CPAP.

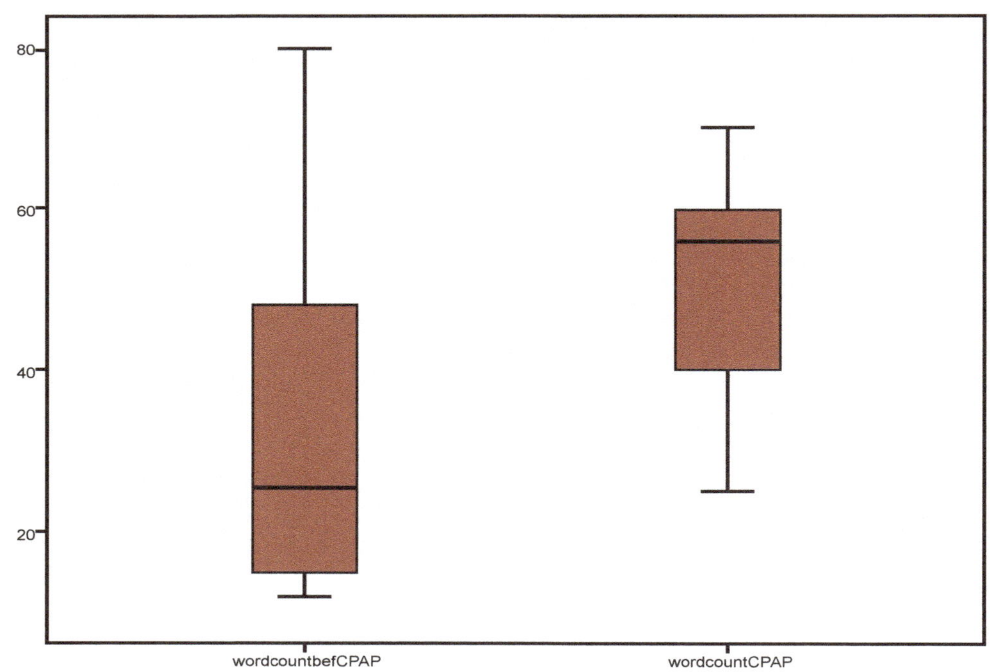

Figure 1: Word count before and under CPAP.

the diferences were non significant, although there was a tendency in women to have more thematic units and to express their dream content in more words then men, both before and under CPAP. Table 2 shows the values of the main parameters in men and in women.

There was a strong negative correlation between the severity of OSAHS expressed by AHI and the percent of REM sleep before CPAP (Pearson's r=- 0,59). The correlations between AHI and age, the word count before CPAP and with the number of thematic units before and after CPAP were non-significant (r<0.2, p>0.05). There was a surprising negative correlation between the AHI and the word count after CPAP (Pearson's r=- 0,66). In contrast with this finding, the percent of REM sleep under CPAP did not show a significant negative correlation with AHI; in other words, REM rebound under CPAP did not correlate with the severity of the condition prior to treatment. Figure 2 shows the scatter plot illustrating the negative correlation between AHI and the percent of REM sleep before CPAP.

Discussions

The possible explanations for the tendency to report dreams with a negative content in untreated sleep apnea would be nocturnal asphyxia on one hand and the tendency of OSAHS patients to be more depressive than other patients on the other hand. Regarding the alternative situation described in the literature (the increase of the negative content of the dreams under CPAP), the possible explanations may be the REM rebound under CPAP (with a more vivid content of the dreams), and a better cognitive function after the nights spent under treatment (with an improved capacity to recall dreams).

Our data are consistent with those in literature showing the increase in dream content under CPAP. There is also a change in the emotional dream content, which may be explained by the better quality of sleep, the lack of asphyxia, or an improved mood in the morning.

Women		Men	
Parameter	Mean ± SD	Parameter	Mean ± SD
Age	61.64 ± 6.25	Age	53.85 ± 11.75
AHI	49 ± 14.47	AHI	54.52 ± 14.27
Word count before CPAP	33.1 ± 24.32	Word count before CPAP	28.8 ± 13.80
Word count under CPAP	47.94 ± 17.37	Word count under CPAP	42.94 ± 14.99
Units before CPAP	1.5 ± 0.71	Units before CPAP	1.26 ± 0.45
Units under CPAP	1.87 ± 0.81	Units under CPAP	1.78 ± 0.91
%REM before CPAP	18.17 ± 5.17	%REM before CPAP	15.52 ± 3.98
%REM under CPAP	26.53 ± 6.56	%REM under CPAP	27.04 ± 6.17

Table 2: Main parameters in men and in women.

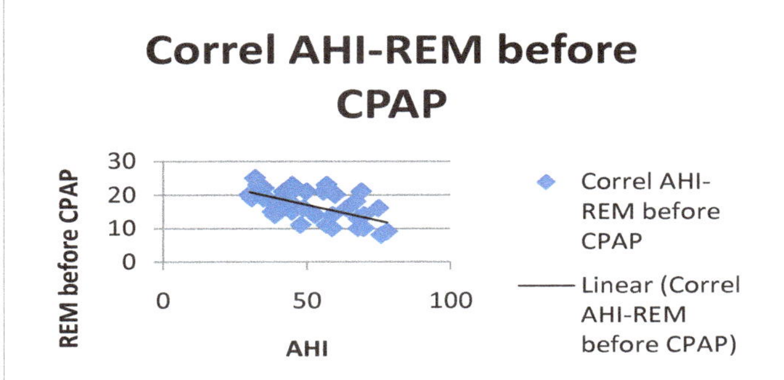

Figure 2: Scatter plot illustrating the correlation between AHI and the percent of REM sleep before CPAP.

The higher percent of the patients who are able to recall their dreams after the first night of therapy may be explained by a better cognitive function after therapy.

The paradoxical results reported by Carrasco et al. [5] is explained by the long extent of the observation period, which exceeds the interval in which REM rebound has been reported at the initiation of CPAP in most of the studies; in the study by Carrasco, dream recall decreased the first months of CPAP and recovered 2 years later [5]

In our study, an interesting aspect of the REM rebound under CPAP is that the percent of REM sleep without CPAP is suboptimal (16.71% REM sleep without CPAP, when the normal amount of REM sleep in adults is between 20% and 25%), while the percent of REM sleep under CPAP is 26,81%, which exceeds the normal range.

The clinical implications of the REM sleep rebound under CPAP may imply an increased severity of sleep disturbed breathing during the titration night, hypothetically requiring a higher therapeutic pressure during the first night of treatment [8].

Another aspect of the REM sleep rebound under CPAP is represented by the improvement in the subjective quality of sleep and an increased early compliance to CPAP [9]. One possible explanation for this association may be represented by an improvement in dream recall and in dream content, which are non-traditional markers of sleep quality. Dream content has been considered a mirror of mental health, especially in the psychoanalysis theory. More research is needed in order to properly assess the potential benefits of CPAP therapy on mental health, which have been so far massively related to an improvement in daytime vigilance, but which may encompass more subtle psychological pathways, such an improvement in dream mentation.

In our study,women presented their dreams using more words and thematic units than men, which is consistent with the general tendency of women to share their dreams more often than men [10]. However, dream sharing is a delicate subject and is influenced by many factors which have not been adressed in this study, such as age, social class and education, factors which might point to class-specific attitudes toward dreams.

Conclusions

There is a rebound in REM sleep associated with an increase in dream recall and a change in dream content at the initiation of treatment for obstructive sleep apnea. The severity of sleep apnea correlates negatively with the percent of REM without therapy and with the increase in word count under CPAP.

References

1. Sleep-related breathing disorders in adults: recommendations for syndrome definition and measurement techniques in clinical research (1999). The Report of an American Academy of Sleep Medicine Task Force. Sleep 22: 667-689.
2. Epstein LJ, Kristo D, Strollo PJ Jr, Friedman N, Malhotra A, et al. (2009) Clinical guideline for the evaluation, management and long-term care of obstructive sleep apnea in adults. J Clin Sleep Med 5: 263-276.
3. Brillante R, Cossa G, Liu PY, Laks L (2012) Rapid eye movement and slow-wave sleep rebound after one night of continuous positive airway pressure for obstructive sleep apnoea. Respirology 17: 547-553.
4. Gross M, Lavie P (1994) Dreams in sleep apnoea patients. Dreaming 4:195-204.
5. Carrasco E, Santamaria J, Iranzo A, Pintor L, De Pablo J, et al. (2006) Changes in dreaming induced by CPAP in severe obstructive sleep apnea syndrome patients. J Sleep Res 15: 430-436.

6. Schredl M, Kraft-Schneider B, Kröger H, Heuser I (1999) Dream content of patients with sleep apnea. Somnologie 3: 319-23.
7. Pagel JF, Kwiatkowski C (2010) The nightmares of sleep apnea: nightmare frequency declines with increasing apnea hypopnea index. J Clin Sleep Med 6: 69-73.
8. Sonka K, Kucerová O, Hoskovec P, Nevsímalová S (1994) Initiation of therapy in the sleep apnea syndrome using continuous positive pressure respiration. Cas Lek Cesk 133: 566-569.
9. Koo BB, Wiggins R, Molina C (2012) REM rebound and CPAP compliance. Sleep Med 13: 864-868.
10. Schredl M (2009) Sharing dreams: sex and other sociodemographic variables. Percept Mot Skills 109: 235-238.

Later Bedtime is Associated with Greater Daily Energy Intake and Screen Time in Obese Adolescents Independent of Sleep Duration

Kristi B Adamo, Shanna Wilson, Kevin Belanger and Jean-Philippe Chaput*

Healthy Active Living and Obesity Research Group, Children's Hospital of Eastern Ontario Research Institute, Ontario, Canada

Abstract

Objective: To examine if sleep timing (combination of bedtime and wake up time) is associated with energy intake and physical activity/sedentary behaviour in obese adolescents.

Methods: Participants included in this cross-sectional examination were 26 (13 females) obese volunteers (BMI ≥ 95th percentile) with a mean age of 13.6 ± 0.5 years and valid data on self-reported sleep, food intake (dietary record), physical activity and sedentary time (accelerometer), screen time (self-reported), and anthropometry (BMI). We categorized participants as "late sleepers" (midpoint of sleep >3:30 a.m., *n*=13) and participants as "normal sleepers" (midpoint of sleep ≤ 2:30 a.m., *n*=13).

Results: As expected, wake-up time and bedtime were different between sleep timing groups ($p<0.01$); however, total sleep duration was the same (9.23 ± 1.14 vs. 9.16 ± 1.28 hours for normal and late sleepers, respectively, $p=0.88$). There was no significant BMI difference between late sleepers and normal sleepers. Total daily caloric intake was 27% higher in late sleepers (425 kcal) compared to normal sleepers ($p=0.04$). Using a linear regression model in the whole sample we observed that later sleep timing was associated with greater total caloric intake, independent of age, sex, BMI, moderate-to-vigorous physical activity (MVPA) and sleep duration ($\beta=368.6$, $p=0.01$). No association was found between sleep timing and MVPA or sedentary time. However, later sleep timing was related to greater screen time, independent of age, sex, BMI and sleep duration ($\beta=105.7$, $p<0.01$).

Conclusion: The present study is the first to report that later bedtime is associated with greater caloric intake and screen time in obese adolescents independent of total sleep duration.

Keywords: Children; Adolescents; Food intake; Obesity; Physical activity; Sleep timing

Introduction

Childhood obesity has been widely identified as a complex condition, with a plethora of factors that are associated with its development. Accumulating evidence suggests that short sleep duration may be an additional determinant of obesity [1,2]. The mechanisms by which short sleep duration influence body weight are under investigation and might involve both sides of the energy balance equation. Experimental sleep restriction has been reported to increase appetite via an up-regulation of appetite-stimulating hormones [3]. Lack of sleep could also lead to weight gain and obesity by increasing the time available for eating and by making the maintenance of a healthy, physically active lifestyle more difficult [4]. In an environment where energy-dense foods are highly palatable and readily available, caloric intake may be directly proportional to the time spent awake, especially if most of wakefulness is spent in screen-based sedentary activities where snacking is common [5]. Furthermore, the increased fatigue and tiredness associated with not having enough sleep may impact overall physical activity participation [6].

In addition to the duration of sleep, sleep timing may also play an important role in energy metabolism and recent studies have set out to investigate the effects of misaligned sleep timing on health [7,8]. For example, an animal model experiment has shown that feeding mice at the "wrong time", i.e. when they are supposed to sleep, can lead to weight gain [9]. Interestingly, a 2011 observational study involving 52 adults has shown that "late sleepers" (midpoint of sleep ≥ 5:30 a.m.) consumed on average 248 more calories per day than "normal sleepers" (midpoint of sleep <5:30 a.m.), with the majority of the excess calories occurring at dinner and after 8:00 p.m. [10]. This finding suggests that greater caloric consumption in the evening may be a behaviour that links later sleep timing to obesity risk. Likewise, two recent cross-sectional studies by Australian researchers have shown that late bedtimes and late wake up times are associated with a higher risk of obesity and poorer diet quality in children and adolescents, independent of sleep duration, physical activity level and sociodemographic characteristics [11,12]. More specifically, children with a later bedtime/later wake time engaged in less Moderate-to-Vigorous Physical Activity (MVPA) and in more screen time compared to a group of early bedtime/early wake time children, despite having similar sleep duration [12]. Similarly, the same authors found that children with a later bedtime/later wake time had a higher Body Mass Index (BMI) Z-score and consumed more nutrient poor foods than the early bedtime/early wake time group [11]. Although the literature is still sparse, these novel findings suggest that sleep timing, particularly time to sleep, is an important factor to consider for health outcomes and behaviours that is distinct and separate from total sleep duration.

A better understanding of children's sleep timing behaviours is thus needed to determine whether children with late-to-bed behaviours engage in more sedentary time and/or consume excess energy, two

***Corresponding author:** Jean-Philippe Chaput, Ph.D, Healthy Active Living and Obesity Research Group, Children's Hospital of Eastern Ontario Research Institute, 401 Smyth Road, Ottawa, Ontario, Canada E-mail: jpchaput@cheo.on.ca

behaviours that may impact body weight. To our knowledge, the present study is the first to investigate sleep timing and its relationship with caloric consumption and activity patterns in a population of obese children and adolescents. The primary objective of this study was to determine whether sleep timing is associated with energy intake and physical activity/sedentary behaviour of obese children and adolescents. We hypothesized that obese children and adolescents with later sleep timing would have greater daily energy intake, lower MVPA and greater sedentary time than those going to bed earlier, independent of total sleep duration and other potential confounding factors.

Subjects and Methods

Participants

A sample of 62 obese children and adolescents aged between 8 and 18 years with a BMI greater than the 95th percentile [13] were recruited from the Children's Hospital of Eastern Ontario (Ottawa, Canada) endocrinology clinic to participate in the Physiological and Psychological Predictors and Determinants of Metabolic Complications of Pediatric Obesity (POC) study between 2008-2010. All new patients visiting the pediatric endocrinology clinic for an obesity assessment were eligible to participate in the POC study and 26 of the original 62 met the eligibility criteria for the current cross-sectional analysis. These included having 5 or more days of self-reported sleep data (time to bed and time to wake), 3 days of complete dietary recording and at least 4 days of valid accelerometer data for assessment of their sleeping, eating and physical activity behaviours, respectively. Further details of the study subjects are displayed in Table 1. The POC protocol was approved by the Children's Hospital of Eastern Ontario's Research Ethics Board and written informed consent (>16 years) or parental consent and child assent (≤ 16 years) were obtained before study initiation as required by the institutional ethics board.

Anthropometric assessment

Weight was measured to the nearest 0.1 kg using a medical grade SECA 634 calibrated digital scale. Standing height was measured to the nearest 0.5 cm using a wall-mounted SECA 222 stadiometer. Body mass index (BMI) was calculated as weight in kilograms divided by height in meters squared and BMI Z- scores were computed. These measurements were performed by trained research assistants according to standardized methods [14].

	Normal sleepers (n=13)	Late sleepers (n=13)	*p* value
Age (years)	13.3 ± 3.1	13.9 ± 2.0	0.53
Sex			0.24
Boys	5 (38)	8 (62)	
Girls	8 (62)	5 (38)	
Height (cm)	157.4 ± 12.0	164.4 ± 11.7	0.15
Body weight (kg)	91.6 ± 27.8	96.4 ± 19.6	0.61
Body mass index (kg/m^2)	36.4 ± 8.1	35.6 ± 6.4	0.77
Wake-up time (hour:min)	7:08 ± 0:41	8:06 ± 0:47	<0.01
Bedtime (hour:min)	21:54 ± 0:34	23:01 ± 0:55	<0.01
Sleep duration (hour)	9.23 ± 1.14	9.16 ± 1.28	0.88
Daily energy intake (kcal/day)	1590 ± 468	2015 ± 543	0.04
% Protein	19.3 ± 5.9	19.2 ± 4.3	0.94
% Carbohydrate	49.6 ± 8.0	48.1 ± 7.1	0.61
% Fat	31.1 ± 7.4	32.7 ± 7.5	0.57
MVPA (min/day)	28.2 ± 10.0	42.9 ± 4.9	0.03
Sedentary time (min/day)	575.6 ± 17.1	560.3 ± 26.4	0.64
Screen time (min/day)	137.5 ± 17.2	225.3 ± 52.4	0.13

Normal sleepers are participants with a midpoint of sleep ≤ 2:30 a.m. and late sleepers are those with a midpoint of sleep > 3:30 a.m.
Statistical significance was assessed by using an independent t-test with continuous variables and by a chi-squared test with categorical variables.

Table 1: Descriptive characteristics of participants (n = 26).

Sleep assessment

Participants were asked to self-report their respective time to sleep and time to wake for a 7-day period, and the average over 7 days was computed (bedtime, wake time, and sleep duration). Previous studies have found good agreement between self-reported sleep timing and objective measures such as actigraphy [11,15].

Classification of sleep timing groups

Midpoint of sleep for each participant was calculated by subtracting half of the total sleep duration from time to wake (e.g., 8:00 a.m. wake time – ½ 10 h slept = 3:00 a.m. midpoint). Participants were categorized a priori into two age-specific groups; children (≤ 12 years) and adolescents (≥ 13 years). The rationale for this stratification is based on the different sleep needs in these two groups [16]. In both age groups, "late sleepers" were defined as having a midpoint of sleep greater than the median and participants with a midpoint of sleep less than or equal to the median were classified as "normal sleepers" for subsequent analyses. The two normal sleep groups, initially stratified by age, were amalgamated into one group (normal sleepers, midpoint of sleep ≤ 2:30 a.m., n=13), and the same procedure was replicated for the late sleepers (midpoint of sleep >3:30 a.m., n=13).

Food intake assessment

All participants were instructed to complete a 3-day dietary record, including 2 week days and 1 weekend day. Participants were shown how to complete the record by the research coordinator who provided instructions about measuring the quantities of ingested foods. Subjects were instructed to log when they ate and what they ate at each meal and snack, during the 3-day period. If time for snack and meals were reported simultaneously, the two meals were merged for consistency. Mean energy and macronutrient intake was calculated using the ESHA food processor SQL dietary analysis software (ESHA Research, USA), with the 2007 Canadian Nutrient File. This method of dietary assessment has been shown to provide a relatively reliable measure of diet in this population [17]. Of note, the 3 days of dietary record data were matched to sleep data for each participant.

Physical activity and sedentary behaviour assessment

Participants were asked to wear an Actical accelerometer over the right side of their hip on an elasticized belt during waking hours for 7 consecutive days. The Actical device measures and records time-stamped movement in all directions and provides an assessment of physical activity level. A valid day was defined as at least 10 hours of wear time; respondents with 4 or more valid days were retained for analyses [18]. For each minute, the level of movement intensity (sedentary, light, and moderate-to-vigorous physical activity - MVPA) was based on published cut-points: sedentary equating to wear-time zeros plus observations less than 100 counts per minute (cpm) [19]; MVPA equating to 1,500 cpm or more [20]. For each child, minutes at each intensity level were summed for each day and averaged for all valid days. Further details on how the MVPA and sedentary time were derived from the accelerometers can be found elsewhere [18,21].

While accelerometers can accurately classify participant's behaviours as sedentary, they do not provide information about the type of sedentary behaviour or context. For this reason, daily screen time values were derived as a mean score of reported time spent watching TV/movies, playing seated videogames and spending time on computers outside of school or homework over a 7 day period. Although self-report measures provide reliable estimates of screen time, their validity remains untested [22].

Statistical analysis

Since there was no statistically significant gender interaction between sleep timing and the outcome variables, data for both sexes were combined to improve clarity and maximize power. Independent *t*-tests were used to test for differences between groups (late sleepers vs. normal sleepers). A chi-squared test was also used to assess statistical significance with categorical variables. Furthermore, we conducted a linear regression analysis to examine the association between sleep timing and daily energy intake, MVPA and sedentary behaviour. In the adjusted analysis, age, sex, BMI, MVPA (when not the outcome) and sleep duration were entered into the model to determine whether the association is independent of these covariates. All statistical analyses were performed using the Statistical Package for Social Science for Windows software (SPSS 20, IBM, USA). A two-tailed p value of less than 0.05 was considered to indicate statistical significance.

Results

Baseline characteristics of participants by sleep timing category are shown in Table 1. The midpoint of sleep for the children ($\leq$ 12 years) was 2:48 a.m., whereas the midpoint of sleep for the adolescents ($\geq$ 13 years) was 3:08 a.m. We observed no significant difference in the anthropometric measurements between sleep timing groups. As expected, time to wake and time to bed were significantly different between child and adolescent groups; however, total sleep duration was not different.

Total daily caloric intake was 27% higher in late sleepers (425 kcal) compared to normal sleepers, p=0.04, with no difference in macronutrient distribution. Figure 1 provides a visual representation of cumulative calorie intake across the day for a sub-sample, n=16, of participants for whom we had complete data on meal timing. Albeit not statistically significant due to the small sample size, this illustrates a tendency for greater food intake later in the evening (after dinner).

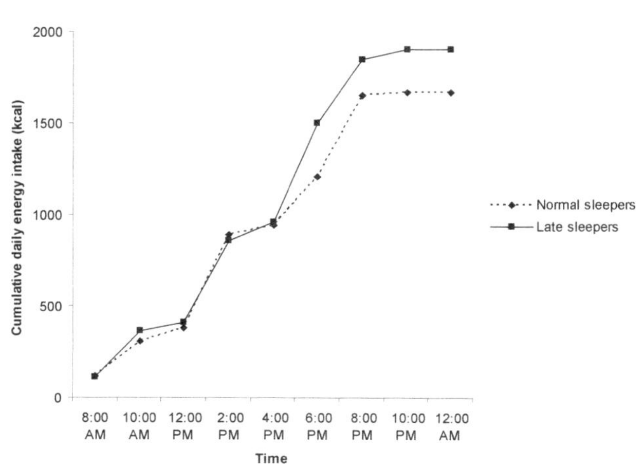

Figure 1: Cumulative daily caloric intake according to sleep timing (n=16 with complete data on meal timing).

MVPA was nevertheless significantly higher in late sleepers; however, late sleepers engaged in 88 min more daily screen time on average, p=0.13, than their counterparts categorized as normal sleepers.

The relationship between sleep timing in the whole sample and daily energy intake is shown in Table 2. We observed that later sleep timing behaviour was associated with greater total caloric intake in this cohort of obese adolescents, independent of sleep duration and other covariates. In the adjusted model (model b), 25% of the variance in daily caloric intake was explained by sleep timing and a 1-hour change in sleep timing was associated with a 369 kcal/day change in energy intake. However, when screen time was entered into the model the association became non- significant. We did not find any association between sleep timing and BMI Z-score (data not shown).

As shown in Table 3, the linear regression analysis did not identify a significant association between sleep timing and daily MVPA or sedentary time in this cohort. Later sleep timing was however related to greater screen time, independent of sleep duration and other covariates, p<0.01. In the adjusted model, 31% of the variance in screen time was explained by sleep timing and a 1-hour change in sleep timing was associated with a 106 min/day change in screen time.

Discussion

Collectively, this study showed that daily caloric intake was 425 kcal higher in late sleepers (midpoint of sleep >3:30 a.m.) compared to normal sleepers (midpoint of sleep ≤ 2:30 a.m.). Furthermore, later sleep timing was associated with greater daily energy intake, independent of sleep duration, BMI, and MVPA; however, the association became non significant after further adjustment for screen time, suggesting that screen time may be a possible mediator of the relationship between sleep timing and increased food consumption. Although sleep timing was not associated with MVPA, we observed that later sleep timing was associated with more screen time regardless of total sleep duration. These findings imply that sleep timing is an important aspect to consider with regards to eating and screen time behaviours in obese children and adolescents and that a narrow focus on sleep duration alone may not be enough.

Our results are concordant with those recently published by other researchers [10-12] showing that later sleep timing is associated with increased food intake and greater screen time engagement. Studies have also repeatedly reported that screen time promotes overconsumption of food [5], suggesting that it may not be surprising to observe a higher food intake later in the day if a large proportion of this time is spent in screen-time sedentary behaviour. However, previous studies in the field have mainly reported that short sleep duration (or experimental sleep restriction) is associated with increased food intake, possibly due to an up-regulation of appetite-stimulating hormones and a longer period of time spent awake [1-3]. The finding that later bedtimes and later wake up times are associated with greater food intake independent of total sleep duration is a novel observation and suggests that sleep timing is also an important additional aspect to consider in the control of energy balance. For instance, a later bedtime likely allows for more unprotected time (i.e. time not spent in school or engaged in a specific activity) for a child or adolescent to access and subsequently consume food or drink.

In contrast to recent findings published by Olds and coworkers [12], we did not find an association of sleep timing with adiposity indices and MVPA in the present study. The most plausible explanation for the lack of association between sleep timing and anthropometric measurements is the fact that the present study was conducted only in an obese sample of children and adolescents, thereby significantly reducing the inter-

	Beta	95% CI	r	p
Unadjusted model	359.8	59.7; 660.0	0.45	0.02
Adjusted model[a]	368.6	101.2; 636.0	0.50	0.01
Adjusted model[b]	141.9	-143.1; 426.8	0.21	0.31

[a]Model adjusted for age, sex, body mass index, moderate-to-vigorous physical activity and sleep duration.
[b]Model adjusted for screen time in addition to age, sex, body mass index, moderate-to-vigorous physical activity and sleep duration.
The beta coefficients represent the change in daily energy intake (kcal) for a 1-hour change in sleep timing.
CI, confidence interval.
N=26.

Table 2: Association between sleep timing and daily energy intake in obese adolescents.

	Beta	95% CI	r	p
MVPA (min/day) Unadjusted model	7.43	-1.88; 16.74	0.40	0.10
	6.36	-1.71; 14.4	0.39	0.11
Sedentary time (min/day) Unadjusted model	11.1	-34.5; 56.8	0.13	0.61
Adjusted model[a]	4.7	-20.9; 30.4	0.10	0.70
Screen time (min/day) Unadjusted model	125.7	42.1; 209.2	0.55	<0.01
Adjusted model[a]	105.7	36.4; 175.1	0.56	<0.01

[a]Model adjusted for age, sex, body mass index, and sleep duration.
The beta coefficients represent the change in moderate-to-vigorous physical activity or sedentary behaviour (min) for a 1-hour change in sleep timing.
MVPA, moderate-to-vigorous physical activity.
N=26.

Table 3: Association of sleep timing with moderate-to-vigorous physical activity and sedentary behaviour in obese adolescents.

individual variability in body size. Additionally, the fact that short sleep duration was the same for both sleep timing groups suggests that sleep duration may be more important in predicting adiposity, as previously reported [1], but that sleep timing may still negatively influence eating and screen time behaviours without necessarily impacting body weight. This observation is reinforced by the fact that late sleepers engaged in more MVPA than normal sleepers, thus suggesting that certain unhealthy behaviours (i.e. greater food intake and screen time) can be compensated for by a greater participation in physical activity so that the net impact on body weight is not different between both sleep timing groups.

Although counterintuitive, the observation showing that late sleepers engaged in more MVPA than normal sleepers is in line with recent studies showing large inter-individual variations in physical activity levels across different sleep patterns [23]. It is possible that physical activity participation is more related to individual motivation than to sleep timing per se. For example, restricted sleep has been shown to increase [24,25], decrease [6,26], or have no effect [27,28] on physical activity level in previous studies. Thus, the higher MVPA in late sleepers compared to normal sleepers can be seen as a balancing force for them; however, adjusting for MVPA did not reduce the association between sleep timing and daily energy intake (i.e. no change in the beta coefficient), suggesting that MVPA is not a major explanatory variable. In contrast, further adjusting for screen time substantially reduced the beta coefficient, suggesting that an important portion of the extra 425 kcal ingested by late sleepers may be attributed to snacking while engaging in screen time. In addition, a projected weekly accumulation of 2,975 extra kilocalories for late sleepers would not be fully compensated for by their approximately 98 extra minutes of weekly MVPA approximating less than 1,000 kcal. The residual positive caloric balance is not inconsequential.

The present study has limitations that warrant discussion. First, the cross-sectional nature of this investigation limits causal inferences. Second, the small sample size and preliminary nature of this study preclude any definitive conclusion and generalization of our findings. This is the first study to explore sleep timing and its relationship with caloric consumption and activity patterns in a population of well-phenotyped obese children and adolescents and the fact that many of our associations were significant despite the small sample suggests that the reported relationships are meaningful and relevant. Third, there are the commonly acknowledged limitations associated with self-reported measures (e.g. recall and social desirability bias). Finally, residual confounding is always a limitation in observational studies and the possibility that some unmeasured variables could influence the reported associations (e.g. maturation, socio-economic status, and family characteristics) is always a possibility.

In summary, the present study shows that later bedtime is associated with greater caloric intake and screen time in obese children and adolescents independent of total sleep duration. These substantial differences suggest that that bedtime is an important factor to consider that is separate and distinct from total sleep duration. Given that the higher energy intake associated with later bedtime appears to be partly explained by screen time, future studies should examine whether reducing screen time can positively influence feeding behaviour of late sleepers.

Acknowledgements

This study was funded by a Canadian Diabetes Association Innovation Grant (#IG-1-07-2307-KA) and equipment was supplied through a CFI /ORF Leaders Opportunity. The funding source had no role in the study design, collection, analysis or interpretation of the data, writing the manuscript, or the decision to submit the paper for publication. Kristi Adamo holds a CIHR New Investigator Award and an MRI Early Researcher Award. Jean-Philippe Chaput holds a Junior Research Chair in Healthy Active Living and Obesity Research. The authors declare no conflict of interest.

References

1. Chaput JP, Tremblay A (2012) Insufficient sleep as a contributor to weight gain: an update. Curr Obes Rep 1: 245-256.
2. Nielsen LS, Danielsen KV, Sørensen TI (2011) Short sleep duration as a possible cause of obesity: critical analysis of the epidemiological evidence. Obes Rev 12: 78-92.
3. Leproult R, Van Cauter E (2010) Role of sleep and sleep loss in hormonal release and metabolism. Endocr Dev 17: 11-21.
4. Chaput JP, Klingenberg L, Sjödin A (2010) Do all sedentary activities lead to weight gain: sleep does not. Curr Opin Clin Nutr Metab Care 13: 601-607.
5. Chaput JP, Klingenberg L, Astrup A, Sjödin AM (2011) Modern sedentary activities promote overconsumption of food in our current obesogenic environment. Obes Rev 12: e12-20.
6. Schmid SM, Hallschmid M, Jauch-Chara K, Wilms B, Benedict C, et al. (2009) Short-term sleep loss decreases physical activity under free-living conditions but does not increase food intake under time-deprived laboratory conditions in healthy men. Am J Clin Nutr 90: 1476-1482.
7. Johnston JD, Frost G, Otway DT (2009) Adipose tissue, adipocytes and the circadian timing system. Obes Rev 10: 52-60.
8. Rüger M, Scheer FA (2009) Effects of circadian disruption on the cardiometabolic system. Rev Endocr Metab Disord 10: 245-260.
9. Arble DM, Bass J, Laposky AD, Vitaterna MH, Turek FW (2009) Circadian

timing of food intake contributes to weight gain. Obesity (Silver Spring) 17: 2100-2102.

10. Baron KG, Reid KJ, Kern AS, Zee PC (2011) Role of sleep timing in caloric intake and BMI. Obesity (Silver Spring) 19: 1374-1381.

11. Golley RK, Maher CA, Matricciani L, Olds TS (2013) Sleep duration or bedtime? Exploring the association between sleep timing behaviour, diet and BMI in children and adolescents. Int J Obes (Lond) 37: 546-551.

12. Olds TS, Maher CA, Matricciani L (2011) Sleep duration or bedtime? Exploring the relationship between sleep habits and weight status and activity patterns. Sleep 34: 1299-1307.

13. Kuczmarski RJ, Ogden CL, Guo SS, Grummer-Strawn LM, Flegal KM, et al. (2002) 2000 CDC Growth Charts for the United States: methods and development. Vital Health Stat 11 : 1-190.

14. The Airlie (VA) Consensus Conference (1988) In: Lohman TG, Roche AF, Martorell R, eds. Standardization of anthropometric measurements. Champaign, IL, Human Kinetics Publishers, pp. 39-80.

15. Lockley SW, Skene DJ, Arendt J (1999) Comparison between subjective and actigraphic measurement of sleep and sleep rhythms. J Sleep Res 8: 175-183.

16. Centers for Disease Control and Prevention (2010) Sleep and sleep disorders. CDC features.

17. Ambrosini GL, O'Sullivan TA, de Klerk NH, Mori TA, Beilin LJ, et al. (2011) Relative validity of adolescent dietary patterns: a comparison of a FFQ and 3 d food record. Br J Nutr 105: 625-633.

18. Colley R, Connor Gorber S, Tremblay MS (2010) Quality control and data reduction procedures for accelerometry-derived measures of physical activity. Health Rep 21: 63-69.

19. Wong SL, Colley R, Connor Gorber S, Tremblay M (2011) Actical accelerometer sedentary activity thresholds for adults. J Phys Act Health 8: 587-591.

20. Puyau MR, Adolph AL, Vohra FA, Zakeri I, Butte NF (2004) Prediction of activity energy expenditure using accelerometers in children. Med Sci Sports Exerc 36: 1625-1631.

21. Colley RC, Garriguet D, Janssen I, Craig CL, Clarke J, Tremblay MS (2009) Physical activity of Canadian children and youth: accelerometer results from the 2007 to 2009 Canadian Health Measures Survey. Health Rep 22: 12-20.

22. Lubans DR, Hesketh K, Cliff DP, Barnett LM, Salmon J, et al. (2011) A systematic review of the validity and reliability of sedentary behaviour measures used with children and adolescents. Obes Rev 12: 781-799.

23. Klingenberg L, Sjödin A, Holmbäck U, Astrup A, Chaput JP (2012) Short sleep duration and its association with energy metabolism. Obes Rev 13: 565-577.

24. Brondel L, Romer MA, Nougues PM, Touyarou P, Davenne D (2010) Acute partial sleep deprivation increases food intake in healthy men. Am J Clin Nutr 91: 1550-1559.

25. Hursel R, Rutters F, Gonnissen HK, Martens EA, Westerterp-Plantenga MS (2011) Effects of sleep fragmentation in healthy men on energy expenditure, substrate oxidation, physical activity, and exhaustion measured over 48 h in a respiratory chamber. Am J Clin Nutr 94: 804-808.

26. St-Onge MP (2013) The role of sleep duration in the regulation of energy balance: effects on energy intakes and expenditure. J Clin Sleep Med 9: 73-80.

27. Bosy-Westphal A, Hinrichs S, Jauch-Chara K, Hitze B, Later W, et al. (2008) Influence of partial sleep deprivation on energy balance and insulin sensitivity in healthy women. Obes Facts 1: 266-273.

28. St-Onge MP, Roberts AL, Chen J, Kelleman M, O'Keeffe M, et al. (2011) Short sleep duration increases energy intakes but does not change energy expenditure in normal-weight individuals. Am J Clin Nutr 94: 410-416.

Abnormal Endocrine and Behavioural Sleep Markers in a Child with Williams Syndrome and Siblings

Dagmara Dimitriou[1,2]*, Anna Sniecinska[3] and Ray K Iles[4]

[1]Department of Psychology and Human Development, Institute of Education, London, United Kingdom, UK
[2]School of Health and Social Science, Middlesex University, London, UK
[3]Faculty of Health, Social Care and Education, Anglia Ruskin University, Chelmsford, UK
[4]Eric Leonard Kruse Foundation for Health Research, Scotland

Abstract

Background: Sleep is critical for optimal child development. However, the role of different variables that influence sleep functioning is still debatable. Children with developmental disorders such as Williams syndrome (WS) suffer from sleep problems throughout their childhood. Little is known about sleep patterns of their siblings.

Methods: Triplets, one of whom has WS and four typically developing (TD) children matched on age (7.8 years old) and gender participated in the study. Sleep was measured using parental sleep questionnaire and actigraphy. Salivary melatonin and cortisol were measured at three time points during the day.

Results: Abnormal sleep patterns, levels of melatonin and cortisol were found in a child with WS and her siblings.

Conclusion: These findings indicate that siblings of children with developmental disorders may also exhibit similar sleep problems. Use of multi-level examination should be adapted by paediatricians to devise sleep management strategies for such children and their families.

Keywords: Williams syndrome; Siblings; Cortisol; Melatonin; Sleep disorders

Introduction

Sleep is a complex behaviour, influenced by a multifaceted interplay between genetic and environmental factors. In particular, induction and maintenance of healthy sleep requires a finely tuned interplay of endocrine, neural and genetic mechanisms with environmental inputs. Accumulating evidence demonstrates that individual sleep EEG patterns are heritable traits [1]. However, environmental factors such as room-sharing, watching TV before bedtime or diet may also play an important role in causal pathways of sleep problems.

High prevalence of sleep problems in developmental disorders such as Williams syndrome (WS) have been reported [2-6]. WS is a genetic disorder caused by the hemizygous microdeletion of some 28 genes on chromosome 7q11.23 [7]. The incidence of WS is approximately 1 in 20,000 live births. The main cognitive characteristics of WS include an IQ levels ranging from 40 to 90, with the majority scoring between 55 and 69; relatively good face recognition and language skills and poor visuo-spatial skills [8]. Children with WS have been reported to suffer from difficulty in settling down at bedtime/falling asleep; prolonged awakenings from sleep and restless sleep. Yet, there are no studies examining causality of their sleep problems and whether their sleep differs from typically developing (TD) siblings. Thus far, studies examining sleep disorders in WS used tools such as questionnaires, actigraphy and/or polysomography. This is the first study to examine sleep profile via analysis of endocrine indicators of sleep patterns, melatonin and cortisol, in the saliva of a child with WS and her siblings. Melatonin (*N*-acetyl-5-methoxytryptamine) is a neurohormone secreted by the pineal gland involved in the regulation of the sleep-wake cycle and plays an important role in neuroprotection in the brain [9]. The secretion of melatonin is inhibited by light, and its level remains low during the daytime [10]. Cortisol (hydrocortisone) is one of the major glucocorticoid hormones secreted by the adrenal cortex. Cortisol levels rise during sleep, rapidly increase after awakening and decrease over the course of the day with nadir early in the sleep period [11-13].

We report cortisol and melatonin profiles of dizygotic female triplets: two of whom are TD, one with WS and typically developing unrelated control children. This is the first study to examine sleep in sibling of a child with WS using multi-level approach, i.e., levels of endocrine markers of sleep-melatonin and/or cortisol, actigraphy, and scores from CSHQ.

Methods

Participants

One female with full WS deletions in the critical region (verified clinically and genetically), two female siblings (Sib1 and Sib2) and 4 TD children matched for chronological age and gender took part in the current study. All children were 7.8 year old. Children in the TD group were not on any current or past medical and did not have any psychiatric or medical diagnosis such as epilepsy and poorly controlled asthma or eczema. Factors such as demographic information, medical and developmental history, and health habits were included as co-variant variables.

At the time of study, the triplets did not suffer from any medical

***Corresponding author:** Dagmara Dimitriou, PhD, Department of Psychology and Human Development, Institute of Education, London, United Kingdom
E-mail: d.annaz@ioe.ac.uk

conditions and were not taking any medications. All children had normal vision. Child with WS and Sib1 are right-handed whereas Sib2 is left-handed.

The triplet family was contacted via the Williams Syndrome Foundation UK. TD children were recruited through local primary schools. Ethical approval was granted by the Institute of Education, University of London Research Ethics Committee and The Williams Syndrome Foundation, UK. Both, parental informed consent and the child's verbal assent were obtained prior to participation.

Measures

Actigraphy: Sleep patterns were measured using actigraphy (movement monitoring), a reliable and valid method for assessing sleep and wake, which shows more than 80% agreement with overnight polysomnographic studies [14].

Each child wore an Actiwatch Mini (CamNTech, Cambridge, UK) on the non-dominant wrist continuously for one week. Data were downloaded to computer and each one-minute epoch was scored as sleep or wake using Sleep Analysis 7 (CamNTech, Cambridge, UK). Sleep start and sleep end were marked as the start and end respectively of a period of 10 or more minutes of immobility. The actigraphy variables of interest are: bed time (time the child is in bed with lights off), time in bed, sleep latency (time from bed time to sleep start), assumed sleep time (time from sleep onset to offset), actual sleep time (assumed sleep minus any periods of wake), night wakings (number of), wake after sleep onset, sleep efficiency (percentage of time spent asleep from sleep onset to offset), moving time (percentage of time spent moving from sleep onset to offset) and fragmentation (an indication of restlessness where a higher figure denotes increased restlessness). In addition, to support analyses of actigraphy data, parents completed a sleep diary recording their child's bed time, getting up time, as well as any daytime naps and night-time awakenings for the duration of the study.

Children's Sleep Habits Questionnaire: Parents completed the Children's Sleep Habits Questionnaire - CSHQ [15]. This is a 45-item caregiver response questionnaire which screens for the occurrence of common sleep problem symptoms in school-aged children. Parents indicate whether each listed characteristic occurs often (5-7 nights per week), sometimes (2-4 nights per week) or rarely (0-1 nights per week) for behaviours such as going to bed (lights out) at the same time each night, sleepwalking, bruxism or snoring. Satisfactory test-retest reliability of CSHQ subscales has been reported for both normal and clinical populations [15].

Melatonin and Cortisol: Levels of melatonin and cortisol were analysed in saliva, collected at three time points: between 4 – 6 pm, evening before going to bed and morning after awakening, using a commercial immunoassays (Salivary Melatonin ELISA - IBL International, Germany; Salivary Cortisol ELISA, Salimetrics Europe, UK). Samples were transported in cardice, centrifuged for 10 min at 3000 rpm, aliquoted and stored at -20°C until analysis. Melatonin in saliva samples (100 µl) were assayed in duplicate by competitive enzyme linked immunosorbent assay (ELISA) with the use of reagents obtained from IBL International, Germany. After adding the substrate, chromophore was formed in inverse proportion to the amount of melatonin and the absorbance was measured by a plate reader (FLUOstar OPTIMA, BMG LABTECH) at 450 nm. The sensitivity of the assay was 0.3 $pgmL^{-1}$.

Levels of cortisol in saliva samples (25 µl) were assayed in duplicate by competitive enzyme immunoassay kit with the use of reagents from Salimetrics Europe, UK. The density of obtained colour was inversely proportional to the amount of cortisol in the analysed sample and the absorbance was measured by a plate reader (FLUOstar OPTIMA, BMG LABTECH) at 450 nm. The sensitivity of the assay was 0.003 μgdL^{-1}.

Although actual levels are recorded, due to the inherent high variability of levels of melatonin and cortisol between individuals and during the day, levels of both hormones were also normalised (set as 100%) based on morning levels of melatonin and cortisol. The usual pattern for melatonin is high at night and low during the day since the synthesis being suppressed by sunlight, in contrast, cortisol is high upon waking and lowering before sleep.

Results

Table 1 presents the results from triplets and matched TD controls on sleep measures and endocrine profiles. Data were analysed using SPSS for Windows, Version 19 (SPSS Inc., Chicago, IL). A number of *t*-tests were carried out followed by inter-group comparisons. Post-hoc comparisons were made using.

Discussion

In line with the previous studies [2,3], the current data based on CSHQ show that the child with WS suffers from sleep problems. However this study also reveals that siblings also suffer from sleep problems, namely, frequent night waking for all three children and daytime sleepiness was shown by the child with WS and Sib1 were

Measures	WS	Sib 1	Sib 2	TD (n=4)
	CSHQ scores			
CSHQ total score	**47**	44	37	39‡
Bedtime resistance	7.0	6.0	6.0	7.0 (1.6)
Sleep onset delay	2.0	3.0	1.0	1.3 (.5)
Sleep duration	4.0	5.0	3.0	3.7 (1.1)
Sleep anxiety	4.0	4.0	4.0	5 (1.2)
Night waking	**6.0**	**5.0**	**5.0**	3.3 (.6)
Parasomnias	7.0	7.0	8.0	8.0 (1.4)
Sleep disordered breathing	3.0	3.0	3.0	3.2 (.5)
Daytime sleepiness	**16.0**	**13.0**	9.0	11.6 (2.5) †
	Actigraphy scores			
Wake time (hr)	**1.85**	**1.25**	**1.73**	0.51*
Actual wake time (%)	**19.07**	**13.33**	**16.77**	5.3*
Actual sleep time (hr)	**7.83**	**8.13**	**8.57**	9.17*
Actual sleep time (%)	**80.93**	**86.67**	**83.23**	94.7*
Sleep latency	**69.33**	**86.67**	22.67	20.33†
Sleep efficiency	**72.3**	**75**	**79.13**	89.97*
	Melatonin			
Afternoon	**0.75**	**0.15**	**0.26**	3.27*
Normalized	**18.47**	**2.64**	**5.96**	99.84*
Evening	**0.15**	**0.15**	**0.7**	12.31*
Normalized	**3.69**	**2.64**	**16.05**	375.45*
Morning	**4.06**	**5.67**	**4.36**	3.28
	Cortisol			
Afternoon	0.1	0.06	**0.31**	0.06
Normalised	**83.33**	**42.85**	**96.87**	25*
Evening	0.05	0.02	0.04	0.03‡
Normalised	**41.66**	14.28	12.5	12.5
Morning	0.12	0.14	0.32	0.24

Significant problems are highlighted in **bold**.
* = Significant difference between TD and all siblings
† = Significant difference between TD and WS and Sib1
‡ = Significant difference between TD and WS

Table 1: Scores on sleep measures, melatonin and cortisol.

reported by parents. More sleep problems and similarities amongst siblings were seen in actigraphy data. Child with WS showed the highest actual wake time, and as a consequence, lowest actual sleep time during the night. Sleep efficiency was also the lowest in this child. The time taken to fall asleep by the child with WS was 69 minutes and her Sib1 showed even higher sleep latency of 86 minutes.

In healthy population, melatonin levels increase before bedtime what is a factor facilitating sleep [10]. This pattern was observed in TD controls, whereas the triplets' melatonin levels were remarkably lower in both the afternoon and evening respectively. Also, cortisol actual levels were lower in the afternoon and evening for controls, siblings and WS individual. However, the normalised cortisol level in the evening did not decrease as much as seen in controls and siblings. Indeed at 46% of morning maxima this is approximately 3 fold higher in the child with WS compared to the unaffected siblings and the TD control.

However, unlike the melatonin normalized levels, normalized cortisol revealed a much more significant difference to controls than the siblings. This may indicate that cortisol is more closely associated with the pathophysiology of sleep disturbance in WS whilst melatonin is more associated with environmental psychophysiology of sleep disturbance in households with WS individuals and unaffected siblings.

Thus far, very few studies have been carried out to analyse endocrine sleep markers in children with developmental disabilities and none of them included individuals with WS and their siblings. The current results confirm that the child with WS indeed has sleep disturbances. Moreover, it demonstrates that this may be a result of mixed aetiology of environmental and pathophysiology since the siblings also displayed clear evidence of sleep disturbance. Abnormal levels of melatonin may be linked to family environmental influence (i.e. lack of night routine and lights out management, one child waking up another etc.) whilst cortisol relates to stress and perhaps a pathophysiology anxiety which is a known feature of WS.

The current study shows that the use of clinical chemistry biomarkers may greatly advance the definition of "caseness" in psychology evaluations [16]. Sleep is a very complex state and can be influenced by multiple factors hence future studies ought to verify impact of home environment on the child's and family cognitive health. Moreover, if we are to establish successful sleep management for children with developmental disorders, careful assessment of family sleep profiles should also be taken [17,18]. What is apparent from sleep literature is that sleep problems have a huge negative impact on academic performance and family functioning as whole. Thus an appropriate intervention would be to train all siblings to adhere to sleep habits routine as early in development as possible [3,19,20].

Acknowledgements

We would like to thank all the parents and children for participating in this study, The UK Williams Syndrome Foundation, UK for their continuous support. This study was funded by the Autour des Williams, France.

References

1. Toth LA (2001) Identifying genetic influences on sleep: an approach to discovering the mechanisms of sleep regulation. Behav Genet 31: 39-46.
2. Annaz D, Hill CM, Ashworth A, Holley S, Karmiloff-Smith A (2011) Characterisation of sleep problems in children with Williams syndrome. Res Dev Disabil 32: 164-169.
3. Ashworth A, Hill CM, Karmiloff-Smith A, Dimitriou D (2013) Cross syndrome comparison of sleep problems in children with Down syndrome and Williams syndrome. Res Dev Disabil
4. Goldman SE, Malow BA, Newman KD, Roof E, Dykens EM (2009) Sleep patterns and daytime sleepiness in adolescents and young adults with Williams syndrome. J Intellect Disabil Res 53: 182-188.
5. Mason TB, Raanan Arens, Jaclyn Sharman, Brooke Bintliff-Janisak, Brian Schultz, et al. (2011) Sleep in children with Williams syndrome. Sleep Med 12:892-827.
6. Youssef NA (2012) ADHD, Sleep Disorders, and other General Medical Conditions: Recommendations for DSM V. J Sleep Disord Ther 1: e106.
7. Chen H (2006) Atlas of genetic diagnosis and counseling, Williams Syndrome. Humana Press:1040-46.
8. Annaz D, Karmiloff-Smith A, Johnson MH, Thomas MS (2009) A cross-syndrome study of Development of holistic face recognition in children with Autism, Down syndrome and Williams syndrome. J Exp Child Psychol 102: 456-486.
9. Clarke M, Crockett S, Sims B (2012) Melatonin Induces Neuroprotection via System Xc Regulation in Neural Stem Cells. J Stem Cell Res Ther 2:120.
10. Claustrat B, Brun J, Chazot G (2005) The basic physiology and pathophysiology of melatonin. Sleep Med Rev 9: 11-24.
11. Rai B, Kaur J (2012) Salivary Stress Markers, Depression, Mood State and Back Pain in Healthy Men in Two Bed Rest Conditions: Validation of Two Models for Human Space Flight. J Aeronaut Aerospace Eng 1:106.
12. Spath-Schwalbe E, Gofferje M, Kern W, Born J, Fehm HL (2003) Sleep disruption alters nocturnal ACTH and cortisol secretory patterns. Biol Psy 29: 575-584.
13. Talbott S (2007) The cortisol connection: Why stress makes you fat and ruins your health- And what you can do about it. (2ndedn), Hunter House.
14. Sadeh A. Hauri P, Kripke D, Lavie P (1995) The role of actigraphy in sleep medicine. Sleep, 18:288-302.
15. Owens JA, Spirito A, McGuinn M (2000) The Children's Sleep Habits Questionnaire (CSHQ): Psychometric properties of a survey instrument for school-aged children. Sleep 23: 1043-1051.
16. Shanker A (2011) Neuroendocrine crosstalk of immunity. J Blood Lymph 1: e105.
17. Baglioni C, Riemann D (2012) Cognitive-Behavioral Treatment for Insomnia Comorbid with Psychiatric Disorders. J Sleep Disorders Ther 1: e112.
18. Singh NK, Bhattacharjee D, Goyal N, Munda SK, Nizamie SH (2012) Perceive Family Environment among Parents, Spouses and Siblings of Alcohol Dependence Patients: A Comparative Study. J Addict Res Ther 3: 126.
19. Field T, Diego M, Delgado J, Medina L (2012) Yoga and Social Support Reduce Prenatal Depression, Anxiety and Cortisol. J Yoga Phys Ther 2: 124.
20. Susan E. Ramsey, Patricia A. Engler, Michael D. Stein, Richard A. Brown, Patricia Cioe, et al. (2011) Effect of CBT on Depressive Symptoms in Methadone Maintenance Patients Undergoing Treatment for Hepatitis C. J Addict Res Ther 2: 109.

A Brief and Selective Review of Treatment Approaches for Sleep Disturbance following Traumatic Brain Injury

Mareen Weber*, **Christian A Webb and William DS Killgore**

McLean Hospital, Harvard Medical School, USA

Abstract

Sleep disturbance often presents as a clinically significant symptom of Traumatic Brain Injury (TBI). Poor sleep may delay recovery, exacerbate psychiatric comorbidities, and even increase suicidal risk among TBI patients. Thus, effective and efficient treatment of sleep disturbance in this population is critical. This review provides a brief, selective, and focused synopsis of several of the more common and empirically tested pharmacological and behavioral approaches and their efficacy in the treatment of sleep disturbance following TBI. Depending on the nature of the injury and the specific sleep-related problems, there may be appropriate uses for pharmacologic interventions such as hypnotic or wake-promoting agents, cognitive-behavioral therapy, sleep hygiene, circadian rhythm modification, or even alternative medicine approaches. Overall, the literature on this important topic is sparse, and existing studies are hampered by relatively small sample sizes, under representation of youth and females, inconsistencies across reports in both time since injury and injury severity. Existing methodological limitations do not currently allow for definitive conclusions regarding the effectiveness of particular treatment approaches. Future research will not only need to address these limitations, but also develop treatment options for children and adolescents, who are currently underrepresented in the literature.

Keywords: Sleep; Traumatic brain injury; Treatment; Therapy; Melatonin; Modafinil; CBT-I; Blue light; Sleep-hygiene

Introduction

Sufficient sleep, both in terms of quantity and quality, is essential for cognitive performance and emotional wellbeing [1], and plays an important role in an individual's overall subjective quality of life [2]. Without sufficient restorative sleep, a person's reaction time is slowed, attentional lapses are more frequent [3,4], and there is an increased risk of work-related injuries and motor vehicle accidents [5]. Lack of sleep affects mood [6], emotional coping capacities [7], and even leads to increased symptoms of anxiety and depression among healthy individuals [8]. At the highest cognitive and emotional levels, sleep loss can degrade decision-making [9,10] and impair complex judgment and reasoning capacities [11,12]. Moreover, insufficient restorative sleep can lead to a number of health-related problems, including greater risk of weight gain and obesity, type 2 diabetes, metabolic problems, and hypertension [13,14]. Thus, regardless of the factors involved, chronically disturbed sleep can have adverse effects on health, emotional wellbeing, and normal cognitive functioning. It is therefore essential for medical practitioners and other clinicians to be aware of the presence of sleep disorders and to provide effective and efficient treatment of these problems when they are identified.

Whereas patients who present with primary sleep complaints, such as insomnia or sleep-related breathing problems, may be easy to identify, there are often clinical situations in which a patient may also have a sleep disorder that goes undiagnosed and untreated because it is not the primary presenting problem. This may often be the case among patients recovering from Traumatic Brain Injury (TBI). Following a TBI, physicians and other practitioners may focus on more overt problems associated with the injury and fail to adequately assess the presence of sleep-related problems in these patients. In fact, recent studies suggest that sleep problems may actually be some of the most common complaints among patients with TBI, with nearly half reporting some insomnia-related problems following their injury [15]. This is particularly troublesome, as sleep may be a vital component of the brain repair and recovery process. For instance, recent animal research suggests that sleep may play a critical role in neural plasticity. Lack of sleep appears to suppress the proliferation of new hippocampal neurons in the dentate gyrus of laboratory animals independent of its effects on circadian disruption or stress hormones [16,17]. Perhaps even more importantly, sleep appears to be essential in the process of neural re growth and regeneration following experimentally induced brain lesions in animals [16,18-20]. For example, rats subjected to experimentally manipulated sleep disturbance following an induced cerebral ischemic stroke showed significantly poorer recovery of function in the post-stroke period compared to those with normal sleep [19]. Thus, emerging evidence suggests that sleep is an important factor in healthy brain development, and plays a vital role in the growth and regeneration of neurons following brain damage.

The role of sleep in recovery from brain injury suggests that treating sleep disturbance in neurological conditions such as TBI might be particularly important in facilitating maximal recovery. Indeed, poor sleep, one of the most frequently reported TBI-related symptoms [21], was shown to complicate recovery from brain injury [22]. The need for effective and efficient treatment protocols in the context of TBI can be assumed to be substantial given the high prevalence and incidence of TBI in both civilian and military personnel – approximately 1.7 million TBIs occur annually in the United States alone [23]. Moreover, approximately 50% of TBI patients report some type of subjective sleep disturbance following their injury [15]. In fact, irrespective of injury

***Corresponding author:** Mareen Weber, McLean Hospital, Harvard Medical School, 115 Mill St, Belmont, MA 02178, USA
E-mail: mweber@mclean.harvard.edu

severity, subjective complaints of poor sleep such as difficulty falling or staying asleep, increased need for daytime naps, excessive daytime sleepiness, or increased fatigue may emerge at any stage following TBI [24]. Furthermore, these complaints appear to increase for up to six weeks following the injury [25] and are often still apparent even 3 years later [26]. Notably, for those patients still in the hospital, sleep maintenance difficulties were most common (81%), while problems with excessive daytime sleepiness were most frequently reported among patients following discharge (73%). In addition to high rates of subjective complaints of insomnia and other sleep problems, TBI patients also show some evidence of objective sleep changes, such as reduced Rapid Eye Movement (REM) sleep and increased stage 2 Non-Rapid Eye Movement (NREM) sleep compared to healthy controls [27]. Another study reported greater slow wave NREM sleep among military veteran patients with TBI compared to veterans with other clinical conditions, and also showed that these patients spent significantly less sleep time awake compared to other groups [28]. However, the evidence for objective sleep problems identified via polysomnography is considerably less consistent than that for subjective complaints [24]. While it is possible that a preexisting subjective sleep problem might worsen following a TBI, a substantial proportion of the sleep disturbances seen following TBI are believed to be a direct result of the injury itself [29].

Matters are complicated by the fact that neither TBI nor sleep disturbance are uniform constructs. The manifestation of TBI can vary greatly depending on the severity of the injury (i.e., mild, moderate, severe), the type of injury (e.g., blunt trauma; open head wound; blast-related; etc.), and the direction of force and location of damage within the brain. Furthermore, these factors may also contribute to the heterogeneous expression of sleep disruption among TBI patients. Some patients may experience higher rates of obstructive sleep apnea, narcolepsy, or periodic limb movements [30,31], while others may experience circadian rhythm disruption such as delayed sleep phase disorder [32]. A recent prospective study using clinician ratings reported that 84% of TBI patients showed evidence of sleep-wake cycle abnormalities at admission to a rehabilitation unit within days after injury, which declined to 66% within one month following their TBI [33]. Interestingly, the severity of sleep disturbance also predicted duration of post-traumatic amnesia. Some patients may experience symptoms consistent with sleep onset insomnia, while others may fall asleep relatively easily but have difficulty maintaining sleep throughout the night. For many, excessive daytime sleepiness or fatigue may be the primary problem [24]. Depending on the nature of the specific sleep disorder, some treatments will be more or less effective, so it is imperative that the clinician conduct a thorough assessment to identify the idiosyncratic sleep problems presented by the patient and tailor treatments to address their particular symptoms or underlying causes.

Within the context of TBI, poor sleep may also exacerbate comorbid psychiatric disorders such as depression or anxiety, or even the experience of pain [25,34]. Of note, insomnia following combat-related mild TBI was shown to predict suicidality [35], highlighting the vital importance of treating sleep disturbance following TBI. These injuries may also be associated with changes in sleep micro- and macro architecture, reduced sleep efficiency, more nighttime awakenings, prolonged sleep onset latency, and increased sleep fragmentation [24], although the clinical significance and reproducibility of many of these changes is uncertain due to the large inconsistencies and methodological limitations across much of the existing literature. Likewise, the empirical evidence of neuropsychological and neurophysiologic correlates of subjective or objective sleep disturbance following TBI is inconsistent at best, and does not allow for the formation of robust conclusions presently [24]. Despite the high prevalence and incidence of subjective sleep disturbance following TBI, the current literature provides little consistent guidance on effective treatment options. Consequently, many clinicians may be generally unaware of the magnitude of the problem of sleep disturbance following TBI and have little information regarding currently accepted treatment approaches. To address this dearth of information, we provide a brief and selective review of the most widely explored treatments for sleep problems following TBI. The present review is not meant to be an exhaustive description or comprehensive evaluation of the scientific literature on sleep treatments. Rather, we selectively reviewed the literature and present a concise overview of the most well-accepted and potentially promising treatments, while highlighting some of the major gaps in the current knowledge about these approaches. These are covered briefly below in the following sections: hypnotic interventions, wake-promoting interventions, Cognitive Behavioral Therapy (CBT) & sleep hygiene, circadian rhythm interventions, and alternative approaches.

Hypnotic interventions

Because patients with TBI often complain of symptoms of insomnia (i.e., problems with sleep onset, sleep maintenance, or delayed sleep phase disorder), there may be occasions where sleep-inducing medications may be prescribed. Such medications may be useful for short-term treatment of sleeplessness. However, the use of sedative-hypnotic agents to promote sleep in adults with TBI is controversial and even discouraged by some, as TBI is often associated with an already high medication burden [36]. More importantly, however, it has been suggested that sleep inducers may potentially delay cognitive recovery from TBI [37] and leave subjective complaints of poor sleep unaffected [38]. In particular, Larson and Zollman [37] reported that typical sleep inducers such as benzodiazepines and atypical gamma-aminobutyric acid (GABA) agonists may be problematic due to their effects on cognitive functioning during peak plasma concentrations and may even impair neuroplasticity. This raises concern that such agents might adversely affect optimal recovery from brain injury. Clearly, patients prescribed such medications should be routinely followed and monitored for safety, effectiveness, and potential effects on recovery. Further research on this topic is greatly needed.

Wake-promoting interventions

For many TBI patients, their primary complaint is fatigue or excessive somnolence during daytime hours. Excessive daytime sleepiness can have a major effect on quality of life and increases the potential for work-related injuries and automobile accidents. Consequently, there may be times when wake-promoting agents might be prescribed to a TBI patient with associated excessive somnolence problems. Modafinil is a wake-promoting agent that is approved for the treatment of excessive daytime sleepiness in narcolepsy, obstructive sleep apnea, or sleep disorder due to shift work. Presumably, modafinil (or its longer acting enantiomer armodafinil) would have a similar wake promoting effect in TBI patients suffering from excessive daytime somnolence. Indeed, a small sample of patients with chronic TBI (severity not reported) and excessive daytime sleepiness showed improved daytime vigilance and normalized nighttime sleep via self-report following five to 13 months of 100-400 mg modafinil administered each morning [39]. In a randomized clinical trial including a small (mostly male) adult sample of individuals with mild and severe TBI at the chronic recovery stage and with subjective excessive daytime sleepiness or fatigue, six weeks of 100-200 mg of morning modafinil significantly reduced subjective daytime sleepiness, but not reports of fatigue compared to placebo [40]. The intervention also improved the objective ability to stay awake in sleep-inducing conditions (i.e., the Maintenance of Wakefulness Test, MWT) and increased sleep latency compared to placebo. Of note, neither the modafinil nor the placebo group produced a clear improvement in subjective ratings of vigilance, suggesting restrictions in modafinil's efficacy in restoring some aspects of cognitive functioning in patients with TBI. This limitation is further supported by two studies in chronic mild to severe TBI and comorbid sleep disturbance (i.e., either narcolepsy, posttraumatic hypersomnia, subjective daytime sleepiness or fatigue) that could not replicate modafinil's beneficial effect on daytime sleepiness, daytime alertness, nighttime sleep or cognitive functioning [30,41]. However, even in healthy individuals, modafinil is often less likely to lead to subjective feelings of arousal (e.g., nervousness, excitation, jitteriness, pounding heart) compared to other types of stimulants such as caffeine [42], potentially leading to a discrepancy between objective and subjective alertness. Thus, there is some limited evidence to support the use of modafinil in aiding objective daytime alertness in TBI patients, but the findings have been inconsistent and further study is clearly needed. More evidence regarding the effects of the longer acting enantiomer, armodafinil, are needed before clear guidelines can be established.

Cognitive behavioral therapy for insomnia (CBT-I)& sleep hygiene

A range of effective non-pharmacological approaches to treating insomnia have been developed, including sleep hygiene education, sleep restriction, stimulus control therapy and relaxation-based interventions [21,43]. One particularly promising approach is Cognitive Behavioral Therapy for insomnia (CBT-I) [44]. CBT-I is a four-to-eight session multi component intervention, which targets factors maintaining insomnia, including both sleep-interfering behaviors and cognitions. CBT-I combines behavioral (e.g., stimulus control, sleep restriction) and cognitive (i.e., restructuring of maladaptive sleep-related cognitions and intrusive pre-sleep thoughts) interventions, as well as incorporating psycho-education regarding sleep. A growing body of evidence supports the efficacy of CBT-I in the treatment of insomnia. Findings from a recently published meta-analysis of randomized controlled trials (RCTs) comparing CBT-I to sleep inducing medications (zopiclone, zolpidem, temazepam, and triazolam) for insomnia suggests that, on average, CBT-I is at least as effective as medications in the treatment of insomnia [45]. Moreover, Mitchell and colleagues reported results indicating that the benefits of CBT-I may be more durable than those of medication.

Given the elevated prevalence of insomnia among individuals who have experienced TBIs, coupled with the growing body of research supporting the efficacy of CBT-I for insomnia, it is surprising that, to our knowledge, only two studies have tested the efficacy of CBT-I associated with TBI [46,47]. These studies provided preliminary evidence that CBT may be an effective intervention for post-TBI insomnia. Although they yielded promising findings, both of these studies were limited by the fact that they relied on single-case experimental designs.

Sleep hygiene approaches may also prove effective for patients with TBI. A recent study from the Department of Veterans Affairs Palo Alto Health Care System (VA PA HCS) reports on the implementation of newly developed sleep hygiene guidelines at their institution [48]. More specifically, the new sleep hygiene program incorporated CBT, exercise, relaxation training, sleep restriction, and stimulus control. A convenience sample of 67 individuals with TBIs admitted to the 18–bed Poly trauma Rehabilitation unit at the VA PA HCS between 2009 (prior to the implementation of the new sleep hygiene guideline) and 2010 (post-implementation) were included in the study. Although not statistically significant, average sleep duration increased slightly from 2009 (M=7.3) to 2010 (M=7.7). However, no change was observed in disability as assessed by a measure of functional independence. Larger, well-designed RCTs are needed to test the efficacy of CBT approaches against credible comparison conditions controlling for placebo-related factors (e.g., treatment outcome expectancies, the passage of time) [49]. Moreover, to the extent that CBT is shown to be an effective treatment for post-TBI insomnia, research will be needed to examine what aspects of this multi component treatment drive improvement (e.g., comparing the full CBT-I package versus a CBT-I intervention which excludes cognitive techniques to examine the incremental benefits, if any, of the cognitive components of treatment). Similar to psychopharmacological interventions, there are no data available on pharmacological interventions in pediatric populations with TBI.

Circadian rhythm interventions

An individual's level of alertness is affected by a number of factors including light exposure, food consumption, and the diurnal fluctuation of melatonin. In healthy individuals, melatonin, a pineal hormone regulated by the hypothalamus, has been shown to influence the timing of the sleep-wake rhythm [50]. Normally, melatonin secretion increases dramatically with the onset of darkness and is believed to prepare the brain for sleep. Melatonin is produced naturally by the body and normally increases in the evening hours as light levels decrease [51]. During sleep, melatonin levels decrease slowly, dropping to their lowest levels in the early morning hours just before natural awakening. For individuals with delayed sleep phase disorder or other problems with sleep onset that may stem from circadian misalignment (i.e., biological circadian phase is out of sync with natural day/night or work schedules), melatonin supplementation may prove beneficial. Timing of melatonin administration is critical, however. Evening administration (i.e., before bedtime) of melatonin leads to an advance in the circadian rhythm (i.e., the person falls asleep earlier in the evening and wakes earlier in the morning), whereas morning administration produces a phase delay (i.e., the person falls asleep later in the night and wakes later in the morning) [52]. For healthy individuals wishing to fall asleep earlier in the evening (i.e., phase advancement), a dose of melatonin (0.3 or 3 mg) taken about 6 to 7 hours before bedtime appears to be effective at producing a phase advance in the circadian rhythm [53].

There may be a role for melatonin in sleep problems in TBI. Some evidence suggests that melatonin may itself be neuro protective in animal models [39,54,55]. Unfortunately, brain injury may affect the cycling or production of melatonin [51]. Due to its involvement in sleep onset, sleep-wake regulation [56], and its putative neuro protective effects, melatonin supplementation has been posited to improve sleep, subsequent daytime alertness, and recovery following TBI in humans. Indeed, one month of daily 5 mg melatonin (time of administration not specified) improved subjective ratings of daytime alertness, sleep quality and sleep onset latency in a small sample of adult men with chronic mild to severe TBI and subjective sleep disturbance [57]. However, objective cognitive functioning did not change, and melatonin did not prove superior to 25 mg tricyclic antidepressant that served as the control intervention. Because these data have not yet been replicated, definitive conclusions are not possible at this stage. To our knowledge, there have been no controlled trials examining the effectiveness of these types of treatments for TBI-related sleep complaints in pediatric samples.

Another method that has recently shown potential efficacy in regulating the circadian rhythm and sleep-wake cycle is morning bright light exposure. Exposure to bright light during the morning hours, especially light in the blue wavelengths, has been shown to suppress daytime melatonin production and produce a phase advancement of the circadian rhythm. Carter et al. combined morning blue-wavelength light therapy with physical exercise and evening melatonin administration to successfully improve the sleep-wake rhythm in a 20-year old veteran who developed major depressive disorder and circadian rhythm sleep disorder following a mild to moderate TBI [58]. Bright light seems particularly promising given its demonstrated ability to improve subjective sleep quality and to increase alertness [59-61]. Comprehensive empirical evidence for its effectiveness in the context of TBI is pending, but emerging evidence by Ponsford et al. [62] suggests that this technique may be effective for improving fatigue in patients with mild to severe TBI. Studies in our own lab are currently ongoing to examine the effectiveness of bright light therapy in improving sleep and post-concussive symptoms in patients with mild TBI. As with most interventions, there are no known studies of light treatment with pediatric populations.

Alternative approaches

Similar to CBT, there are surprisingly few data on other non-pharmacological treatments in the literature. Acupuncture proved to be of some effectiveness in one recent study, as subjective sleep quality and objective cognitive functioning associated with chronic TBI (severity not disclosed) improved compared to pre-treatment, but not for the control group who did not receive the intervention [63]. Similarly, single-case studies suggest biofeedback to be effective to treat insomnia following TBI with comorbid posttraumatic stress disorder [64]. However, as systematic clinical trials are pending, there are currently not enough data to argue in favor of routine application of either acupuncture or biofeedback.

Conclusion and Future Directions

Overall, there is surprisingly little data on the efficacy of pharmacological and non-pharmacological treatment options for sleep disturbance following TBI. Published data have thus far focused exclusively on adult populations. Given that TBI is highly prevalent in children and adolescents [65], this is particularly problematic. The existing research literature in adult TBI is scant and fraught with methodological limitations. Most studies have included predominantly male populations and tend to ignore TBI severity. There are several reasons why it is imperative that future research begins to include information about TBI severity as a matter of course. In particular, brain damage and its behavioral correlates, including cognitive functioning, disability status, and awareness of TBI-related deficits have been shown to vary with TBI severity. This means that some treatment protocols might be more appropriate, and potentially more effective, for individuals with mild than severe TBI. For example, severe TBI may significantly affect meta cognition and self-reflection, which in turn may impede an efficient and effective implementation of CBT. In contrast, TBI severity may be less likely to moderate the efficacy of non-pharmacological approaches such as bright light therapy, although this currently remains an open question. Clearly, systematic studies are needed to establish the extent to which TBI severity might influence therapy outcome. Thus, for the field to move forward, treatment protocols need not only be developed for children and adolescents with sleep disturbance following TBI, but also tested in more balanced samples representing both sexes and carefully considering TBI severity.

In sum, the present brief and very selective review suggests that the extant literature on treatments for sleep problems among individuals with TBI is extremely limited. Non-pharmacologic approaches such as CBT, sleep hygiene, light therapy, and perhaps circadian influencing supplements such as melatonin appear to have some potential to improve sleep in this population. Comprehensive animal models of the effects of TBI on sleep disruption and larger, well-designed placebo controlled trials in humans are greatly needed before firm treatment recommendations can be supported.

References

1. Killgore WD (2010) Effects of sleep deprivation on cognition. Prog Brain Res 185: 105-129.
2. Pilcher JJ, Ginter DR, Sadowsky B (1997) Sleep quality versus sleep quantity: relationships between sleep and measures of health, well-being and sleepiness in college students. J Psychosom Res 42: 583-596.
3. Dinges DF, Pack F, Williams K, Gillen KA, Powell JW, et al. (1997) Cumulative sleepiness, mood disturbance, and psychomotor vigilance performance decrements during a week of sleep restricted to 4-5 hours per night. Sleep 20: 267-277.
4. Lim J, Dinges DF (2008) Sleep deprivation and vigilant attention. Ann N Y Acad Sci 1129: 305-322.
5. Gander PH, Marshall NS, Harris RB, Reid P (2005) Sleep, sleepiness and motor vehicle accidents: a national survey. Aust N Z J Public Health 29: 16-21.
6. Penetar D, McCann U, Thorne D, Kamimori G, Galinski C, et al. (1993) Caffeine reversal of sleep deprivation effects on alertness and mood. Psychopharmacology (Berl) 112: 359-365.
7. Killgore WD, Kahn-Greene ET, Lipizzi EL, Newman RA, Kamimori GH, et al. (2008) Sleep deprivation reduces perceived emotional intelligence and constructive thinking skills. Sleep Med 9: 517-526.
8. Kahn-Greene ET, Killgore DB, Kamimori GH, Balkin TJ, Killgore WD (2007) The effects of sleep deprivation on symptoms of psychopathology in healthy adults. Sleep Med 8: 215-221.
9. Killgore WD, Balkin TJ, Wesensten NJ (2006) Impaired decision making following 49 h of sleep deprivation. J Sleep Res 15: 7-13.
10. McKenna BS, Dickinson DL, Orff HJ, Drummond SP (2007) The effects of one night of sleep deprivation on known-risk and ambiguous-risk decisions. J Sleep Res 16: 245-252.
11. Killgore WD, Killgore DB, Day LM, Li C, Kamimori GH, et al. (2007) The effects of 53 hours of sleep deprivation on moral judgment. Sleep 30: 345-352.
12. Olsen OK, Pallesen S, Eid J (2010) The impact of partial sleep deprivation on moral reasoning in military officers. Sleep 33: 1086-1090.
13. Killick R, Banks S, Liu PY (2012) Implications of sleep restriction and recovery on metabolic outcomes. J Clin Endocrinol Metab 97: 3876-3890.
14. Zimberg IZ, Dâmaso A, Del Re M, Carneiro AM, de Sá Souza H, et al. (2012) Short sleep duration and obesity: mechanisms and future perspectives. Cell Biochem Funct 30: 524-529.
15. Mathias JL, Alvaro PK (2012) Prevalence of sleep disturbances, disorders, and problems following traumatic brain injury: a meta-analysis. Sleep Med 13: 898-905.
16. Mueller AD, Mear RJ, Mistlberger RE (2011) Inhibition of hippocampal neurogenesis by sleep deprivation is independent of circadian disruption and melatonin suppression. Neuroscience 193: 170-181.
17. Mueller AD, Pollock MS, Lieblich SE, Epp JR, Galea LA, et al. (2008) Sleep deprivation can inhibit adult hippocampal neurogenesis independent of adrenal stress hormones. Am J Physiol Regul Integr Comp Physiol 294: R1693-1703.
18. Gao B, Cam E, Jaeger H, Zunzunegui C, Sarnthein J, et al. (2010) Sleep disruption aggravates focal cerebral ischemia in the rat. Sleep 33: 879-887.
19. Zunzunegui C, Gao B, Cam E, Hodor A, Bassetti CL (2011) Sleep disturbance impairs stroke recovery in the rat. Sleep 34: 1261-1269.
20. Nakanishi H, Sun Y, Nakamura RK, Mori K, Ito M, et al. (1997) Positive correlations between cerebral protein synthesis rates and deep sleep in Macaca mulatta. Eur J Neurosci 9: 271-279.
21. Zeitzer JM, Friedman L, O'Hara R (2009) Insomnia in the context of traumatic brain injury. J Rehabil Res Dev 46: 827-836.

22. Mahmood O, Rapport LJ, Hanks RA, Fichtenberg NL (2004) Neuropsychological performance and sleep disturbance following traumatic brain injury. J Head Trauma Rehabil 19: 378-390.

23. Bruns J Jr, Hauser WA (2003) The epidemiology of traumatic brain injury: a review. Epilepsia 44 Suppl 10: 2-10.

24. Orff HJ, Ayalon L, Drummond SP (2009) Traumatic brain injury and sleep disturbance: a review of current research. J Head Trauma Rehabil 24: 155-165.

25. Chaput G, Giguère JF, Chauny JM, Denis R, Lavigne G (2009) Relationship among subjective sleep complaints, headaches, and mood alterations following a mild traumatic brain injury. Sleep Med 10: 713-716.

26. Cohen M, Oksenberg A, Snir D, Stern MJ, Groswasser Z (1992) Temporally related changes of sleep complaints in traumatic brain injured patients. J Neurol Neurosurg Psychiatry 55: 313-315.

27. Schreiber S, Barkai G, Gur-Hartman T, Peles E, Tov N, et al. (2008) Long-lasting sleep patterns of adult patients with minor traumatic brain injury (mTBI) and non-mTBI subjects. Sleep Med 9: 481-487.

28. Capaldi VF 2nd, Guerrero ML, Killgore WD (2011) Sleep disruptions among returning combat veterans from Iraq and Afghanistan. Mil Med 176: 879-888.

29. Kempf J, Werth E, Kaiser PR, Bassetti CL, Baumann CR (2010) Sleep-wake disturbances 3 years after traumatic brain injury. J Neurol Neurosurg Psychiatry 81: 1402-1405.

30. Castriotta RJ, Atanasov S, Wilde MC, Masel BE, Lai JM et al. (2009) Treatment of sleep disorders after traumatic brain injury. J Clin Sleep Med 5: 137-144.

31. Verma A, Anand V, Verma NP (2007) Sleep disorders in chronic traumatic brain injury. J Clin Sleep Med 3: 357-362.

32. Ayalon L, Borodkin K, Dishon L, Kanety H, Dagan Y (2007) Circadian rhythm sleep disorders following mild traumatic brain injury. Neurology 68: 1136-1140.

33. Nakase-Richardson R, Sherer M, Barnett SD, Yablon SA, Evans CC, et al. (2013) Prospective Evaluation of the Nature, Course, and Impact of Acute Sleep Abnormality After Traumatic Brain Injury. Arch Phys Med Rehabil .

34. Lew HL, Pogoda TK, Hsu PT, Cohen S, Amick MM, et al. (2010) Impact of the "polytrauma clinical triad" on sleep disturbance in a department of veterans affairs outpatient rehabilitation setting. Am J Phys Med Rehabil 89: 437-445.

35. Bryan CJ, Clemans TA, Hernandez AM, Rudd MD (2013) Loss of consciousness, depression, posttraumatic stress disorder, and suicide risk among deployed military personnel with mild traumatic brain injury. J Head Trauma Rehabil 28: 13-20.

36. Collen J, Orr N, Lettieri CJ, Carter K, Holley AB (2012) Sleep disturbances among soldiers with combat-related traumatic brain injury. Chest 142: 622-630.

37. Larson EB, Zollman FS (2010) The effect of sleep medications on cognitive recovery from traumatic brain injury. J Head Trauma Rehabil 25: 61-67.

38. Cantor JB, Bushnik T, Cicerone K, Dijkers MP, Gordon W, et al. (2012) Insomnia, fatigue, and sleepiness in the first 2 years after traumatic brain injury: an NIDRR TBI model system module study. J Head Trauma Rehabil 27: E1-14.

39. Teitelman E (2001) Modafinil for narcolepsy. Am J Psychiatry 158: 970-971.

40. Kaiser PR, Valko PO, Werth E, Thomann J, Meier J, et al. (2010) Modafinil ameliorates excessive daytime sleepiness after traumatic brain injury. Neurology 75: 1780-1785.

41. Jha A, Weintraub A, Allshouse A, Morey C, Cusick C, et al. (2008) A randomized trial of modafinil for the treatment of fatigue and excessive daytime sleepiness in individuals with chronic traumatic brain injury. J Head Trauma Rehabil 23: 52-63.

42. Killgore WD, Rupp TL, Grugle NL, Reichardt RM, Lipizzi EL, et al. (2008) Effects of dextroamphetamine, caffeine and modafinil on psychomotor vigilance test performance after 44 h of continuous wakefulness. J Sleep Res 17: 309-321.

43. Morin CM, Bootzin RR, Buysse DJ, Edinger JD, Espie CA, et al. (2006) Psychological and behavioral treatment of insomnia:update of the recent evidence (1998-2004). Sleep 29: 1398-1414.

44. Perlis ML, Jungquist C, Smith MT, Posner D (2005) Cognitive behavioral treatment of insomnia: A session-by-session guide (Vol. 1). Springer, New York.

45. Mitchell MD, Gehrman P, Perlis M, Umscheid CA (2012) Comparative effectiveness of cognitive behavioral therapy for insomnia: a systematic review. BMC Fam Pract 13: 40.

46. Ouellet MC, Morin CM (2004) Cognitive behavioral therapy for insomnia associated with traumatic brain injury: a single-case study. Arch Phys Med Rehabil 85: 1298-1302.

47. Ouellet MC, Morin CM (2007) Efficacy of cognitive-behavioral therapy for insomnia associated with traumatic brain injury: a single-case experimental design. Arch Phys Med Rehabil 88: 1581-1592.

48. Perlis ML, McCall WV, Jungquist CR, Pigeon WR, Matteson SE (2005) Placebo effects in primary insomnia. Sleep Med Rev 9: 381-389.

49. De La Rue-Evans L, Nesbitt K, Oka RK (2013) Sleep hygiene program implementation in patients with traumatic brain injury. Rehabil Nurs 38: 2-10.

50. Chase JE, Gidal BE (1997) Melatonin: therapeutic use in sleep disorders. Ann Pharmacother 31: 1218-1226.

51. Shekleton JA, Parcell DL, Redman JR, Phipps-Nelson J, Ponsford JL, et al. (2010) Sleep disturbance and melatonin levels following traumatic brain injury. Neurology 74: 1732-1738.

52. Lewy AJ, Ahmed S, Jackson JM, Sack RL (1992) Melatonin shifts human circadian rhythms according to a phase-response curve. Chronobiol Int 9: 380-392.

53. Mundey K, Benloucif S, Harsanyi K, Dubocovich ML, Zee PC (2005) Phase-dependent treatment of delayed sleep phase syndrome with melatonin. Sleep 28: 1271-1278.

54. Maldonado MD, Murillo-Cabezas F, Terron MP, Flores LJ, Tan DX, et al. (2007) The potential of melatonin in reducing morbidity-mortality after craniocerebral trauma. J Pineal Res 42: 1-11.

55. Ates O, Cayli S, Gurses I, Yucel N, Iraz M, et al. (2006) Effect of pinealectomy and melatonin replacement on morphological and biochemical recovery after traumatic brain injury. Int J Dev Neurosci 24: 357-363.

56. Rajaratnam SMW, Cohen DA, Rogers NL (2009) Melatonin and melatonin analogues. Sleep Med Clin 4: 179-193.

57. Kemp S, Biswas R, Neumann V, Coughlan A (2004) The value of melatonin for sleep disorders occurring post-head injury: a pilot RCT. Brain Inj 18: 911-919.

58. Carter KA, Lettieri CJ, Pena JM (2010) An unusual cause of insomnia following IED-induced traumatic brain injury. J Clin Sleep Med 6: 205-206.

59. Smith MR, Revell VL, Eastman CI (2009) Phase advancing the human circadian clock with blue-enriched polychromatic light. Sleep Med 10: 287-294.

60. Santhi N, Aeschbach D, Horowitz TS, Czeisler CA (2008) The impact of sleep timing and bright light exposure on attentional impairment during night work. J Biol Rhythms 23: 341-352.

61. Viola AU, James LM, Schlangen LJ, Dijk DJ (2008) Blue-enriched white light in the workplace improves self-reported alertness, performance and sleep quality. Scand J Work Environ Health 34: 297-306.

62. Ponsford JL, Ziino C, Parcell DL, Shekleton JA, Roper M, et al. (2012) Fatigue and sleep disturbance following traumatic brain injury--their nature, causes, and potential treatments. J Head Trauma Rehabil 27: 224-233.

63. Zollman FS, Cyborski C, Duraski SA (2010) Actigraphy for assessment of sleep in traumatic brain injury: case series, review of the literature and proposed criteria for use. Brain Inj 24: 748-754.

64. McLay RN, Spira JL (2009) Use of a portable biofeedback device to improve insomnia in a combat zone, a case report. Appl Psychophysiol Biofeedback 34: 319-321.

65. McKinlay A, Grace RC, Horwood LJ, Fergusson DM, Ridder EM, et al. (2008) Prevalence of traumatic brain injury among children, adolescents and young adults: prospective evidence from a birth cohort. Brain Inj 22: 175-181.

Acromegaly and Sleep Disordered Breathing

Muhammed Emin Akkoyunlu and Fatih Yakar*

Bezmialem Vakif University Medical Faculty, Department of Pulmonary Medicine, Istanbul, Turkey

Abstract

Acromegaly is the result of oversecretion of growth hormone and IGF-1 and the disease can affect several organ systems. Sleep Disordered Breathing (SDB) is a frequent disease in acromegaly patients. The mechanism of SDB is somewhat different in acromegaly patients than SDB in normal population. Although central apneas can be seen, obstructive apneas according to structural changes complicate the course of the disease. Treatment of SDB is as important as the treatment of acromegaly. In this review, we searched the medical literature and summarized the etiology, pathogenesis, mechanism of SDB development and treatment of SDB in acromegaly patients.

Keywords: Acromegaly; Sleep disordered breathing; Obstructive apnea; Central apnea; Positive airway pressure

Introduction

Sleep Disordered Breathing (SDB) is a common disorder characterized by fragmented sleep due to recurrent episodes of apnea and hypopnea [1]. Two different kinds of apnea can be seen in patients; obstructive and central. Obstructive Sleep Apnea (OSA) occurs as a result of obstruction at the upper airways but Central Sleep Apnea (CSA) ensues in the absence of rib cage and abdominal movements which is a sign of loss of ventilatory drive [2]. Although SDB affects 2-4% [3] of the normal population its prevalence can increase in specific patient groups or diseases. Especially patients with endocrine diseases like acromegaly, hypothyroidism, diabetes and Cushing's syndrome are more prone to have SDB [2].

Acromegaly is a rare disease (estimated prevalence is 1:140,000-250,000) that affect both sexes and cause abnormal growth of bony structures, visceral organs and soft tissues due to over production of Growth Hormone (GH) and insulin like growth factor (IGF-1) after closure of epiphyseal plates [4,5]. The presence of SDB in acromegaly was described at the 19th century first by Roxburg and Collins [6]. They described heavy snoring and daytime sleepiness in an acromegaly patient. To date, retrospective and prospective studies have shown the presence of SDB in acromegaly patients and reported prevalence roughly 60% [7-19]. High body mass index, neck circumference, GH and IGF1 levels, older age, and increased index-finger circumference are known predictors of SDB in acromegaly [20]. Also, narcolepsy [21], cheyne stokes respiration in sleep [22] and restless leg syndrome [23] were reported in acromegaly patients.

Mechanisms of SDB in Acromegaly

There are different kinds of presumptive mechanisms to cause SDB in acromegaly. These are changes in bony structures and soft tissues (hypertrophy and edema), obesity/overweight, mechanical alterations of the upper airway and alterations at neuromuscular control of ventilation [24]. The main triggering point is the increased levels of GH and IGF-1. Many studies showed higher frequencies of SDB in active acromegalic patients with a positive correlation with GH and IGF-1 levels [9,13,17,24], but van Haute et al. [19] couldn't observe this correlation. The two types of apnea may be seen in acromegaly; obstructive apnea and central apnea. Although obstructive apnea is more frequent, some studies indicate higher level of GH and IGF-1 levels in central apnea [10].

Changes in Bony Structures and Soft Tissues

Because obstructive apneas are more frequent, skeletal abnormalities are initially incriminated. Several anatomical abnormalities can occur in acromegalic patients; Hochban et al. [25] showed a dorsocaudal rotation of the mandible which leads to posterior displacement of the tongue, more vertical bony growth of the face which causes narrowing of the bony frame work of the nasopahrynx. However, these findings were not supported by other investigators. Also, in the study of Dostalova et al. [26] skeletal abnormalities in acromegaly patients with SDB were different from those in apneic patients without acromegaly and they reported the role of soft tissue changes be more important in obstructive apneas of acromegaly [26]. Although anatomical deformities can cause apneas, they are not sufficient to explain the whole course.

Growth hormone and IGF-1 regulates metabolism and body composition [27]. Due to over secretion of these hormones in acromegaly, an increase in body water and lean body mass cause altered body composition [28]. These changes in soft tissue can occur locally or generally. Local changes are deposition of glycosaminoglycan and collagen, and tissue edema [1]. Also, Kamenicky et al. [29], showed that tissue edema is due to increased renal sodium reabsorption, by direct stimulation of epithelial sodium channel by GH and IGF-I, which causes generalized edema. Patients with generalized edema also have a high prevalence of SDB, and this may be related to repositioning of the fluid from the lower extremities to the neck while the patient is lying, casing pharyngeal obstruction [30,31]. The soft tissue swelling of the upper airways leads to obstruction in acromegalic patients [16,27,32]. Edematous and polypoid nasal mucosa can block nasal passages and can cause altered sleep quality [33].

The increase in the size of the pharyngeal structures either due to depositions or edema can be shown by Magnetic Resonance Imaging (MRI). MRI, compared with radiographs, has the advantage

***Corresponding author:** Fatih YakarBezmialem Vakif University, Medical Faculty, Department of Pulmonolgy, 34093 Fatih-Istanbul, Turkey,
E-mail: fyakar@yahoo.com

of more precise delineation of the tongue volume [34]. Herrmann et al. [14], studied tongue volume by use of MRI and reported 36% greater in acromegalics than control patients and showed decrement in the signal intensity of the tongue after acromegaly treatment which indicates water/edema resolution. van Haute et al. [19] showed serious downsizing in thickness of the tongue, soft palate, pharyngeal walls and the opening of oropharyngeal space after treatment in one patient with MRI.

Rosenow et al. [20] reported a relatively high frequency of SDB in patients with acromegaly, with a positive correlation with GH/IGF1 levels, age, neck and index-finger circumference as measures of soft tissue hypertrophy. Interestingly, in this study, index finger circumference greater than or equal to 8.5 cm was associated with frequency of desaturations [35].

Mechanical Alterations

Changes in the structural component of the pharynx, tongue and bones with hypertrophy of parapahryngeal and retropharyngeal soft tissue deteriorate the patency of the upper airways. Isono et al. [36], compared acromegaly patients with and without OSAS, and found that the former group have more collapsible airways. Patients in this study were not obese and body mass indices were lower than 27 kg/m^{2}. Also, our study [37] revealed similar findings that acromegaly patients with and without OSAS have similar BMIs.

Obesity/Overweight

Some studies reported that excessive weight is associated with SDB in acromegaly patients [1,24], but also SDB can manifest independent of weight in acromegaly [35]. Although there are not sufficient evidence in the studies, increase of weight can be a risk factor of SDB development in acromegaly.

Central Nervous System Changes

The frequency of central apnea is increased in acromegaly patients. Grunstein et al. [10] reported central apnea in 20% of the 54 acromegalic patients. The suspected mechanism for increased central apnea was GH and IGF-1 induced central chemosensitivity to hypercapnia. Somatostatin, also known as growth hormone-inhibiting hormone, is a peptide hormone which controls the secretion of GH and affects neurotransmissions. Grunstein et al. [38] postulated that the loss of the inhibitory pathway of somatostatin causes loss of regulation on the central respiratory control in the brainstem and hypothalamus [10]. On the other hand, upper airway closure with inhibition of ventilation and increased ventilatory gain are other potantial etiologies for central sleep apnea development [39].

Consequences of SDB in Acromegaly

Cardiovascular complications

Cardiovascular complications are the major cause of mortality and morbidity in acromegaly. The risk of cardiovascular complications increases even in mild OSAS [40,41]. These complications may occur both due to the direct affect of acromegaly on myocardium (hypertrophy, myopathy or arrhythmias) and affect of SDB on cardiovascular system. Repeated hypoxia/reperfusions cause oxidative stress, inflammation, tissue injury and eventually lead to hypertension, coronary artery disease, arrhythmia and heart failure [42]. Also, SDB affects the limbic system (amygdala and hippocampus) and leads to dysregulation of blood pressure [43]. Coronary artery disease prevalence changes between 3 to 37% in different series, arrhythmias were present in 40% of subjects and arterial hypertension was reported in 30-405 of patients [24].

Neurocognitive complications

The frequency of SDB (between 20 and 80% of patients) in acromegaly is greater than in normal population. Owing to fragmented sleep, these patients suffer from daytime sleepiness, poor memory, loss of concentration, irritability, increased risk of accidents and depression [24,44-48].

Endocrine complications

The relationship between endocrine disease and SDB is complex. While some endocrine problems can cause SDB, also SDB can lead to endocrine diseases with probable mechanisms of hypoxemia, hypercapnia, and fragmented sleep [2]. Nocturnal awakenings cause cortisol and catecholamine release and eventually hormonal axis alteration. Increased cortisolemia is a risk factor for metabolic syndrome [49]. Moreover, GH exhibits lipolytic and insulin resistance effects and IGF-1 cause anti-lipolysis and insulin sensitivity [28]. Dysregulation of glucose and lipid metabolisms, due to excessive GH and IGF-1, are present in acromegaly patients with SDB. In the study of van Haute et al. [18], AHI was significantly higher in diabetic acromegaly patients. Davi et al. [11], had similar findings; in their study, AHI of diabetic patients was higher than non-diabetics, and hormonally uncontrolled acromegalic patients were overweighed, IGF-1 levels and diabetes frequency were higher than hormonally controlled patients.

Treatment

Treatment of acromegaly patients with SDB should be directed towards both acromegaly and sleep problem. It is postulated that if the acromegaly can be controlled, due to hormonal and structural changes, SDB will regress. But the effect of acromegaly control on the course of SDB is controversial [11,18,34,50]. Some studies have shown that SDB can remain even after complete hormonal treatment of acromegaly because of permanent structural changes [1,11,24]. In our study, we have shown some regression in the severity of SDB but there was no reduction in the necessity of positive airway pressure (PAP) therapy [37]. Consistent with our results, ACCP Sleep Medicine Board advice respiratory specialists to remain vigilant for evaluating the patients for PAP therapy [51].

Acromegaly treatment

Control of GH and IGF-1 secretion is the currently available main goal of the treatment in acromegaly. Optimal treatment should normalize GH/IGF-1 levels, preserve normal pituitary functions, prevent recurrence, be effective for long term, and relieve comorbidities (cardiovascular and metabolic complications) [24]. Although there is no single perfect treatment modality to control the disease, three treatment options for acromegaly are present; medical, surgical or radiotherapy.

– Surgery allows removal of the adenoma or reduction of the tumoral mass. It is cost effective and most of the patients are treated with surgery due to rapid initiation. However, large tumor size and invasive tumors, high levels of circulating GH during preoperative period, are harbingers of surgical failure [18, 24,52,53]. Overall cure rate of transsphenoidal surgery is 44-76% [54].

– Radiotherapy reduces tumor volume and GH/IGF-1 values but onset of action is slow and hypopituitarism may develop. After improvements in surgical techniques popularity of radiotherapy decreased [55-57].

– Pharmacotherapy can be started as first line therapy, especially in patients with contraindications to surgery, or can be applied following surgery or radiotherapy. Dopamine agonists, somatostatin receptor ligands and GH receptor antagonist (pegvisomant) are the currently available drugs for pharmacotherapy [24].

SDB treatment

Treatment strategies of acromegaly may help to relive the symptoms of SDB. Surgical treatment of acromegaly can improve sleep-disordered breathing. Cadieux et al. [58] treated two acromegaly patients with tracheostomy, successfully. In the study of Mickelson et al. [59] they reported that transsphenoidal hypophysectomy or transsphenoidal hypophysectomy and radiation treatment of acromegaly improved SDB, but also reported that uvulopalatopharyngoplasty did not improve SDB. Some studies showed significant improvement or cure after adenomectomy [18,60], while others found persisting nocturnal problems [61].

Many studies reported that SDB symptoms and severity in acromegaly patients improved with pharmacotherapy [13,62,63]. Octreotide and pegvisomant treatments have demonstrated improvement in patients with acromegaly and SDB [13,35,50,58,63]. Although hormone control strategies may reduce the severity, SDB does not completely disappear in acromegaly patients. In our recent study, 14 acromegaly patients had SDB and 12 of the cohort had indication of PAP therapy. After 6 months of acromegaly remission, 11 of 12 patients remained to be indicated for PAP therapy [37].

Conclusion

SDB may develop in acromegaly patients due to direct excessive hormonal activity on central nervous system (inhibition of somotostatinergic pathways), structural changes (soft tissue and bony structure) or aberration in the regulation of metabolism. Treatment of acromegaly may relieve SDB course but does not cure. In all acromegaly patients with SDB, treatment strategies for SDB must be planned concomitantly with acromegaly treatment.

References

1. Attal P, Chanson P (2010) Endocrine aspects of obstructive sleep apnea. J Clin Endocrinol Metab 95: 483-495.
2. Bottini P, Tantucci C (2003) Sleep apnea syndrome in endocrine diseases. Respiration 70: 320-327.
3. Durán J, Esnaola S, Rubio R, Iztueta A (2001) Obstructive sleep apnea-hypopnea and related clinical features in a population-based sample of subjects aged 30 to 70 yr. Am J Respir Crit Care Med 163: 685-689.
4. Chanson P, Salenave S (2008) Acromegaly. Orphanet J Rare Dis 3: 17.
5. Blanco Pérez JJ, Blanco-Ramos MA, Zamarrón Sanz C, Souto Fernández A, Mato Mato A, et al. (2004) [Acromegaly and sleep apnea]. Arch Bronconeumol 40: 355-359.
6. Roxburgh R, Collis AJ (1896) Notes on a Case of Acromegaly. Br Med J 2: 63-65.
7. Buyse B, Michiels E, Bouillon R, Bobbaers H, Demedts M (1997) Relief of sleep apnoea after treatment of acromegaly: report of three cases and review of the literature. Eur Respir J 10: 1401-1404.
8. Rosenow F, McCarthy V, Caruso AC (1998) Sleep apnoea in endocrine diseases. J Sleep Res 7: 3-11.
9. Weiss V, Sonka K, Pretl M, Dostálová S, Klozar J, et al. (2000) Prevalence of the sleep apnea syndrome in acromegaly population. J Endocrinol Invest 23: 515-519.
10. Grunstein R, Ho K, Sullivan C (1991) Sleep apnoea in acromegaly. Ann Intern Med 121: 527–562.
11. Davi' MV, Dalle Carbonare L, Giustina A, Ferrari M, Frigo A, et al. (2008) Sleep apnoea syndrome is highly prevalent in acromegaly and only partially reversible after biochemical control of the disease. Eur J Endocrinol 159: 533-540.
12. Hart TB, Radow SK, Blackard WG, Tucker HS, Cooper KR (1985) Sleep apnea in active acromegaly. Arch Intern Med 145: 865-866.
13. Herrmann BL, Wessendorf TE, Ajaj W, Kahlke S, Teschler H, et al. (2004) Effects of octreotide on sleep apnoea and tongue volume (magnetic resonance imaging) in patients with acromegaly. Eur J Endocrinol 151: 309-315.
14. Hochban W, Ehlenz K, Conradt R, Brandenburg U (1999) Obstructive sleep apnoea in acromegaly: the role of craniofacial changes. Eur Respir J 14: 196-202.
15. Ip MS, Tan KC, Peh WC, Lam KS (2001) Effect of Sandostatin LAR on sleep apnoea in acromegaly: correlation with computerized tomographic cephalometry and hormonal activity. Clin Endocrinol (Oxf) 55: 477-483.
16. Pekkarinen T, Partinen M, Pelkonen R, Iivanainen M (1987) Sleep apnoea and daytime sleepiness in acromegaly: relationship to endocrinological factors. Clin Endocrinol (Oxf) 27: 649-654.
17. Perks WH, Horrocks PM, Cooper RA, Bradbury S, Allen A, et al. (1980) Sleep apnoea in acromegaly. Br Med J 280: 894-897.
18. Sze L, Schmid C, Bloch KE, Bernays R, Brändle M (2007) Effect of transsphenoidal surgery on sleep apnoea in acromegaly. Eur J Endocrinol 156: 321-329.
19. van Haute FR, Taboada GF, Corrêa LL, Lima GA, Fontes R, et al. (2008) Prevalence of sleep apnea and metabolic abnormalities in patients with acromegaly and analysis of cephalometric parameters by magnetic resonance imaging. Eur J Endocrinol 158: 459-465.
20. Rosenow F, Reuter S, Deuss U, Szelies B, Hilgers RD, et al. (1996) Sleep apnoea in treated acromegaly: relative frequency and predisposing factors. Clin Endocrinol (Oxf) 45: 563-569.
21. Barnes AJ, Pallis C, Joplin GF (1979) Acromegaly and narcolepsy. Lancet 2: 332-333.
22. Laroche C, Festal G, Poenaru S, Caquet R, Lemaigre D, et al. (1976) [A case of periodic respiration in a patient with acromegaly]. Ann Med Interne (Paris) 127: 381-385.
23. Cannavò S, Condurso R, Ragonese M, Ferraù F, Alibrandi A, et al. (2011) Increased prevalence of restless legs syndrome in patients with acromegaly and effects on quality of life assessed by Acro-QoL. Pituitary 14: 328-334.
24. Scacchi M, Cavagnini F (2006) Acromegaly. Pituitary 9: 297-303.
25. Dostalova S, Sonka K, Smahel Z, Weiss V, Marek J, et al. (2001) Craniofacial abnormalities and their relevance for sleep apnoea syndrome aetiopathogenesis in acromegaly. Eur J Endocrinol 144: 491-497.
26. Freda PU, Shen W, Heymsfield SB, Reyes-Vidal CM, Geer EB, et al. (2008) Lower visceral and subcutaneous but higher intermuscular adipose tissue depots in patients with growth hormone and insulin-like growth factor I excess due to acromegaly. J Clin Endocrinol Metab 93: 2334-2343.
27. Dimopoulou C, Sievers C, Wittchen HU, Pieper L, Klotsche J, et al. (2010) Adverse anthropometric risk profile in biochemically controlled acromegalic patients: comparison with an age- and gender-matched primary care population. Pituitary 13: 207–214.
28. Kamenicky P, Viengchareun S, Blanchard A, Meduri G, Zizzari P, et al. (2008) Epithelial sodium channel is a key mediator of growth hormone-induced sodium retention in acromegaly. Endocrinology 149: 3294-3305.
29. Chiu KL, Ryan CM, Shiota S, Ruttanaumpawan P, Arzt M, et al. (2006) Fluid shift by lower body positive pressure increases pharyngeal resistance in healthy subjects. Am J Respir Crit Care Med 174: 1378-1383.
30. Shiota S, Ryan CM, Chiu KL, Ruttanaumpawan P, Haight J, et al. (2007) Alterations in upper airway cross-sectional area in response to lower body positive pressure in healthy subjects. Thorax 62: 868-872.
31. Dostálová S, Smahel Z, Sonka K (1998) Craniofacial abnormalities in sleep apnoea syndrome. Acta Chir Plast 40: 49-53.
32. Cheung NW, Boyages SC (1997) Increased incidence of neoplasia in females with acromegaly. Clin Endocrinol (Oxf) 47: 323-327.
33. Berg C, Wessendorf TE, Mortsch F, Forsting M, Teschler H, et al. (2009)

Influence of disease control with pegvisomant on sleep apnoea and tongue volume in patients with active acromegaly. Eur J Endocrinol 161: 829-835.

34. Vorona RD (2009) Sleep, sleep disorders and the endocrine system. ACCP Sleep Medicine Board Review: (4thedn), Published by American College of Chest Physician Nortbrook USA 163-165.

35. Isono S, Saeki N, Tanaka A, Nishino T (1999) Collapsibility of passive pharynx in patients with acromegaly. Am J Respir Crit Care Med 160: 64-68.

36. Akkoyunlu ME, Ilhan MM, Bayram M, Tasan E, Karaköse K, et al. (2013) Sleep Apnea in Acromegaly Toraks Dernegi 16. Annual Congress.

37. Grunstein RR, Ho KY, Berthon-Jones M, Stewart D, Sullivan CE (1994) Central sleep apnea is associated with increased ventilatory response to carbon dioxide and hypersecretion of growth hormone in patients with acromegaly. Am J Respir Crit Care Med 150: 496-502.

38. Grunstein RR, Ho KK, Sullivan CE (1994) Effect of octreotide, a somatostatin analog, on sleep apnea in patients with acromegaly. Ann Intern Med 121: 478-483.

39. Lavie P, Herer P, Peled R, Berger I, Yoffe N, et al. (1995) Mortality in sleep apnea patients: a multivariate analysis of risk factors. Sleep 18: 149-157.

40. Shahar E, Whitney CW, Redline S, Lee ET, Newman AB, et al. (2001) Sleep-disordered breathing and cardiovascular disease: cross-sectional results of the Sleep Heart Health Study. Am J Respir Crit Care Med 163: 19-25.

41. Bradley TD, Floras JS (2009) Obstructive sleep apnoea and its cardiovascular consequences. Lancet 373: 82-93.

42. Emin Akkoyunlu M, Kart L, Kılıçarslan R, Bayram M, Aralasmak A, et al. (2013) Brain Diffusion Changes in Obstructive Sleep Apnoea Syndrome. Respiration.

43. Al Lawati NM, Patel SR, Ayas NT (2009) Epidemiology, risk factors, and consequences of obstructive sleep apnea and short sleep duration. Prog Cardiovasc Dis 51: 285-293.

44. Malhotra A, White DP (2002) Obstructive sleep apnoea. Lancet 360: 237-245.

45. Lindberg E, Carter N, Gislason T, Janson C (2001) Role of snoring and daytime sleepiness in occupational accidents. Am J Respir Crit Care Med 164: 2031-2035.

46. Harris M, Glozier N, Ratnavadivel R, Grunstein RR (2009) Obstructive sleep apnea and depression. Sleep Med Rev 13: 437-444.

47. Akkoyunlu ME, Altin R, Kart L, Atalay F, Örnek T, et al. (2013) Investigation of obstructive sleep apnoea syndrome prevalence among long-distance drivers from Zonguldak, Turkey. Multidisciplinary Respiratory Medicine. 8:10

48. Buckley TM, Schatzberg AF (2005) On the interactions of the hypothalamic-pituitary-adrenal (HPA) axis and sleep: normal HPA axis activity and circadian rhythm, exemplary sleep disorders. J Clin Endocrinol Metab 90: 3106-3114.

49. Freedman NS (2009) Positive Airway Pressure Therapy for Obstructive Sleep Apnea Syndrome: The Bordsand Beyond. ACCP Sleep Medicine Board Reivew: (4thedn), Published by American College of Chest Physician Nortbrook, USA 293-312.

50. Abosch A, Tyrrell JB, Lamborn KR, Hannegan LT, Applebury CB, et al. (1998) Transsphenoidal microsurgery for growth hormone-secreting pituitary adenomas: initial outcome and long-term results. J Clin Endocrinol Metab 83: 3411-3418.

51. Colao A, Ferone D, Marzullo P, Lombardi G (2004) Systemic complications of acromegaly: epidemiology, pathogenesis, and management. Endocr Rev 25: 102-152.

52. Sheppard MC (2003) Primary medical therapy for acromegaly. Clin Endocrinol (Oxf) 58: 387-399.

53. Wass JA (2003) Radiotherapy in acromegaly: a protagonists viewpoint. Clin Endocrinol (Oxf) 58: 128-131.

54. Barkan AL (2003) Radiotherapy in acromegaly: the argument against. Clin Endocrinol (Oxf) 58: 132-135.

55. Thorner MO (2003) Controversy: radiotherapy for acromegaly. Clin Endocrinol (Oxf) 58: 136-137.

56. Cadieux RJ, Kales A, Santen RJ, Bixler EO, Gordon R (1982) Endoscopic findings in sleep apnea associated with acromegaly. J Clin Endocrinol Metab 55: 18-22.

57. Mickelson SA, Rosenthal LD, Rock JP, Senior BA, Friduss ME (1994) Obstructive sleep apnea syndrome and acromegaly. Otolaryngol Head Neck Surg 111: 25-30.

58. Lamberts SW, van Koetsveld P, Hofland L (1989) A close correlation between the inhibitory effects of insulin-like growth factor-I and SMS 201-995 on growth hormone release by acromegalic pituitary tumours in vitro and in vivo. Clin Endocrinol (Oxf) 31: 401-410.

59. Pelttari L, Polo O, Rauhala E, Vuoriluoto J, Aitasalo K, et al. (1995) Nocturnal breathing abnormalities in acromegaly after adenomectomy. Clin Endocrinol (Oxf) 43: 175-182.

60. Colao A, Pivonello R, Auriemma RS, De Martino MC, Bidlingmaier M, et al. Efficacy of 12-month treatment with the GH receptor antagonist pegvisomant in patients with acromegaly resistant to long-term, high-dose somatostatin analog treatment: effect on IGF-I levels, tumor mass, hypertension and glucose tolerance. European Journal of Endocrinology 154:467–477.

61. Higham CE, Trainer PJ (2008) Growth hormone excess and the development of growth hormone receptor antagonists. Exp Physiol 93: 1157-1169.

62. Tolis G, Angelopoulos NG, Katounda E, Rombopoulos G, Kaltzidou V, et al. (2006) Medical treatment of acromegaly: comorbidities and their reversibility by somatostatin analogs. Neuroendocrinology 83: 249-257.

63. Chanson P, Timsit J, Benoit O, Augendre B, Moulonguet M, et al. (1986) Rapid improvement in sleep apnoea of acromegaly after short-term treatment with somatostatin analogue SMS 201-995. Lancet 1: 1270-1271.

Permissions

All chapters in this book were first published in JSDT, by OMICS International; hereby published with permission under the Creative Commons Attribution License or equivalent. Every chapter published in this book has been scrutinized by our experts. Their significance has been extensively debated. The topics covered herein carry significant findings which will fuel the growth of the discipline. They may even be implemented as practical applications or may be referred to as a beginning point for another development.

The contributors of this book come from diverse backgrounds, making this book a truly international effort. This book will bring forth new frontiers with its revolutionizing research information and detailed analysis of the nascent developments around the world.

We would like to thank all the contributing authors for lending their expertise to make the book truly unique. They have played a crucial role in the development of this book. Without their invaluable contributions this book wouldn't have been possible. They have made vital efforts to compile up to date information on the varied aspects of this subject to make this book a valuable addition to the collection of many professionals and students.

This book was conceptualized with the vision of imparting up-to-date information and advanced data in this field. To ensure the same, a matchless editorial board was set up. Every individual on the board went through rigorous rounds of assessment to prove their worth. After which they invested a large part of their time researching and compiling the most relevant data for our readers.

The editorial board has been involved in producing this book since its inception. They have spent rigorous hours researching and exploring the diverse topics which have resulted in the successful publishing of this book. They have passed on their knowledge of decades through this book. To expedite this challenging task, the publisher supported the team at every step. A small team of assistant editors was also appointed to further simplify the editing procedure and attain best results for the readers.

Apart from the editorial board, the designing team has also invested a significant amount of their time in understanding the subject and creating the most relevant covers. They scrutinized every image to scout for the most suitable representation of the subject and create an appropriate cover for the book.

The publishing team has been an ardent support to the editorial, designing and production team. Their endless efforts to recruit the best for this project, has resulted in the accomplishment of this book. They are a veteran in the field of academics and their pool of knowledge is as vast as their experience in printing. Their expertise and guidance has proved useful at every step. Their uncompromising quality standards have made this book an exceptional effort. Their encouragement from time to time has been an inspiration for everyone.

The publisher and the editorial board hope that this book will prove to be a valuable piece of knowledge for researchers, students, practitioners and scholars across the globe.

List of Contributors

Scott G Williams
Department of Medicine, Womack Army Medical Center, Fort Bragg, North Carolina, USA
Department of Medicine, Uniformed Services University, Bethesda, Maryland, USA

Christopher J Lettieri
Pulmonary, Critical Care and Sleep Medicine, Walter Reed National Military Medical Center, Bethesda, Maryland, USA
Department of Medicine, Uniformed Services University, Bethesda, Maryland, USA

José Carlos Pereira Jr
Departamento de Pediatria – Faculdade de Medicina de Jundiaí, Jundiaí, SP, Brazil

Marcia Pradella-Hallinan
Departamento de Psicobiologia - Universidade Federal de São Paulo, Brazil

Yi-jun Ge and Gui-hai Chen
Department of Neurology, the First People's Hospital of Chenzhou, China

Lan Xia
Department of Neurology, the Second Affiliated Hospital of Anhui Medical University, China

Fang Wang
Department of Neurology, the First Affiliated Hospital of Anhui Medical University, China

Sohil A Khan
School of Pharmacy, Griffith University, Gold Coast, Australia
Mater Research Institute, Mater Health Services, South Brisbane, Australia
Griffith Health Institute, Griffith University, Gold Coast, Australia

Treasure M McGuire
Mater Research Institute, Mater Health Services, South Brisbane, Australia
School of Pharmacy, The University of Queensland, Woolloongabba, Australia

Helen S Heussler
Mater Research Institute, Mater Health Services, South Brisbane, Australia
Deparrment of Respiratory and Sleep Medicine, Mater Children's Hospital, Mater Health Services, South Brisbane, Australia
School of Medicine, The University of Queensland, Herston, Australia

Maria Luisa Sacchetti, Maria Teresa Di Mascio, Silvia Ottaviani, Danilo Toni and Marco Fiorelli
Department of Neurology and Psychiatry, Sapienza University, Rome, Italy

Giacomo Della Marca
Sleep Unit, Institute of Neurology, Catholic University, A. Gemelli, Rome, Italy

Antonio Minni
Department of Sensory Organs, Sapienza University of Rome, Rome, Italy

Barry G Fields, Sharon Schutte-Rodin and Megin Myers
Center for Sleep and Circadian Neurobiology, Division of Sleep Medicine, University of Pennsylvania, USA

Michael L. Perlis
Center for Sleep and Circadian Neurobiology, Division of Sleep Medicine, University of Pennsylvania, USA
Department of Psychiatry, University of Pennsylvania Medical Center, Philadelphia, Pennsylvania, USA

Shittu RO
Department of Family Medicine, Kwara State Specialist Hospital, Nigeria

Issa BA and Olanrewaju GT
Department of Behavioral Sciences, University of Ilorin Teaching Hospital, Nigeria

Odeigah LO
Department of Family Medicine, University of Ilorin Teaching Hospital, Nigeria

Sule AG
Department of Family Medicine, Ahmadubello University, Teaching Hospital, Nigeria

Sanni MA
Department of Hematology, Kwara State Specialist Hospital, Nigeria

Uthman MB and Aderibigbe SA
Department of Epidemiology and Community Health, University of Ilorin Teaching Hospital, Nigeria

Nyamngee AA
Department of Medical microbiology and parasitology, College of Health, Sciences, University of Ilorin, Nigeria

Oommen Nainan
Graded Specialist-Orthodontics & Dentofacial Orthopedics, Naval Institute of Dental Sciences, India

Jayan B
Department of Dental Surgery, Armed Forces Medical College, India

Chopra SS
Classified Specialist-Orthodontics & Dentofacial Orthopedics, Corps Dental Unit, India

Mukherjee M
Classified Specialist-Periodontology, Military Dental centre, India

Athanasia Pataka
Department of Respiratory Medicine, Respiratory Failure Unit, G. Papanikolaou Hospital, University of Thessaloniki, Thessaloniki, Greece

Kathy Sexton Radek
Suburban Pulmonary and Sleep Associates, 700 E Ogden Avenue, Suite 201, Westmont, IL 60559 Elmhurst College, USA

Julie Kaprelian
The Chicago School of Professional Psychology, Merchandise Mart, 13th Floor, Chicago, IL, USA

Kenneth Blum
Department of Psychiatry, University of Florida, McKnight Brain Institute, USA
Impact genomics, Inc., Lederoch, Pennsylvania, USA

Marlene-Oscar-Berman
Departments of Psychiatry and Anatomy & Neurobiology, Boston University School of Medicine, and Boston VA Healthcare System, Boston, USA

William Downs B
Impact genomics, Inc., Lederoch, Pennsylvania, USA

Eric R Braverman
Department of Psychiatry, University of Florida, McKnight Brain Institute, USA
Department of Clinical Neurology, Path Research Foundation, USA

Florian Kreuk, Kristina Dushaj, Courtney Truesdell and Mona Li
Department of Clinical Neurology, Path Research Foundation, USA

Scott Jones and John Giordano
Department of Holistic Medicine, National Institute for Holistic Addiction Studies, USA

Joan Borsten
Department of Addiction Research & Therapy, Malibu Beach Recovery Center, USA

Thomas Simpatico
Human Integrated Services Unit University of Vermont Center for Clinical & Translational Science, College of Medicine, USA

Debmayla Barh
Institute of Integrative Omics & Applied Biotechnology, India

Margaret A Madigan
Impact genomics, Inc., Lederoch, Pennsylvania, USA
Department of Clinical Neurology, Path Research Foundation, USA
Department of Personalized Genomics, IGENE LLC., USA

Stephen Schoenthaler
Department of Holistic Medicine, National Institute for Holistic Addiction Studies, USA
Department of Sociology, California State University, USA

Deirdre A. Conroy and Edward D. Huntley
University of Michigan, Department of Psychiatry, 4250 Plymouth Road, Ann Arbor, MI 48109, USA

Gruber Reut
McGill University, Montreal, Quebec, Canada
Attention, Behavior and Sleep Lab, Douglas Mental Health University Institute, Quebec, Canada

Bergmame Lana
McGill University, Montreal, Quebec, Canada
Attention, Behavior and Sleep Lab, Douglas Mental Health University Institute, Quebec, Canada

Tatyana Mollayeva
Toronto Rehabilitation Institute, 550 University Avenue, Rm 11207, Toronto, Ontario M5G 2A2, Canada

Tetyana Kendzerska
Institute of Health Policy, Management and Evaluation University of Toronto, 155 College Street, Suite 425 Toronto, Canada

Shirin Mollayeva
University of Toronto, Canada

Angela Colantonio
Saunderson Family Chair in Acquired Brain Injury Research, Toronto Rehabilitation Institute, University of Toronto, Canada
Domenico Maurizio Toraldo
Department of Rehabilitation, Unit Care Respiratory, ASL/Lecce, Italy

Francesco De Nuccio and Giuseppe Nicolardi
Laboratory of Human Anatomy and Neuroscience, Department of Biological and Environmental Sciences and Technologies, University of Salento, Italy

Salvatore Mauro
Laboratory of Genetic, "Vito Fazzi", ASL Lecce, Italy

Francesco Spirito
Division of Cardiovascular disease, City of Lecce Hospital, Lecce, Italy

Alessandro Distante
ISBEM Research Institute, Medical School of University of Pisa, Pisa, Italy

Alberto Caprioglio
Associated Professor and Head, Department of Orthodontics, School of Dentistry, University of Insubria, Italy

Alessandro Ollà, Gian Marco Abbate and Federico Migliori
DDS, Department of Orthodontics, School of Dentistry, University of Insubria, Italy

Franca Marino
Assistant Professor, Centre of Research in Medical Pharmacology, School of Dentistry, University of Insubria, Italy

Carlo Mangano
Assistant Professor, Department of Oral Surgery, School of Dentistry, University of Insubria, Italy

Marco Cosentino
Associated Professor and Head, Centre of Research in Medical Pharmacology, School of Medicine, University of Insubria, Italy

Luana Nosetti
Assistant Professor, Department of Pediatrics, School of Medicine, University of Insubria, Italy

Massoud Daheshia, David Bradshaw, John Perri and Gilbert Seda
Department of Pulmonary and Critical Care Medicine, Naval Medical Center San Diego, San Diego, CA 92134, USA

Carolyn H Welsh
Denver Veterans Affairs Medical Center, Denver, Colorado, USA

Markus Dworak
Harvard Medical School, West Roxbury, MA, USA

Alfred Wiater
Department of Pediatrics, Hospital Cologne Porz/ Rhine, Cologne, Germany

Xi Han
Department of Neurosurgery, Huashan Hospital, Fudan University, China

Ping Sheng and Yan Dong
Neuroscience center, Second Military Medical University, China
Department of Neurosurgery, Second Military Medical University, China

Chengguang Huang, Mingkun Yu and Lijun Hou
Department of Neurosurgery, Second Military Medical University, China
Neuroscience center, Second Military Medical University, China

Inderjeet S Brar
Affinity Medical Center, Massillon, OH, USA

Ramakant Sharma
Louis Stokes Cleveland VA Medical Center, Cleveland, OH, USA

Gaurav Khanna
University of Cincinnati, Cincinnati, OH, USA

Dennis Auckley
MetroHealth Medical Center, Case Western Reserve University, Cleveland, OH, USA

Nuntigar Sonsuwan
Department of Otolaryngology, Chiang Mai University, Chiang Mai, 50200, Thailand

Sutida Ameiam
Uttaradit Hospital, Uttaradit, Thailand

Kittisak Sawanyawisuth
Department of Medicine, Faculty of Medicine, Khon Kaen University, Khon Kaen, 40002, Thailand

Jinhui Chiang and Ryan Chiang
Chinese Medicine Clinic, I-I-Tang (IIT), Taiwan

Nalan Demir
Department of Chest Diseases, School of Medicine, Ankara University, Ankara, Turkey

Oğuz Köktürk and Tansu Ulukavak Ciftçi
Department of Chest Diseases, School of Medicine, Gazi University, Sleep Medicine Unit, Ankara, Turkey

Ozlem Gülbahar and Neslihan Celik Bukan
Department of Biochemistry, School of Medicine, Gazi University, Ankara, Turkey

Kenan Köse
Department of Statistics, School of Medicine, Ankara University, Ankara, Turkey

Catherine Lamblin, François Jouniaux, François Codron and Thibaut Gentina
Hôpital Privé La Louvière, Générale de Santé, Lille, France

Elodie Gentina
Skema Business School - Université de Lille, MERCUR Research, France

Aiman Tulaimat
Cook County Health and Hospital Systems, Division of Pulmonary, Critial Care, and Sleep Medicine, USA

Swathy Puthalapattu
Division of Pulmonary and Critical Care Medicine, Emory University School of Medicine, Atlanta, Georgia, USA

Jesse Roman-Rodriguez and Rafael L Perez
University of Louisville, Louisville, Kentucky, USA
Louisville Veterans Affairs Medical Center, Louisville, Kentucky, USA

Srinivas Bhadriraju
Baylor College of Medicine, Houston, Texas, USA

Octavian C Ioachimescu
Atlanta Veterans Affairs Medical Center, Atlanta, Georgia, USA
Division of Pulmonary and Critical Care Medicine, Emory University School of Medicine, Atlanta, Georgia, USA

Chia-Mo Lin
Fu-Jen University Medical College and ShinKong Wu Ho-Su Hospital Sleep Center, Taipei, Taiwan

Hsiao-Yean Chiu RNMS
Taipei Medical University, Taipei Taiwan
Christian Guilleminault Stanford University Sleep Medicine Division, Stanford, CA, USA

Veronica Eguiguren and Marcela Smurra
Hospital Tornú, Argentina

Susana Blanco
Faculty of Engineering, University of Belgrano-CONICET, Argentina

Cecilia DiRisio
Dosimetry Laboratory and Medical Technology, Faculty of Engineering, University of Belgrano, Argentina

Shittu RO, Odeigah LO and Sule AG
Department of Family Medicine, Kwara State Specialist Hospital, Nigeria

Issa BA and Olanrewaju GT
Department of Behavioral Sciences, University of Ilorin Teaching Hospital, Nigeria

Sanni MA
Department of Hematology, Kwara State Specialist Hospital, Nigeria

Aderibigbe SA
Department of Epidemiology and Community Health, University of Ilorin Teaching Hospital, Nigeria

Michael J Hasselberg, Anton P Porsteinsson and Lisa Boyle
Department of Psychiatry, University of Rochester School of Medicine and Dentistry, 601 Elmwood Ave., Rochester, NY 14642, USA

Kathy P Parker
University of Rochester School of Nursing, 255 Crittenden Blvd., Rochester, NY 14642, USA

Carl Stepnowsky and Zia Agha
Health Services Research & Development Unit, Veterans Affairs San Diego Healthcare System, San Diego, CA, USA
Department of Medicine, University of California, San Diego, USA

Tania Zamora and Christine Edwards
Health Services Research & Development Unit, Veterans Affairs San Diego Healthcare System, San Diego, CA, USA

Lin Liu
Health Services Research & Development Unit, Veterans Affairs San Diego Healthcare System, San Diego, CA, USA
Department of Family and Preventive Medicine, University of California, San Diego, USA

Saban-Hakki Onen
Hospices Civils de Lyon, Hôpital Antoine Charial, Centre Gériatrique de Médecine du Sommeil, F-69340 Francheville, France
Inserm U1028, Université Lyon1, F-69373 Lyon Cedex 08, France

Virgine Dauphinot
Hospices Civils de Lyon, CMRR Biostatistiques, Hôpital des Charpennes, F-69100 Villeurbanne, France

Nalaka S Gooneratne
Center for Sleep and Circadian Neurobiology and Division of Sleep Medicine, School of Medicine, University of Pennsylvania, Philadelphia, PA, USA
Division of Geriatric Medicine, School of Medicine, University of Pennsylvania, Philadelphia, PA, USA

Ghislaine Watchueng
Hospices Civils de Lyon, Hôpital Antoine Charial, Centre Gériatrique de Médecine du Sommeil, F-69340 Francheville, France

Jian-Sheng Lin
Inserm U1028, Université Lyon1, F-69373 Lyon Cedex 08, France

Fannie Onen
CHU Bichat Claude Bernard, APHP, Service de Gériatrie, F-75018 Paris, France
INSERM U669, Université Paris Descartes, 75014 Paris, France

Gowri Raman
Center for Clinical Evidence Synthesis, Institute for Clinical Research and Health Policy Studies, Tufts Medical Center, Tufts University School of Medicine, Boston, MA, USA

Yuan Zhang
School of Nursing, University of Massachusetts, Lowell, MA, USA

Vincent J Minichiello
Department of Family Medicine, University of Wisconsin, Madison, WI, USA

Carolyn D'Ambrosio
Pulmonary, Critical Care and Sleep Medicine Division, Tufts Medical Center, Tufts University School of Medicine, Boston, MA, USA

Chenchen Wang
Center for Integrative Medicine, Division of Rheumatology, Tufts Medical Center, Tufts University School of Medicine, Boston, MA, USA

Ashish Kumar U
3rd Year MBBS Student, Father Muller Medical College, Kankanady, Mangalore, Karnataka, India

Princy Louis Palatty
Department of Pharmacology, Father Muller Medical College, Kankanady, Mangalore, Karnataka, India

Mohammad Torabi Nami
Department of Neuroscience, School of Advanced Medical Science and Technology, Shiraz University of Medical Sciences, Shiraz, Iran

Karkare K, Sinha S, Taly AB and Rao S
Departments of Neurology and Biostatistics, National Institute of Mental Health and NeuroSciences (NIMHANS), Bangalore

Christie Racine, Natasha J. Williams, Ferdinand Zizi and Girardin Jean-Louis
Center for Healthful Behavior Change, Department of Population Health, NYU Langone Medical Centre, NY, USA

Kaushal Kalra
Department of Family Practice, SUNY Downstate Medical Centre, NY, USA

Mirnova Ceide
Albert Einstein College of Medicine of Yeshiva University, Department of Psychiatry and Behavioural Sciences, NY, USA

Mauro V Mendlowicz
Department of Psychiatry and Mental Health, Universidade Federal Fluminense, NY, USA
Institute of Psychiatry, Universidade Federal do Rio de Janeiro, NY, USA

Sinziana Lovin
University Lower Danube, Faculty of Medicine, Galati, Romania

Carmen Rusu
Psychotherapy practice, Galati Romania

Mihai Mutica
Hospital of Pychiatry, Galati, Romania

Anamaria Necula
Hospital of Pneumology, Timisoara, Romania

Costinela Georgescu
University Lower Danube, Faculty of Medicine, Galati, Romania

Kristi B Adamo, Shanna Wilson, Kevin Belanger and Jean-Philippe Chaput
Healthy Active Living and Obesity Research Group, Children's Hospital of Eastern Ontario Research Institute, Ontario, Canada

Dagmara Dimitriou
Department of Psychology and Human Development, Institute of Education, London, United Kingdom, UK
School of Health and Social Science, Middlesex University, London, UK

Anna Sniecinska
Faculty of Health, Social Care and Education, Anglia Ruskin University, Chelmsford, UK

Ray K Iles
Eric Leonard Kruse Foundation for Health Research, Scotland

Mareen Weber, Christian A Webb and William DS Killgore
McLean Hospital, Harvard Medical School, USA

Muhammed Emin Akkoyunlu and Fatih Yakar
Bezmialem Vakif University Medical Faculty, Department of Pulmonary Medicine, Istanbul, Turkey

Index